PSYCHIATRY
UPDATE

AMERICAN PSYCHIATRIC ASSOCIATION

Annual Review

Vol. 4

EDITED BY ROBERT E. HALES, M.D.
ALLEN J. FRANCES, M.D.

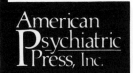
American Psychiatric Press, Inc.

1400 K Street, N.W.
Washington, DC
1985

American Psychiatric Press, Inc.

1400 K STREET, N.W.
WASHINGTON, D.C. 20005

Typeset by VIP Systems, Alexandria, VA
Manufactured by Fairfield Graphics, Fairfield, PA

Psychiatry Update: Volume 4
ISSN 0736-1866
ISBN 0-88048-239-7 (hardbound with CME Supplement)
ISBN 0-88048-039-4 (pbk.)

Printed and bound in the United States of America.

To Dianne
Who makes everything in life worthwhile

R.E.H.

To my mother and father, and my brother, Richard

A.J.F.

PSYCHIATRY UPDATE: VOLUME I
The American Psychiatric Association Annual Review (1982)

Lester Grinspoon, M.D., Editor

The Psychiatric Aspects of Sexuality
Virginia A. Sadock, M.D., Preceptor

The Schizophrenic Disorders
Robert Cancro, M.D., Med.D.Sc., Preceptor

Depression in Childhood and Adolescence
Henry H. Work, M.D., Preceptor

Law and Psychiatry
Alan A. Stone, M.D., Preceptor

Borderline and Narcissistic Personality Disorders
Otto F. Kernberg, M.D., Preceptor

PSYCHIATRY UPDATE: VOLUME II
The American Psychiatric Association Annual Review (1983)

Lester Grinspoon, M.D., Editor

New Issues in Psychoanalysis
Arnold M. Cooper, M.D., Preceptor

Geriatric Psychiatry
Ewald W. Busse, M.D., Preceptor

Family Psychiatry
Henry Grunebaum, M.D., Preceptor

Bipolar Illness
Paula J. Clayton, M.D., Preceptor

Depressive Disorders
Gerald L. Klerman, M.D., Preceptor

PSYCHIATRY UPDATE: VOLUME III
The American Psychiatric Association Annual Review (1984)

Lester Grinspoon, M.D., Editor

Brief Psychotherapies
Toksoz Byram Karasu, M.D., Preceptor

Children at Risk
Irving Philips, M.D., Preceptor

Consultation-Liaison Psychiatry
Zbigniew J. Lipowski, M.D., Preceptor

Alcohol Abuse and Dependence
George E. Vaillant, M.D., Preceptor

The Anxiety Disorders
Donald F. Klein, M.D., Preceptor

PSYCHIATRY UPDATE: THE AMERICAN PSYCHIATRIC ASSOCIATION ANNUAL REVIEW, VOLUME 4 (1985)

Robert E. Hales, M.D. and Allen J. Frances, M.D., Editors

An Introduction to the World of Neurotransmitters and Neuroreceptors
Joseph T. Coyle, M.D., Section Editor

Neuropsychiatry
Stuart C. Yudofsky, M.D., Section Editor

Sleep Disorders
David J. Kupfer, M.D., Section Editor

Eating Disorders
Joel Yager, M.D., Section Editor

The Therapeutic Alliance and Treatment Outcome
John P. Docherty, M.D., Section Editor

PSYCHIATRY UPDATE: THE AMERICAN PSYCHIATRIC ASSOCIATION ANNUAL REVIEW, VOLUME 5 (1986)

Allen J. Frances, M.D. and Robert E. Hales, M.D., Editors

Schizophrenia
Nancy C. Andreasen, M.D., Ph.D., Section Editor

Drug Abuse and Drug Dependence
Robert B. Millman, M.D., Section Editor

Adolescent Psychiatry
Carolyn Robinowitz, M.D. and Jeanne Spurlock, M.D., Section Editors

Personality Disorders
Robert M. A. Hirschfeld, M.D., Section Editor

Psychotherapeutic Management of Medical Conditions
David Spiegel, M.D. and W. Stewart Agras, M.D., Section Editors

Group Psychotherapy
Irvin D. Yalom, M.D., Section Editor

PSYCHIATRY UPDATE: THE AMERICAN PSYCHIATRIC ASSOCIATION ANNUAL REVIEW, VOLUME 6 (1987)

Robert E. Hales, M.D. and Allen J. Frances, M.D., Editors

Unipolar Affective Disorders
Jan Fawcett, M.D., Section Editor

Advances in Laboratory and Diagnostic Techniques
John M. Morihisa, M.D. and Solomon H. Snyder, M.D., Section Editors

DSM-III (Revised)
Robert L. Spitzer, M.D., Section Editor

Violence and the Violent Patient
Kenneth Tardiff, M.D., Section Editor

Psychiatric Epidemiology
Myrna M. Weissman, Ph.D., Section Editor

Psychopharmacology Drug Interactions and Side Effects
Philip A. Berger, M.D. and Leo E. Hollister, M.D., Section Editors

American Psychiatric Association
ANNUAL REVIEW
Volume 4

Editorial Advisory Board

CONTENTS

Introduction

Now that we have the "Annual Review," I wonder how we ever got along without it. It fills the wide gap between the information presented in our excellent array of journals and that presented in such encyclopedic tomes as the *Comprehensive Textbook* and the *American Handbook*. As, if not more, timely than journal articles, and more focused and manageable to read than the voluminous texts—it presents us each year with five specific topic areas that are of great current interest, often because of the research recently generated within them.

The idea for the *Annual Review* was that of Lester Grinspoon, immediate past chairman of the American Psychiatric Association's Scientific Program Committee, whose many creative ideas have immensely enriched our annual meeting. Dr. Grinspoon ably edited the series through its first three volumes and reminded us how hungry we have become for high quality, in-depth monographic material. He has been succeeded as editor by Robert E. Hales and Allen J. Frances and after my initial reading of the book, I can reassure the reader that they have upheld the high standards set by Dr. Grinspoon.

This fourth volume has beautifully captured the excitement and promise of the field of psychiatry as it now exists. Just read Robert Post's chapter on the future of interfaces between psychiatry and neurology and see if your pulse doesn't quicken. Those who really want to dig into the leading edges of neuro-transmitter research will be rewarded by this rich and complex section. As our population over 65 doubles by the year 2030, it behooves us to become better equipped to diagnose, treat and care for the elderly mentally ill—and Stuart Yudofsky's excellent section on neuropsychiatry is a good beginning. Sleep and eating disorders are also comprehensively presented and while some boundaries may be imprecisely drawn, such as anorexia and bulimia, the presentation of syndromes in each is sophisticated but practical. Finally, lest you surmise that everything exciting is taking place in the neuronal synapses—John Docherty's section on the therapeutic alliance will correct that impression.

What is clear throughout the book is the progress we have made as a field in moving from a clinical art to a clinical science. This is true whether we are talking about the fact that the tremendously rapidly-advancing field of research concerning neurotransmitters and their interactions with receptors has direct clinical impact on the development of more specific psychotropic medications; or that the rapprochement between psychiatry and neurology has direct bearing on the increasing clinical proximity of both practitioners and the way we conceptualize the disorders from which our patients suffer; or that the expanding amount of exciting research in sleep disorders has immediate clinical bearing on our understanding and treatment of these disorders; or that our expanding knowledge about eating disorders helps us day to day in dealing with these terribly troublesome entities; or that a better understanding of the intricacies of the psychotherapeutic relationship assist us in many ways in a multiplicity of therapeutic endeavors.

It is clear to me after my first reading that I will have to dip into Volume 4 of the *Annual Review* again and again—to look up specific syndromes and their treatment as I encounter them clinically, to brush up on my always-failing memory concerning neurotransmitters, and to remind myself from time to time, that I'm not the only psychiatrist who thinks great things are happening and will continue to happen in our field.

I look forward to rereading the *Annual Review*—and to hearing its authors present firsthand at the 138th annual meeting of the American Psychiatric Association in Dallas, Texas in May 1985. My congratulations to the authors, section editors, and editorial board, but especially to the two chief editors. If this tome is any indication, the next three should be as exciting as the first three.

John A Talbott, M.D.

Professor of Psychiatry
Cornell University Medical College

President
American Psychiatric Association

Foreword

by Robert E. Hales, M.D. and Allen J. Frances, M.D.

Volume 4 of the *American Psychiatric Association Annual Review* of psychiatry marks the beginning of our tenure as coeditors of this series. We would like to acknowledge our gratitude to Lester Grinspoon, M.D., the originator and founding Editor of the *Annual Review*. The excellence of Dr. Grinspoon's three Volumes provided us with a model and simplified the task of attracting the very best Section Editors and chapter contributors for Volume 4.

The fact that modern psychiatry is a discipline of such remarkable breadth, diversity, and emerging new knowledge presents continual challenge and opportunity. It is clear that there will never be a shortage of fascinating topics for consideration, but it is less clear how best to apportion space and emphasis. We have settled on a plan for the next several years that should provide comprehensive and timely coverage of major areas of interest, while allowing space for more narrowly defined specialty topics in which new developments are especially interesting. We will complete a thorough review of major psychiatric topics every five years. Each volume will include one or more sections in three broad areas: psychopathology, a psychiatric specialty, and a psychiatric treatment. Every other year, a topic in child psychiatry will be chosen.

The process of assembling and editing Volume 4 of the *Annual Review* has been a special pleasure and education for us. The widening boundaries of psychiatry are perhaps best reflected in the topical distance that is travelled between the first and last sections of this book. We begin with the fascinating exploration of the transmission of information at the neuronal synapse and conclude with equally fascinating new findings regarding the central importance of the therapeutic alliance in various patient-therapist encounters. A modern practitioner must remain familiar with a vast array of knowledge spanning neurobiological, psychodynamic, cognitive and behavioral therapies, and social systems approaches. A major goal in our selection of topics and in instructions to contributors has been to provide a broad, comprehensive and integrative perspective that does full justice to the many points of view, and research methods that enrich our field.

Volume 4 consists of five subject areas in which there have recently emerged especially interesting data with direct and important implications for clinical practice. Dr. Joseph Coyle's section on Neurotransmitters and Neuroreceptors crisply summarizes the revolutionary expansion in our understanding of the mechanics of neurotransmitter and neuroreceptor interactions in both normal and psychopathological brain functioning. Dr. Stuart Yudofsky's Neuropsychiatry section highlights brain–behavior interactions as they present in a variety of clinical conditions. The sections on Sleep and Eating Disorders, edited by Drs. David Kupfer and Joel Yager, respectively, address increasingly common clinical disorders, the diagnosis and treatment of which have been recently

---

advanced by exciting new physiological understanding and the development of psychological and biological treatment approaches. Finally, Dr. John Docherty's section on the Therapeutic Alliance summarizes newly acquired research findings in what is essentially the oldest and perhaps most essential clinical issue: the vicissitudes of the doctor-patient relationship.

A number of people have made this book possible. John Talbott, M.D., President of the American Psychiatric Association, provided us with overall editorial assistance and wrote the eloquent introduction to this Volume. We also received much help from our Editorial Advisory Board: Judy Gold, M.D., Fred Guggenheim, M.D., John Morihisa, M.D., Alan Pollack, M.D., Carolyn Robinowitz, M.D. and Betty Small, M.D. The Medical Director of the American Psychiatric Association, Melvin Sabshin, M.D., greatly assisted us with the conceptualization and organization of this Volume. Many people at the American Psychiatric Press, Inc., provided meticulous editing of the entire manuscript and thoughtful attention to the numerous details associated with successful publication of this book: especially Ron McMillen, General Manager of APPI; Hermine Dlesk, Editorial Assistant; Tim Clancy, Editor; Eve Nelson Shapiro, Technical Editor; and Jane Todaro, Secretary. Sandy Landfried, our Administrative Assistant, deserves our gratitude and significant recognition for coordinating all the many editorial meetings and correspondence, involving not only this Volume but future Volumes of the *Annual Review* series. Her patience and persistence were invaluable in successfully accomplishing this project.

The staff of the Office of Education of the American Psychiatric Association, especially Mr. Michael Miller, greatly assisted us with the Continuing Medical Education pamphlet available in connection with Volume 4. This CME package is introduced particularly for the benefit of those who may not have had the opportunity to attend the Psychiatry Update session at the American Psychiatric Association Annual Meeting in Dallas, Texas.

We thank our departmental Chairmen, Colonel Harry Holloway, M.D., USA, and Dr. Robert Michels, for their guidance and assistance. Most importantly, we are grateful to our wives, Dianne and Vera, for their encouragement with this project and other work regarding the Annual Meeting.

We are pleased to present to you the *American Psychiatric Association Annual Review: Volume 4*. We hope that you will find the numerous changes we instituted to be in keeping with the spirit of the previous three Volumes and that we have provided you with a clinically useful update in the field of psychiatry. We hope that you will enjoy and learn from it.

Contributors

Richard Abrams, M.D.
Professor and Vice Chairman, Department of Psychiatry and
Behavioral Sciences, University of Health Sciences/The Chicago
Medical School

Huda Akil, Ph.D.
Associate Professor, Department of Psychiatry,
University of Michigan, Ann Arbor

Arthur H. Auerbach, M.D.
Assistant Professor of Psychiatry,
University of Pennsylvania School of Medicine

David Bear, M.D.
Assistant Professor of Psychiatry, Harvard Medical School;
Section of Neurology in Psychiatry,
New England Deaconess Hospital

Susan J. Blumenthal, M.D.
Research Psychiatrist, Center for Studies of Affective Disorders;
Clinical Research Branch, National Institute of Mental Health

Joseph T. Coyle, M.D.
Director of Child Psychiatry; Professor of Psychiatry,
Neuroscience, Pharmacology, and Pediatrics,
The Johns Hopkins University School of Medicine

Ian Creese, Ph.D.
Professor of Neuroscience, The School of Medicine,
University of California, San Diego

John P. Docherty, M.D.
Chief, Psychosocial Treatments Research Branch,
National Institute of Mental Health

Elke D. Eckert, M.D.
Associate Professor of Psychiatry, University of Minnesota

Salvatore J. Enna, Ph.D.
Professor of Pharmacology, Neurobiology and Anatomy,
University of Texas at Houston School of Medicine

Milton Erman, M.D.
Assistant Professor of Psychiatry,
University of Texas Health Science Center, Dallas;
Medical Director, Sleep/Wake Disorders Center,
Presbyterian Hospital of Dallas

Todd Wilk Estroff, M.D.
Research Facilities, Fair Oaks Hospital, Summit, New Jersey

Susan J. Fiester, M.D.
Visiting Scientist, Psychosocial Treatments Research Branch,
National Institute of Mental Health

Allen J. Frances, M.D.
Vice-Chairperson, Scientific Program Committee,
American Psychiatric Association;
Associate Professor of Psychiatry,
Cornell University Medical College;
Director, Outpatient Division,
New York Hospital, Payne Whitney Psychiatric Clinic

Roy Freeman, M.D.
Instructor in Neurology, Harvard Medical School;
Section of Neurology, New England Deaconess Hospital

Paul E. Garfinkel, M.D.
Professor of Psychiatry, University of Toronto;
Chief, Department of Psychiatry, Toronto General Hospital

David M. Garner, Ph.D.
Director of Research, Department of Psychiatry,
Toronto General Hospital;
Associate Professor of Psychiatry, University of Toronto

James Gibbs, M.D.
Associate Professor of Psychiatry,
Cornell University Medical College;
Edward W. Bourne Behavioral Research Laboratory,
The New York Hospital-Cornell Medical Center,
Westchester Division

J. Christian Gillin, M.D.
Professor of Psychiatry, University of California
School of Medicine, San Diego

Mark S. Gold, M.D.
Director of Research, Fair Oaks Hospital, Summit, New Jersey;
Director of Research, Psychiatric Institute of Delray,
Delray Beach, Florida

Jack A. Grebb, M.D.
Medical Staff Associate, Neuropsychiatry Branch,
National Institute of Mental Health;
Intramural Research Program,
Saint Elizabeths Hospital, Washington, D.C.

Mark Greenberg, Ph.D.
Instructor in Psychiatry, Harvard Medical School;
Section of Psychiatry, New England Deaconess Hospital

Robert E. Hales, M.D.
Chairperson, Scientific Program Committee,
American Psychiatric Association;
Assistant Professor of Psychiatry,
Uniformed Services University of the Health Sciences,
Bethesda, Maryland

Dianna E. Hartley, Ph.D.
Assistant Professor of Psychology,
Langley Porter Psychiatric Institute,
University of California, San Francisco

Peter J. Hauri, Ph.D.
Professor of Psychiatry, Dartmouth Medical School

Mardi Horowitz, M.D.
Professor of Psychiatry, University of California, San Francisco

Paul Isaacs, Ph.D.
Research Fellow, Department of Psychiatry,
Toronto General Hospital

Aaron Janowsky, Ph.D.
Clinical Neuroscience Branch,
National Institute of Mental Health

Lissy F. Jarvik, M.D., Ph.D.
Department of Psychiatry, UCLA Neuropsychiatric Institute

Dilip V. Jeste, M.D.
Chief, Unit on Movement Disorders and Dementia,
Neuropsychiatry Branch; National Institute of Mental Health
Intramural Research Program; Saint Elizabeths Hospital,
Washington, D.C.

Enrico E. Jones, Ph.D.
Associate Professor, Department of Psychology,
University of California, Berkeley

Ismet Karacan, M.D., D.Sc. (Med.)
Professor of Psychiatry and Director, Sleep Disorders and
Research Center, Baylor College of Medicine;
Associate Chief of Staff for Research and Development,
Veterans Administration Medical Center, Houston

Jeffrey E. Kelsey, B.S.
Department of Psychiatry, University of Michigan, Ann Arbor

Sidney Kennedy, M.B., B.Ch.
Assistant Professor, Department of Psychiatry,
University of Toronto

Janice L. Krupnick, M.S.W.
Clinical Assistant Professor, Department of Psychiatry,
Georgetown School of Medicine

David J. Kupfer, M.D.
Professor and Chairman of Psychiatry, University of Pittsburgh
School of Medicine; Department of Psychiatry,
Western Psychiatric Institute and Clinic

Juan F. Lopez, M.D.
Department of Psychiatry, University of Michigan, Ann Arbor

Lester Luborsky, Ph.D.
Professor of Psychology in Psychiatry, University of
Pennsylvania School of Medicine

Charles Marmar, M.D.
Assistant Professor of Psychiatry,
University of California, San Francisco

Wallace B. Mendelson, M.D.
Chief, Unit on Sleep Studies, Clinical Psychobiology Branch,
National Institute of Mental Health

James E. Mitchell, M.D.
Associate Professor of Psychiatry, University of Minnesota

Constance A. Moore, M.D.
Assistant Professor of Psychiatry; Associate Director, Sleep
Disorders and Research Center; Director, Human Sexuality
Program; Baylor College of Medicine, Texas Medical Center

Steven M. Paul, M.D.
Chief, Clinical Neuroscience Branch,
National Institute of Mental Health

Robert M. Post, M.D.
Chief, Biological Psychiatry Branch,
National Institute of Mental Health

A.L.C. Pottash, M.D.
Research Facilities, Fair Oaks Hospital, Summit, New Jersey

Richard L. Pyle, M.D.
Assistant Professor of Psychiatry, University of Minnesota

Stephen L. Read, M.D.
Veterans Administration Medical Center, West Los Angeles

Charles F. Reynolds III, M.D.
Associate Professor of Psychiatry and Neurology;
Director, Sleep Evaluation Center; Western Psychiatric Institute
and Clinic, University of Pittsburgh School of Medicine

Howard P. Roffwarg, M.D.
Professor of Psychiatry; Director, Sleep Study Unit;
University of Texas Health Science Center
and Presbyterian Hospital, Dallas

A. John Rush, M.D.
Betty Jo Hay Professor of Psychiatry;
Director, Affective Disorders Unit,
University of Texas Health Science Center, Dallas

Michael J. Sateia, M.D.
Assistant Professor of Psychiatry, Dartmouth Medical School;
Medical Director, Dartmouth-Hitchcock Sleep Disorders Center

David Schiff, B.A.
New England Deaconess Hospital, Department of Psychiatry,
Harvard Medical School

James E. Shipley, M.A., M.D.
Assistant Professor of Psychiatry; Postdoctoral Fellow in Clinical
Research, Sleep Evaluation Center; Western Psychiatric Institute
and Clinic, University of Pittsburgh School of Medicine

Frederick Sierles, M.D.
Associate Professor and Director of Undergraduate Training,
Department of Psychiatry and Behavioral Sciences,
University of Health Sciences/The Chicago Medical School

Jonathan M. Silver, M.D.
New York State Psychiatric Institute

Phil Skolnick, Ph.D.
Laboratory of Bioorganic Chemistry, National Institute on
Arthritis, Diabetes, Digestive and Kidney Diseases,
Bethesda, Maryland

Gary W. Small, M.D.
Department of Psychiatry and Biobehavioral Sciences,
University of California, Los Angeles;
Neuropsychiatric Institute and West Los Angeles
Veterans Administration Medical Center, Brentwood Division

Gerard P. Smith, M.D.
Professor of Psychiatry, Cornell University Medical College;
Edward W. Bourne Behavioral Research Laboratory,
The New York Hospital-Cornell Medical Center,
Westchester Division

Michael Strober, Ph.D.
Associate Professor of Psychiatry;
Director, Teenage Eating Disorders Program,
Department of Psychiatry and Biobehavioral Sciences,
UCLA School of Medicine

I

An Introduction to the World of Neurotransmitters and Neuroreceptors

ection

I

An
ntroduction
o the World
f Neuro-
ransmitters
nd
Neuroreceptors

Contents

Section I

An Introduction to the World of Neurotransmitters and Neuroreceptors

Introduction

by Joseph T. Coyle, M.D., Section Editor

Psychopharmacologic drugs represent a major and powerful treatment modality in clinical psychiatry. While many of the commonly used psychotropic medications were discovered serendipitously, basic research over the last decade has provided compelling evidence that these drugs exert their therapeutic effects and cause many of their side effects by altering chemical neurotransmission in the brain. While this research has been conducted, there has also been an explosion in knowledge about the fundamental processes involved in chemical neurotransmission associated with a rapidly expanding list of substances that serve as neurotransmitters in the brain.

These advances provide a foundation for the rational approach toward the use of psychotropic medications in clinical psychiatry. Our burgeoning understanding of the fundamental mechanisms of action of psychotropic drugs is leading to the development of new drugs with more specific effects and fewer side effects. Furthermore, insights developed from the therapeutic effects of psychotropic drugs, coupled with a clear understanding of their molecular sites of action in the brain, have led to the formulation of hypotheses that neurotransmitter disturbances may be responsible for certain major mental disorders.

The following chapters are intended to introduce the clinician to the recent advances in brain research in neurotransmitters. We have focused on those neurotransmitter systems that are clearly implicated in psychotropic drug action: norepinephrine and antidepressants, dopamine and neuroleptics, gamma-amino butyric acid and anxiolytics/sedatives, acetylcholine and anticholinergics, and endorphins and narcotics. We hope that these chapters will provide a foundation for the reader to understand and pursue future research findings in this emerging, important area of psychiatry.

Chapter 1

Introduction to the Pharmacology of the Synapse

by Joseph T. Coyle, M.D.

DISCOVERY OF THE PSYCHOTROPICS

The major advance in psychiatry since 1950 has been the introduction of effective medications for the treatment of serious psychiatric disorders. Within the 15 years between 1951 and 1966, the antipsychotic neuroleptics, tricyclic antidepressants, benzodiazepines and lithium were added to the armamentarium of therapies available to psychiatrists. The implementation of these drugs was associated with a remarkable decline in the number of patients requiring chronic institutional care in the United States. The majority of patients who were able to be deinstitutionalized because of the new psychotropic medications did suffer from schizophrenia; but a significant number undoubtedly had affective disorders. Psychotropics are now among the most widely prescribed class of medications, with approximately one person in five receiving this class of drug.

It should be emphasized that the discovery of each class of psychotropic medication was almost always serendipitous. Thus, chlorpromazine was developed as an antihistamine and was noted to exhibit "tranquilizing effects" on agitated, psychotic patients. Imipramine was synthesized as an analogue of chlorpromazine but was shown to have mood elevating effects on depressed patients. The monoamine oxidase inhibitors were developed from the observation of the euphoriant effects of certain antitubercular drugs. While lithium was discovered by Cade in the search for an antidote to an hypothesized toxin responsible for manic psychosis, the experimental basis for selecting lithium derived from its toxic properties in guinea pigs that were unrelated to its therapeutic effects. In other words, the progenitors of our current psychotropic medications and, in many cases, still the most frequently used drugs, were discovered not by design but by chance.

In the 1960s, clinical investigators sought objective methods to assess the clinical efficacy of psychotropic medications. The task was particularly difficult because the pathologic bases of psychiatric disorders were unknown; and the mechanisms of action of the drugs were obscure. This concerted effort led to the implementation of "placebo controlled, double blind" design for psychotropic drug evaluation. Placebo treatment controlled for the possibility that the patient's involvement in a therapeutic relationship might affect the course of the disorder, or that the disorder might spontaneously remit during the period

The author receives support from an NIMH Career Development Award (MH00125) and a grant from the Surdna Foundation.

of treatment. "Double blind" referred to the fact that neither the investigator nor the patient knew whether active drug was being administered; this strategy prevented potential biases for or against pharmacotherapy that might color either the reaction of the patient or the evaluation of the clinician. Clinical studies based upon these techniques provided compelling evidence of the efficacy of neuroleptics in treating the acute symptoms of schizophrenic psychosis, of tricyclic antidepressants in relieving the symptoms of endogenous depression, and of lithium in stabilizing the mood disturbances in manic-depressive disorder.

Since dosage (both of placebo and active drug) was adjusted according to clinical response in the majority of the studies, optimal dosage requirements were also determined. Furthermore, during this exploratory phase, several structurally related drugs were examined in clinical trials but were determined to be ineffective. Thus, these studies generated an important data base for the structural activity relationships among the various classes of psychotropic drugs in their therapeutic potency. In other words, the clinical studies provided critical information about the efficacy and potency of the various psychotropic medications that was invaluable for probing their basic mechanisms of action in fundamental studies. The last 15 years has been a time in which these clinical observations have been taken back to the laboratory to clarify the mechanisms of action of the various classes of psychotropic medications.

NEUROTRANSMITTERS AND PSYCHOTROPICS

Armed with the extensive information on the clinical profiles of the major classes of psychotropic medications, investigators were able to proceed with basic studies to uncover their mechanisms of action. An underlying assumption of these studies was that there should be a close correspondence between therapeutic efficacy and the effects on the fundamental properties of neurons. Adherence to this principle was essential, because the complex structure of the drugs and their lipophilic properties could affect a variety of cell functions if the drugs were at sufficiently high concentrations. Indeed, early studies demonstrated that phenothiazines, for example, altered membrane fluidity, mitochondrial function and the activity of the neuronal sodium pump; but these cellular alterations occurred at concentrations many magnitudes above those associated with therapeutic effect, and did not exhibit any correlation between clinical potency of the various phenothiazines and these effects. In other words, phenothiazines devoid of antipsychotic activity were as effective as those with antipsychotic effects. The finding that emerged repeatedly from the basic investigations was that clinical efficacy appeared to correlate best with alterations in the processes involved in chemical neurotransmission.

What has evolved from tentative proposals initially put forward ten to 15 years ago, and has been sustained by the progressive accumulation of evidence, is that the primary mechanisms of action of the major classes of psychotropic medications—including neuroleptics, antidepressants, analgesics and anxiolytics/hypnotics—involve selective alterations of specific forms of chemical neurotransmission. On a basic level, these findings have prompted an ever widening search to identify the neurotransmitters utilized by neuronal pathways in the brain, and have led to an explosion of information revealing the complexity and diversity of chemically encoded information processing in the brain. At the clinical level, clarification of the mechanisms of interactions of the drugs with specific neurotransmitter systems has led to the generation of hypotheses that disruption in these processes may play a role in the pathophysiology of the various psychiatric disorders responsive to the drugs. Accordingly, psychiatrists now confront both in the literature as well as in clinical practice an increasing emphasis upon understanding the role of neurotransmitter dysfunction in the diagnosis and treatment of psychiatric disorders.

GENERAL PRINCIPLES OF SYNAPTIC NEUROTRANSMISSION

Cellular Anatomy of the Neuron

The neuron is a cell that is highly specialized, both anatomically as well as biochemically, to carry out the fundamental role of processing information. Being a cell, each neuron contains a nucleus, which possesses the entire genetic endowment. Thus, in this sense, the neuron is an autonomous living unit capable of synthesizing all components required for independent life. However, in contrast to many other cell types, such as those of the liver, mucosa, or hemopoetic system (which are capable of cell division throughout life), the high degree of differentiation and specialization of the neuron generally precludes cell division once the neuron is mature. Lack of regenerative properties of neurons has obvious implications for the irreversible effects of damage to the nervous system.

The neuron can be divided into four anatomical components: the cell body or "soma"; the dendrites; the axon; and the synapse (Figure 1). The cell body of the neuron contains the nucleus, which possesses the full complement of chromosomes. The cell body is the site at which synthesis of virtually all proteins and other structural components of the neurons takes place. These processes are controlled by the transcription of information from the DNA within the nucleus through messenger RNA (mRNA); this information is transported to sites adjacent to the nucleus, where the mRNA is translated to synthesize structural and metabolic proteins. The size of the neuronal cell body, which includes its biosynthetic machinery, is roughly proportional to the extent of the projection of axons and terminals of the neuron. It should be emphasized that only a very small percentage of the neuronal cell volume is contained within the cell body, with the bulk of cell volume distributed through the axonal and dendritic arbor. For this reason, the metabolic and synthetic demands upon the neuronal cell body are remarkable, as the neuronal cell body sustains the rest of the neuron. Materials synthesized within the cell body are then transported down the axons and dendrites; conversely, breakdown products of metabolic and structural proteins in the axons and dendrites are transported back to the cell body for processing.

The axon is a fine tubular extension from the neuronal cell body down which impulses flow to the nerve terminals. The neuron emits only one axon, the length of which varies from less than a millimeter for interneurons to over a meter for motor neurons innervating the extremities. The axon, as it approaches its field of innervation, may branch to varying degrees, depending upon the

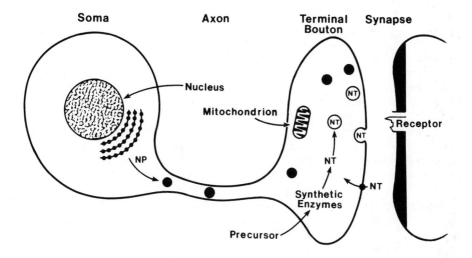

Figure 1. Schematic representation of the neuron. The figure presents the main structural components of the neuron (not shown in scale) emphasizing those aspects involved in chemical neurotransmission. NP = neuropeptide; NT = neurotransmitter.

number of neurons with which it makes synaptic contacts. Some neurons may have very specific and restricted contacts, whereas the axons of other neurons (such as the nigrostriatal dopaminergic neurons) may arborize tremendously to contact millions of neurons in their terminal field of innervation.

The dendrites are multiple tubular extensions of the neuronal cell body that serve as the primary structure for the reception of synaptic contacts from other neurons. Relay neurons may have very sparse dendritic extensions consistent with a very limited synaptic input from other neurons. Neurons involved in integrative functions, such as the pyramidal cells in the cerebral cortex, have very extensive dendritic "trees" that receive synaptic input from thousands of neurons. The synapse is a specialized structure at which the nerve terminal makes contact with the receptive portion of the adjacent neuron (Figure 1). The synapse consists of an outpouching of the terminal aspects of the axon known as a "bouton," which is firmly attached to the dendritic membrane of the adjacent neuron by synaptic specializations. The membrane at the synapse is markedly enriched with receptors that respond to the neurotransmitter released by the terminal bouton. The terminal bouton itself contains a number of cellular structures that allow it to remain metabolically and functionally rather independent from the neuronal cell body. Thus, it contains mitochondria—the power packs of the cell that generate cellular energy from metabolism of glucose, the enzymes involved in the synthesis and degradation of the neurotransmitter, and storage vesicles that maintain substantial concentrations of neurotransmitter in a protected state—ready for release on demand. When brain tissue is disrupted by gentle homogenization in isotonic sucrose solution, the synapse with the terminal bouton and the adjacent postsynaptic membrane specialization are sheared off to form "synaptosomes," which have been exploited for studying fundamental aspects of synaptic neurotransmission.

Electrogenic Properties of Neurons

A fundamental property of all neurons is the excitable nature of their membrane, which confers the ability to generate and transmit a wave of electrochemical depolarization. This property derives from the specialized nature of the membrane, which maintains a voltage gradient and possesses voltage sensitive ion channels. Intercallated in the neuronal membrane is an energy dependent ion pump that secretes two ions of sodium for every potassium ion pumped into the neuron. This uneven distribution of ions—with high intracellular potassium and low extracellular potassium in the face of high extracellular sodium and low intracellular sodium—results in a voltage difference between the outside and the inside of the neuron of approximately -70 mV. When the neuronal membrane is depolarized by the opening of sodium channels associated with excitatory receptors, the voltage difference across the membrane falls. When the voltage difference is reduced below -35 mV, this causes voltage dependent sodium channels adjacent to the excitatory synapse to open, generating an "action potential." This localized depolarization spreads along the dendrite, past the cell body and down the axon as adjacent voltage dependent sodium channels are opened, much like a line of falling dominoes. Thus, the transmittal of information from the receptive area of the neuron down the axons to its terminals occurs by means of electrochemical communication.

The neuronal dendrites are continuously summating all the excitatory and inhibitory inputs to determine whether a neuron will generate an action potential. This decision is an all or none process; and, when the balance is struck towards depolarization (for example, -35 mV), an action potential is generated. The innervation to the neuron is not random but, rather, is highly organized. Excitatory inputs are generally concentrated at the distal ends of dendrites, whereas the inhibitory inputs are located primarily at the proximal end of dendrites and around the cell body. This spatial distribution means that inhibitory input plays a predominant role in determining whether a neuron will generate an action potential. Inhibitory receptors are coupled with chloride channels. With the influx of chloride resulting from activation of inhibitory receptors, the voltage difference across the neuronal membrane becomes greater (-70 mV to -90 mV), so that a greater level of depolarization will be required to reduce the voltage difference across the membrane to generate an action potential.

Chemical Neurotransmission

Whereas the transmittal of information from one end of the neuron to the other involves electrochemical mechanisms, the transmittal of information between neurons at the synapse depends upon chemical messengers known as neurotransmitters. Neurotransmitters are information-charged molecules that are synthesized by neurons from innocuous precursors such as amino acids. The neuron uses the same neurotransmitter throughout all its synaptic connections and, thus, the neurotransmitter can be considered the "language of communication" for the neuron. The neurotransmitter utilized by a neuron confers on that neuron a high degree of biochemical specialization. Thus, the neuron possesses the biosynthetic machinery for forming the neurotransmitter; it contains substantial stores of the neurotransmitter within vesicles at the nerve terminal ready for release when action potential reaches the nerve terminal; and it possesses the biochemical processes required to rapidly terminate the action of the neurotransmitter after release into the synaptic cleft. Neurons usually are endowed with the capabilities to synthesize only one type of neurotransmitter, although there are exceptions which will be discussed below. Neurons grouped together to serve common functions generally use the same neurotransmitter; thus, the few thousand neurons whose cell bodies are localized within the locus ceruleus use norepinephrine as their neurotransmitter. During the last decade, the number of substances in the brain and in the periphery thought to serve as neurotransmitters has increased markedly, and over 30 substances have now been identified as potential neurotransmitters (Table 1).

Receptors

The information contained within the neurotransmitter is translated by highly specific receptors. The receptor can be divided into two essential components: The first is the recognition site, which lies on the outer membrane of the neuron and is likely concentrated at areas of synaptic contacts; the second is the transducer, which is activated by the binding of the neurotransmitter to the recognition site and produces the physiologic effects. The recognition sites exhibit remarkably high specificity for binding the relevant neurotransmitter: Subtle alterations in the structure of the neurotransmitter molecule, such as changes in its three-dimensional orientation, can result in drastic loss of affinity for the receptor recognition site. It appears that receptor recognition sites can be coupled with different types of transducers, depending upon the circumstances, but the association of the receptor with a certain type of transducer generally predominates.

Table 1. Putative Neurotransmitters in the Brain

Biogenic Amines	Neuropeptides
Acetylcholine	Angiotensin
Dopamine	Beta-Endorphin
Norepinephrine	Bombesin
Epinephrine	Bradykinin
Histamine	Cholecystokinin
Serotonin	Corticotropin Releasing Factor
	Dynorphin
	Gastrin
Amino Acids	Leucine-Enkephalin
Aspartic Acid	Methionine-Enkephalin
Gamma-Amino Butyric Acid	Vasoactive Intestinal Peptide
Glutamic Acid	Somatostatin
Glycine	Substance-P
Homocysteine	Thyrotropin Releasing Factor
Taurine	Vasopressin

The transducers linked to neurotransmitter receptors can be divided into two broad classes: those that are ion channels and regulate the passage of ions through the neuronal membrane, and those that are linked to enzymatic processes within the neuron. The receptors coupled to ion channels alter the basic electrophysiologic characteristics of the neuron, affecting the decision to generate an action potential. Receptors coupled to enzymes, such as adenyl cyclase, result in long-term alterations in neuronal characteristics that may modulate the neuron's response to its excitatory or inhibitory inputs.

Glia

Although generally ignored in the considerations of neuropsychopharmacology, glia—the cells that sustain neurons—clearly play an important role in synaptic neurotransmission. In fact, there are more glial cells in the brain than nerve cells, and they serve many different roles. They provide the myelin sheath that serves as the insulation to accelerate the velocity of conduction of action potentials down axons. Other glial cells envelop the neuronal cell bodies and may play a role in sustenance and nutrition. It is becoming evident that glial cells also affect neurotransmission by inactivating released neurotransmitters, and by providing certain neurons with precursors for synthesizing their neurotransmitters. Neurotransmitter-specific receptors of some types, such as the beta-adrenergic receptor, are found on glia; and, thus, it appears that neurons may communicate with their associated glia via neurotransmitters. Nevertheless, the neuropsychopharmacologic implications of these interactions with glia remain poorly understood at the present time.

NEUROTRANSMITTERS

One of the most intense and actively expanding areas of research in brain sciences is the identification and characterization of the substances used as neurotransmitters in the brain and in the peripheral nervous system. Historically, the first neurotransmitters were identified in studies conducted on peripheral sympathetic and parasympathetic neurons. Thus, Loewi identified "vagus stuff" in the heart, which was subsequently demonstrated to be acetylcholine released by the vagal nerve; and Von Euler and his colleagues characterized "symphatin," which proved to be norepinephrine, the primary neurotransmitter of sympathetic neurons. The determination of the role of acetylcholine and norepinephrine as neurotransmitters in the peripheral autonomic system led in the 1950s to studies demonstrating the existence of these substances within the brain. With the elaboration of the concept of chemical neurotransmission, investigators began to focus on the central nervous system to identify the putative neurotransmitters. These studies led to the proposal that several amino acids serve as neurotransmitters that are uniquely localized to the brain, at least in mammals. During the last decade, peptide hormones originally identified in the peripheral neurons, especially in the gastrointestinal tract, have been shown to be localized in brain neurons.

Neurotransmitter Criteria

Because of the immense complexity of the central nervous system and the reactivity of neurons to a variety of chemical stimuli, the task of demonstrating that a substance may serve as a neurotransmitter is methodologically quite complicated. Rigid criteria have been established for determining whether a substance is a neurotransmitter; and, currently, only a few substances have satisfied all these criteria for brain neurons. These criteria include the following: The neuron must have the capability of synthesizing the substance; the substance must be released from the neuronal terminals when they are depolarized; exogenous application of the substance to receptive neurons must mimic the effects of the substance released from the nerve terminals; and drugs that antagonize the effects of the exogenous substance on receptive neurons must also specifically antagonize the effects of the substance released from the nerve terminals. With the development of sensitive and specific biochemical and immunological techniques to visualize substances at the cellular level and to detect their release in extremely small amounts, it has been possible to satisfy the first two criteria for over 30 substances (see Table 1). However, the complexity of the neuronal connections and the extremely fine structures involved in synaptic contacts make it especially difficult to probe the actions of putative neurotransmitters at the level of identified synapses. For this reason, it has been much more difficult to satisfy the latter two criteria for most putative neurotransmitters. As alternative strategies, investigators have attempted to demonstrate neurophysiologic, neurochemical and behaviorial effects specifically associated with the action of putative neurotransmitters placed in brain regions containing the substance; and they have attempted to demonstrate that activation of the neurons containing the substance produces effects similar to those of the exogenous substance, and that both can be antagonized by specific drugs.

Neurotransmitter Types

The putative neurotransmitters can be divided into three major categories: biogenic amines, amino acids and neuropeptides. These categories reflect, in part, relative concentrations of the neurotransmitters, their anatomical localization and possibly their functional role. The biogenic amine neurotransmitters—including dopamine, norepinephrine, epinephrine, serotonin, acetylcholine and histamine—are found in micromolar (10^{-6} M) concentrations in major brain areas, although considerable regional variation in concentration does exist. The neurons that utilize the biogenic amines usually have their cell bodies located in the reticular core within the brainstem, which has traditionally been known as the reticular activating system. These neurons provide relatively diffuse innervation throughout the neuroaxis, including the limbic system and the cerebral cortex. The concentration of the amino acid neurotransmitters, including glutamic acid, aspartic acid, gamma amino butyric acid (GABA) and glycine is in the millimolar (10^{-3} M) range. These neurotransmitters appear to be involved in the communication of very discrete excitatory or inhibitory effects, and may serve as the basis for primary transmittal of "hard" information within the nervous system. The neuropeptides are generally found in nanomolar (10^{-9} M) concentrations within major brain regions and typically have a very irregular distribution in the brain; thus, certain brain regions may contain substantial concentrations of a particular neuropetide, while others may be devoid of the substance. Many of the neuropeptides have been associated with specific functions, such as regulation of the release of pituitary hormones, although anatomic studies suggest a broader role in brain function. Nevertheless, the broad brain distribution of the various neuropeptides and their neurophysiologic effects precludes a simple and inclusive description of their functions.

An important distinction between the neuropeptides, on the one hand, and the biogenic amine and amino acid neurotransmitters, on the other, is their mechanism of synthesis. The biogenic amines and amino acid neurotransmitters conform much more closely to the classical concept of the metabolic disposition of the neurotransmitters. Thus, the availability of these neurotransmitters for release is controlled at the level of the nerve terminal. Although the enzymes involved in the synthesis of these neurotransmitters are formed in the cell body and transported to the nerve terminals, the synthesis of the neurotransmitters themselves is regulated entirely at the level of the nerve terminal. In other words, rapid changes in the rate of release of these neurotransmitters can be compensated for by local synthesis of new neurotransmitters from the precursors that are taken up into the nerve terminal. In contrast, the neuropeptides are synthesized at the level of the cell body by translation from mRNA, much like any other neuronal protein. Precursor neuropeptides are then transported down the axon to the nerve terminal where they are processed to form the active neuropeptide, which is available for release at the synapse. There is little evidence that neuropeptides, once released, can be recycled by re-uptake into the nerve terminal, unlike the biogenic amines and the amino acid neurotransmitters. Furthermore, to restore levels of neuropeptides released at the nerve terminals, additional precursor peptides must be formed within the cell body and then transported down to the nerve terminal. This difference between the two major classes of neurotransmitters suggests that neuropeptides may be less amenable to sustained release.

Co-localization

It has long been thought that neurons utilize one and only one neurotransmitter. This principle has been designated Dale's law, although in defense of this eminent investigator, he proposed that the same neurotransmitter is used throughout the axonal extensions of a neuron. Evidence has been mounting in recent years that more than one neurotransmitter may be contained in and released by a specific neuron. Generally, the combination involves a simple neurotransmitter (biogenic amine or amino acid) and a neuropeptide as the co-transmitter. Although the functional advantage of co-transmitters remains poorly understood, it appears (in a few simple systems examined in the periphery) that the amine neurotransmitter serves a specific signal function; the neuropeptide co-transmitter appears to serve a long-term modulatory function on adjacent cells. The fact that neurons may contain and release more than one transmitter markedly increases the complexity of neurocommunication within the brain. Instead of approximately 30 potential neurotransmitters, one must consider the approximate combination of all possible neurotransmitters—about 435. In fact, data developed thus far indicate little consistency in co-localization with some dopamine neurons containing cholecystokinin and others devoid of this neuropeptide, and some noradrenergic neurons containing enkephalins and others containing different neuropeptides. By combining the effects of the simple neurotransmitter and the co-localized neuropeptide that would have a fairly restricted brain localization, there is the possibility of more discrete pharmacologic manipulation of neuronal function.

MECHANISM OF ACTION OF PSYCHOTROPIC DRUGS

The biochemical processes involved in effective synaptic neurotransmission represent the potential sites of pharmacologic intervention to either enhance or attenuate the action of a given neurotransmitter. These processes, which are vulnerable to pharmacologic manipulation, include enzymes involved in the synthesis or catabolism of the neurotransmitter, uptake and storage processes, and the receptors that mediate or modulate synaptic neurotransmission.

The dopaminergic neuronal system is currently among the best characterized with regard to pharmacological manipulation of their function, and serves as an instructive example of the multiple sites where drugs might act to selectively alter chemical neurotransmission (see Figure 2). In terms of interfering with dopaminergic neurotransmission, a number of sites have been exploited. The amino acid analogues alpha–methyl–tyrosine and alpha–methyldopa (Aldomet) serve as competitive inhibitors of the enzymes in the synthesis pathway for dopamine and can, in sufficient quantities, reduce the availability of releasable dopamine. Dopamine is stored in vesicles at the nerve terminal; this vesicular storage process is selectively and potently inhibited by reserpine (Serpasil), which depletes dopamine stores. Released dopamine stimulates postsynaptic receptors to exert its effects. Dopamine receptors can be blocked by neuroleptic drugs such as haloperidol and chlorpromazine. On the other hand, dopaminergic neurotransmission can be enhanced at several different sites. Administration of the precursor amino acid, L-dopa, will enhance the synthesis of

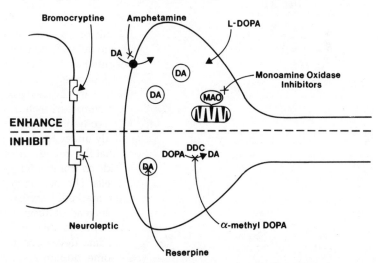

Figure 2. Sites of drug action that alter dopaminergic neurotransmission. Drugs that enhance dopaminergic neurotransmission are presented in the upper half of the schematic synapse; those drugs, whose net effect is to reduce dopaminergic neurotransmission, are presented in the lower half. Drugs that stimulate a process are presented as arrows (→); those that inhibit a process are presented as crosses (✗).

dopamine. Drugs such as bromocriptine have direct agonist effects at dopamine receptors and therefore can stimulate the receptors regardless of dopamine release. The action of dopamine in the synaptic cleft can be prolonged by such stimulant drugs as cocaine, methylphenidate and amphetamine, which inhibit the uptake-inactivation of dopamine; and monoamine oxidase inhibitors also potentiate the action of dopamine by impairing its enzymatic degradation. Such principles can be applied to other neurotransmitters, as will be reviewed in the following chapters of this section.

CONCLUSION

The elucidation of the mechanisms of action of neuropsychotropic drugs that are effective in relieving the symptoms of various psychiatric and neurologic disorders have led logically to the implication that disruption in the function of the affected neurotransmitter systems may be involved in the basic pathophysiology of the disorders. While conclusive evidence of a selective abnormality in a specific neurotransmitter system in the etiology of a psychiatric disorder remains to be developed, there is indirect evidence to support the role of such an abnormality in a number of disorders, including schizophrenia, affective disorders, anxiety disorders and attention deficit disorders. Future studies involving analysis of brains of patients who have died with these disorders, as well as recently developed *in vivo* techniques such as positron emission tomography, will be required to better delineate the potential role of neurotransmitters in the etiology of major psychiatric disorders.

Chapter 2

Dopamine and Antipsychotic Medications

by Ian Creese, Ph.D.

Pharmacological evidence has suggested an association of central nervous system (CNS) dopaminergic neuronal dysfunction in the etiology of schizophrenia. Chronic abuse of stimulants such as amphetamine, which are known to enhance dopaminergic activity in the brain, can lead to the development of a paranoid psychosis that is almost indistinguishable from classic paranoid schizophrenia. An acute amphetamine administration will exacerbate the symptomatology of a schizophrenic and initiate a recurrence of psychosis in a schizophrenic in remission (Creese, 1983b). However, schizophrenic symptomatology can be reduced by the administration of reserpine (which depletes brain dopamine) and by the antipsychotic neuroleptic drugs such as haloperidol and chlorpromazine (which act by blocking dopamine postsynaptic receptors), thereby decreasing dopamine's actions in the brain.

ANTIPSYCHOTIC MEDICATIONS: A HISTORY OF THE RESEARCH

Before the twentieth century, with neither knowledge of disease processes nor the mechanisms of drug action, the discovery of therapeutic drugs proceeded entirely by chance. Even in recent years the discovery of chlorpromazine's antipsychotic activity was serendipitous. The use of animal models to test drugs heralded a new era in pharmaceutical research, but, unfortunately, results obtained in experimental animals cannot always be applied to man. In the search for a pharmacological therapy for schizophrenia, a satisfactory animal model of established relevance to the human psychopathology is lacking. For example: It is difficult to discern the similarity between the mechanism that causes a neuroleptic to reduce schizophrenic symptoms, and the mechanism that stops a rat from jumping up on a pole to avoid an electric shock (a common screen for antipsychotic agents). Such screening techniques have been empirically shown to correlate with pharmacologic potency in the treatment of schizophrenia. Whether a common biochemical or physiological substrate exists for these superficially dissimilar actions is much more difficult to establish. Such animal behaviors are mediated by many neurochemical and neuroanatomical systems that may or may not be a part of the pathophysiology of schizophrenia.

Phenothiazines

The impressive clinical success of the phenothiazines in the treatment of schizophrenia sparked many inquiries into the biochemical effects of these drugs. Medicinal chemists subjected the phenothiazine molecule to many remodelings:

The resulting compounds varied in their clinical efficacy. Considering only a few of the many derivatives, fluphenazine (with a fluoride-substituted A ring) is about ten times more potent than chlorpromazine (with a chloride-substituted A ring) as an antipsychotic. Chlorpromazine is many times more potent than promazine (with no substitution on the A ring), a phenothiazine nearly devoid of antipsychotic activity. However, promazine, like the efficacious phenothiazines, possesses a full complement of antihistamine and other side effects. These results were of great importance to pharmacologists and biochemists. Such a series of drugs, with different potencies as antipsychotics but with similar pharmacologic effects, can now be tested in any biochemical system which might be thought to be involved in their therapeutic action. When the correct *in vitro* system is investigated, the same relative potencies of the various drugs must be maintained. A drug such as promazine is "the exception that proves the rule": it possesses all the nonspecific actions of the phenothiazines, with none of the critical aspects responsible for the antipsychotic property of the rest of their family. Therefore, any biochemical or behavioral test that finds promazine to be equal to or more potent than chlorpromazine, definitely cannot be involved in the mechanism of action of antipsychotic, neuroleptic drugs; and could probably not be related directly to the schizophrenic process. In the late 1950s and early 1960s, Janssen introduced a new series of neuroleptic agents—the butyrophenones—that demonstrated the same behavioral and clinical effects as the phenothiazines. Haloperidol is a typical member of this class, and is similar in potency to fluphenazine.

Receptor Theory of Drug Action

Much early research focused on potential presynaptic mechanisms of drug action as sites responsible for psychiatric disease. However, recent technical developments have allowed postsynaptic mechanisms to be investigated, both in relation to the mechanism of drug action, and to direct assay of receptors in postmortem CNS tissue taken from patients with psychiatric disease. Early in this century, Ehrlich and Langley advanced the receptor theory of drug action (Parascandola, 1981). Nowhere has their original "lock and key" theory proved more apt than in the case of CNS neurotransmitter receptors and the psychoactive drugs that act on them. For example: Although there are many possible sites of action for a neuroleptic drug in the CNS, electrophysiological, pharmacological, and behavioral studies have provided evidence that their actions are mediated by direct binding to neurotransmitter receptors as antagonists. However, the elucidation of the entire cascade of events leading from receptor occupancy to behavioral or emotional response presents scientific and philosophical problems now beyond comprehension. Much of modern psychopharmacology has been based on the hypothesis that a single biochemical deficit may explain global mental and behavioral disturbances, and thus be a target for simple and rational pharmacological therapy. Therefore, by identifying the single *initial* event of neurotransmitter or drug action (which is often conserved over a wide phylogenetic range) these difficulties can be obviated. It is this elimination of other variables—accomplished by the direct assay of receptor occupancy— that has made the newly developed technique of neurotransmitter receptor radioligand binding so valuable to our understanding of psychoactive drugs' biochemical mechanisms of action, and the role these receptors may play in the etiology of psychiatric diseases. This is especially true because most receptors are stable in postmortem tissue as long as the tissue is rapidly chilled and frozen after death and can readily be examined.

Dopamine Receptor Research

By 1970, research suggested that the most likely mechanism of action of neuroleptic drugs was the blockade of postsynaptic dopamine receptors. However, no biochemical method for the study of dopamine receptors had been developed and it was therefore impossible to test this hypothesis directly. In 1972, neuroleptic pharmacology was thrown into disarray when "the" dopamine receptor was first biochemically identified. Greengard and associates demonstrated that homogenates of rat corpus striatum would accumulate cyclic adenosine monophosphate (cAMP) when exposed to dopamine (Kebabian et al, 1972). Certain neurotransmitter and hormone receptors on the cell surface are linked to the intracellular enzyme, adenylate cyclase. Binding of the appropriate neurotransmitter/hormone to the receptor activates the adenylate cyclase, which converts ATP to cAMP. The transient increase in the intracellular levels of cAMP, the "second messenger," causes the physiological response resulting from the binding of the neurotransmitter to its receptor.

Phenothiazine neuroleptics were potent, competitive inhibitors of the activation of adenylate cyclase by dopamine; and a similarity was seen in their pharmacological potencies as dopamine antagonists in animals, in their antipsychotic activity in man and in their influences on the dopamine-sensitive adenylate cyclase. This, of course, supported the hypothesis that neuroleptic action is mediated by blocking dopamine receptors (Iversen, 1975). There were, however, marked discrepancies for butyrophenones and other neuroleptics. For example: Haloperidol, which clinically and pharmacologically is ten to 100 times more potent than chlorpromazine, appeared weaker than, or at best equal to, chlorpromazine in its influences on the dopamine-stimulated adenylate cyclase (Creese et al, 1978). Furthermore, the most potent butyrophenone, spiroperidol (or spiperone)—which is about five times more potent than haloperidol in intact animals and in controlling schizophrenia—was weaker than haloperidol and chlorpromazine in inhibiting dopamine's stimulation of adenylate cyclase. More recently, benzamide antipsychotics such as sulpiride have been found to be altogether devoid of inhibitory potency at this receptor (Creese et al, 1983).

These discrepancies raised the possibility that butyrophenones might not block dopamine receptors at all, but rather act in some other system and influence dopaminergic activity indirectly. This would account for the marked difference in chemical structure between phenothiazines and butyrophenones despite their pharmacological similarities. An alternative hypothesis, which was not considered initially, is that more than one type of dopamine receptor exists. Thus, butyrophenones could exhibit low affinity at the receptors responsible for eliciting an increase in cAMP, while they would exhibit higher potencies at those dopamine receptors responsible for most of their behavioral and clinical effects. This hypothesis stimulated radioligand binding studies with ^{3}H–neuroleptics to search for the "neuroleptic receptor" and, perhaps, a second type of dopamine receptor. Before discussing these exciting studies in more detail, a short discussion of the anatomy of dopamine systems is in order.

ANATOMY OF DOPAMINERGIC SYSTEMS

The nigrostriatal pathway accounts for approximately 70 percent of the total brain content of dopamine, and has become an obvious focus of research (Figure 1). The existence of the nigrostriatal pathway was strongly implied by the observations of Hornykiewicz (1966), who demonstrated that patients with Parkinson's disease display a concomitant loss of dopamine in the striatum or basal ganglia, along with the degeneration of cells in the substantia nigra, pars compacta. The other major dopamine pathways originate from a group of cells in the ventrotegmental area surrounding the interpeduncular nucleus, and innervate the olfactory tubercle, adjacent limbic areas, and the anterior cortical structures. They are called the mesolimbic and mesocortical systems, respectively. The substantia nigra and ventrotegmental dopamine cell groups are frequently referred to as the A–9 and A–10 nuclear groups, respectively, following the original designation by Dahlstrom and Fuxe (1964) in their pioneering fluorescence in histochemical studies. However, since the introduction of more sensitive histologic techniques, it is becoming clear that the dopamine systems are more complex than originally thought (Moore and Bloom, 1978).

Of the other dopamine pathways, the tubero-hypophysial system has received the most attention. Dopamine from this hypothalamic cell group is released into the portal blood system where it is carried to the anterior pituitary and inhibits prolactin release from mammotrophs (Weiner and Ganong, 1978).

The role of these various pathways in schizophrenia is not known. A reasonable hypothesis, however, is that the nigrostriatal pathway, which is part of the extrapyramidal motor system, is involved in the motoric symptoms seen in some

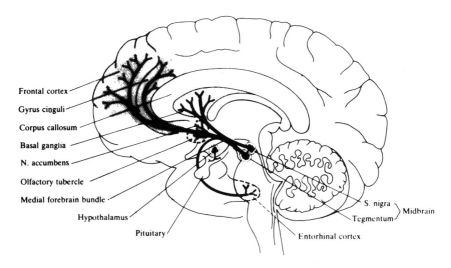

Figure 1. The principal dopamine projections in the human brain.

forms of schizophrenia (catatonia) and the parkinsonian side effects of neuro-leptic drugs. The mesolimbic and mesocortical pathways, brain areas classically associated with intellectual function and emotions, are involved in the more cardinal psychiatric symptoms of the disease. The elevation in prolactin levels caused by neuroleptic drugs is the result of dopamine receptor blockade in the anterior pituitary.

RADIOLIGAND BINDING STUDIES

Since 1973, the availability of neurotransmitters or drugs radioactively labeled to extremely high specific activities (>10 Ci/mmol) with ^{125}I or more generally ^{3}H, has allowed the quantitation of receptor bound drug to many of the known neurotransmitter receptors. The assays themselves are quite simple (Bennett, 1984). A small volume of homogenized brain tissue or purified synaptosomal membranes is added to nanomolar quantities of the ^{3}H–drug or ligand as it is called. After incubation for sufficient time to allow equilibrium to be reached between the association and dissociation of the ^{3}H–ligand with the receptor sites, the ^{3}H–ligand bound to the membranes is separated from that remaining free in solution by one of several methods. The most popular, because of its speed and convenience, is by filtration under reduced pressure over glass fiber filters. The amount of ^{3}H–ligand trapped on the filters is thus a direct measure of the amount of drug occupying sites on the membranes.

A major problem, the understanding of which enabled successful quantitation of neuroleptic binding to CNS dopamine receptors, was that of "nonspecific binding." In contrast to the "specific binding" of the radiolabeled neuroleptic to bona fide dopamine receptors, a portion of the labeled ligand is both trapped by the membranes and bound in a relatively nonspecific fashion to other cellular components. This "nonspecific" binding is not displaceable by an excess of nonradioactive drug or other similar drugs which interact at dopamine receptors (Yamamura et al, 1984). Such nonspecific binding sites, in general, have much lower affinity for the radiolabeled neuroleptic than the dopamine receptors themselves; but because they so vastly outnumber the specific dopamine recep-tor sites, nonspecific binding can nonetheless account for a significant fraction of the total ^{3}H–ligand bound. Nonspecific binding must be measured in some way and subtracted from the total binding if the amount of specific dopamine receptor binding is to be accurately determined. Binding assays are therefore always done in replicates where one set of samples contains tissue and ^{3}H–ligand to give total binding, and another otherwise identical set contains, in addition, a high concentration of unlabeled competing drug known to bind to dopamine receptors, and thus completely displace all specific dopamine receptor binding of the radioligand. The amount of binding to true dopamine receptors is therefore always determined indirectly, by the subtraction of nonspecific from total ^{3}H–ligand receptor binding.

An accurate way to determine the crucial specific dopamine receptor binding sites responsible for a neuroleptic drug's action from its "nonspecific" binding sites is that of isomeric specificity. If activity of a neuroleptic is exhibited *in vivo* by only one of its optical or geometric isomers, then a similar difference in isomeric activity must also be exhibited by the *in vitro* receptor system responsible for mediating its action. For example, the neuroleptic, butaclamol, exists as optical isomers. Only (+)butaclamol is antischizophrenic and exhibits neuroleptic activity in animal models; (−)butaclamol is inactive. (+)Butaclamol displaces ^{3}H–neuroleptic binding to brain membranes at very low concentrations while, in contrast, a 10,000-fold higher concentration of (−)butaclamol is required to displace ^{3}H–neuroleptic binding (Creese, 1983a). This suggests that the selective, high affinity displacement by (+)butaclamol represents binding to receptors responsible for neuroleptic action.

Such binding assays allow the determination of more than just the presence or absence of a particular neurotransmitter receptor in a tissue sample. With a fixed quantity of tissue, increasing the amount of labeled ligand will increase the amount of ligand bound until there are no more empty receptors to be occupied. This "saturation" is approached in a smooth hyperbolic curve with increasing ligand concentration. When linearized by the Scatchard equation, the saturation data can easily be used to obtain both the absolute number of sites (per gram of tissue or milligram of protein), and the affinity of these sites for the ligand. Affinity is expressed as the "K_D"—that concentration of ligand required to half saturate the receptors—and, in general, is directly related to potency. By including varying concentrations of a competing drug in the presence of a fixed concentration of labeled ligand, the affinity of an unlabeled drug for a receptor population can also be determined.

The *in vitro* radioligand binding technique thus provides an excellent testing system with which to screen for other active drugs that bind to the same receptor. This method is not only sensitive and specific, but also rapid and inexpensive. Only milligram quantities of a new drug need be synthesized for study, and there are no special isotopic requirements, as all studies are based not on the direct measurement of the binding of the experimental drug itself but rather on its displacement of a radioactive, commercially available ligand whose pharmacology is known in detail. Thus, the interactions of a drug with an entire battery of neurotransmitter receptor systems can be assessed within a few hours. Such receptor-binding/drug screening techniques have many beneficial characteristics. They enable detailed structure-activity relationships to be examined unencumbered by variations in absorption or metabolism. This is an obviously efficient way to focus on the pharmacologically active portions of a molecule and direct further synthetic programs, as well as provide insight into the possible structural characteristics of receptors (Creese, 1984).

Early dopamine receptor binding studies utilized the butyrophene ^{3}H–haloperidol and later ^{3}H–spiroperidol (Creese et al, 1983; Seeman, 1980). Not surprisingly, both drugs bind to membranes from many brain regions. In the corpus striatum, the brain region receiving the greatest dopamine innervation, the binding was greatly enriched. Among neurotransmitters and their pharmacologic agonists, only dopaminergic drugs displaced the ^{3}H–butyrophenones from their binding sites, suggesting that they might indeed be labeling dopamine receptors. As already mentioned, the recently introduced neuroleptic butaclamol exists as optical isomers, of which only the (+) isomer has pharmacological activity as an antipsychotic agent and dopamine antagonist. If ^{3}H–butyrophenone binding sites are indeed the receptor sites responsible for the pharmacological activity of butaclamol, then only its clinically active isomer should be potent in displacing the ^{3}H–ligand binding. Indeed (+) butaclamol inhibits the ^{3}H–butyrophenone binding with distinct high (nanomolar) and low (micromolar) affinity components. The inactive isomer displays only low affinity competition of ^{3}H–butyrophenone binding.

The affinities of neuroleptics of diverse chemical structures for striatal dopamine receptors labeled with ^{3}H–butyrophenones correlate closely with their antipsychotic potencies in man (Creese et al, 1976; Seeman et al, 1976) (Figure 2). It is quite striking that one can predict clinical potencies from *in vitro* effects of drugs, since average clinical doses vary quite markedly among patients. Moreover, clinical potencies are affected by variable absorption, metabolism and penetration of drugs into the brain. Presumably, over the wide range of drugs investigated, these factors tend to equalize. The close correlation between neuro-

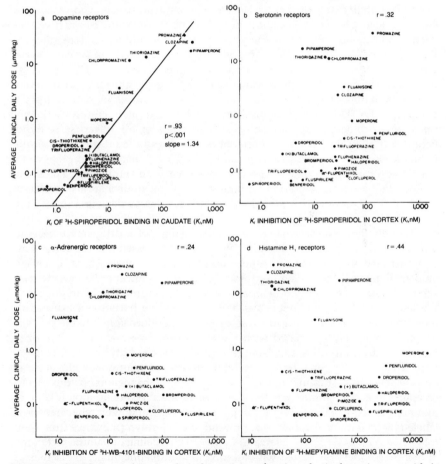

Figure 2. Correlations of *in vivo* clinical potencies of antipsychotic drugs in man with *in vitro* receptor affinities at (a) dopaminergic D–2 receptors; (b) serotonergic S–2 receptors; (c) adrenergic alpha–1 receptors; and (d) histaminergic H–1 receptors. Reprinted from The American Journal of Psychiatry 137:1518, 1980. Copyright © 1980, The American Psychiatric Association. Reprinted by permission.

leptic drugs' clinical potencies and affinities for dopamine receptors is by no means fortuitous. Studies of the potencies of neuroleptics in competing for alpha-adrenergic, serotonergic 5HT–2, histaminergic H–1 (Peroutka and Snyder, 1980) (Figure 2), opiate, and muscarinic cholinergic receptors demonstrate no correlation at all with their clinical potencies as antipsychotic agents (Creese, 1983).

Because the clinical activity of drugs is difficult to quantify, it is desirable to relate binding properties of neuroleptics with their pharmacological actions in animals where *in vivo* activity can be more objectively determined (Creese, 1983b; Creese et al, 1976). Apomorphine, a directly acting dopamine agonist, induces a stereotyped motor behavior in rodents consisting of sniffing, licking and gnawing. Psychopharmacological studies have demonstrated that this derives from stimulation of dopamine receptors in the corpus striatum and/or nucleus accumbens. The ability of neuroleptics to block apomorphine-induced sterotyped behavior also predicts the clinical potencies of these drugs as antipsychotic agents, and has been used by the pharmaceutical industry as a screening test (Janssen and Van Bever, 1978). Amphetamine also elicits a similar stereotyped motor behavior, by causing a direct release of dopamine and blockade of dopamine reuptake in the striatum. Blockade of these amphetamine effects also predicts clinical activities of neuroloptics. Accordingly, potencies of neuroleptics in competing for ^{3}H–haloperidol binding correlate extremely closely with their potencies in blocking apomorphine and amphetamine-induced stereotyped behavior ($r > 0.9$). In addition, neuroleptics are among the most effective antiemetics known. They are thought to act by blocking dopamine receptors in the chemoreceptor trigger zone in the postrema area of the brainstem. The ability of neuroleptics to prevent apomorphine-induced emesis in dogs also correlates well with their affinities for ^{3}H–haloperidol binding sites in the striatum (Creese et al, 1976).

Although these studies have compared bovine striatal dopamine receptor affinity to drug effects in other animals and then to man, recent studies have demonstrated that striatal dopamine receptors are quite similar in all species studied (Seeman, 1980). The impressive correlation between the clinical, anti-schizophrenic actions of neuroleptics and their blockade of dopamine receptors labeled with ^{3}H–butyrophenones is more striking than has been observed for any other biochemical effect of these drugs. It therefore seems likely that this action is intimately associated with the antischizophrenic effects of the drug. However, drug affinities at ^{3}H–butyrophenone binding sites do not correlate with drug affinities in interactions with the dopamine stimulated adenylate cyclase, clearly distinguishing two subtypes of dopamine receptors. Those receptors linked to stimulation of cAMP formation have been termed D–1 dopamine receptors—their behavioral function is as yet unknown. Those receptors labeled by ^{3}H–butyrophenones have recently been termed D–2 dopamine receptors (Creese et al, 1983; Kebabian and Calne, 1979). In many locations, activation of D-2 receptors is associated with an inhibition of adenylate cyclase activity.

Receptor Supersensitivity—Implications for Tardive Dyskinesia

Behavioral changes following specific lesions of the nigrostriatal dopamine pathway suggest that postsynaptic dopamine receptors in the corpus striatum become supersensitive to dopamine after removal of their normal innervation. For example, bilateral injections of the selective neurotoxin 6–hydroxydopamine, which kills dopamine cell bodies in the substantia nigra, mimics the degeneration that occurs in Parkinson's disease. Rats lesioned with 6-hydroxydopamine display increased stereotyped behavioral responses to apomorphine, a dopamine receptor agonist, and respond to previously subthreshold doses. These behaviorally supersensitive rats exhibit a twofold increase in ^{3}H–haloperidol binding to D–2 receptors in the striatum. Thus, the increase in D–2 receptors corresponds with a concomitant increase in behavioral "supersensitivity" (Creese et al, 1977).

Such "up regulation" of receptors, as it is termed, is a common feature of most receptor systems when the endogenous ligand is removed. Supersensitivity of dopamine receptors has considerable clinical implications in both neurology and psychiatry. It is thought that the ability of L-dopa to alleviate symptoms of Parkinson's disease derives, in part, from supersensitivity of the dopamine receptors (induced by the degeneration of the nigrostriatal pathway) in the brains of these patients. Recent studies have investigated ^{3}H–haloperidol binding in post mortem brains from patients who have died with Parkinson's disease (Lee et al, 1978). Both the putamen and caudate nuclei of the striatum demonstrated about 50 percent increases in ^{3}H–haloperidol binding. However, no increase was seen in patients on L-dopa therapy. In fact, animal studies have shown that L-dopa treatment can reverse both behavioral and biochemical manifestations of dopamine receptor supersensitivity (Seeman, 1980; Friedhoff et al, 1977). This finding may relate to the "on-off" phenomenon seen with L-dopa therapy in Parkinson's disease, when refractory periods to L-dopa's beneficial effects occur. This is thought to result from a "down regulation" of the "up regulated" receptors caused by the dopaminergic denervation in this disease. It has thus been suggested that the stopping of L-dopa therapy for an intermittent time will allow these "down regulated" receptors to increase in sensitivity, so that the patient becomes sensitive to L-dopa therapy once more.

Tardive dyskinesia is a major complication of the long-term treatment of schizophrenic patients with neuroleptic drugs, that frequently worsens when the neuroleptic dose is lowered or terminated (Baldessarini and Tarsy, 1979). Increasing the dose of neuroleptic may temporarily alleviate symptoms, but the dyskinesia soon reappears after this temporary reversal. The dyskinesia can be exacerbated by dopamine agonists, such as L-dopa. To provide an animal model of tardive dyskinesia, rats and mice have been treated chronically with neuroleptic drugs. Such treatments may produce abnormal movements in rodents but always lead to an enhanced sensitivity to the motor stimulant effects of apomorphine. As has already been mentioned, lesioning the nigrostriatal dopamine pathway also produces an enhanced sensitivity to dopamine receptor agonists, which is thought to result from a dopamine receptor supersensitivity following denervation. Thus, speculation has linked the development of tardive dyskinesia to an iatrogenic supersensitivity of dopamine receptors following their prolonged blockade by chronic neuroleptic administration (Baldessarini and Tarsy, 1977). Some investigators have suggested that "tardive psychosis" can also occur following chronic neuroleptic treatment (Chouinard and Jones, 1980).

A true receptor supersensitivity appears to accompany the behavioral supersensitivity to dopamine agonists following denervation; therefore, it appeared reasonable to test the hypothesis that chronic receptor blockade with neuroleptic drugs in rats might also be related to a receptor supersensitivity (Creese et al, 1983; Creese and Sibley, 1981). Rats have been treated from three weeks to over one year with neuroleptics. Following the termination of the chronic treatment there is a highly significant 20 to 70 percent increase in the number of D–2 receptors. This increase in the number of butyrophenone D–2 receptors is consistent with the behavioral supersensitivity to apomorphine in rats treated with a similar dose schedule of neuroleptics. These results therefore suggest that tardive dyskinesia might similarly result from an increase in a population of D–2 receptors. It is interesting that even after long treatments, the behavioral and receptor changes in rates are still reversible a few weeks following drug withdrawal, while in tardive dyskinesia they are not.

Must tardive dyskinesia always be a concomitant of chronic neuroleptic treatment? Some recent animal experiments suggest that it may be controllable by pharmacologic means. Concurrent lithium treatment blocks both the behavioral supersensitivity to chronic neuroleptic treatment in rats and decreases the receptor supersensitivity that normally would occur (Klawans et al, 1977; Pert et al, 1978). In other animal studies, L-dopa treatment was similarly able to reverse the increase in ^{3}H–dopamine binding caused by chronic haloperidol treatment, and reverse the behavioral effects of up-regulated receptors following chronic neuroleptic treatment (Seeman, 1980; Friedhoff et al, 1977). These results have led to the suggestion that L-dopa treatment might be useful in modulating up-regulated dopamine receptors in man following chronic neuroleptic therapy.

Dopamine Receptor Changes in Schizophrenia

As we have already discussed, much pharmacologic evidence suggests that schizophrenia may involve a hyperactivity in dopamine systems. All drugs that ameliorate the symptoms of schizophrenia are antagonists of dopamine receptors. Dopamine releasing agents such as amphetamine or methylphenidate can induce a schizophrenia-like psychosis in normal subjects and can exacerbate the symptoms of schizophrenia. However, studies of dopamine metabolites in cerebrospinal fluid (CSF) in acute schizophrenia and in post mortem brains have failed to reveal evidence of increased dopamine turnover, although increased concentrations of dopamine itself have been observed in certain areas of basal ganglia (Mackay et al, 1982). It remains possible that there is a disturbance of dopaminergic processes at the level of the postsynaptic receptor.

Four studies have provided support for this hypothesis in reporting significant (50 to 200 percent) increases in post mortem ^{3}H–butyrophenone binding in the brains of schizophrenic patients (Crow et al, 1978; Lee and Seeman, 1980; Lee et al, 1978; Mackay et al, 1980). However, most of these schizophrenics had been previously treated with antipsychotic medication. It is therefore unclear whether the observed receptor increase is a primary cause of the disease process or simply iatrogenic—for example, the result of chronic neuroleptic treatment. Three studies addressing this question have yielded contradictory results. A recent study (Mackay et al, 1980, 1982) suggests that the elevation in dopamine receptors observed in the schizophrenic brain is the result of neuroleptic treatment. In this study, brain tissue was obtained post mortem from patients diagnosed as psychotic. The case histories of all patients showed that previously they had received at least three years of neuroleptic treatments. However, a few of these patients had received no neuroleptic medication for a month or more before death. The density of ^{3}H–spiroperidol binding sites was significantly raised in the psychotic group in both the caudate nucleus and nucleus accumbens. This increase was limited to the patients who were receiving neuroleptic medication up until death. Patients who had been free of neuroleptic drugs for at least one month before death did not show increases in ^{3}H–spiroperidol binding sites. However, such a rapid reversal of a neuroleptic induced upregulation of dopamine receptors would be surprising, especially in light of the fact that tardive dyskinesia is often thought to be irreversible. In contrast, in the post mortem series of Crow et al (1978) where an increase B_{max} for ^{3}H–spiroperidol was observed in the caudate nucleus, five out of 20 cases apparently had not received neuroleptic drugs for at least one year before death. Though still present, the increase in B_{max} was not as great in this group. This was also true for a number of "drug free" cases reported by Lee et al (1978). These findings suggest that dopamine receptor supersensitivity might be associated with schizophrenic illness rather than with the drugs used to treat it. Crow and colleagues have refined these studies even further (Crow et al, 1981; Cross et al, 1983). They have shown that the D–2 receptor increase is the same, regardless of whether or not the patients demonstrated tardive dyskinesia. Furthermore, Huntington's disease patients, who also received chronic neuroleptics for their movement disorder, did not evidence a D–2 increase. The implications of this particular result are unclear, however, since the striatal degeneration which occurs in Huntington's disease is associated with a loss of D–2 receptors.

In a further refinement, Crow (1982) has suggested that schizophrenia may be divided into two distinct diagnostic and etiologic categories. Type I schizophrenia is associated with an increased proportion of positive symptoms, such as hallucinations, has a good prognosis and responds to neuroleptic treatment. Type II schizophrenia is associated with the negative symptoms of affective flattening and poverty of speech, is not ameliorated by neuroleptics and has a poor prognosis. These patients evidence such signs of structural brain damage as enlarged ventricles. Crow suggests that Type I schizophrenia is associated with increased D–2 receptors, while Type II is not. This could account for the occasional finding of no increase in D–2 receptors in schizophrenics in some studies. It is interesting that D–1 receptors neither appear to be increased prior to drug treament, nor to be increased in schizophrenics who have enhanced D–2 receptors (Crow et al, 1981). However, in a recent study, evidence suggests that D–1 receptors may exhibit enhanced coupling to adenylate cyclase (Memo et al, 1983). The implications of this finding are unclear, as the function of D–1 receptors is unknown. These results are both exciting and tantalizing: The demonstration that a psychiatric illness is the result of a deficit in receptor regulation would markedly change current psychiatric concepts and have a major clinical impact.

NEUROLEPTIC SIDE EFFECTS ARE DUE TO RECEPTOR INTERACTIONS

It must be emphasized that few drugs are absolutely specific in their interactions with any one neurotransmitter receptor; and at therapeutic dose levels, they may interact with many different receptors. In some cases, this can lead to undesirable side effects; in other cases an interaction with another neurotransmitter system appears to be able to counteract unwanted side effects that result from interactions with the primary therapeutic site of action of the drug. Chronic drug treatments can also give rise to a therapeutic response or to a spectrum of side effects that do not occur following acute dosage. This often appears to be mediated by way of changes in receptor properties, including those initially responsible for the therapeutic efficacy of the drug (as has already been discussed for tardive dyskinesia).

Neuroleptics, Autonomic Side Effects, and Alpha-Adrenergic Receptors

Autonomic sympatholytic effects such as orthostatic hypotension and sedation are among the untoward actions of neuroleptic drugs. These side effects have been attributed to blockade of central and peripheral alpha-noradrenergic receptors (Peroutka et al, 1977), but direct quantitative evaluation of alpha-receptor blockade in the CNS by these agents was not feasible before the advent of receptor binding assays. Recently it has become possible to label the alpha-noradrenergic receptors with a specific antagonist that has been designated ^{3}H–WB4101. Most neuroleptics are highly potent in competing for ^{3}H–WB4101 binding to alpha-receptor sites in the rat brain (Peroutka et al, 1977). The most potent drug is the butyrophenone, droperidol, whose K_i value for inhibiting ^{3}H–WB4101 binding is 0.7 nM. All the commonly used neuroleptics display K_i values under 50 nM, putting them in the same range of potency as the classic alpha-adrenergic antagonists phentolamine and phenoxybenzamine, whose K_i values are 3.6 and 4.0 nM, respectively. Thus the neuroleptics, as a general class, are approximately equal in potency to alpha-noradrenergic receptor and dopaminergic receptor antagonists.

Although the neuroleptics are potent inhibitors of alpha-noradrenergic receptor binding, their relative potencies differ markedly from their relative activities in inhibiting ^{3}H–butyrophenone binding. As therapeutic brain levels of neuroleptics may be expected to correspond to the drug concentrations required for optimal blocking of dopamine receptors, the clinical propensity of neuroleptics to block alpha-noradrenergic receptors would be related, not to their absolute potencies as alpha-noradrenergic receptor blockers, but to the ratio of their potencies as alpha-noradrenergic receptor antagonists and to their potencies as dopamine receptor antagonists. Drugs with low ratios would be expected to elicit a substantial amount of alpha-noradrenergic receptor blockade at blood and brain levels of the drug required for adequate dopamine receptor blockade. In contrast, drugs with high ratios would be employed clinically at the very low dose levels required to secure dopamine receptor blockade and, in general, would be less likely to elicit side effects associated with alpha-noradrenergic receptor blockade. Butyrophenones such as haloperidol and spiroperidol, and piperazine phenothiazines such as fluphenazine and trifluoperazine, display ratios (K_i ^{3}H–WB4101 binding/K_i ^{3}H–haloperidol binding) greater than 8 and have a relatively low propensity to elicit hypotension and sedation. In contrast, promazine and clozapine have ratios of less than 0.2 and have the greatest tendency to cause orthostatic hypotension and sedation. In general, the finding that alkylamino and piperidine phenothiazines are more sedating and hypotensive than are the piperazine agents is manifested in the lower ratios of the former drugs; while the butyrophenones tend to be relatively nonsedating and have a low incidence of orthostatic hypotension and, correspondingly, have substantially higher ratios.

Neuroleptics, Extrapyramidal Parkinsonian Side Effects, and Muscarinic-Cholinergic Receptor Binding

Some of the most frequent side effects of neuroleptic therapy are the parkinsonian extrapyramidal side effects of rigidity and akinesia. In fact, these side effects are so common that it has been generally thought that antipsychotic activity and extrapyramidal side effects are inexorably linked. Recently two drugs, clozapine and thioridazine, have attracted a good deal of clinical and biochemical attention. These antipsychotics have a much lower incidence of extrapyramidal side effects than are associated with other neuroleptics. The fact that one can obtain effective antischizophrenic activity without extrapyramidal side effects led to the hypothesis that extrapyramidal side effects and antipsychotic activity might be mediated by distinct dopamine receptors with slightly differing drug specificities in different regions of the brain.

Since the striatum is part of the extrapyramidal motor system, it is thought that the parkinsonian side effects are probably associated with dopamine receptor blockade in the striatum. The mesolimbic areas of the forebrain (nucleus accumbens, olfactory tubercle, amygdala, and frontal cerebral cortex) are classically associated with emotional behavior; thus, these areas appear to be likely candidates for mediating the antipsychotic activity of neuroleptics. However, the results of studies to date (both radioreceptor and biochemical) have been conflicting, and have not provided much evidence to support this hypothesis. The fact that the relative affinities of clozapine and thioridazine for ^{3}H–haloperidol binding sites in bovine striatum in relation to other neuroleptics correspond reasonably well with their clinical potencies, indicates that these drugs probably exert their antischizophrenic effects by a mechanism similar to the other antipsychotic agents, and that the dopamine receptors labeled by ^{3}H–butyrophenones do not differ appreciably between different brain regions (Creese et al, 1976).

If, then, clozapine and thioridazine produce their antipsychotic effects by the same mechanisms as other neuroleptic agents, why is it that when given in therapeutic antischizophrenic doses, these drugs do not produce the same incidence of extrapyramidal side effects? Two series of recent studies may provide an answer.

It is well known that concurrent administration of anticholinergic drugs is especially effective in antagonizing the extrapyramidal side effects of neuroleptics, without apparently reducing their antipsychotic action (Snyder et al, 1974). The therapeutic efficacy of the anticholinergics apparently reflects a balance in the corpus striatum between dopamine and acetylcholine involved in motor control. Thus, antagonizing the effects of acetylcholine is equivalent to enhancing those of dopamine, and vice versa. If neuroleptics vary in their anticholinergic properties, they may well vary in their propensities to induce extrapyramidal side effects. In studies of the binding of ^{3}H–quinuclidinyl benzilate (QNB), a potent antagonist of muscarinic cholinergic receptors) to striatal membrane preparations, this hypothesis was confirmed. Clozapine, which is almost devoid of extrapyramidal side effects, has the greatest affinity for muscarinic receptors, quite close to that of classic anticholinergic agents. Thioridazine, which elicits almost as few extrapyramidal symptoms as clozapine, is the second most potent antagonist. The alkylamino phenothiazines, whose moderate incidence of extrapyramidal actions is greater than that of thioridazine, have correspondingly less affinity for the acetylcholine receptor. Piperazine phenothiazines and the butyrophenones, whose frequency of extrapyramidal side effects is greatest, have the least affinity for the muscarinic receptors (Miller and Hilley, 1974; Snyder et al, 1974). According to this hypothesis, the simultaneous blockade of acetylcholine receptors by drugs such as clozapine and thioridazine antagonizes their extrapyramidal side effects. Because of their negligible anticholinergic activity at normal doses, drugs such as haloperidol elicit many more extrapyramidal side effects. Some drugs, such as pimozide, are relatively weak at cholinergic receptors, and their lack of extrapyramidal side effects may be related to their slower onset of action (Laduron and Leysen, 1979). However, screening of potentially useful antipsychotic drugs for muscarinic receptor affinity may provide a simple *in vivo* predictor of their propensities to induce extrapyramidal side effects.

A recent series of electrophysiological studies has taken a more sophisticated approach (Chiodo and Bunney, 1983; White and Wang, 1983a). As reviewed below, the results of their studies suggest that chronic dopamine receptor blockade with neuroleptics markedly alters the activity of dopamine neurons, which contributes to their neurologic side effects. Their starting point is a somewhat controversial clinical observation—the antipsychotic activity of neuroleptic drugs and their concomitant parkinsonian side effects do not occur instantaneously. Dynamic changes must occur in the dopamine systems to explain the temporal characteristics of the clinical response. Using rats, the studies compare the acute versus chronic effects of neuroleptics on the electrophysiological activity of two dopamine pathways—the nigrostriatal system originating from the substantia nigra (A–9), and the cortico-limbic systems originating from the ventral tegmentum (A–10).

Extracellular recordings of neuronal activity were made in the A–9 and A–10 areas of the rat brain. Acute administration of chlorpromazine and haloperidol has been shown to increase both the firing rate of dopamine neurons and the number of active dopamine neurons that can be identified in the A–9 and A–10 areas. It was originally thought that this increase in dopaminergic activity occurred because of reduced inhibitory feedback from the striatum to the dopaminergic cell bodies in a homeostatic attempt to overcome the postsynaptic dopamine receptor blockade (Carlsson and Lindquist, 1963). It is now known that, in addition to this mechanism, neuroleptics also block dopamine receptors on dopamine terminals in the striatum, and dopamine receptors found on the dopamine neuronal cell bodies themselves in the A–9 and A–10 areas (Roth, 1979). These "autoreceptors" are functionally inhibitory in that dendritically released dopamine inhibits dopamine neuron firing; and in terminal areas, released dopamine inhibits both its synthesis and further release. It is not surprising, then, that all the antipsychotic drugs, both classical and atypical, increased the number of dopamine cells that could be found as the recording electrode was lowered through circumscribed regions of the A–9 and A–10 areas. White and Wang were able to find a dissociation with just acute treatment: They found that clozapine and thioridazine increased the number of dopamine neurons firing in the A–10 area but not in the A–9 area. By contrast, the nonantipsychotic metaclopramide, which can cause extrapyramidal side effects, increased activity in the A–9 area but not in the A–10 area.

This dissociation became even more pronounced following chronic (three to four week) neuroleptic administration. Both groups of investigators have previously shown that chronic treatment with classic neuroleptics results in the almost complete silencing of dopamine neurons, in contrast to their acute activation. This appears to be the result of the neurons going into depolarization block, since they can be reactivated by iontophoretic application of GABA, an inhibitory neurotransmitter, but not by the excitant glutamate (Bunney and Grace, 1978; White and Wang, 1983b). Both research groups found very few active dopamine neurons in either A–9 or A–10 areas following chronic treatment with haloperidol or chlorpromazine. It is important to note that chronic clozapine and thioridazine treatment leads to a reduced number of active dopamine neurons in only the A–10 area; while metaclopramide, which causes extrapyramidal side effects but lacks antipsychotic activity, provides a double dissociation by decreasing the number of active dopamine neurons in the A–9 area but not changing the number of active neurons in the A–10 area.

What do these results suggest happens clinically when a neuroleptic is given? Postsynaptic D–2 dopamine receptors are directly blocked by neuroleptics, thereby decreasing dopamine's synaptic action. Homeostatic mechanisms increase the firing rate of dopamine neurons with a consequent increase in the synaptic release of dopamine. The functional outcome of this is to decrease the effective receptor blockade by the neuroleptic and reduce both its antipsychotic and extrapyramidal side effects. With time, however, dynamic changes take place. The homeostatic mechanisms fail as the dopamine neurons go into depolarization block and synaptic dopamine release is reduced. The effective blockade of postsynaptic dopamine receptors increases, maximizing the antipsychotic effect of the drug and also its parkinsonian extrapyramidal side effects. Since the atypical neuroleptics such as clozapine and thioridazine do not produce depolarization block of the A–9 area, dopamine is still released in the striatum, overcoming to some extent the blockade of receptors there. Hence, these drugs do not produce the same degree of extrapyramidal side effects; however, they effectively block activity in the A–10 area, giving rise to their antipsychotic activity. Unfortunately, the mechanism responsible for this differential effect is unknown.

SIMPLE, SENSITIVE AND SPECIFIC RADIORECEPTOR ASSAY FOR BLOOD NEUROLEPTIC LEVELS

The failure of many patients to respond to standard doses of a neuroleptic appears to be related, at least in part, to a failure to attain adequate blood and hence brain levels of the drug. Clearly, the physician wants to administer high enough doses to reach therapeutic levels, even in patients who absorb the drug poorly or who are extremely rapid metabolizers. On the other hand, the physician needs to utilize the lowest effective dose of neuroleptic, because the likelihood of eliciting tardive dyskinesia probably increases as a function of increasing the dose. For these reasons, it would be desirable to monitor patient blood levels of neuroleptics routinely. Until recently, this has not been feasible because available techniques were either too complicated for routine clinical application, or they did not measure all of the different neuroleptics and their active metabolites in everyday use.

It is well established that neuroleptic drugs (or their therapeutically active metabolites) are clinically efficacious in proportion to their potency in blocking brain D–2 receptors. Thus, it is possible to directly measure neuroleptic levels in plasma or serum by their inhibition of ^{3}H–haloperidol or ^{3}H–spiroperidol binding to D–2 receptors in a sample of rat or bovine caudate membrane (Creese and Snyder, 1977; Tune et al, 1980). No extraction procedure is necessary, as small volumes (15–30μl) of plasma or serum do not interfere with binding; and neuroleptics compete with ^{3}H–butyrophenone binding at much lower concentrations than the usual therapeutic blood levels.

The radioreceptor assay has several advantages and may be routinely conducted for large patient populations. The assay is selective for neuroleptics and can therefore be utilized in patients receiving other drugs (Creese et al, 1981). Among other drug classes, only the dopaminergic ergots and a few tricyclic antidepressants (Lader, 1980) compete significantly in these assays. However, these agents are not usually prescribed for schizophrenics. Metabolites of neuroleptic that are therapeutically active will be detected in this assay, because they, too, compete for dopamine receptor binding. This is a major advantage of the radioreceptor assay, since some metabolites produced *in vivo* are active in blocking dopamine receptor activity (Creese et al, 1981); yet these metabolites would have to be individually identified to be detected by fluorimetric or spectrometric/chromatographic methods. In addition, the procedure is highly sensitive. With haloperidol, as little as 2.5 ng/ml of total serum haloperidol can be readily detected (Creese and Snyder, 1977). This radioreceptor assay offers the potential for routine application to all patients receiving neuroleptics. The procedure is sensitive and simple to perform. As many as a hundred assays can be conducted in three hours by one technician. Since the clinical potencies of neuroleptics are well correlated with their affinities for D–2 receptors, the sensitivity of the assay is greater for drugs that are employed therapeutically at lower doses.

The radioreceptor assay detects metabolites that compete for dopamine receptor binding and that are therefore therapeutically active (Freedberg et al, 1979). For instance, a substantial portion of the therapeutic activity of chlorpromazine may be attributed to its metabolite, 7–hydroxychlorpromazine, which has almost as much affinity for dopamine receptors as chlorpromazine itself. Since blood levels of 7–hydroxychlorpromazine vary widely among patients and are often higher than those of chlorpromazine, measuring chlorpromazine alone is unlikely to provide the most effective indicator of a patient's level of antischizophrenic drug activity. A similar situation exists for thioridazine and its metabolite mesoridazine. The clinical studies thus far published indicate that the radioreceptor assay of total serum neuroleptic activity does have good predictive value in terms of the presence or absence of a therapeutic response, or the production of side effects (Burnett et al, 1980; Calil et al, 1979; Cohen et al, 1980a,b,c; Rosenblatt et al, 1979; Tune et al, 1980a,b).

It is hoped that utilization of this application of the radioligand binding technique will make it possible to better control the degree of blockade of dopamine receptors by dopamine antagonist drugs. This has great clinical utility, particularly insuring that patients are not overmedicated and thereby more likely to develop untoward side effects. There is recent evidence to suggest a "therapeutic window" may exist with high blood levels of neuroleptic associated with a diminution in response (Kucharski et al, 1984). Thus, the common clinical practice of escalating the dosage in the instance of a poor clinical response might be questionable, if a poor response can also be associated with too high a neuroleptic blood level. Patients with tardive dyskinesia may have higher serum blood levels of neuroleptic than do other patients (Jeste et al, 1979). This could result from the longer hospitalization common to these patients (Kucharski et al, 1980); longer hospitalization may indicate a history of poor therapeutic response and hence higher neuroleptic dose regimens.

FUTURE DIRECTIONS

A new technique, positron emission tomography (PET), gives hope that many of the questions relating to receptor changes in psychiatric disease can be resolved in the near future (Wagner et al, 1983). With this technique, ligands are made with a very energetic and short-lived positron emitting substitutions such as ^{11}C or ^{77}Br. These ligands can be given to patients and the binding study conducted *in vivo*, the receptor binding of the drug being visualized by the computerized PET images. Thus, acute and drug-free patients will soon be able to be investigated without the requirement of death! These studies are still in their early developmental phase (Wagner et al, 1983; Crowley et al, 1983; Welch et al, 1983), but they give every hope of being a most successful and relatively noninvasive technique.

REFERENCES

Baldessarini RJ, Tarsy D: Relationship of the actions of neuroleptic drugs to the pathophysiology of tardive dyskinesia. Int Rev Neurobiol 21:1, 1979

Bennett JP Jr: Methods in binding studies, in Neurotransmitter Receptor Binding. Edited by Yamamura HI, Enna SJ, Kuhar MJ. New York, Raven Press, 1984

Bjorklund A, Lindvall O: Dopamine in dendrites of substantia nigra neurons: suggestions for a role in dendritic terminals. Brain Res 83:531-537, 1975

Bunney BS, Grace AA: Acute and chronic haloperidol treatment: comparison of effects on nigral dopaminergic cell activity. Life Sci 23:1715-1728, 1978

Bunney BS, Walters JR, Roth RH, et al: Dopaminergic neurons: effects of antipsychotic drugs and amphetamine on single cell activity. J Pharmacol Exp Ther 185:560-571, 1973

Burnett GB, Prange AJ Jr, Wilson IC, et al: Adverse effects of anticholinergic antiparkinsonian drugs in tardive dyskinesia: an investigation of mechanism. Neuropsychobiology 6:109-120, 1980

Calil HM, Avery DH, Hollister LE, et al: Serum levels of neuroleptics measured by dopamine radioreceptor assay and some clinical observations. Psychiatry Res 1:39-44, 1979

Carlsson A, Lindqvist M: Effect of chlorpromazine or haloperidol on formation of 3–

methoxytyramine and normetanephrine in mouse brain. Acta Pharmacol Toxicol 20:140-144, 1963

Chiodo LA, Bunney BS: Typical and atypical neuroleptics: differential effects of chronic administration on the activity of A9 and A10 midbrain dopaminergic neurons. J Neurosci 3:1607-1619, 1983

Chouinard G, Jones BD: Neuroleptic-induced supersensitivity psychosis: clinical and pharmacologic characteristics. Amer J Psychiatry 137:16, 1980

Cohen BM, Herschel M, Miller E, et al: Radioreceptor assay of haloperidol tissue levels in the rat. Neuropharmacology 19:663-668, 1980a

Cohen BM, Lipinski JF, Harris PQ, et al: Clinical use of the radioreceptor assay for neuroleptics. Psychiatry Res 1:173-178, 1980b

Cohen BM, Lipinski JF, Pope HG, et al: Neuroleptic blood levels and therapeutic effect. Psychopharmacology 70:191-193, 1980c

Crawley JCW, Smith T, Veall N, et al: Dopamine receptors displayed in living human brain with ^{77}Br-p-bromospiperone. The Lancet II:975, 1983

Creese I: Receptor interactions of neuroleptics, in Neuroleptics: Neurochemical, Behavioral and Clinical Perspectives. Edited by Coyle JT, Enna SJ. New York, Raven Press, 1983a

Creese I: Stimulants: Neurochemical, Behavioral and Chemical Perspectives. New York, Raven Press, 1983b

Creese I: Receptor binding as a primary drug screening device, in Neurotransmitter Receptor Binding. Edited by Yamamura HI, Enna SJ, Kuhar MJ. New York, Raven Press, 1984

Creese I, Sibley DR: Receptor adaptations to centrally acting drugs. Annu Rev Pharmacol Toxicol 21:357-391, 1981

Creese I, Snyder SH: A novel, simple and sensitive radioreceptor assay for antischizophrenic drugs in blood. Nature 270:180-182, 1977

Creese I, Burt DR, Snyder SH: Dopamine receptor binding predicts clinical and pharmacological potencies of antischizophrenic drugs. Science 192:481-483, 1976

Creese I, Burt DR, Snyder SH: Dopamine receptor binding enhancement accompanies lesion-induced behavioral supersensitivity. Science 197:596, 1977

Creese I, Burt DR, Snyder SH: Biochemical actions of neuroleptic drugs: focus on the dopamine receptor, in Handbook of Psychopharmacology, vol 10. Edited by Iversen LL, Iversen SD, Snyder SH. New York, Plenum Press, 1978

Creese I, Lader S, Rosenberg B: A radioreceptor assay for neuroleptic drugs, in Clinical Pharmacology in Psychiatry-Neuroleptic and Antidepressant Research. Edited by Usdin E, Dahl SG, Gram LF, et al. New York, Macmillan Press, 1981

Creese I, Sibley DR, Hamblin MW, et al: The classification of dopamine receptors: relationship to radioligand binding. Annu Rev Neurosci 6:43-71, 1983

Crow TJ: The biology of schizophrenia. Experientia 38:1275-1282, 1982

Crow TJ, Owen F, Cross AJ, et al: Letters to the Editor. The Lancet I:36, 1978

Cross AJ, Crow T, Ferrier IN, et al: Dopamine receptor changes in schizophrenia in relation to the disease process and movement disorder. J Neural Transm 18:265-272, 1983

Dahlstrom A, Fuxe K: Evidence for the existence of monoamine-containing neurons in the central nervous system. I. Demonstration of monoamines in the cell bodies of brain stem neurons. Acta Physiol Scand Suppl 62, 232:1-55, 1964

Freedberg KA, Innis RB, Creese I, et al: Antischizophrenic drugs: differential plasma protein binding and therapeutic activity. Life Sci 24:2467-2474, 1979

Friedhoff AJ, Bonnet K, Rosengarten H: Reversal of two manifestations of dopamine receptor supersensitivity by administration of L-dopa. Chemistry, Pathology and Pharmacology 16:411, 1977

Hornykiewicz O: Dopamine and brain function. Pharmacology Research 18:925-964, 1966

Iversen LL: Dopamine receptors in the brain. Science 188:1084-1089, 1975

Jansen PAJ, VanBever WFM: Structure activity relationships of the butyrophenones and biphenylbutylpiperidines, in Handbook of Psychopharmacology, vol. 10. Edited by Iversen LL, Iversen SD, Snyder SH. New York, Plenum Press, 1978

Jeste DV, Rosenblatt JR, Wagner RL, et al: High serum levels in tardive dyskinesia. New Engl J Med 301:1184, 1979

Kebabian JW, Calne DB: Multiple receptors for dopamine. Nature 277:93-96, 1979

Kebabian JW, Petzold GL, Greengard P: Dopamine-sensitive adenylate cyclase in caudate nucleus of rat brain and its similarity to the "dopamine receptor". Proc Natl Acad Sci USA 79:2145-2149, 1972

Klawans HL, Weiner WJ, Nausieda PA: The effect of lithium on an animal model of tardive dyskinesia. Prog Neuropsychopharmacol 1:53-60, 1977

Kucharski LT, Smith JM, Dunn DD: Tardive dyskinesia and hospital discharge. J Nerv Ment Dis 168:215-218, 1980

Kucharski LT, Alexander P, Tune L, et al: Serum neuroleptic concentrations and clinical response: a radioreceptor assay investigation of acutely psychotic patients. Psychopharmacology 82:194-198, 1984

Lader, SR: A radioreceptor assay for neuroleptic drugs in plasma. J Immunoassay, 1:57-75, 1980

Laduron P, Leysen JE: Is the low incidence of extrapyramidal side-effects of antipsychotics associated with antimuscarinic properties? J Pharmacol, 30:120-122, 1979

Lee T, Seeman P: Elevation of brain neuroleptic/dopamine receptors in schizophrenia. Am J Psychiatry 137:191-197, 1980

Lee T, Seeman P, Rajput A, et al: Receptor basis for dopaminergic supersensitivity in Parkinson's disease. Nature 273:59-61, 1978a

Lee T, Seeman P, Tourtellotte W, et al: Binding of ^{3}H–neuroleptics and ^{3}H–apomorphine in schizophrenic brains. Nature 274:897-900, 1978b

Mackay AVP, Bird ED, Spokes EG, et al: Dopamine receptors and schizophrenia: drug effect or illness? The Lancet II:915-916, 1980

Mackay AVP, Iversen LL, Rossor M, et al: Increased brain dopamine and dopamine receptors in schizophrenia. Arch Gen Psychiatry 39:991, 1982

Memo M, Kleinman JE, Hanbauer I: Coupling of dopamine D_1 recognition sites with adenylate cyclase in nuclei accumbens and caudatus of schizophrenics. Science 221:1304-1307, 1983

Miller RJ, Hiley CR: Anti-muscarinic properties of neuroleptics and drug-induced Parkinsonism. Nature, 248:596-597, 1974

Moore RY, Bloom FE: Central catecholamine neuron systems: anatomy and physiology of the dopamine systems. Annu Rev Neurosci 1:129-169, 1978

Parascandola J: Origns of the receptor theory, in Towards Understanding Receptors, Edited by Lamble JW. New York, Elsevier/North Holland, 1981

Peroutka SJ, Snyder SH: Relationship of neuroleptic drug effects at brain dopamine, serotonin, alpha-adrenergic and histamine receptors to clinical potency. Am J Psychiatry 137:1518-1522, 1980

Peroutka SJ, U'Prichard DC, Greenberg DA, et al: Neuroleptic drug interactions with norepinephrine alpha-receptor binding sites in rat brain. Neuropharmacology, 16:549-556, 1977

Pert A, Rosenblatt J, Swit C, et al: Long term treatment with lithium prevents the development of dopamine receptor supersensitivity. Science 201:171-173, 1978

Rosenblatt JE, Pert CB, Colison J, et al: Measurement of serum neuroleptic concentration by radioreceptor assay: concurrent assessment of clinical psychosis ratings. Comm Psychopharmacol, 3:153-158, 1979

Roth RH: Dopamine autoreceptors: pharmacology, function and comparison with postsynaptic dopamine receptors. Comm Psychopharmacol 3: 429-445, 1979

Seeman P: Brain dopamine receptors. Pharmacol Rev 32:229-313, 1980

Seeman P, Lee T, Chau-Wong M, et al: Antipsychotic drug doses and neuroleptic/dopamine receptors. Nature 261:717-719, 1976

Snyder SH, Banerjee SP, Yamamura HI, et al: Drugs, neurotransmitters and schizophrenia. Science 184:1243-1253,1974

Tune LE, Creese I, Coyle JT, et al: Low neuroleptic serum levels in patients receiving fluphenazine decanoate. Am J Psychiatry 137:80-82, 1980a

Tune LE, Creese I, DePaulo JR, et al: Clinical state and serum neuroleptic levels measured by radioreceptor assay in schizophrenia. Am J Psychiatry, 137:187-190, 1980b

Wagner HN Jr, Burns HD, Dannals RF, et al: Imaging dopamine receptors in the human brain by positron tomography. Science 221:1264-1266, 1983

Weiner RI, Ganong WF: Role of brain monoamines and histamine in regulation of anterior pituitary secretion. Physiol Rev 58:905-976, 1978

Welch MJ, Kilbourn MR, Mathias CJ, et al: Comparison in animal models of ^{18}F-spiroperidol and ^{18}F-haloperidol: potential agents for imaging the dopamine receptor. Life Sci 33:1687-1693, 1983

White FJ, Wang RY: Differential effects of classical and atypical antipsychotic drugs on A9 and A10 dopamine neurons.Science 221:1054-1056, 1983a

White FJ, Wang RY: Comparison of the effects of chronic haloperidol treatment on A9 and A10 dopamine neurons in the rat. Life Sci 32:983-993, 1983b

Yamamura HI, Enna SJ, Kuhar MJ: Neurotransmitter Receptor Binding. New York, Raven Press, 1978; 2nd edition, 1984

Chapter 3

Monoaminergic Neurotransmitters and Antidepressant Drugs

by Steven M. Paul, M.D., Aaron Janowsky, Ph.D. and Phil Skolnick, Ph.D.

Central monoamine containing neurons have been thought to be critically involved in the pharmacological actions of a variety of psychotropic drugs, including antidepressants, antipsychotics, psychomotor stimulants and anxiolytics. Indeed, the evidence that such a small and highly discrete collection of monoamine containing perikarya (comprising less than five percent of the brain's neurons) may mediate the mood elevating properties of antidepressants is rather compelling. Over the past few years, however, it has become apparent that the activity of any given single neurotransmitter system may well depend on the inhibitory and excitatory influences of neighboring systems, and thus it may be too simplistic to attribute the drug induced normalization of a complex pathophysiologic syndrome, like depression, to a change in the "level" or "activity" of only one neurotransmitter. It is more likely that drug induced alterations in monoaminergic neurons result in compensatory changes in a number of interacting neurotransmitter systems and, in fact, the delayed time course of antidepressant action in man is more consistent with a perturbation in one or more homeostatic mechanisms. This review will focus on alterations in monoaminergic neurotransmission as a kind of "final common pathway" for the antidepressant activity of chemically dissimilar antidepressants, as well as electroconvulsive therapy (ECT). Since much of the evidence that will be presented involves a description of drug induced changes in synaptic biochemical events, the reader is referred to Chapter One, "Introduction to the Pharmacology of the Synapse," by Joseph Coyle, for an explanation of the basic principles of chemical neurotransmission.

Deciphering the neurochemical events mediating the therapeutic actions of psychotropic drugs in man is problematic because of the obvious difficulties inherent in studying the human brain, and because of the lack of appropriate peripheral and/or *in vitro* model systems. Accordingly, most of the studies designed to elucidate the mechanisms of action of antidepressants are carried out in laboratory animals and an attempt is made to extrapolate this data to man. Antidepressants, particularly the tricyclic antidepressants, produce a variety of pharmacological effects, and it has therefore been especially difficult to decipher which of their neurochemical actions are directly related to their therapeutic properties. In fact, it can be argued that there is, at present, a great deal more known about the biochemical actions of antidepressants which mediate their major side effects (such as sedation, orthostatic hypotension, dry mouth, blurred vision, constipation, and so forth), than there is about those mechanisms that subserve their therapeutic (namely, mood elevating) properties. Nonetheless, in this chapter we will attempt to focus on the possible actions of antidepressants that have been thought to underlie their therapeutic actions and, specifically, those that involve monoaminergic neurotransmission.

Among the earliest evidence that antidepressants may work through an action on monoaminergic neurotransmission was the clinical observation that iproniazid, a monoamine oxidase inhibitor, had a "psychic energizing" effect in patients with tuberculosis (Loomer et al, 1957). Subsequent clinical studies in depressed patients have consistently substantiated that a variety of chemically unrelated monoamine oxidase inhibitors are effective antidepressants. These findings, coupled with the observation that reserpine (which depletes both central and peripheral catecholamines and indoleamines) produces a syndrome in many individuals that closely resembles endogenous depression, formed the basis of the "catecholamine theory of affective disorders"—a hypothesis which is still of great heuristic value (Bunney and Davis, 1965; Schildkraut, 1965). The "catecholamine hypothesis" continues to influence contemporary research efforts on depression and the mode of action of antidepressants; albeit much more sophisticated, questions concerning the interaction of antidepressants with both catecholamine and indoleamine neurotransmitter systems are being pursued. These studies have more recently focused on both the acute and chronic effects of antidepressants on neurotransmitter receptors and thus, indirectly, on the "turnover" of the neurotransmitter itself.

DIRECT EFFECTS OF ANTIDEPRESSANTS ON MONOAMINERGIC NEURONS: REUPTAKE AND RECEPTORS

Shortly after the discovery of the now well-known neuronal uptake process for catecholamines (Potter and Axelrod, 1963), it was shown that tricyclic antidepressants, such as imipramine and desipramine, were quite potent in blocking the reuptake of exogenously administered or endogenously released catecholamines into presynaptic nerve terminals (Iverson, 1974). These effects were clearly shown to occur *in vivo* and at pharmacologically relevant doses of the antidepressants. The inhibition of presynaptic uptake produced by tricyclic antidepressants would theoretically increase the availability of norepinephrine and/ or serotonin in the synapse and thus at the receptor—a finding that would be consistent with the "catecholamine hypothesis" of depression. In later studies the tertiary amine tricyclic antidepressants, such as imipramine and amitriptyline, were found to be quite potent in blocking serotonin uptake, while their corresponding secondary amines (desipramine and nortriptyline) were more potent in blocking norepinephrine uptake (Koe, 1976). Clinically, however, there is virtually no difference in the therapeutic potency of these drugs (Klein et al, 1980); therefore it is difficult to attribute the therapeutic actions of these agents to their effects in blocking catecholamine or indoleamine uptake. Moreover, the inhibition of uptake produced by tricyclic antidepressants occurs immediately after drug administration, while the therapeutic effects of virtually all antidepressants require at least one and perhaps several weeks to develop. Despite these caveats, there are still some investigators who believe that the inhibition of norepinephrine and/or serotonin uptake is the initial and critical event mediating the therapeutic actions of these drugs. However, the recent development of many novel antidepressants that do not block catecholamine or indoleamine uptake, and the demonstration that several rather potent uptake inhibitors are devoid of antidepressant activity (Zis and Goodwin, 1979), makes such a hypothesis far less tenable.

A resurgence of interest in the possible relationship between altered presynaptic catecholamine and/or indoleamine uptake and the pathophysiology of depression has been sparked by the recent demonstration of high affinity binding sites for [^{3}H] imipramine in rat and human brain, as well as platelets (Raisman et al, 1979; Paul et al, 1980). These binding sites, which were initially thought to represent specific "receptors" for the tricyclic antidepressants (Raisman et al, 1979), have since been shown to be associated with the uptake or transport mechanism for serotonin in both brain and platelet membranes (Langer et al, 1980; Paul et al, 1981a). Similar high affinity binding sites for [^{3}H] desipramine have also been demonstrated in brain tissue from a variety of species, including man (Rehavi et al, 1982); and, not surprisingly, these have been shown to be structurally associated with the norepinephrine uptake system. Thus, the high affinity [^{3}H] imipramine and [^{3}H] desipramine binding sites in the brain can be thought of as specific drug recognition sites mediating the inhibition of serotonin and norepinephrine uptake respectively by tricyclic antidepressants and chemically related drugs (Paul et al, 1984). The pharmacological significance of these binding sites with respect to the therapeutic actions of antidepressants (and to their ability to inhibit biogenic amine uptake) is questionable. Nevertheless, the ability to quantitate these binding sites in platelets and post mortem brain tissue using radioligands has provided a valuable tool for examining the biogenic amine uptake system in depression. Although a detailed analysis of the pharmacological and biochemical characteristics of these binding sites and their relationship to the monoaminergic uptake mechanisms is beyond the scope of this review, a few important findings should be noted.

First, several investigators have reported that the pharmacological and biochemical characteristics of the [^{3}H] imipramine binding sites in brain and platelet membranes are quite similar (Rehavi et al, 1980), if not identical. Second, a number of clinical studies have found a decreased density (that is, number) of [^{3}H] imipramine binding sites in platelets from severely depressed patients compared to age- and sex-matched controls (Briley et al, 1980; Paul et al, 1981b). The decrease in the number of platelet [^{3}H] imipramine binding sites appears to be a state dependent phenomenon—normalizing with recovery both following ECT or tricylic antidepressant treatment (Suranyi-Cadotte et al, 1983). Finally, several independent groups have now reported a decrease in the number of [^{3}H] imipramine binding sites in post mortem brain tissue from patients who have committed suicide, compared to those succumbing from a variety of nonpsychiatric disorders (Stanley et al, 1982; Paul et al, 1984). These results are reminiscent of earlier findings demonstrating a decrease in the V_{max} of serotonin uptake in platelets from depressed patients (Tuomisto and Tukiainen, 1976), as well as a decrease in serotonin metabolites in post mortem brain tissue from persons who have committed suicide (Bourne et al, 1968). Taken together, these data suggest that an alteration in the neuronal uptake of serotonin is either involved in, or results from, some forms of depression.

As mentioned previously, antidepressant drugs (especially tricyclic antidepressants) are pharmacologically rather "nonspecific" compounds and are capable of interacting with many neurotransmitter receptors. In at least two cases such interactions appear to be quite relevant in explaining the pharmacological properties of these drugs. Many tricyclic antidepressants, for example, are quite potent antihistaminic agents and have been shown to be relatively potent antagonists of both types of histamine receptors (H_1 and H_2). Further, it has been suggested that the antagonism of H_2-sensitive adenylate cyclase in the brain by tricyclic antidepressants may be related to their therapeutic properties (Kanof and Greengard, 1978). More recent studies, however, have shown that other psychotropic drugs, including many neuroleptics (which are presumably devoid of antidepressant activity), are much more potent than the tricyclic antidepressants in inhibiting H_2 receptors; and that the latter, in fact, have a much higher affinity for the other class of histamine (H_1) receptors (Richelson, 1978). In this regard, several tricyclic antidepressants (for example, doxepin and amitriptyline) are among the most potent H_1 antagonists known; and many others are of comparable potency to clinically employed antihistaminic agents, such as brompheniramine. Although the affinity of most tricyclic antidepressants for H_1 receptors is quite high, there is still a discrepancy between their relative potencies in blocking H_1 receptors and their therapeutic potencies as antidepressants. In contrast, there is an excellent correlation between the sedative effects of various antidepressants as derived from either animal screening tests (Hall and Ogren, 1981) or from clinical studies (Ogren et al, 1981), and the potency of these drugs in blocking H_1 receptors. It is likely that the antihistaminic properties of tricyclic antidepressants (while unrelated to their therapeutic actions) are at least, in part, responsible for their sedative effects.

In addition to H_1 receptors, many tricyclic antidepressants also bind with high affinity to alpha (α) adrenoceptors and, specifically, to the α_1 subtype. U'Prichard and co-workers (1978) have studied a series of tricyclic antidepressants (and other psychotropic drugs) for their ability to bind to α_1-adrenoceptors, and have found that virtually all commonly used tricyclic antidepressants have relatively high affinities for α_1-adrenoceptors; but that the tertiary amines—doxepin, amitriptyline, and imipramine—are considerably more potent than are the secondary amine derivatives. In examining a series of antidepressants, these authors have also observed relatively good correlations between α_1 adrenoceptor affinity and their sedative/hypotensive properties (U'Prichard et al, 1978). Moreover, for six of the most commonly used tricyclic antidepressants, the affinities of these compounds for α_1 adrenoceptors parallels their efficacy in reducing psychomotor agitation in agitated, depressed patients; or, conversely, in producing psychomotor activation in motorically retarded depressed patients (Snyder and Peroutka, 1984). Because of the limited number of drugs tested, these data should be interpreted cautiously; but they do suggest that an interaction of tricyclic antidepressants with α_1 adrenoceptors may be related to some of the therapeutic effects of these drugs (for example, the ability to reduce agitation in certain depressed patients); and certainly such information could be of clinical use.

Direct effects of antidepressants on other monoaminergic neurotransmitter receptors, including those for dopamine (D_2) and serotonin ($5HT_1$ and $5HT_2$) have been reported (Hauger and Paul, 1983; Snyder and Peroutka, 1984). However, these effects appear to be idiosyncratic in that only a few drugs are active at either receptor. Furthermore, in most cases these interactions occur at relatively high concentrations and, thus, it is questionable whether they occur during treatment with pharmacologically relevant doses. With the possible exception of the α_1 adrenoceptor, there is little evidence that a direct interaction of antidepressants with either pre- or postsynaptic receptor or reuptake mechanisms is responsible for their therapeutic activity.

CHRONIC EFFECTS OF ANTIDEPRESSANTS ON MONOAMINERGIC NEURONS: β-ADRENERGIC AND SEROTONERGIC RECEPTORS

The time lag between administration of antidepressants (tricyclic antidepressant, monoamine oxidase inhibitors, or ECT) and the onset of therapeutic activity (Klein et al, 1980) has prompted considerable effort to define the neurochemical effects of chronic (as opposed to acute) administration of these drugs. More recent studies have focused on the chronic effects of antidepressants on post-synaptic monoaminergic receptors.

Vetulani and Sulser (1975) were the first to demonstrate that chronic (but not acute) administration of various antidepressants to rats reduces the activity of the norepinephrine stimulated adenylate cyclase in the limbic forebrain. Activation of adenylate cyclase results in an increase in intracellular cyclic adenosine monophosphate (cAMP), and the latter has been shown to be an important "second messenger" mediating the physiological effects of various hormones and neurotransmitters. The stimulation of brain adenylate cyclase by norepinephrine is at least partially mediated by β-adrenoceptors (Sulser et al, 1978); and subsequently, several researchers have shown that the actual number of forebrain β-adrenoceptors is also reduced following chronic administration of antidepressants (Banerjee et al, 1977). In addition, a reduction in the number of β-adrenoceptors was observed not only with typical tricyclic antidepressants but also with monoamine oxidase inhibitors and the atypical antidepressants, iprindole and mianserin (Sulser et al, 1978). Thus, chemically diverse and unrelated antidepressants are all capable of decreasing the density of β-adrenoceptors, and/or the responsiveness of the β-adrenoceptor coupled adenylate cyclase system, following chronic administration. By contrast, other drugs that share common pharmacological properties with the tricyclic antidepressants, such as various anticholinergic and antihistaminergic agents, all fail to produce similar changes in β-adrenoceptor function. Other neurotransmitter receptors—including muscarinic-cholinergic, histaminergic, and dopaminergic receptors—are not consistently altered during chronic administration of antidepressants to animals, thereby supporting the selectivity of antidepressants for the β-adrenoceptor system (Hauger and Paul, 1983).

The time course of the antidepressant induced decrease in β-adrenoceptors in animals is in keeping with the delayed therapeutic effects of these drugs in man. It is interesting that both electroconvulsive treatment (ECT) and REM sleep deprivation (which are both clinically effective antidepressants) decrease cerebral β-adrenoceptors in animals somewhat faster than is observed with the chemical antidepressants (Sulser et al, 1978; Bergstrom and Kellar, 1978; Mogilnicka et al, 1980)—a finding that may be related to their relatively rapid anti-depressant effects in man. It is noteworthy that administration of both chemical and nonchemical (ECT, REM sleep deprivation) antidepressants results in β-adrenoceptor desensitization; and, with a time course that parallels their clinical actions.

The most obvious explanation for the decrease in brain β-adrenoceptors following chronic antidepressant administration is that all of these drugs somehow increase the intrasynaptic concentration of norepinephrine. Indeed, chemical or electro-lytic lesions of the noradrenergic neurons that project to the forebrain completely prevent the decrease in β-adrenoceptors produced by antidepressants (Wolfe et al, 1978; Janowsky et al, 1982a). Therefore, a presynaptic site of action for anti-depressants seems likely. For the very potent norepinephrine uptake blockers, such as desipramine and nortriptyline, this action could occur by an inhibition of presynaptic uptake. Even drugs such as iprindole—which fail to block cate-cholamine uptake—are capable of increasing the synaptic levels of norepineph-rine, and, thus, other as yet unknown presynaptic mechanisms must be evoked.

One possible mechanism that has been proposed to explain the presynaptic actions of antidepressants involves the regulation of norepinephrine release, which is partially controlled by presynaptic α-adrenergic "autoreceptors." Stud-ies have shown that the presynaptic α_2 "autoreceptor" adjusts the neuronal firing rate to correspond to the synaptic concentration of the transmitter. An increase in the intrasynaptic concentration of norepinephrine results in "feed-back inhibition" of neurotransmitter release via activation of presynaptic α_2 adrenoceptors. This "feedback inhibition," if unaltered, would theoretically retard the development of antidepressant induced desensitization of β-adrenoceptors by reducing the synaptic concentration of norepinephrine. Previous studies in both the peripheral (Crews and Smith, 1978) and central (Spyraki and Fibiger, 1980) nervous systems have shown that chronic, but not acute, administration of many antidepressants reduces presynaptic α_2-receptor inhibition, resulting in an enhanced release of norepinephrine. Thus, many antidepressants apparently increase the intrasynaptic concentration of norepinephrine (and thus decrease postsynaptic β-adrenoceptors) by first desensitizing presynaptic α_2 "autorecep-tors." Since acute administration of some tricyclic antidepressants appears to directly activate presynaptic α_2 "autoreceptors" on neurons of the locus ceru-leus, thus preventing enhanced release of norepinephrine (Cedarbaum and Aghajanian, 1976; Svensson and Usdin, 1978), several groups have investigated whether concomitant administration of α-adrenergic blockers will accelerate the development of β-adrenoceptor desensitization following antidepressant treat-ment. It is interesting that both phenoxybenzamine and yohimbine have been reported to decrease the time lag of cerebral β-adrenoceptor desensitization observed following administration of both tricyclic antidepressants and mono-amine oxidase inhibitors (Crews et al, 1981; Johnson et al, 1980). Whether α-adrenoceptor blockers accelerate the therapeutic effects of antidepressants in depressed patients is still not known, but such a study would be of both practical and theoretical interest.

In addition to reducing the number of central β-adrenoceptors, antidepres-sants also appear to alter the number of serotonin receptors in various forebrain regions. The ascending serotonergic projections from the midbrain, therefore, represent another important monoaminergic neurotransmitter system that is affected by antidepressants. As is the case with alpha and beta adrenoceptors, there are at least two subtypes of serotonin receptors, designated $5HT_1$ and $5HT_2$. Serotonin receptors in the frontal cortex can be labelled with [^{3}H]-spiro-peridol, and these are primarily of the $5HT_2$ subtype. Snyder and his collaborators (Peroutka et al, 1981) have provided evidence that $5HT_2$ receptors mediate many of the behavioral effects of drugs that increase central serotonin function. In related studies, Peroutka and Snyder (1980) have shown that chronic administration of antidepressants to rats decreases the number of $5HT_2$ receptors in the brain, and with some drugs this reduction is quite dramatic. Since acute administration of antidepressants fails to alter $5HT_2$ receptors, it is unlikely that this decrease is due to residual drugs present in the membrane preparation. These authors also argue that most antidepressants are far more potent in reducing $5HT_2$ receptors than β-adrenoceptors (with the possible exception of desipramine, which is more effective in reducing β-adrenoceptors). Though some antidepressants (for example, imipramine and pargyline) can also reduce the other subclass of serotonergic receptor, most antidepressants have no effect on $5HT_1$ receptors, suggesting that desensitization of $5HT_2$ receptors may be more relevant to their therapeutic effects.

The mechanisms responsible for the antidepressant induced decrease in $5HT_2$ receptors are far less clear than are those mediating the reduction in β-adrenoceptors. In fact, destruction of central serotonergic neurons with the neurotoxin 5,7 dihydroxytryptamine, fails to alter the decrease in $5HT_2$ receptors seen after chronic administration of antidepressants (Tang et al, 1981). Furthermore, chronic administration of mianserin (a purported $5HT_2$ antagonist and putative antidepressant) reduces $5HT_2$ receptors in the cortex; a curious phenomenon, given that receptor antagonists generally produce "up-regulation" of their respective receptors. It is therefore uncertain whether serotonin plays a role in regulating the number or affinity of $5HT_2$ receptors, and whether the effects of chronic antidepressant treatment are mediated via pre- or postsynaptic mechanisms. In addition, some discrepancies exist in relating the antidepressant induced changes in central $5HT_2$ receptors to the clinical effects of these drugs. For example, ECT, in contrast to all chemical antidepressants, actually increases the number of $5HT_2$ receptors in various brain regions (Kellar et al, 1981). While at first glance such data seem incompatible with a common mechanism of antidepressant action, it is not necessarily inconsistent, in that the "physiological" effects of increased or decreased $5HT_2$ receptor density on "functional" serotonergic activity are still unclear. More recently, Mikuni and Meltzer (1983) have shown relatively potent effects of several phenothiazines, including chlorpromazine, in reducing cortical $5HT_2$ receptors following chronic administration. While it may be argued that certain phenothiazines have antidepressant activity in some patients, these data contrast with the marked selectivity of antidepressants for reducing β-adrenergic receptor function.

Recent evidence also suggests that a functional linkage exists between the noradrenergic and serotonergic neurotransmitter systems that is especially evident in mediating the antidepressant induced alterations in β-adrenoceptors. When the serotonergic system is destroyed by lesioning with the specific neurotoxin 5,7 dihydroxytryptamine, chronic administration of antidepressants fails to reduce the number of cortical β-adrenoceptors (Janowsky et al, 1982b). Furthermore, the affinity of β-adrenoceptors for agonists (such as norepinephrine), but not antagonists is altered by serotonergic denervation (Manier et al, 1983); the latter apparently "uncoupling" the receptor from the adenylate cyclase complex. Conversely, destruction of the noradrenergic system with 6–hydroxydopamine markedly reduces the ability of several antidepressants (including ECT) to enhance serotonin mediated behaviors in rats (Green and Deakin, 1980; Grahame-Smith et al, 1983). In a sense, these findings unify several major hypotheses of depression and the mechanism of action of antidepressants. They also highlight the difficulty in isolating a drug effect to a specific neurotransmitter system, since there are apparently subtle and permissive interactions between systems.

The alterations in monoaminergic neurotransmission produced by antidepressants may also be subject to changes in the hormonal milieu of the organism. Adrenocorticotropin hormone (ACTH), for example, has been shown to accelerate the development of β-adrenoreceptor desensitization produced by certain antidepressants, and this effect is apparently independent of the release of adrenal steroids (Kendall et al, 1982). Previous investigators, however, have shown that adrenal steroids retard the development of β-adrenoceptor supersensitivity in the hippocampus of rats lesioned with 6–hydroxydopamine (Roberts and Bloom, 1981). Ovarian steroids have also been shown to influence the decrease in $5HT_2$ receptors produced by chronic administration of imipramine to rats. Ovariectomy abolishes the imipramine induced decrease in $5HT_2$ receptors, and this effect is reversed by estradiol and/or progesterone administration (Kendall et al, 1981). Thus, the hormonal changes that occur in postmenopausal women may profoundly influence the efficacy of antidepressants; and the possible therapeutic effects of hormone replacement and concomitant antidepressant treatment should be explored more carefully in these patients. These results also serve to emphasize one of the major shortcomings of research in animals and the extrapolation of animal data to man: Some would argue that human psychopathological conditions can never be reliably mimicked in animals, and therefore the critical neurochemical effects of antidepressants may not be apparent in a presumably healthy rat; although this is a very difficult argument to test experimentally, it is noteworthy that animal models do have good predictive value in drug screening tests for novel antidepressants. Furthermore, both the behavioral and biochemical effects of reserpine (a known depressogenic compound in man) are reliably reversed by virtually all antidepressants in animal models.

MISCELLANEOUS MECHANISMS

Rapid progress in delineating and understanding the mechanisms of chemical neurotransmission is prompting even more sophisticated studies on the neurochemical effects of antidepressants. Menkes and coworkers, for example (1983), have recently reported that chronic (but not acute) administration of various antidepressants to rats facilitates the activation of brain adenylate cyclase by a stable analogue of guanosine 5'–triphospate. These results suggest that antidepressants may produce their effects at a site distal to the receptor by promoting the interaction of the regulatory and catalytic subunits of adenylate cyclase. Such an effect might result in an enhanced responsiveness to a variety of neurotransmitters whose physiological actions are mediated by way of the adenylate cyclase system.

Recent studies on the mechanisms of action of lithium have also implicated a completely different "second messenger" system in the action of antidepressants. It is now generally accepted that the hydrolysis of phosphatidylinositol (or polyphosphoinositides) to various inositol-phosphates is coupled to a number of neurotransmitter receptors (for example, muscarinic-cholinergic, α-adrenergic, serotonergic, and so forth) (Berridge et al, 1982). Allison and Blisner (1976) were the first to observe that pharmacologically relevant doses of lithium specifically inhibit the enzyme inositol–1–phosphatase, resulting in a decrease in the recycling of inositol to phosphatidylinositol. Theoretically, the effect of lithium would serve to decrease the turnover of phosphatidylinositol and, thus, the physiological effects of receptors that are linked to this system. It is as yet unclear whether other antidepressants alter neurotransmitter mediated phosphatidylinositol turnover, but studies are in progress in a number of laboratories to answer this question.

CONCLUSIONS

Antidepressants appear to interact with monoaminergic neurotransmitters in animals and under pharmacologically relevant conditions. The most consistent neurochemical changes common to most, if not all, antidepressants (tricyclic antidepressants, monoamine oxidase inhibitors, ECT) involve chronic "adaptational" alterations in the number of β-adrenergic and serotonergic ($5HT_2$) receptors. The "desensitization" of postsynaptic β-adrenergic and $5HT_2$ receptors following chronic antidepressant treatment is most likely mediated by an as yet unidentified presynaptic action on neurotransmitter "turnover." Neurotransmitter systems also seem to interact with each other, and it is clear that the serotonergic system plays a permissive role in mediating antidepressant induced changes in the noradrenergic system, and vice versa. It is unlikely, therefore, that the mood elevating properties of antidepressants will be solely attributable to a change in a single neurotransmitter. However, that the initial actions of antidepressant treatments may involve alterations in monoamine neurotransmission is well supported by the data.

REFERENCES

Allison JH, Blisner ME: Inhibition of the effect of lithium on brain inositol by atropine and scopolamine. Biochem Biophys Res Commun 68:1332-1338, 1976

Banerjee SP, Kung LS, Riggi SJ, et al: Development of beta-adrenergic subsensitivity by antidepressants. Nature 268:455-456, 1977

Bergstrom DA, Kellar KJ: Effect of electroconvulsive shock on monoaminergic receptor binding sites in rat brain. Nature 278:464-466, 1979

Berridge MJ, Downes CP, Hanley MR: Lithium amplifies agonist-dependent phosphatidylinositol responses in brain and salivary glands. Biochem J 206:587-595, 1982

Bourne HR, Bunney WE Jr, Colburn RW, et al: Noradrenaline, 5–hydroxytryptamine and 5–hydroxindoleacetic acid in hindbrains of suicidal patients. Lancet 2:805-808, 1968

Briley MS, Langer SZ, Raisman R, et al: Tritiated imipramine binding sites are decreased in platelets of untreated depressed patients. Science 209:303-305, 1980

Bunney WE Jr, Davis JM: Norepinephrine in depressive reactions: a review. Arch Gen Psychiatry 13:483-494, 1965

Cedarbaum JM, Aghajanian G: Noradrenergic neurons of the locus coeruleus: inhibition by epinephrine and activation by the alpha antagonist piperoxane. Brain Res 112:413-419, 1976

Crews FT, Smith CB: Presynaptic alpha receptor subsensitivity after long-term antidepressant treatment. Science 202:322-324, 1978

Crews FT, Paul SM, Goodwin FK: Acceleration of β-receptor desensitization in combined administration of antidepressants and phenoxybenzamine. Nature 290:787-789, 1981

Green AR, Deakin JFW: Brain noradrenaline depletion prevents ECS-induced enhancement of serotonin- and dopamine-mediated behavior. Nature 285:232-233, 1980

Grahame-Smith DG, Cowen PJ, Green AR, et al: β-adrenoceptor agonists enhance the functional activity of brain 5–hydroxytryptamine: relationship to antidepressant activity, in Clinical Pharmacology in Psychiatry. Edited by Gram LF, Usdin E, Dahl S, et al, London, MacMillan Press, Ltd., 1983

Hall H, Ogren SO: Effects of antidepressant drugs on different receptors in the brain. Eur J Pharmacol 70:393-407, 1981

Hauger RL, Paul SM: Neurotransmitter receptor plasticity: alterations by antidepressants and antipsychotics. Psychiatric Annals 13(5):399-407, 1983

Iversen LL: Uptake: mechanism for neurotransmitter amines. Biochem Pharmacol 23:1927-1935, 1974

Janowsky AJ, Steranka LR, Sulser F: Role of neuronal signal input in the down-regulation of central noradrenergic receptor function by antidepressant drugs. J Neurochem 39:290-292, 1982a

Janowsky AJ, Okada F, Applegate C, et al: Role of serotonergic input in the regulation of the β-adrenoceptor coupled adenylate cyclase system in brain. Science 218:900-901, 1982b

Johnson RW, Reisine T, Spotnitz S, et al: Effects of desipramine and yohimbine on α_2 and β_2-adrenoceptor sensitivity. Eur J Pharmacol 67:123-127, 1980

Kanof PD, Greengard P: Brain histamine receptors as targets for antidepressant drugs. Nature 272:329-333, 1978

Kellar KJ, Cascio CS, Butler JA, et al: Differential effects of electroconvulsive shock and antidepressant drugs on serotonin–2 receptors in rat brain. Eur J Pharmacol 69:515-518, 1981

Kendall DA, Stancel GM, Enna SJ: Imipramine: effect of ovarian steroids on modifications in serotonin receptor binding. Science 211:1183-1185, 1981

Kendall DA, Duncan R, Slopis J, et al: Influence of adrenocorticotropin hormone and yohimbine on antidepressant induced declines in rat brain neurotransmitter receptor binding and function. J Pharmacol Exp Therap 222:566-571, 1982

Klein DF, Gittelman R, Quitkin F, et al: Diagnosis and Drug Treatment of Psychiatric Disorders: Adults and Children. Baltimore, Williams and Wilkins, 1980

Koe K: Molecular geometry of inhibitors of the uptake of catecholamines and serotonin in synaptosomal preparations of rat cortex. J Pharmacol Exp Ther 199:649-661, 1976

Langer SZ, Moret C, Raisman R, et al: High affinity [^{3}H] imipramine binding in rat hypothalamus: association with uptake of serotonin but not of norepinephrine. Science 210:1133-1135, 1980

Loomer HP, Saunders JC, Kline NS: Clinical and pharmacodynamic evaluation of iproniazid as psychic energizer. Psychiatry Research Rep 8:129-141, 1957

Manier DH, Okada F, Janowsky A, et al: Serotonergic denervation changes binding characteristics of beta-adrenoreceptors in rat cortex. Eur J Pharmacol 86:137-139, 1983

Menkes DB, Rasenick MM, Wheeler MA, et al: Guanosine triphosphate activation of brain adenylate cyclase: enhancement by long-term antidepressant treatment. Science 219:65-67, 1983

Mikuni MK, Meltzer HY: Reduction of serotonin–2 receptors in rat cerebral cortex after subchronic administration of imipramine, chlorpromazine, and the combination thereof. Life Sci 34:87-92, 1984

Mogilnicka E, Arbilla S, Depoortere H, et al: Rapid–eye–movement sleep deprivation decreases the density of ^{3}H–dihydroalprenolol and ^{3}H–imipramine binding sites in the rat cerebral cortex. Eur J Pharmacol 65:289-292, 1980

Ogren SO, Cott JM, Hall H: Sedative/anxiolytic effects of antidepressants in animals. Acta Psychiatr Scand 63 (Suppl 290):277-288, 1981

Paul SM, Rehavi M, Skolnick P, et al: Demonstration of specific high affinity binding sites for [^{3}H] imipramine on human platelets. Life Sci 26:953-959, 1980

Paul SM, Rehavi M, Rice KC, et al: Does high affinity [^{3}H] imipramine binding label serotonin reuptake sites in brain and platelet. Life Sci 28:2753-2760, 1981a

Paul SM, Rehavi M, Skolnick P, et al: Depressed patients have decreased binding of tritiated imipramine to platelet serotonin "transporter." Arch Gen Psychiatry 38:1315-1317, 1981b

Paul SM, Rehavi M, Skolnick P, et al: High affinity binding of antidepressants to biogenic amine transport sites in human brain and platelet, in Studies in Depression in Neurobiology of Mood Disorders, vol. 1. Edited by Post RM, Ballenger JC. Baltimore, Williams and Wilkins, 1984

Peroutka SJ, Snyder SH: Long term antidepressant treatment decreases spiroperidol-labeled serotonin receptor binding. Science 210:88-90, 1980

Peroutka SJ, Lebovitz RM, Snyder SH: Two distinct central serotonin receptors with different physiological functions. Science 212:827-829, 1981

Potter LT and Axelrod, J: Studies on the storage of norepinephrine and effect of drugs. J Pharmacol Exp Therap 140:199-206, 1963

Raisman R, Briley M, Langer SZ: Specific tricyclic antidepressant binding sites in rat brain. Nature 281:148-150, 1979

Rehavi M, Paul SM, Skolnick P, et al: Demonstration of specific high affinity binding sites for [^{3}H] imipramine in human brain. Life Sci 26:2273-2279, 1980

Rehavi M, Skolnick P, Brownstein MJ, et al: High affinity binding of [^{3}H] desipramine to rat brain: a presynaptic marker for noradrenergic uptake sites. J Neurochem 38:889-895, 1982

Richelson E: Tricyclic antidepressants block histamine H_1 receptors of mouse neuroblastoma cells. Nature 274:176-177, 1978

Roberts DCS, Bloom FE: Adrenal steroid induced changes in β-adrenergic receptor binding in rat hippocampus. Eur J Pharmacol 74:37-41, 1981

Schildkraut JJ: Catecholamine hypothesis of affective disorders: review of supporting evidence. Am J Psychiatry 122:509-522, 1965

Snyder SH, Peroutka SJ: Antidepressants and neurotransmitter receptors, in Neurobiology of Mood Disorders, Vol 1. Edited by Post RM, Ballenger JC. Baltimore, Williams and Wilkins, 1984

Spyrakic C, Fibiger HC: Functional evidence for subsensitivity of noradrenergic α-receptors after chronic desipramine treatment. Life Sci 27:1863-1867, 1980

Stanley M, Virgilio J, Gershon S: Tritiated imipramine binding sites are decreased in the frontal cortex of suicides. Science 216:1337-1339, 1982

Sulser F, Vetulani J, Mobley PL: Mode of action of antidepressant drugs. Biochem Pharmacol 27:257-261, 1978

Suranyi-Cadotte BE, Wood PL, Nair NPV, et al: Normalization of platelet [^{3}H] imipramine binding in depressed patients. Eur J Pharmacol 85:351-357, 1983

Svensson TH, Usdin T: Feedback inhibition of brain noradrenalin neurons by tricyclic antidepressants: α-receptor mediation. Science 202:1089-1091, 1978

Tang SW, Seeman P, Kwam S: Differential effect of chronic desipramine and amitryptyline treatment on rat brain adrenergic and serotonergic receptors. Psychiatry Res 4:129-138, 1981

Tuomisto J, Tukiainen E: Decreased uptake of 5–hydroxytryptamine in blood platelets from depressed patients. Nature 262:596-598, 1976

U'Prichard DC, Greenberg DA, Sheehan PP, et al: Tricyclic antidepressants: therapeutic properties and affinity for alpha-noradrenergic receptor binding sites in the brain. Science 199:197-198, 1978

Vetulani J, Sulser F: Action of various antidepressant treatments reduces reactivity of noradrenergic cyclic AMP generating systems in limbic forebrain. Nature 257:495-496, 1975

Wolfe BB, Harden TK, Sporn JR, et al: Presynaptic modulation of beta-adrenergic receptors in rat cerebral cortex after treatment with antidepressants. J Pharmacol Exp Ther 207:446-457, 1978

Zis AP, Goodwin FK: Novel antidepressants and the biogenic amine hypothesis of depresion: the case of iprindole and mianserin. Arch Gen Psychiatry 36:1097-1107, 1979

This chapter was written by the authors in their private capacities. No official support or endorsement by NIMH is intended or should be inferred.

Chapter 4

The Cholinergic Systems in Psychiatry

by Joseph T. Coyle, M.D.

One of the ironies of psychopharmacology is that the role of central cholinergic neurons in the pathophysiology of neuropsychiatric disorders has only been appreciated in the last few years, despite the fact that acetylcholine was demonstrated to be a neurotransmitter over 60 years ago (Loewi, 1921). In fact, it is safe to state that more is known about the organization of central endorphin systems, which were first identified less than a decade ago, than is known about the central cholinergic neurons. The primary reason for this slow advance in understanding brain cholinergic processes is that neuroanatomic methods for precisely identifying cholinergic neurons were not available until quite recently. Consequently, the development of immunocytochemical procedures for visualizing the cholinergic neurons, and the application of quantitative neurochemical procedures for measuring cholinergic markers in the brain, have led over the last five years to a resurgence of interest in central cholinergic neurons. Recent findings implicate the cholinergic neurons in Alzheimer's Dementia (Coyle et al, 1983), Down's syndrome (Price et al, 1982), Parkinson's syndrome (Whitehouse et al, 1983) and even schizophrenia (Stevens, 1982).

BIOCHEMISTRY OF THE CHOLINERGIC NEURON

Choline Acetyltransferase

Cholinergic neurons are endowed with the ability to synthesize, store and release acetylcholine as their neurotransmitter (Figure 1). Acetylcholine is formed within the neurons by the enzyme, choline acetyltransferase (Rossier, 1977). This enzyme transfers an acetyl group from acetyl Coenzyme–A to choline by the formation of an ester bond between the two precursors. Choline itself is found in remarkably high concentrations within the brain; and, aside from its role as a precursor to acetylcholine, choline serves several other functions: most notably, it is a major constituent of cellular membranes. It appears that the bulk of the brain choline is synthesized in the liver and is actively transported into the brain, although recent studies suggest that choline synthesis does occur *de novo* within the brain.

Choline Uptake

The cholinergic neurons possess a specific, high affinity uptake process for choline, which actively transports the precursor into the cholinergic axons and terminals (Kuhar et al, 1973). Inhibition of the uptake process interferes with acetylcholine synthesis: This finding indicates that the intraneuronal availability

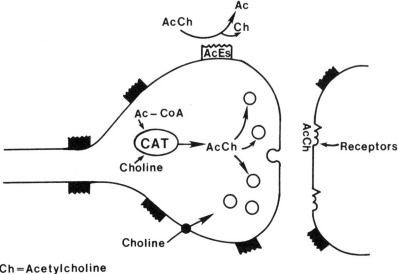

AcCh = Acetylcholine
CAT = Choline Acetyltransferase
AcEs = Acetylcholine Esterase

Figure 1. Schematic representation of a cholinergic synapse.

of choline is a rate limiting step in acetylcholine synthesis. Consistent with this hypothesis, inhibition of the synthetic enzyme choline acetyltransferase has little impact on acetylcholine synthesis until the enzyme activity is reduced by greater than 85 percent, indicating that choline acetyltransferase activity is in considerable excess of that required to maintain the levels of the neurotransmitter. Additional evidence of the important role played by the uptake process for choline is the fact that the velocity of uptake is dependent upon the antecedent history of the activity of the cholinergic neurons. Thus, when cholinergic neurons are relatively inactive, the velocity of choline uptake is low; and, after a period of intense activity associated with increased release of acetylcholine, the velocity of choline uptake increases significantly.

Acetylcholinesterase

Acetylcholinesterase is the enzyme that catalyzes the hydrolytic inactivation of acetylcholine. Several different molecular forms of the enzyme (isozymes) are found throughout the body, and one form is actively secreted into the cerebrospinal fluid (CSF) (Brimijoin, 1983). The broad cellular distribution of acetylcholinesterase, including localization on red blood cell membranes, indicates that it is not restricted to cholinergic neurons, unlike choline acetyltransferase or the choline high affinity uptake process. Nevertheless, histochemical studies to visualize this enzyme reveal that cholinergic neurons are markedly enriched with acetylcholinesterase (Shute and Lewis, 1967). In addition, areas of synaptic contact between cholinergic nerve terminals and muscle in the periphery or other neurons in the brain are also enriched with acetylcholinesterase. The high activity of acetylcholinesterase concentrated in the synaptic cleft ensures that acetylcholine will be rapidly inactivated after release at the synapse. Pharmacologic inhibition of acetylcholinesterase potentiates cholinergic neurotransmission by prolonging the survival of acetylcholine released at the synapse. Under extreme conditions, such as poisoning with insecticides with potent acetylcholinesterase inhibitory action, serious central and peripheral toxic effects reflect the unopposed cholinergic neurotransmission.

Acetylcholine Receptors

The effects of acetylcholine are mediated by receptors on the cells receiving synaptic input from the cholinergic neurons. Over 70 years ago, pharmacologists (Dale, 1914) distinguished two types of acetylcholine receptors on the basis of their response to agonists and their sensitivity to antagonists (Table 1). The receptors at the neuromuscular junction respond to the acetylcholine analogue, nicotine, are antagonized by d-tubocurarine, and are therefore designated "nicotinic receptors." In contrast, receptors mediating the effects of acetylcholine at smooth muscles in the heart and in the gut are activated by muscarine, are antagonized by atropine, and are consequently designated "muscarinic receptors." These distinctions have generally held up over the years and have recently been verified by molecular neurobiologic approaches. Nevertheless, while there is evidence of distinct muscarinic and nicotinic acetylcholine receptors in the brain, the complexity of the physiologic and pharmacologic effects of acetylcholine in the brain preclude a simplified dichotomy.

MUSCARINIC RECEPTOR. The muscarinic acetylcholine receptor mediates the effects of acetylcholine released by peripheral parasympathetic neurons innervating smooth muscle (gut, iris, heart, and the like) and glandular structures (lacrimal, salivary, sweat, among others). Muscarinic receptors also play a major, if not dominant, role in mediating the effects of acetylcholine in the central nervous system (CNS), especially in the basal ganglia and in the cortical-limbic regions. The muscarinic receptors exert their physiologic effects by interacting with at least two transducers. In many cells, stimulation of muscarinic receptors results in an activation of the intracellular enzyme, guanalate cyclase, which forms cyclic guanalate monophosphate (GMP) as its "second messenger" (Goldberg and Haddox, 1977). The increased intracellular concentration of cyclic GMP affects a variety of metabolic processes that are catalyzed by elevated levels of cyclic GMP. Muscarinic receptors may also be coupled to potassium channels.

Table 1. Acetylcholine Receptors

Type	Agonists	Antagonists	Distribution
Nicotinic	Nicotine	D-Tubocurarine	Striate Muscles Autonomic Ganglia Brain Stem
Muscarinic	Muscarine	Atropine	Smooth Muscles Glands Forebrain

With activation of these receptors, pores in the neuronal membrane close, preventing the egress of potassium from the neuron, thereby enhancing its excitability (Krnjevic and Ropert, 1982). Both stimulation of guanalate cyclase and inhibition of potassium currents appear to have as their primary effects modulation of neuronal excitability.

Considerable information has been developed about the precise localization of muscarinic receptors in the brain through the use of ligand binding autoradiographic techniques (Kuhar and Yamamura, 1976). This method takes advantage of the fact that certain muscarinic receptor antagonists bind to the receptor with remarkably high specificity and affinity. The drug quinuclidinyl benzilate, for example, once bound to the muscarinic receptor, dissociates with a half-life of several hours. With this method, histologic sections obtained from a frozen brain and affixed to a microscopic slide are incubated in physiologic saline containing highly radioactive quinuclidinyl benzilate. After extensive washing to remove traces of the radioactive drug not bound to muscarinic receptors (which rapidly diffuse from the tissue section), the sections are covered with a photographic emulsion. After a suitable period of exposure to allow the radioactive drug to interact with the photographic emulsion, the slides are developed. When the sections are viewed through a microscope, the silver grains precipitated by the radioactivity emitted by quinuclidinyl benzilate can be seen overlying the neurons bearing muscarinic receptors. As shown in the section through the monkey brain (Figure 2), muscarinic receptors are found in high density in the corpus striatum and have an uneven laminar distribution in the cerebral cortex.

NICOTINIC RECEPTOR.   The best characterized receptor in neurobiology is the nicotinic receptor, which mediates the effects of acetylcholine released at the terminals of motor neurons innervating voluntary muscles. Advantage has been taken of the fact that the nicotinic receptor is found in extremely high density in the electric organ of such fish as Torpedo. The receptor has been purified to homogeneity; its amino acid sequence has been determined; and its molecular structure has been rigorously defined (Figure 3). The receptor is a polymer of five peptides with a total molecular weight of approximately 250,000 daltons. The receptor is a funnel-shaped macromolecular complex with a central pore that serves as the sodium channel. The funnel extends through the entire thickness of the neuronal membrane and the outer lips, rises above the exterior of the membrane and possesses two recognition sites to which acetylcholine binds (Stroud, 1983). With highly specific antibodies directed against the subunits of the nicotinic receptor, it has been possible to demonstrate its molecular topology and the close chemical similarities of the nicotinic receptors in the Torpedo fish, rat, cow and man.

Injection of purified nicotinic receptor into experimental animals to produce antiserum against the receptor results in the development of a myasthenia gravis-like syndrome (Drachman, 1978). These findings and related studies provide compelling evidence that myasthenia gravis is an autoimmune disease, in which antibodies are produced in man that bind to components of the nicotinic receptor at the neuromuscular junction. The binding of the antibodies to the nicotinic receptor and the subsequent cross-linking of the receptors by the antibodies not only interferes with their function, but also markedly enhances their rate of

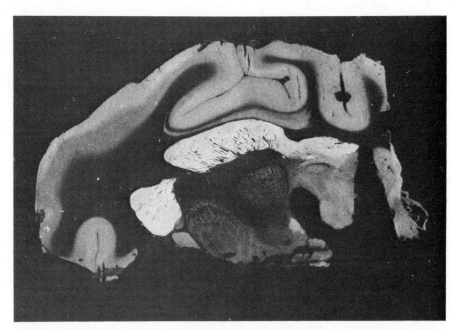

Figure 2. Autoradiographic visualization of muscarinic receptors in monkey brain. Parasagital section through the monkey brain was prepared for autoradiographic visualization of muscarinic receptors. Receptor density is proportionate to lightness as viewed by dark field illumination. Note high density of muscarinic receptors in caudate and putamen, moderate density in neocortex and absence of receptors in white matter. (Courtesy of M.J. Kuhar, Ph.D.)

degradation. Antibodies specific for the subunits of the nicotinic receptor have also been used recently to demonstrate presence of nicotinic receptor components on brain neurons.

THE ANATOMY OF CHOLINERGIC NEURONS

As noted above, one aspect of the study of cholinergic neurons that has significantly lagged behind other areas of investigation is the development of precise methods for delineating their anatomic distribution in the brain. Indirect methods for mapping putative cholinergic neurons have been based upon histochemical techniques to visualize acetylcholinesterase, the enzyme that hydrolyzes acetylcholine (Shute and Lewis, 1967). Although this enzyme is markedly enriched in cholinergic neurons, it is also found on other neuronal types, as well as neurons receiving cholinergic innervation. Thus, this method cannot yield unequivocal results. Within the last few years, a number of laboratories have been able to develop highly specific antibodies against choline acetyltransferase. As this enzyme confers upon the neuron the ability to synthesize acetylcholine, it serves as the most specific enzyme marker for cholinergic neurons. With these specific antibodies, it is now possible to visualize and map cholinergic neuronal systems with a high degree of confidence by immunocytochemical techniques (Mesulam et al, 1983). On the basis of localization and function, four distinct

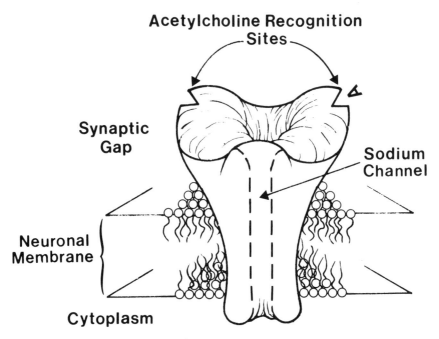

Acetylcholine Recognition Sites

Synaptic Gap

Sodium Channel

Neuronal Membrane

Cytoplasm

Figure 3. Three-dimensional view of the nicotinic acetylcholine receptor. A = acetylcholine.

cholinergic neuronal systems can be identified that are relevant to psychiatry, either because of their involvement in the pathophysiology of neuropsychiatric disorders, or because they may be affected by psychotropic medications (Figure 4).

Parasympathetic Neurons

An important component of the autonomic nervous system is the parasympathetic nervous system that utilizes acetylcholine as its primary neurotransmitter. The parasympathetic neurons develop from the embryonic neural crest cells that also give rise to the sensory neurons, the sympathetic noradrenergic neurons and peptidergic neuronal systems localized in the gut. Developmental neurobiologic studies indicate that trophic factors released by target sites of innervation play a critical role in determining the differentiation of the embryonic neural crest cells into parasympathetic cholinergic neurons, as opposed to sympathetic noradrenergic neurons. The cholinergic parasympathetics generally have their cell bodies located in ganglia near their sites of innervation, whereas the noradrenergic sympathetics have their ganglia located close to the midline.

The parasympathetic neurons provide innervation to smooth muscle in the gut, heart and iris, as well as to various glandular structures. Muscarinic acetylcholine receptors generally mediate the effects of acetylcholine on parasympathetically innervated cells. Recent studies have indicated that neurons may contain a neuropeptide in addition to the amine neurotransmitter (Hokfelt et al, 1980). The cholinergic parasympathetics, for example, innervating the sali-

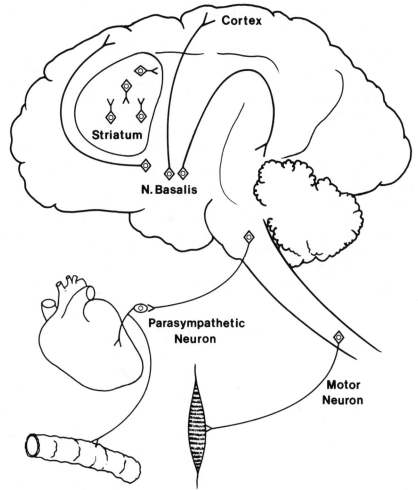

Figure 4. Major cholinergic neuronal systems.

vary gland contain the neuropeptide vasoactive intestinal peptide (VIP). Physiologic studies indicate that acetylcholine released by the parasympathetic terminals stimulate the secretion of saliva, whereas the co-released VIP dilates the smooth muscles on blood vessels to augment blood flow.

Motor Neurons

The motor neurons, which innervate the voluntary (for example, striate) musculature, have their cell bodies located in the ventral horn of the spinal cord or in nuclear groupings in the brain stem (such as the motor components of the cranial nerves). The cell bodies of the motor neurons are quite large and project axons that may extend over a meter or more to innervate the voluntary muscles. Nicotinic receptors, described above, mediate the effects of acetylcholine at the neuromuscular junction. Activation of the nicotinic receptors by acetylcholine opens their sodium channels, resulting in muscle membrane depolarization and muscular contraction.

Striatal Local Circuit Neurons

Local circuit neurons have very abbreviated axonal arbors and innervate other neurons in close proximity to their own cell body. Cholinergic local circuit neurons have been identified in the various regions of the brain, but the most relevant group are those found in the basal ganglia—for example, the caudate and putamen. Those cholinergic neurons are of an intermediate size and represent approximately one percent of the neuronal cell bodies in the basal ganglia. Nevertheless, they provide a remarkably dense innervation to the basal ganglia, so that the concentration of acetylcholine and the specific activity of choline acetyltransferase are several-fold higher than any other major brain region. The predominant postsynaptic effects of acetylcholine in the basal ganglia are mediated by muscarinic acetylcholine receptors, analogous to those responsive to peripheral parasympathetic cholinergic neurons.

Considerable evidence indicates that the nigrostriatal dopaminergic input to the basal ganglia plays an inhibitory role in regulating the activity of the cholinergic neurons in the basal ganglia. Thus, as indicated in Figure 5, enhanced dopaminergic activity inhibits the release of acetylcholine, and therefore atten-

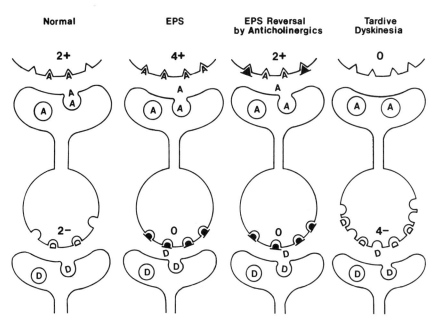

Figure 5. Drug interactions in the striatum. The synaptic relationship between the nigrostriatal dopaminergic terminals and striatal cholinergic neurons is presented. Dopamine (D) inhibits the activity of acetylcholine (A) releasing interneurons in the striatum by activating dopamine receptors. Neuroleptics (▲) block the dopamine receptors, resulting in increased activity of cholinergic neurons and the emergence of acute extrapyramidal side effects. These can be counteracted by anticholinergic drugs (▲). In tardive dyskinesia, there is an increase in density and supersensitivity of the dopamine receptors.

uates the stimulation of postsynaptic muscarinic receptors; in contrast, reduction in dopamine receptor stimulation disinhibits the cholinergic neurons and augments the stimulation of postsynaptic muscarinic receptors. Of course, dopamine neurons likely innervate noncholinergic neurons in the basal ganglia, and mechanisms involved in the control of cholinergic neuronal activity in this region, are undoubtedly more complex than the original "balance hypothesis" between dopamine and acetylcholine.

Basal Forebrain Cholinergic Complex

A group of exceptionally large neuronal cell bodies, overlying the hypothalamus and located within the ventral and the medial aspects of the globus pallidus, extend forward over several centimeters to the septum and make up the basal forebrain cholinergic complex. The caudal aspects of the complex consist of a portion of the substantia innominata known as the nucleus basalis of Meynert. More anteriorly, these cholinergic neuronal cell bodies are grouped within the diagonal band of Broca and the medial septal nucleus. These neuronal cell bodies stain intensely for acetylcholinesterase and have recently been shown to contain choline acetyltransferase by immunocytochemical methods (Mesulam et al, 1983). Selective lesions of these neuronal cell bodies in the basal forebrain complex, both in rats and in primates, result in marked reductions in cholinergic markers in the cortex, hippocampus and limbic system; thus, the basal forebrain complex provides 70 to 90 percent of the cholinergic innervation to these regions (McKinney et al, 1983).

Retrograde tracing techniques have clarified the topographic organization of the basal forebrain cholinergic projections to the cortex. With this technique, a small amount of tracer, such as a fluorescent dye, is injected into an area of nerve termination, which in these studies were highly discrete regions of the cortex. The dye is taken up by the terminals and transported down the axons to the cell bodies of origin. After a suitable delay, the experimental animal is sacrificed, and the site of injection and the labeled cell bodies in the basal forebrain are identified. The presence of the fluorescent dye in neuronal cell bodies indicates that the labeled neurons send axons to innervate the area receiving the injection. This technique has revealed that the basal forebrain cholinergic neurons send axons to innervate the cerebral cortex and limbic system in a topographically organized fashion. Cholinergic neurons, with cell bodies located in the caudal aspects of the complex within the ventral and medial aspects of the globus pallidus, innervate the frontal cortex; in contrast, neuronal cell bodies located in the anterior aspects of the complex within the medial septum and diagonal band project to the temporal cortex and the hippocampal formation. The cholinergic cell bodies of the basal forebrain complex are located in the reticular core and receive inputs from extensive areas of the brain, including the other aminergic components of the reticular core.

The precise role played by the basal forebrain cholinergic projections remains, in large part, poorly defined at the present time. Considerable evidence derived from pharmacologic studies, as well as the effects of lesions on the cholinergic pathways innervating the hippocampal formation, suggests that the septal and diagonal band cholinergic neurons play a critical role in certain aspects of memory. Interference with their integrity or function rather selectively impairs working memory, an intermediate stage between immediate registration and long-term memory; thus, while immediate recall of information is unaffected, the ability to remember information several minutes later is disrupted, along with subsequent incorporation of this information into long-term memory (Drachman, 1978). Neurophysiologic correlates of these processes appear to be associated with theta rhythms generated by activation of the septo-hippocampal cholinergic projection (Mitchell et al, 1982). Interference with cholinergic function in the cortex proper is associated with desynchronization of the cortical EEG; and these neurons are thought to play a role in modulating sleep, as is the case for the noradrenergic and serotonergic projections to the cortex. There is also evidence from clinical psychopharmacologic studies that central cholinergic neurons, presumably those projecting to limbic regions, are involved in regulation of mood (Davis et al, 1978). Therefore, drugs that block central muscarinic acetylcholine receptors result in euphoria, while drugs that enhance central cholinergic neurotransmission produce depressive symptoms.

CLINICAL ASPECTS OF CHOLINERGIC NEURONS

Extrapyramidal Disorders

As noted above, cholinergic interneurons provide a remarkably dense innervation of the basal ganglia, such as the caudate and putamen. These two brain structures (together known as the striatum) play an important role, along with the cerebellum, in modulating motor activity. The basal ganglia are designated the "extrapyramidal system" to distinguish them from the cortical output (pyramidal cells) that directly controls motor function. In addition, the basal ganglia are interconnected with the limbic system and receive diffuse innervation from virtually all areas of the cerebral cortex, which implicates the basal ganglia in cognitive and affective processes.

PARKINSON'S SYNDROME. That anticholinergic drugs might affect the symptoms of extrapyramidal disorders, especially Parkinson's syndrome, has been appreciated for over a century. Parkinson's syndrome is a group of disorders characterized clinically by involuntary tremor, rigidity and bradykinesia; and pathologically by the degeneration of the nigrostriatal dopaminergic pathway. It is reported that Charcot used the extract of belladonna, which contains the muscarinic receptor blocker hyoscine, to effectively treat patients with Parkinson's disease. In this century a number of drugs with a variety of structures, including atropine-like analogues, phenothiazines and antihistamines, were also found to be effective in reducing the symptoms of Parkinson's syndrome, especially the tremor. Using the guinea pig ileum as a bioassay for muscarinic cholinergic activity, Ahmed and Marshall (1962) demonstrated a close correlation between the clinical efficacy of these drugs in Parkinson's disease and their potency in blocking the acetylcholine-induced contraction of the ileum. They concluded that the property these drugs shared, and the property that accounted for their antiparkinsonian effects, was their ability to block muscarinic receptors.

The anticholinergics, however, presented two important limitations. First, their effects were restricted primarily to the tremor, whereas the bradykinesia and rigidity were much less responsive. Second, they had a very narrow therapeutic-to-toxic ratio and caused distressing peripheral parasympathetic side effects, as well as delirium. With the discovery by Hornykiewicz and his colleagues (Ehinger and Hornykiewicz, 1960) that the pathophysiology of Parkinson's syndrome results from a selective degeneration of the nigrostriatal dopaminergic pathway, L-dopa therapy and the more recently introduced direct dopamine receptor agonists have largely supplanted anticholinergics in the treatment of Parkinson's disease. L-dopa, which as the precursor for dopamine enhances its synthesis, has a broader therapeutic efficacy than the anticholinergics and, in particular, improves the bradykinesia and rigidity—the more disabling symptoms of the disorder (Calne et al, 1979).

NEUROLEPTICS. The antipsychotic neuroleptic drugs have as their molecular mechanism of therapeutic action blockade of central dopamine receptors (Creese et al, 1976). The antipsychotic action of neuroleptics is thought to derive from alterations in dopaminergic neurotransmission in the cortex and limbic system. Nevertheless, neuroleptics have equal access to dopamine receptors in the striatum, and thereby produce a reversible, pharmacologic dopaminergic "denervation" of the striatum (Figure 5). This mechanism accounts for the extrapyramidal side effects that occur with neuroleptic drugs. As listed in Table 2, the clinical manifestations of these side effects include various aspects of parkinsonian-like symptoms such as bradykinesia, rigidity and tremor, as well as acute dystonic reactions and akathisia.

There seems to be remarkable variation among individuals in their susceptibility to develop extrapyramidal side effects with neuroleptic treatment, since the presence and severity of these neurologic symptoms do not correlate well with the dosage or blood level of the neuroleptic (Tune and Coyle, 1982). This variation may reflect inherent individual differences in the ability of the nigrostriatal dopaminergic pathway to adapt to postsynaptic dopamine receptor blockade. Anticholinergic drugs reverse the neuroleptic-induced extrapyramidal side effects. As indicated above, loss of dopaminergic inhibitory influences over the striatal cholinergic interneurons results in their disinhibition and enhanced release of acetylcholine. Thus, the anticholinergic drugs redress this functional cholinergic imbalance by attenuating the excessive stimulation of the postsyn-

Table 2. Neuroleptic-Induced Extrapyramidal Side Effects: Role of Anticholinergic Drugs

Symptom	Anticholinergic Effects
Dystonic Reaction	Marked Improvement
Pseudo-Parkinsonism	Modest to Marked Improvement
Tremor	
Rigidity	
Bradykinesia	
Facial Immobility	
Akathisia	Modest Improvement
Acute Dyskinesia	Modest Improvement
Tardive Dyskinesia	Exacerbation

aptic muscarinic cholinergic receptors in the striatum. While patients vary considerably in their ability to absorb and metabolize the anticholinergic drugs, the serum levels of anticholinergic drugs correlate well with the reduction in acute extrapyramidal side effects.

DYSKINESIAS. Dystonia musculorum deformans is a group of disorders with symptomatic onset, typically in childhood or adolescence, that involves a persistent contraction of various muscle groups. As the disorder progresses, it can result in disabling and painful contortions. The symptoms of this disorder resemble the acute dystonic reactions that can occur with neuroleptic treatment. Fahn (1983) has reported that substantial doses of anticholinergic drugs can reduce the symptoms in many patients suffering from dystonia musculorum deformans.

Huntington's Disease and tardive dyskinesia are two extrapyramidal disorders in which the motor symptoms reflect an apparent excess of striatal dopaminergic neurotransmission. In Huntington's Disease, a hereditary disorder transmitted as an autosomal dominant, there is a progressive degeneration of the neurons within the striatum, including the cholinergic neurons and the striatonigral GABAergic neurons; the nigrostriatal dopaminergic pathway remains intact. This selective pattern of neuronal loss results in a functional excess of striatal dopaminergic influence, which is symptomatically manifest by the choreoathetotic movement disorder characteristic of Huntington's Disease. That impaired cholinergic neurotransmission contributes to the symptomatic manifestations of Huntington's Disease has been demonstrated by the fact that drugs that block muscarinic receptors exacerbate the movement disorder; and drugs that potentiate cholinergic neurotransmission (such as the acetylcholinesterase inhibitor physostigmine) can attenuate the symptoms (Ringel et al, 1973).

Tardive dyskinesia is a relatively irreversible movement disorder that occurs in patients receiving neuroleptic treatment. Typically, the onset of the disorder involves oral and buccal dyskinesia, facial grimacing and, in extreme cases, lordotic posturing and restless movements of the extremities. Epidemiologic studies suggest that age, lifetime neuroleptic dose, preexisting brain damage and female sex are risk factors for the development of tardive dyskinesia. Prolonged administration of neuroleptics to experimental animals results in a drug-induced denervation supersensitivity of dopamine receptors in the striatum manifest by an increase in dopamine receptor number and sensitivity (Figure 5). Thus, the response of striatal cholinergic neurons to the basal release of dopamine is markedly augmented, resulting in excessive inhibition. Pharmacologic strategies that attenuate dopaminergic neurotransmission, either by depleting dopamine stores with tetrabenazine or by blocking dopamine receptors with neuroleptics, attenuate the movement disorder. Anticholinergic drugs that reduce the symptoms of acute extrapyramidal side effects by further impairing striatal cholinergic neurotransmission exacerbate the symptoms of tardive dyskinesia. Conversely, administration of drugs that enhance cholinergic neurotransmission, such as the acetyl cholinesterase inhibitor, physostigmine, or the acetylcholine precursor, choline, have been shown to reduce the symptoms of tardive dyskinesia (Jeste and Wyatt, 1979).

Dementia

ALZHEIMER'S DISEASE. Recent studies have provided compelling evidence of the critical role played by cholinergic neurons located in the basal forebrain that innervate the cerebral cortex and hippocampus in the pathophysiology of Alzheimer's type dementia. Neuropathologic findings indicate that 60 percent or more of the individuals over the age of 65 who suffer from dementia exhibit the neuropathology described in the much rarer disorder, presenile dementia of the Alzheimer type (Terry and Davies, 1980). The pathologic stigmata, diagnostic of Alzheimer's disease, include neuritic plaques and neurofibrillary tangles. Neuritic plaques consist of a central core of amyloid, a proteinaceous deposit, surrounded by dystrophic neurons. Neuritic plaques appear to be intimately related to the pathophysiology of the dementia, since the density of plaques in the cortex correlates with the severity of cognitive impairments measured in individuals prior to death. Neurofibrillary tangles are intraneuronal accumulations of highly cross-linked protein fibers.

Studies in recent years have provided compelling evidence that dysfunction of forebrain cholinergic neurons are involved in the pathophysiology of Alzheimer's dementia (Table 3). Drachman (1977) demonstrated that low doses of drugs that block central muscarinic receptors, when administered to young healthy adults, reproduced the cognitive deficits observed in the elderly. Thus, he proposed that impaired cholinergic neurotransmission might contribute to the symptoms of senile dementia. In the mid 1970s, a number of laboratories undertook studies to measure the levels of markers associated with the specific neurotransmitter systems in the cerebral cortex and hippocampus in the brains of patients who had died with pathologically confirmed Alzheimer's dementia. These studies revealed striking and selective reductions in the presynaptic markers for cholinergic neurons in the cerebral cortex and hippocampal formation. Thus, the activity of choline acetyltransferase, the enzyme that synthesizes acetylcholine, was reduced by 60 to 90 percent, depending upon the area studied; and acetyl cholinesterase, the enzyme that catalyzes hydrolysis of acetylcholine, was also reduced considerably (Terry and Davies, 1980). Sims and his colleagues (1983), using cortical samples obtained at biopsy, demonstrated that high affinity uptake process for choline, another marker for cholinergic terminals, was markedly decreased in activity as well as in the ability of the cortical

Table 3. Neurotransmitter Deficits in Alzheimer's Disease

Neurotransmitter	Cell Bodies	Reduction
Acetylcholine	Nucleus Basalis	Severe
Norepinephrine	Locus Ceruleus	Variable
Serotonin	Raphe Nuclei	Minimal
Vasoactive Intestinal Peptide (VIP)	Cortex	None
Cholecystokinin	Cortex	None
Somatostatin	Cortex	Moderate
γ-Amino Butyric Acid	Cortex	None

slices to synthesize acetylcholine *in vitro*. In contrast, markers for neurons known to be located within the cerebral cortex, such as the GABAergic neurons, and cholecystokinin and vasoactive intestinal peptide (VIP) containing neurons, remain within the range of normals.

The reduction in cholinergic markers in the cortex is consistent with the degeneration of the basal forebrain cholinergic system (Coyle et al, 1983). Recent studies have demonstrated a striking loss of the large cholinergic cell bodies located in the basal forebrain complex and a commensurate reduction in the activity of choline acetyltransferase within the nucleus basalis. Analysis of other neurotransmitter systems in post mortem brain from patients with pathologically confirmed Alzheimer's dementia suggest that some may also be affected but not to the extent of the cortical cholinergic projections. Somatostatin, a neuropeptide localized primarily in cortical intrinsic neurons, is reduced by approximately 50 percent in cortex and hippocampus in Alzheimer's dementia. Inconsistent alterations in the presynaptic markers for the cortical noradrenergic neurons have been reported with some studies describing marked reductions and others finding negligible changes. Bondareff et al (1982) have recently demonstrated that the locus ceruleus, the cell bodies of origin of the cortical noradrenergic pathway, exhibits substantial cell loss, especially in those patients with earlier age of onset of symptoms. Thus, it is apparent that other neurotransmitter defined systems are involved to a variable extent in Alzheimer's dementia, although results thus far indicate that the cortical cholinergic projections are the most consistently and severely affected. Furthermore, the demonstration that neuritic plaques (one of the critical neuropathologic features of Alzheimer's dementia) are enriched with acetylcholinesterase activity, provides an intriguing link among the impairment of cognitive functions, a diagnostic neuropathologic alteration and the synaptic neurochemical abnormalities in Alzheimer's dementia (Struble et al, 1982).

PHARMACOTHERAPY. The demonstration of the cortical cholinergic deficits in Alzheimer's dementia led logically to the hypothesis that potentiation of cholinergic neurotransmission would attenuate the symptoms of the disorder. Indeed, Sitaram et al (1980) demonstrated in young adults that the muscarinic receptor antagonist, scopolamine, impaired working memory and that arecholine, a centrally active agonist at cholinergic receptors, enhanced performance on this memory task; furthermore, those individuals most sensitive to scopolamine exhibited the greatest potentiation in performance by arecholine. While the results in clinical studies with patients suffering from Alzheimer's dementia have been rather variable, recent, well-controlled studies indicate that administration of physostigmine or physostigmine and choline produced statistically significant improvements in the performance of these patients on memory tasks (Thal et al, 1983; Mohs and Davis, 1982). Nevertheless, these studies have not indicated that this pharmacologic intervention radically alters the clinical state of the individual. Thus, while results of these investigations further implicate the role of cholinergic neurons in the pathophysiology of Alzheimer's dementia, the clinical utility of these pharmacologic strategies remains unclear.

OTHER DEMENTIAS. There are numerous other causes for dementia aside from Alzheimer's disease; and the specificity of the role of cholinergic dysfunction in the symptomatic manifestations of these disease processes remains an important consideration (Table 4). Down's syndrome, or trisomy 21, is associated with a remarkably high incidence, if not a universal prevalence, of Alzheimer's type of pathology in the brains of those who live through the third decade. Post mortem analysis has revealed marked reductions in the activity of choline acetyltransferase in the cerebral cortex and degeneration of nucleus basalis neurons in a limited number of aged Down's individuals that have been studied (Price et al, 1982). Up to 50 percent of patients suffering from Parkinson's disease develop dementia; the brains of many demented Parkinsonian patients exhibit both a high density of neuritic plaques in cortex as well as loss of the cholinergic neuronal cell bodies in the nucleus basalis (Whitehouse et al, 1983). Thus, these two disorders demonstrate an intriguing extension of the correlation between certain aspects of Alzheimer's type of neuropathology and degeneration of the cortical cholinergic pathways. In contrast, Huntington's disease, which is associated with a progressive dementia that does not exhibit either the apraxis and aphasias or the neuropathologic alterations characteristic of Alzheimer's dementia, is not associated with reductions in choline acetyltransferase in the cortex or degeneration of nucleus basalis cholinergic cell bodies.

Anticholinergic Effects of Psychotropic Medications

A number of psychotropic medications have significant anticholinergic effects through blocking muscarinic receptors. These properties of the drugs contribute to significant and potentially serious side effects by interfering with peripheral parasympathetic or central cholinergic neurotransmission. The drugs used to treat the extrapyramidal side effects associated with neuroleptic treatment (with the exception of amantadine) have, as their primary mechanism of action, blockade of central muscarinic receptors. While the anticholinergic properties of commonly used antiparkinsonian drugs such as benztropine mesylate (Cogentin), trihexyphenidyl hydrochloride (Artane) or biperiden (Akineton) are well accepted, the anticholinergic action of other agents such as diphenhydramine (Benadryl), whose primary mechanism of action is blockade of histamine receptors, is often less appreciated. Diphenhydramine has achieved some favor for treating acute extrapyramidal side effects, especially dystonic reactions, because the sedating side effects associated with its antihistaminic properties has a relaxing effect on the patient—although the primary mechanism for reduction of the extrapyramidal side effect is through blockade of central muscarinic receptors.

The significant anticholinergic properties of other psychotropic agents used to treat psychiatric disorders can, unfortunately, be neglected. As a class, the

Table 4. Cholinergic Deficits in Cortex in Dementia

Disorder	Plaques	Cholinergic Losses
Alzheimer's Dementia	Yes	Yes
Aged Down's Syndrome	Yes	Yes
Parkinson's Disease with Dementia	Often	Yes
Huntington's Disease	None	None

tricyclic antidepressants exhibit substantial but variable anticholinergic effects. Amitriptyline (Elavil) and doxepin (Sinequan) exhibit substantial muscarinic blocking activity, whereas nortriptyline (Aventyl) and protriptyline (Vivactil) have substantially weaker anticholinergic effects. The anticholinergic properties of these drugs are responsible for many of their peripheral and central side effects. Thus, blockade of peripheral parasympathetic muscarinic receptors is responsible for the impairment in visual accommodation, dry mouth, constipation and difficulty in urination that occur with tricyclic antidepressant treatment. Interference with central cholinergic neurotransmission, particularly in the cortex and limbic system, may result in flagrant confusional states or, at a more subtle level, impairments in recent memory. The anticholinergic properties of tricyclic antidepressants clearly have additive effects with other anticholinergic drugs, including over-the-counter drugs, classical antiparkinsonian drugs and certain neuroleptic medications.

The anticholinergic properties of neuroleptic medication are much more variable. The less potent neuroleptics such as thioridazine (Mellaril) and, to a lesser extent, chlorpromazine (Thorazine) exhibit significant muscarinic receptor blocking activity, whereas the more potent neuroleptics such as fluphenazine (Prolixin) and haloperidol (Haldol) have rather weak anticholinergic action. The anticholinergic effect of thioridazine may account for the significantly lower incidence of acute extrapyramidal side effects seen with this drug, as opposed to therapeutically equivalent doses of incisive neuroleptics. In other words, the intrinsic anticholinergic activity of thioridazine assists in countering the extrapyramidal-inducing effects of the dopamine receptor blocking activity of the neuroleptic in the striatum (Snyder et al, 1974). This advantage must be weighed against the potential disadvantage of exposing individuals, who do not develop extrapyramidal side effects, to the unnecessary anticholinergic effects of the drug.

Aside from the pharmacodynamic changes associated with aging, clinical and preclinical findings suggest that aged individuals may be more susceptible to the anticholinergic properties of drugs. Blockade of peripheral parasympathetic function may be associated with toxic megacolon, severe urinary retention or striking tachycardia in elderly patients. Furthermore, elderly individuals appear to be much more vulnerable to impairments in central cholinergic function that result in toxic confusional states. These vulnerabilities must be considered along with the fact that elderly individuals are much more likely to be receiving a larger number of prescribed and proprietary drugs than younger individuals, and that many of these drugs may have significant anticholinergic effects (antiparkinson drugs, over-the-counter drugs, antihistamines and antidepressants).

CONCLUSION

The last decade has been a period of increasing appreciation of the anatomy and physiology of cholinergic neurotransmission. Aside from the well-defined role of cholinergic neurons in peripheral parasympathetic function, recent studies have illuminated the neuroanatomic organization and functional characteristics of the central cholinergic neurons that project to the cerebral cortex, hippocampus and limbic system. These studies have implicated dysfunction of central cholinergic neurons in the pathophysiology of Alzheimer's dementia and the cognitive impairments associated with anticholinergic drugs. In addition, the critical role played by striatal cholinergic neurons in the pathophysiology of extrapyramidal disorders, and the extrapyramidal side effects induced by neuroleptic medication, is better understood. As one looks toward the future, it is apparent that the potential role of central cholinergic neuronal systems in the pathophysiology of neuropsychiatric disorders and strategies to correct cholinergic deficits will represent a major thrust in psychopharmacologic research.

REFERENCES

Ahmed A, Marshall PB: Relationship between anti-acetylcholine and anti-tremorine activity in antiparkinsonian and related drugs. Br J Pharmacol 18:247-254, 1962

Bondareff W, Mountjoy CQ, Roth M: Loss of neurons of origin of the adrenergic projection to cerebral cortex (nucleus locus ceruleus) in senile dementia. Neurology 32:164-168, 1982

Brimijoin S: Molecular forms of acetylcholinesterase in brain, nerve and muscle: nature, localization and dynamics. Prog Neurobiol 21:291-322, 1983

Calne DB, Kebabian J, Sibergeld E, et al: Advances in the neuropharmacology of parkinsonism. Ann Intern Med 90:219-229, 1979

Coyle JT, Price DL, DeLong MR: Alzheimer's disease: a disorder of cholinergic innervation of cortex. Science 219:1184-1190, 1983

Creese I, Burt DR, Snyder SH: Dopamine receptor binding predicts clinical and pharmacological potencies of antischizophrenic drugs. Science 192:481-483, 1976

Dale HH: The action of certain esters and ethers of choline and their relation to muscarine. J Pharmacol Exp Ther 6:147-190, 1914

Davis KL, Berger PA, Hollister LE, et al: Physostigmine in mania. Arch Gen Psychiatry 35:119-122, 1978

Drachman DA: Memory function in man: does the cholinergic system have a specific role? Neurology 27:783-790, 1977

Drachman DA: Myasthenia gravis. N Engl J Med 298:136-142, 1978

Ehinger H, Hornykiewicz O: Verteilung von noradrenalin und dopamin (3-hydroxytryramin) des gehirn des menchen und ihr verhalten bei erkrankungen des extrapyramidalen systems. Klin Wochenschr 38:1236-1239, 1960

Fahn S: High dose anticholinergic therapy in dystonia. Neurology 33:1255-1261, 1983

Goldberg N, Haddox MK: Cyclic GMP metabolism and involvement in biological regulation. Annu Rev Biochem 46:823-896, 1977

Hokfelt T, Johansson O, Ljungdahl A, et al: Peptidergic neurones. Nature (Lond) 284:515-521, 1980

Jeste D, Wyatt RJ: In search of treatment for tardive dyskinesia. Review of the literature. Schizophr Bull 5:251-263, 1979

Krnjevic K, Ropert N: Electrophysiological and pharmacological characteristics of facilitation of hippocampal population spiras by stimulation of the medial septum. Neuroscience 7:2165-2183, 1982

Kuhar MJ, Yamamura HI: Localization of cholinergic muscarinic receptors in rat brain by light microscopic radioautography. Brain Res 110:229-243, 1976

Kuhar MJ, Sethy VH, Roth RH, et al: Choline: selective accumulation by central cholinergic neurons. J Neurochem 20:581-593, 1973

Loewi O: Uber humorale Ubertragbarkeit der Herznervenwin Kung. Pfbig Arch ges Physiol 189:239-242, 1921

McKinney M, Coyle JT, Hedreen JC: Topographic analysis of the innervation of the rat neocortex and hippocampus by the basal forebrain cholinergic system. J Comp Neurol 217:103-121, 1983

Mesulam M-M, Mufson EG, Levely AI, et al: Cholinergic innervation of cortex by the basal forebrain: cytochemistry and cortical connections of the septal area, diagonal band nuclei, nucleus basalis (substantia innominata) and hypothalamus in the rhesus monkey. J Comp Neurol 214:170-197, 1983

Mitchell SJ, Rawlins JNP, Steward O, et al: Medial septal area lesions disrupt rhythm and cholinergic staining in medial entorhinal cortex and produce impaired radial arm maze behavior in rats. J Neurosci 2:292-302, 1982

Mohs RC, Davis KL: Signal detectability analysis of the effect of physostigmine on memory in patients with Alzheimer's disease. Neurobiol Aging 3:105-110, 1982

Price DL, Whitehouse PJ, Struble RG, et al: Alzheimer's disease and Down's syndrome. Ann NY Acad Sci 396:145-164, 1982

Ringel SP, Guthrie A and Klawans HL: Current treatment of Huntington's chorea. Adv Neurol 1:797-804, 1973

Rossier J: Choline acetyltransferase: a review with special reference to its cellular and subcellular localization. Int Rev Neurobiol 20:283-337, 1977

Shute CCD, Lewis PR: The ascending cholinergic reticular system: neocortical, olfactory and subcortical projections. Brain 90:497-522, 1967

Sims NR, Bowen DM, et al: Metabolic processes in Alzheimer's disease: adenine nucleotide content and production of $^{14}CO_2$ from [U–^{14}C] glucose *in vitro* in human neocortex. J Neurochem 41:1329-1334, 1983

Sitaram N, Weingartner H, Gillin J: Human serial learning: enhancement with arechdine and choline and impairment with scopolamine. Science 201:274–276, 1978

Snyder SL, Greenberg D, Yamamura HI: Antischizophrenic drugs and brain cholinergic receptors. Arch Gen Psychiatry 31:58-61, 1974

Stevens JR: Neuropathology of schizophrenia. Arch Gen Psychiatry 39:1131-1139, 1982

Stroud RM: Acetylcholine receptor structure. Neuroscience Commentaries 1:124-138, 1983

Struble RG, Cork LC, Whitehouse PJ, et al: Cholinergic innervation in neuritic plaques. Science 216:413-415, 1982

Terry RD, Davies P: Dementia of the Alzheimer type. Annu Rev Neurosci 3:77-95, 1980

Thal LJ, Field PA, Masur DM, et al: Oral physostigmine and lecithin improve memory in Alzheimer's disease. Ann Neurol 13:491-496, 1983

Tune L, Coyle JT: Acute extrapyramidal side-effects: serum levels of neuroleptics and anticholinergics. Psychopharmacology 75:9-15, 1982

Whitehouse PJ, Hedreen JC, White CL, et al: Basal forebrain neurons in dementia of Parkinson's disease. Ann Neurol 13:243-248, 1983

Chapter 5

γ-Aminobutyric Acid (GABA), Pharmacology and Neuropsychiatric Illness

by S.J. Enna, Ph.D.

Amino acids are found in abundance in all tissues, including the central nervous system (CNS). These organic molecules are the basic constituents of protein, and are formed as by-products of intermediary metabolism. In the past, little thought was given to the possibility that they may also serve as neurotransmitters. In recent years it has been discovered that a number of amino acids induce a neurotransmitter-like response when applied directly to nerve tissue (Enna, 1979). Some amino acids also meet the other criteria associated with neurotransmitters, such as storage and accumulation in nerve endings, and a synaptic localization of the enzymes associated with their synthesis and degradation. Four of the amino acids found to have these properties have received special consideration: γ-aminobutyric acid (GABA); glycine; L-glutamic acid; and L-aspartic acid. GABA and glycine decrease neuronal activity by causing a hyperpolarization of nerve cells (Enna, 1979; Enna and Gallagher, 1983); for this reason they are considered inhibitory neurotransmitter substances. L-glutamic and L-aspartic acids appear to be excitatory neurotransmitters, because they increase cell firing by depolarizing nerve tissue (Coyle, 1980). A major hindrance to a more complete characterization of these transmitters has been the lack of drugs capable of selectively manipulating these systems: For example, while glutamic and aspartic acid antagonists have been discovered, they do not readily cross the blood-brain barrier (Coyle, 1980). In contrast, relatively selective and systemically active glycine and GABA antagonists have been identified (Enna, 1979). These drugs are potent convulsants, supporting the hypothesis that glycine and GABA mediate inhibitory influences in the brain. Although glycine agonists have not been found, a number of drugs are known to activate GABAergic transmission (Enna, 1983). These developments have led to a more complete characterization of the neurophysiologic and pharmacologic characteristics of GABA.

GABA was first identified in the mammalian CNS over 30 years ago (Roberts and Frankel, 1950). While there was evidence suggesting that GABA is a neurotransmitter at the crustacean neuromuscular junction, many scientists were reluctant to accept the idea that it served a similar function in the mammalian brain. Among the reasons for this hesitation was the observation that the concentration and distribution of brain GABA are much greater than are more traditional neurotransmitter substances. Moreover, while GABA induces an electrophysiological response, this action appeared to be nonselective. It was not until the 1960s that conclusive evidence was obtained to support the hypoth-

Table 1. Some Amino Acid Neurotransmitter Candidates

Compound	Structure	Electrophysiological Response
γ-Aminobutyric acid (GABA)	$H_2N–CH_2–CH_2–CH_2–\overset{\displaystyle O}{\overset{\|}{C}}OH$	Inhibition
Glycine	$H_2N–CH_2–\overset{\displaystyle O}{\overset{\|}{C}}OH$	Inhibition
L-Glutamic acid	$HO\overset{\displaystyle O}{\overset{\|}{C}}–CH_2CH_2–CH–\overset{\displaystyle O}{\overset{\|}{C}}OH$	Excitation
L-Aspartic acid	$HO\overset{\displaystyle O}{\overset{\|}{C}}–CH_2–CH–\overset{\displaystyle O}{\overset{\|}{C}}OH$ $\quad\quad\quad\overset{\|}{N}H_2$	Excitation

esis that GABA is a neurotransmitter in higher species. Most important was the discovery of drugs—in particular bicuculline and picrotoxin—that can selectively antagonize the neurophysiologic response to this amino acid (Curtis and Johnston, 1974).

Research during the past 20 years has shown that GABA plays a major role in the action of a variety of psychotherapeutic agents; and there are indications that alterations in GABAergic transmission may account for the symptoms of a number of neuropsychiatric disorders (Enna, 1981). The aim of this chapter is to summarize the laboratory and clinical data relating to GABA neurobiology and pharmacology. It is hoped that this discussion will demonstrate the importance of GABA in clinical medicine, as well as the potential impact that further development in this area may have on the management of a number of neurologic and psychiatric illnesses.

NEUROBIOLOGICAL CHARACTERISTICS

Neurochemistry

GABA is synthesized from the amino acid glutamic acid, by the enzyme glutamic acid decarboxylase (GAD) (Table 1). This reaction occurs within CNS neurons, making GAD a useful marker for GABAergic elements. Like other neurotransmitters, GABA is stored in nerve terminals and dendrites and is released into the synaptic cleft following depolarization of the cell (Iversen et al, 1971). The released GABA attaches to receptors located on the external surface of adjacent neurons. Following receptor activation, the GABA molecules are either reaccumulated into GABAergic terminals or glia, or are metabolized (Iversen and Kelly, 1975) (Figure 1). There are at least two sodium-dependent GABA transport sites in brain tissue. It is thought that the transporter having a higher affinity

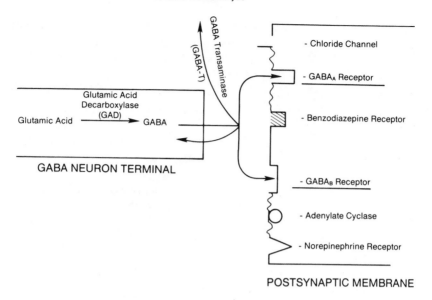

Succinic Semialdehyde

GABA Transaminase (GABA-T)

- Chloride Channel
- GABA_A Receptor
- Benzodiazepine Receptor
- GABA_B Receptor
- Adenylate Cyclase
- Norepinephrine Receptor

Glutamic Acid $\xrightarrow{\text{Glutamic Acid Decarboxylase (GAD)}}$ GABA

GABA NEURON TERMINAL

POSTSYNAPTIC MEMBRANE

Figure 1. Schematic representation of a GABA synapse.

(greater attraction) for GABA is most important for conserving this transmitter in nerve endings. The GABA, which accumulates into glia and which diffuses away from the synaptic region, is accessible to the enzyme GABA transaminase (GABA–T) and converted to succinic semialdehyde, a neurobiologically inactive substance.

An understanding of these metabolic processes is important for a proper appreciation of the drugs influencing GABAergic activity. For example: Agents that inhibit GAD will reduce the amount of GABA in the brain and decrease GABAergic transmission; conversely, drugs that inhibit GABA–transaminase (GABA–T) increase the concentration of GABA, thereby enhancing GABAergic tone. The re-uptake site represents another target for drug action. Compounds inhibiting sodium-dependent transport of GABA into neurons and glia prolong the sojourn of GABA in the synaptic cleft, thereby increasing the response to a given amount of released transmitter. Similarly, drugs enhancing GABA release would facilitate the action of this substance, while agents inhibiting release should diminish GABAergic activity.

While there are no drugs known that selectively influence GABA release, compounds have been found to inhibit GABA synthesis, metabolism and re-uptake (Table 2). Isonicotinic acid hydrazide (INH) inhibits both GAD and GABA–T, thereby increasing or decreasing the brain content of GABA, depending upon the dose administered (Sawaya et al, 1978). INH inhibits the activity of both GAD and GABA–T by antagonizing the action of pyridoxal phosphate (vitamin B_6), an essential co-factor for these enzymes. At a dose that inhibits GABA synthesis, INH decreases GABAergic transmission and provokes seizure activity. Nipecotic acid inhibits high affinity GABA transport into neurons and glia

(Johnston et al, 1976). While nipecotic acid does not readily cross the blood-brain barrier, ester derivatives are active in laboratory tests (Brehm et al, 1979). Nipecotic acid esters have anticonvulsant and sedative properties, supporting the hypothesis that inhibition of GABA transport enhances the efficacy of this inhibitory transmitter system. While neither INH nor nipecotic acid are used to treat CNS disorders, agents such as these have provided valuable insights into the pharmacological and functional characteristics of GABAergic transmission.

Distribution

Neurons either containing or responsive to GABA are found throughout the mammalian CNS (Enna et al, 1975). While GABA concentrations are greatest in extrapyramidal areas, significant levels are found in the cerebral cortex, the limbic system, cerebellum, brainstem and spinal cord. The cell bodies of dopamine, norepinephrine and serotonin neurons have a more discrete localization, and virtually all of their nerve terminals emanate from groups of cells located in the mesencephalic-pontine area. In contrast, GABA neurons are present in

Table 2. Effect of Various Drugs on GABAergic Transmission

Drug	Mechanism of Action	Effect on GABA Transmission	Primary Response or Clinical Use
Isonicotinic acid hydrazide (INH)	Inhibition of GAD (at high doses)	Decrease	Seizures
Valproic acid	Inhibition of GABA–T	Increase	Anticonvulsant
Nipecotic acid	Inhibition of GABA Uptake	Increase	Anticonvulsant
Benzodiazepines	Indirect activation of $GABA_A$ Receptors	Increase	Anxiolytics and Hypnotics
Baclofen	Direct Activation of $GABA_B$ Receptors	Increase	Muscle Relaxant
Progabide	Direct Activation of $GABA_A$ and $GABA_B$ Receptors	Increase	Anticonvulsant
THIP	Direct Activation of $GABA_A$ Receptors	Increase	Analgesic (?)
Bicuculline	Direct Inhibition of $GABA_A$ Receptors	Decrease	Seizures
Barbiturates	Interaction with $GABA_A$ Receptor Chloride Channel	Increase	Hypnotic

virtually all brain regions, with most of these possessing relatively short axon projections terminating on neurons in the vicinity of the cell body (interneurons). Only a few relatively long GABA projections linking separate brain regions, such as those between the corpus striatum and the substantia nigra (Staines et al, 1980), have been identified. This type of innervation may have functional and, therefore, clinical significance. Given their diffuse pattern of innervation arising from a small number of neuronal cell bodies, dopamine, norepinephrine and serotonin systems appear to exert a broad, modulating influence over neurons in the brain and spinal cord. In contrast, the large number of GABAergic neurons scattered throughout the CNS indicates that GABA is more likely to participate in a greater variety of regionally specific functions.

It should be noted that GABA neurons are found only in the CNS. While small amounts of GABA have been detected in peripheral organs and blood (Ferkany et al, 1978; Taniguchi et al, 1982), there is no real evidence suggesting that GABA serves a physiological role in peripheral tissue. Because the more classical neurotransmitters are involved in peripheral autonomic function as well as in CNS activity, psychotherapeutics (neuroleptics and antidepressants) that influence these transmitters provoke side effects associated with modifications in autonomic nervous system activity, such as hypo- or hypertension and constipation. Because GABA is not present to any appreciable degree in peripheral tissue, GABAergic drugs may have few, if any, peripheral side effects associated with their use. While the autonomic nervous system may be modified by an action of drugs on central regulatory mechanisms, these effects may be less pronounced than they might be for agents that directly influence ganglionic transmission, or that interact with transmitter receptors on peripheral tissues.

Receptor Properties

A great deal of research has been aimed at defining the biochemical, physiological and pharmacological properties of GABA receptor sites in the brain (Enna, 1983). Current data suggest at least two pharmacologically and functionally distinct receptors for this neurotransmitter (Bowery, 1983) (Figure 1). $GABA_A$ receptors are localized to dendrites and cell bodies, and represent a macromolecular complex consisting of at least two distinct components. One component is that portion of the receptor to which GABA attaches and which is referred to as the receptor recognition site. The interaction of GABA with this site modifies the second component, which regulates membrane permeability to chloride ions. Depending upon the concentration gradient for chloride, this ion will either enter or exit the cell following activation of the recognition site, resulting in an alteration in the polarity of the neuron. For most CNS neurons, the extracellular concentration of chloride ion is significantly greater than intracellular levels. Therefore, activation of $GABA_A$ receptor recognition sites results in an influx of chloride, causing a hyperpolarization of the cell and a decrease in neuronal activity (Enna and Gallagher, 1983). Thus, the two most fundamental components of the $GABA_A$ receptor complex are the recognition site and an associated chloride ion channel. Some $GABA_A$ receptors may also possess a third constituent, the benzodiazepine site (discussed below), the activation of which increases the sensitivity of the recognition site to GABA (Guidotti, 1982).

Less is known about the molecular characteristics of $GABA_B$ receptors. There is evidence that some GABA$_B$ receptors are located on nerve terminals containing other transmitter substances such as glutamic acid, norepinephrine, serotonin, and dopamine (Bowery, 1983). Activation of GABA$_B$ receptors diminishes the release of these transmitters. It has also been discovered that a population of GABA$_B$ receptors influences receptor responses to other neurotransmitters (Karbon et al, 1984): For example, stimulation of norepinephrine receptors causes an increase in the synthesis of cyclic nucleotides (Enna and Strada, 1983). This is thought to be due to a coupling between norepinephrine receptors and the enzyme adenylate cyclase, so that receptor activation increases the activity of the enzyme which, in turn, catalyzes the conversion of ATP to cyclic AMP (cAMP) (Figure 2). While the precise role of cAMP in neurotransmission is not yet defined, it may influence a variety of cellular activities, including regulating the ion permeability of the neuronal membrane. Selective GABA$_B$ receptor agonists, such as β–p–chlorophenyl GABA (baclofen), a drug used to treat spasticity, enhance the cAMP response to norepinephrine and other neurotransmitters in brain tissue slices (Figure 2). Thus, when rat brain cerebral cortex is incubated with increasing concentrations of norepinephrine, the conversion of ATP to cAMP increases approximately tenfold. By itself the ($-$) isomer of baclofen has little effect on cAMP formation, but it dramatically amplifies the response to a given concentration of norepinephrine (Figure 2). This interaction is found only with the ($-$) isomer of baclofen, the clinically active constituent, whereas ($+$)

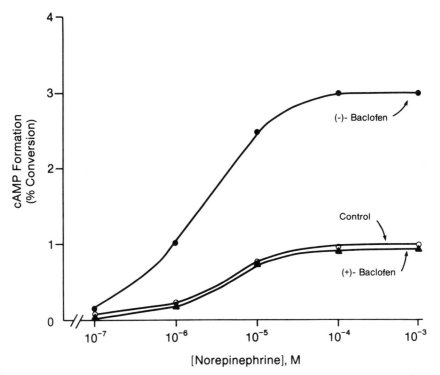

Figure 2. Effect of baclofen on norepinephrine stimulated cAMP accumulation in rat brain cerebral cortex.

baclofen is inactive both in this assay and as a therapeutic agent (Figure 2). Inasmuch as GABA$_A$ receptor agonists do not potentiate this response to catecholamines, this action appears to be mediated by a separate group of GABA receptors (Karbon et al, 1984). These data, suggesting that GABA modifies the neuronal response to other transmitters, have a number of important clinical implications that will be discussed later in this chapter.

GABA$_A$ and GABA$_B$ receptors are differentiated primarily on the basis of pharmacologic selectivity. While GABA activates both sites, certain GABA analogues are selective for either of the two receptors. The GABA receptor antagonists bicuculline and picrotoxin block only GABA$_A$ receptor responses. No drugs have been found to inhibit GABA$_B$ receptors. The identification of multiple classes of GABA receptors suggests additional targets for drug action; the further characterization of the GABA receptor family could lead to the development of more selective therapeutic agents.

Functional Activity

Activation of GABA$_A$ receptors modifies chloride ion permeability, resulting in a hyperpolarization of the neuron and a diminution in neuronal activity (Enna and Gallagher, 1983). Drugs that activate GABA$_A$ receptors (agonists) have a behavioral pharmacologic profile similar to that of CNS depressants. That is, GABA$_A$ agonists are sedating, they increase seizure threshold and cause skeletal muscle relaxation (Enna, 1981). Inhibition of GABA$_A$ receptors, either by direct-acting antagonists or by inhibition of GABA synthesis, results in seizures. Activation of GABA$_B$ receptors also causes skeletal muscle relaxation and sedation. However, GABA$_B$ agonists are poor anticonvulsants in man (Terrence et al, 1983). Thus, while there are some similarities among the behavioral and clinical responses to GABA$_A$ and GABA$_B$ receptor stimulants, their differences support the theory that these receptors mediate somewhat different physiological responses.

GABA DYSFUNCTION AND NEUROPSYCHIATRIC ILLNESSES

Neurologic Disorders

There is a growing body of evidence to support a link between GABAergic dysfunction and a variety of neurological diseases (Enna, 1981) (Table 3). A number of studies have shown a significant reduction in basal ganglia GAD activity, as well as a significant reduction in the concentration of cerebrospinal fluid (CSF) GABA, in the brains of patients who have died with Huntington's disease (Perry et al, 1973; Enna et al, 1977). These data suggest a loss of GABA-containing neurons. Because the basal ganglia are important for regulating movement, this deficiency may account for some of the motor abnormalities characteristic of this illness.

Extrapyramidal GAD activity and GABA levels are generally decreased in Parkinson's disease, and there is a significant reduction in the number of GABA receptors in the substantia nigra (Hornykiewicz et al, 1976; Lloyd et al, 1977). This latter loss is probably due to the degeneration of the nigrostriatal dopamine

Table 3. Relationship Between GABA and Neuropsychiatric Disorders

Condition	Evidence	Reference
DEMONSTRATED		
Huntington's Disease	Decrease in GAD activity throughout basal ganglia	Perry et al, 1973
Parkinson's Disease	Decrease in GABA$_A$ receptors in substantia nigra	Lloyd et al, 1977
Epilepsy	Decrease in GAD activity and GABA$_A$ receptors in a focal brain area and decrease in CSF GABA content	Ribak et al, 1979 Lloyd et al, 1981 Wood et al, 1979
POSTULATED		
Anxiety	Benzodiazepine interaction with GABA$_A$ receptors	Olsen and Enna, 1983
Affective Illness	Some antidepressants modify GABA$_A$ receptor binding and GABA agonists may have antidepressant activity	Maggi and Enna, 1980 Morselli et al, 1980
Schizophrenia	Anatomical relationship between GABA neurons and mesolimbic dopamine system	Garbutt and van Kammen, 1983

cells that contain GABA receptor recognition sites. Because these GABAergic abnormalities are probably not primary manifestations of the disorder, it is not known whether these alterations contribute to the symptoms of the disease. Inasmuch as Parkinson's patients suffer from a degeneration of nigral dopaminergic neurons, it could be argued that a decrease in nigral GABA activity may be beneficial, since GABA appears to exert an inhibitory influence on this dopamine pathway (Scheel-Kruger, 1983).

Much research has been directed toward defining the possible relationship between GABA and epilepsy (Enna and Beutler, 1984). Biochemical studies reveal a significant reduction in GABA, GAD activity and GABA receptor binding in the area of an epileptic focus (Ribak et al, 1979; Ross and Craig, 1981; Lloyd et al, 1981) (Table 3). Because inhibitory influences are important in preventing the spread of seizure activity, a reduction in GABAergic function may signify an impairment of inhibitory mechanisms in the focal area. There have also been reports of a reduction in cerebrospinal fluid (CSF) GABA with certain types of epilepsy, lending further support to the hypothesis that a decrease in GABAergic transmission could be responsible for the generation of seizures (Wood et al, 1979).

Based on these and other studies, it now appears certain that modifications in GABAergic function account for the symptoms of some neurologic disorders. While the primacy of the GABA abnormality is difficult to establish, these findings suggest that manipulation of this system could prove beneficial in the management of some central nervous system illnesses. Indeed, given the ubiquitous distribution of GABA neurons, it is likely that most neurodegenerative disorders involve some change in GABAergic function.

Psychiatric Disorders

Evidence supporting a GABA involvement in psychiatric illness is less direct than is evidence supporting a GABA involvement in neurologic disorders. Because anxiolytics appear to act through GABA receptors (Malick et al, 1983), it is possible that some types of anxiety result from a modification in this transmitter pathway. However, there are no data to directly link a change in either pre- or postsynaptic GABAergic function with anxiety states.

Chronic administration of lithium modifies $GABA_A$ receptor binding in certain regions of the rat brain (Maggi and Enna, 1980). If a similar change occurs in man, it is conceivable that this receptor alteration may contribute to the therapeutic response. There have also been preliminary reports suggesting that GABA receptor agonists may have antidepressant potential, and that GABA–T inhibitors may be effective in the treatment of mania (Morselli et al, 1980; Emrich et al, 1981). While the data are not yet substantial enough to firmly link GABA with affective illness, they are sufficient to encourage further investigation.

It has been hypothesized that GABA agonists may be beneficial in the treatment of schizophrenia (Garbutt and van Kammen, 1983) (Table 3). This proposal is partially based on the finding that GABA decreases the activity of the mesolimbic dopamine pathway, a system thought to be important for mediating some symptoms of this disorder (Pearlson and Coyle, 1983). Because antipsychotics diminish brain dopaminergic function through blockade of dopamine receptors, GABA agonists may be able to accomplish the same thing by inhibiting the activity of dopamine neurons. However, preliminary clinical trials indicate that GABA agonists have either no effect, or worsen the symptoms, of schizophrenia (Garbutt and van Kammen, 1983).

GABA PHARMACOLOGY

Anxiolytics and Sedative-Hypnotics

Some of the most compelling evidence to support a role for GABA in CNS function is derived from studies aimed at defining the mechanism of action of sedative-hypnotic agents (Malick et al, 1983). To fully appreciate the clinical implications of this research, it is important to remember that sedation, sleep and general anesthesia represent different degrees of CNS depression. For much of this century, the barbiturates were the most popular drugs for manipulating CNS activity. Low doses were prescribed as "daytime-sedatives" for the management of anxiety, while higher doses were given to encourage sleep (hypnotic effect). Still higher doses, or more potent agents, were needed for general anesthesia, the deepest level of CNS depression. Beyond general anesthetic doses, these and other depressants suppress the brain centers regulating respiration and blood pressure, resulting in death. Therefore, the clinically defined states of sedation, sleep and general anesthesia can be viewed as a continuum representing various stages of CNS depression.

A major problem with using barbiturates to relieve anxiety is that they also cause a significant amount of sedation. Because of this, it was believed that sedation (which may be defined as a decrease in motor activity and mental acuity) was necessary to calm anxious patients. This concept changed radically in the early 1960s with the introduction of the benzodiazepines (Librium and Valium) since, at the proper dose, these drugs relieve anxiety without causing a marked sedation in most patients. This observation represented a major breakthrough in the clinical management of anxiety, as well as an advance in the research in the biology of this condition. The benzodiazepines also differ from the barbiturates and other sedative-hypnotics in that they are very poor general anesthetics, even at extremely high doses. While other hypnotics induce all levels of CNS depression, the benzodiazepines are unique because they are unable to suppress brain activity much beyond the level of hypnosis. The benzodiazepines, therefore, appear able to selectively reduce anxiety with a much greater therapeutic index than are the barbiturates, meprobamate, chloral hydrate and other hypnotics; for these reasons, they rapidly gained popularity as sedative-hypnotics. Indeed, because these drugs relieve anxiety without significantly depressing the CNS, their designation as sedatives did not accurately describe the clinical response in anxious patients. Therefore, the term "anxiolytic" entered the medical lexicon to convey the notion of a drug that selectively reduces the discomfort associated with anxiety.

These clinical observations stimulated research aimed at defining the mechanism of action of benzodiazepines, because it was believed that a better understanding of these drugs could lead to a better definition of the biological mechanisms causing anxiety. While it was found that the benzodiazepines, as well as the barbiturates, modified brain neurotransmitter activity, investigators were unable to identify a particular neurochemical response that could account for the differences in their clinical profiles (Enna, 1982). GABA is among the neurotransmitter systems influenced, with GABAergic activity being enhanced by both barbiturates and benzodiazepines (Olsen and Enna, 1983). Further work has indicated that these drugs do not directly stimulate the GABA receptor recognition site, but rather indirectly facilitate GABAergic function. However, neither the benzodiazepines nor the barbiturates have any significant effect on GABA synthesis, degradation, release or re-uptake.

Recent experiments have revealed that the barbiturates influence GABA neurotransmission by interacting with the $GABA_A$ receptor-coupled chloride channel (Figure 1). It appears that the barbiturates attach to a region of the neuronal membrane in close proximity to the chloride channel; and when the GABA recognition site is activated by endogenous GABA, the channel remains open for a longer time than normal. This prolongs the response to GABA and enhances the functional activity of the receptor. The benzodiazepines do not act at the same site as barbiturates, although they too enhance the response to

GABA. Rather, benzodiazepines attach to specific sites on the neuronal membrane that are coupled to the GABA receptor recognition site (Figure 1). Attachment of the benzodiazepines increases the affinity, or attraction, of the receptor site for GABA, enabling the receptor to respond to smaller concentrations of this neurotransmitter. Thus, while the barbiturates and benzodiazepines both enhance GABAergic transmission, they do so by different mechanisms.

These molecular findings are important for understanding the differences in the clinical actions of these drugs. That is, while all $GABA_A$ receptors appear to be associated with a chloride ion channel, only some have an associated benzodiazepine recognition site. Because of this, barbiturates, and possibly other hypnotics, activate virtually all $GABA_A$ receptor systems; the benzodiazepines influence only a select group of $GABA_A$ receptors, yielding a distinct clinical response. These data may also explain why the barbiturates are more complete CNS depressants than are the benzodiazepines: By influencing a larger number of inhibitory receptors, barbiturates can cause a more substantial reduction in brain activity. In addition, because the benzodiazepines are more selective as anxiolytics, it would seem that at least a portion of those GABA receptors possessing a benzodiazepine component mediate the anxiety response. This has led to speculation that anxiety may be due to an underactivity of a select group of GABAergic neurons or GABA receptors, while sedation may result from the activation of a different population of these receptors. If this hypothesis is correct, it may be possible to develop a GABA agonist that is selective for only those receptors associated with anxiety. Such a drug may not be a CNS depressant and, unlike the benzodiazepines and barbiturates, may not interact with alcohol and other hypnotics. Therefore, it could be a much safer agent for the management of anxious patients.

The discovery of a specific benzodiazepine binding component in the brain raises the interesting question of whether there may be some endogenous chemical that normally interacts with this site (Paul et al, 1980). In other words, these data may indicate that the brain contains an endogenous anxiolytic that normally acts to modify the sensitivity of a select population of GABA receptors. It is equally possible that the endogenous agent is an anxiogenic substance that may be important for maintaining alertness. In the latter case, the benzodiazepines would be antagonists of the natural transmitter. The identification of an endogenous anxiogenic or anxiolytic would be useful in the design of new psychotherapeutic drugs. The existence of such an agent would, in addition, suggest that some forms of anxiety may be due to an alteration in the synthesis, release or metabolism of this substance. In any event, studies on the mechanism of action of the benzodiazepines have provided new insights into the clinical relevance of the GABA transmitter system, and have conclusively demonstrated its relationship to the action of an important group of therapeutic agents.

Antiepileptics

The clinical data suggesting a GABAergic dysfunction in some forms of epilepsy are not surprising, given the fact that a decrease in GABA transmission is known to induce seizure activity (Table 2). For example, both of the $GABA_A$ receptor antagonists, bicuculline and picrotoxin, are potent convulsants. By preventing the increase in chloride transport induced by GABA receptor activation, these substances decrease the firing threshold for CNS neurons, and increase their rate of discharge. Conditions or drugs which inhibit GAD activity, and therefore GABA synthesis, also induce seizures in laboratory animals and man. Such findings have led to the proposal that GABAergic drugs may be useful in the treatment of epilepsy.

Just as barbiturates have been a mainstay in antiepileptic drug therapy (Krall et al, 1978), benzodiazepines have been widely used to control certain types of seizures (Browne and Penry, 1973). While the benzodiazepines are limited in their utility because tolerance develops to their antiepileptic action, they are the drugs of choice for treating acute conditions such as status epilepticus, and for the short-term management of grand mal seizures when other medications have failed. Given the mechanism of action of barbiturates and benzodiazepines, these data support the hypothesis that an increase in GABAergic activity may be beneficial in the management of seizures.

Two newer antiepileptics also appear to work through the GABA system (Chapman et al, 1982; Morselli et al, 1980). Valproic acid inhibits GABA transaminase, the enzyme responsible for the degradation of GABA (Figure 1 and Table 2); the concentration of neuronal GABA and, presumably, the functional activity of this inhibitory system are thereby increased. There is some debate as to whether this neurochemical action of valproic acid completely explains its clinical effectiveness, but it now provides the most plausible explanation for its actions. Valproic acid is effective in the treatment of both grand mal and petit mal epilepsies, unlike other antiepileptic medications (Grant, 1976). Because valproic acid may be a more generalized activator of GABAergic transmission than either the barbiturates or benzodiazepines, it could be argued that this type of action provides a greater range of antiepileptic efficacy. Another drug, progabide, is a direct acting GABA receptor agonist that is also reported to be a broad-spectrum antiepileptic (Morselli et al, 1980). This compound and its metabolites attach to both $GABA_A$ and $GABA_B$ receptor recognition sites, mimicking the action of GABA.

In summary, both clinical and basic pharmacological data suggest that modifications in GABAergic transmission influence seizure threshold. Therefore, there will be a continuing effort to exploit these findings for developing safer and more efficacious antiepileptic medications.

CLINICAL POTENTIAL OF GABA AGONISTS AND ANTAGONISTS

Several studies suggest that GABA agonists induce an analgesic effect in laboratory animals (Kendall et al, 1982). It should be noted that the GABA agonist analgesic profile is remarkably similar to that observed with opiates. Because these drugs do not display many of the side effects associated with opiates— such as respiratory depression, reduction of gastrointestinal motility, and an increase in intracranial pressure—GABA agonists may be useful alternatives to the opiates in the management of pain. One of the difficulties associated with GABA analgesia is that the analgesic dose is nearly identical to the sedative dose. However, data suggest that the analgesic action of GABA agonists is unrelated to their sedative properties, posing the possibility of developing a GABA analgesic with little or no sedative activity (Kendall et al, 1982).

Because modifications in GABA transmission may be associated with extra-pyramidal disorders, it has been postulated that GABAergic drugs may be useful in treating patients with these conditions. Unfortunately, there are few clinical studies to support this hypothesis. For example, while progabide is reportedly effective in some Huntington subjects (Morselli et al, 1980), most GABAergic drugs have had no significant effect in treating this disorder (Tell et al, 1981). It is possible that these failures are due to the fact that Huntington's disease is characterized by a loss of many different neuronal types, only one of which is GABAergic.

It is unlikely that GABA agonists would be useful in the treatment of Parkinson's disease, given the fact that the GABA system is inhibitory on nigral dopamine neurons. Clinical trials support this supposition, with GABA agonists being either inactive or worsening the symptoms of the disorder (Bartholini et al, 1979). If it can be demonstrated that GABA receptors in the substantia nigra are pharmacologically different from those located in other brain regions, it may be possible to develop region-specific GABA receptor antagonists that could be used to treat this disorder. Such a drug would release the normal brake on the nigrostriatal dopamine system, maximizing the activity of those neurons remaining in the brain affected by Parkinson's disease.

GABA agonists have been reported to be of some benefit in the treatment of tardive dyskinesia (Tamminga et al, 1979). It is believed that this disorder may be caused by supersensitive dopamine receptors in the corpus striatum. Neuroleptics are known to induce this syndrome, presumably because the long-term blockade of striatal dopamine receptors ultimately leads to a supersensitive state in this brain area (Jenner and Marsden, 1983). Indeed, the potential for this side effect is the major limiting factor in the use of neuroleptics. It seems reasonable to conclude that by inhibiting the activity of the nigrostriatal dopamine system, GABA agonists diminish the striatal dopaminergic tone, reducing the dyskinesia. Although clinical trials have been promising, further studies are needed to establish the efficacy of GABA agonist therapy in this disorder.

Because $GABA_B$ receptor activation may influence the activity of other neurotransmitter systems, there is speculation that $GABA_B$ agonists or antagonists may be useful in the treatment of affective illness and schizophrenia. For example: If the primary action of $GABA_B$ receptor-activation is inhibition of norepinephrine, dopamine and serotonin release, then $GABA_B$ antagonists may be effective antidepressants, since depression is thought to be caused by an underactivity of these biogenic amine transmitter systems (Fuller, 1981). On the other hand, if the primary response to a $GABA_B$ agonist is enhancement of monoaminergic receptor activity (Figure 2), these drugs, either alone or in combination with standard antidepressants, may be therapeutic. Schizophrenia appears to be characterized by an overactivity of the dopaminergic system in brain limbic areas (Pearlson and Coyle, 1983); therefore, if $GABA_B$ receptor activation amplifies the receptor response to dopamine, a $GABA_B$ antagonist might be used to treat this disorder. It should be noted that the $GABA_B$ agonist baclofen has been found to be ineffective in treating schizophrenia and, in fact, causes schizophrenic-like symptoms in some patients (Davis et al, 1976). This finding supports the hypothesis that an antagonist for this GABA receptor might be beneficial in the treatment of this disorder.

SUMMARY AND CONCLUSIONS

Thirty years of experimentation have shown that GABA is a major inhibitory neurotransmitter in the CNS. Activation of GABA pathways leads to depression of the CNS; inhibition causes stimulation and seizures. GABAergic transmission can be enhanced in a variety of ways: Benzodiazepines and barbiturates potentiate GABA receptor activity indirectly; valproic acid increases GABA transmission by inhibiting the catabolism of this amino acid. The distribution of GABA in the mammalian CNS is so widespread that it seems possible that we have only begun to fully exploit this system for therapeutic gain. The recent identification of multiple types of pharmacologically distinct GABA receptors is important in this regard. Just as the discovery of cholinergic (nicotinic and muscarinic) and noradrenergic (α_1, α_2, β_1, β_2) receptor subtypes has led to the development of therapeutically useful agents, so the characterization of pharmacologically and functionally distinct GABA receptors should prove beneficial in the treatment of mental illness. Studies have provided us with reason to hope that further work can lead to the discovery of novel agents for the treatment of depression, schizophrenia and pain. GABAergic drugs may have further advantages, because this transmitter appears to have little or no function outside the CNS; therefore, these agents may induce fewer side effects than contemporary psychotherapeutic drugs. These findings with the GABA system have also demonstrated the general importance of amino acid transmitters in regulating brain function. All these advances indicate that CNS pharmacology is entering a new era with the development of drugs capable of modifying the action of these chemicals in the brain.

REFERENCES

Bartholini G, Lloyd KG, Worms P, et al: GABA and GABAergic medication: relation to striatal dopamine function and parkinsonism, in Advances in Neurology, vol. 24. Edited by Poirier LJ, Sourkes TL, Bedard PJ. New York, Raven Press, 1979

Bowery NG: Classification of GABA receptors, in The GABA Receptors. Edited by Enna SJ. Clifton, NJ, Humana Press, 1983

Brehm L, Krogsgaard-Larsen P, Jacobsen P: GABA uptake inhibitors and structurally related "pro-drugs", in GABA-Neurotransmitters. Edited by Krogsgaard-Larsen P, Scheel-Kruger J, Kofod H. Copenhagen, Munksgaard, 1979

Browne TR, Penry JK: Benzodiazepines in the treatment of epilepsy: a review. Epilepsia 14:277-310, 1973

Chapman A, Keane PE, Meldrum BS, et al: Mechanism of anticonvulsant action of valproate. Prog Neurobiol 19:315-359, 1982

Coyle JT: Excitatory amino acid receptors, in Neurotransmitter Receptors, Part 1: Amino Acids, Peptides and Benzodiazepines. Edited by Enna SJ, Yamamura HI. New York, Chapman and Hall, 1980

Curtis DR, Johnston GAR: Amino acid transmitters in the mammalian central nervous system. Rev Physiol Biochem Pharmacol 69:97-188, 1974

Davis KL, Holllister LE, Berger PA: Baclofen in schizophrenia. The Lancet June 5:1245, 1976

Emrich HM, v. Zerssen D, Kissling W, et al: On a possible role of GABA in mania: therapeutic efficacy of sodium valproate, in GABA and Benzodiazepine Receptors. Edited by Costa E, diChiara G, Gessa GL. New York, Raven Press, 1981

Enna SJ: Amino acid neurotransmitter candidates. Annual Reports in Medicinal Chemistry 14:41-50, 1979

Enna SJ: Neuropharmacological and clinical aspects of γ-aminobutyric acid (GABA), in Neuropharmacology of Central Nervous System and Behavioral Disorders. Edited by Palmer G. New York, Academic Press, 1981

Enna SJ: The role of neurotransmitters in the pharmacologic actions of benzodiazepines, in Biology of Anxiety. Edited by Mathew R. New York, Bruner/Mazel, 1982

Enna SJ (ed): The GABA Receptors. Clifton, NJ, Humana Press, 1983

Enna SJ, Beutler JA: The GABA receptor as a site for antiepileptic drug action, in Epilepsy and GABA Receptor Agonists: Basic and Therapeutic Research. Edited by Morselli P, Lloyd KG. New York, Raven Press, in press.

Enna SJ, Gallagher JP: Biochemical and electrophysiological characteristics of mammalian GABA receptors. Int Rev Neurobiol 24:181-212, 1983

Enna SJ, Kuhar MJ, Snyder SH: Regional distribution of postsynaptic receptor binding for γ-aminobutyric acid (GABA) in monkey brain. Brain Res 93:168-174, 1975

Enna SJ, Stern LZ, Wastek GJ, et al: Cerebrospinal fluid GABA variations in neurological disorders. Arch Neurol 34:683-685, 1977

Enna SJ, Strada SJ: Postsynaptic receptors: recognition sites, ion channels and second messengers, in Clinical Neurosciences, vol. 5. Edited by Rosenberg R, Grossman R, Schochet S, et al. New York, Churchill Livingstone, 1983

Ferkany JW, Smith LA, Seifert WE, et al: Measurement of gamma-aminobutyric acid (GABA) in blood. Life Sci 22:2121-2128, 1978

Fuller RW: Enhancement of monoaminergic neurotransmission by antidepressant drugs, in Antidepressants: Neurochemical, Behavioral and Clinical Perspectives. Edited by Enna SJ, Malick JB, Richelson E. New York, Raven Press, 1981

Garbutt JC, van Kammen DP: The interaction between GABA and dopamine: implications for schizophrenia. Schizophrenia Bull 9:336-353, 1983

Grant RHE: The management of epilepsy. Scott Med J 21:11-22, 1976

Guidotti A: Molecular mechanisms in the interaction between benzodiazepines and γ-aminobutyric acid receptors, in Pharmacological and Biochemical Aspects of Neurotransmitter Receptors. Edited by Yoshida H, Yamamura H. New York, Wiley, 1982

Hornykiewicz O, Lloyd KG, Davidson L: The GABA system and function of the basal ganglia in Parkinson disease, in GABA in Nervous System Function. Edited by Roberts E, Chase T, Tower D. New York, Raven Press, 1976

Iversen LL, Kelly JS: Uptake and metabolism of γ-aminobutyric acid by neurons and glial cells. Biochem Pharmacol 24:933-938, 1975

Iversen LL, Mitchell JF, Srinivasan V: The release of γ-aminobutyric acid during inhibition of the cat visual cortex. J Physiol (Lond) 212:519-534, 1971

Jenner P, Marsden CD: Neuroleptics and tardive dyskinesia, in Neuroleptics: Neurochemical, Behavioral and Clinical Perspectives. Edited by Coyle JT, Enna SJ. New York, Raven Press, 1983

Johnston GAR, Stephanson AL, Twitchin B: Uptake and release of nipecotic acid by rat brain slices. J. Neurochem 16:83-87, 1976

Karbon EW, Duman RS, Enna SJ: $GABA_B$ receptors and norepinephrine-stimulated cAMP production in rat brain cortex. Brain Res 306:327–332, 1984

Kendall DA, Browner M, Enna SJ: The antinociceptive effect of GABA agonists: evidence for a cholinergic involvement. J Pharmacol Exp Ther 220:482-487, 1982

Krall RL, Penry JK, Kupferberg HJ, et al: Antiepileptic drug development. I. History and a program for progress. Epilepsia 19:393-408, 1978

Lloyd KG, Munari C, Bossi L, et al: Biochemical evidence for the alterations of GABA-mediated synaptic transmission in pathological brain tissue (stereo EEG or morphological definition) for epileptic patients, in Neurotransmitters, Seizures and Epilepsy. Edited by Morselli P, Lloyd KG, Löscher W, et al, New York, Raven Press, 1981

Lloyd KG, Shemen L, Hornykiewicz O: Distribution of high affinity sodium-independent ^{3}H–γ-aminobutyric acid (^{3}H–GABA) binding in the human brain: alterations in Parkinson's disease. Brain Res 127:269-278, 1977

Maggi A, Enna SJ: Regional alterations in rat brain neurotransmitter systems following chronic lithium treatment. J Neurochem 34:888-892, 1980

Malick JB, Enna SJ, Yamamura HI: Anxiolytics: Neurochemical, Behavioral and Clinical Perspectives. New York, Raven Press, 1983

Morselli PL, Bossi L, Henry JF, et al: On the therapeutic action of SL 76002, a new GABA-mimetic agent: preliminary observations in neuropsychiatric disorders. Brain Res Bull 5:411-414, 1980

Olsen RW, Enna SJ: GABA and anxiolytics, in Anxiolytics: Neurochemical, Behavioral and Clinical Perspectives. Edited by Malick JB, Enna SJ, Yamamura HI. New York, Raven Press, 1983

Paul S, Marangos P, Skolnick P: CNS benzodiazepine receptors: is there an endogenous-ligand, in Psychopharmacology and Biochemistry of Neurotransmitters. Edited by Yamamura H, Olsen R, Usdin E. New York, Elsevier-North Holland, 1980

Pearlson G, Coyle JT: The dopamine hypothesis and schizophrenia, in Neuroleptics: Neurochemical, Behavioral and Clinical Perspectives. Edited by Coyle JT, Enna SJ. New York, Raven Press, 1983

Perry TL, Hansen S, Kloster M: Huntington's chorea, deficiency of γ-aminobutyric acid in brain. N Engl J Med 288:337-342, 1973

Ribak CE, Harris AB, Vaugh JE, et al: Inhibitory GABAergic nerve terminals decrease at sites of focal epilepsy. Science 205:211-214, 1979

Roberts E, Frankel S: γ-aminobutyric acid in brain: its formation from glutamic acid. J Biol Chem 187:55-63, 1950

Ross SM, Craig CR: γ-aminobutyric acid concentration, 1–glutamic 1–decarboxylase activity, and properties of the γ-aminobutyric acid postsynaptic receptor in cobalt epilepsy in the rat. J Neurosci 1:1388-1396, 1981

Sawaya C, Horton R, Meldrum B: Transmitter synthesis and convulsant drugs: effects of pyridoxal phosphate antagonists and allylglycine. Biochem Pharmacol 27:475-481, 1978

Scheel-Kruger J: The GABA receptor and animal behavior, in The GABA Receptors. Edited by Enna SJ. Clifton, NJ, Humana Press, 1983

Staines WA, Nagy JI, Vincent SR, et al: Neurotransmitters contained in the efferents of the striatum. Brain Res 194:391-402, 1980

Tamminga CA, Crayton JW, Chase TN: Improvement in tardive dyskinesia after muscimol therapy. Arch Gen Psychiatry 36:595-598, 1979

Taniguchi H, Murakami K, Yoshioka M, et al: GABA and insulin in pancreatic islets, in Problems in GABA Research. Edited by Okada Y, Roberts E. Amsterdam, Excerpta Medica, 1982

Tell G, Bohlen P, Schechter PJ, et al: Treatment of Huntington disease with γ-acetylenic GABA, an irreversible inhibitor of GABA transaminase: increased CSF GABA and homo-carnosine without clinical amelioration. Neurology 31:207-21, 1981

Terrence CF, Fromm GH, Roussan MS: Baclofen: its effect on seizure frequency. Arch Neurol 40:28-29, 1983

Wood JH, Hare TA, Glaeser BS, et al: Low cerebrospinal fluid γ-aminobutyric acid content in seizure patients. Neurology 29:1203-1208, 1979

Chapter 6

Neuropeptide Biology: Basic and Clinical Lessons From the Opioids

by Stanley J. Watson, Ph.D., M.D., Jeffrey E. Kelsey, B.S., Juan F. Lopez, M.D. and Huda Akil, Ph.D.

Peptides are powerful, biologically active substances with numerous roles in psychiatry, neurology and the neurosciences. This chapter reviews the basic structure, functions and biology of peptides, with particular emphasis on the ACTH and beta–endorphin peptide families. It discusses the evidence for ACTH and beta–endorphin regulation disturbances in endogenous depression, and identifies possible sites in the hypothalamic-pituitary-adrenal (HPA) axis for these disturbances. Emphasis is placed on findings from current popular laboratory tests, such as the dexamethasone suppression test (DST).

AMINO ACIDS, PEPTIDES AND PEPTIDE BONDS

Amino acids are ". . . the basic structural units of proteins. An amino acid consists of an amino group, a carboxyl group, a hydrogen atom, and a distinctive R group bonded to a carbon atom, which is called the alpha-carbon. . . ." (Stryer, 1981, p. 13). Figure 1 illustrates the primary structure of a prototypical amino acid.

A peptide is, in brief, a "short" chain of amino acids. Peptides have the same structure as proteins; that is, they are polymers of amino acids. The difference is that peptides contain less than 100 amino acids, while proteins contain more than 100 amino acids.

A peptide bond (Figure 2) is produced with the chemical bonding of two amino acids and the liberation of a water molecule. Biologically active peptides

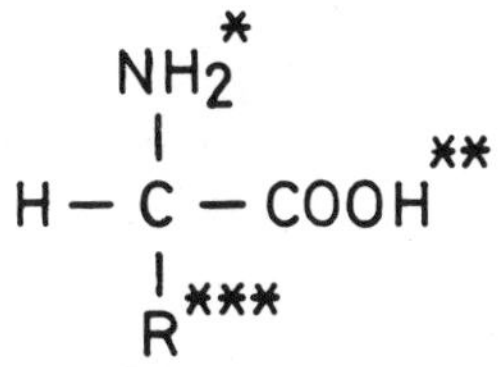

$$\overset{*}{NH_2}$$
$$|$$
$$H - C - COOH^{**}$$
$$|$$
$$\underset{R}{R}^{***}$$

* Amino Group; ** Carboxyl Group; *** R-Side Group

Figure 1. Primary structure of an amino acid.

This work was supported by NIMH Grant #MH36168 and NIDA Grant #DA02265 to SW and HA; Neuroscience Training Grant #MH14279-07 to JK.

are constructed from a series of amino acid residues coupled with peptide bonds. Biologically produced peptides contain only the 20 naturally occurring L–amino acids, while man-made peptides can contain D–amino acids and their congeners.

The Functions of Peptides

These "small" proteins can play a wide variety of roles. Peptides may function as neurotransmitters, neuromodulators and hormones. Neurotransmitters communicate discrete information at the synapse; neuromodulators exert a wide sphere of influence that alters neuronal sensitivity to other neurotransmitters; and hormones are released into the general circulation to diffusely affect the function of many cell types.

The potential of a simple five amino acid peptide can be appreciated by considering the number of possible sequence combinations: With 20 amino acids as candidates for each position, and five positions, there are 3,200,000 possible combinations. Even at this level, with a simple pentapeptide, it is clear that the amount of information contained in a peptide is enormous.

The actions of neuropeptides are mediated through specific receptor proteins located on the surface of the cell. The peptide structure is designed to activate one receptor type and not another.

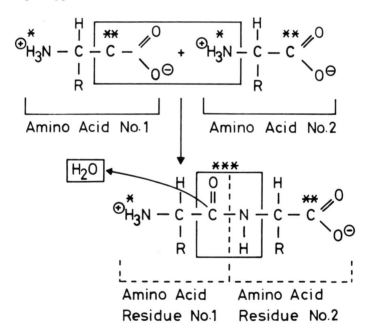

✱ Amino Group; ✱✱ Carboxyl Group; ✱✱✱ Peptide Bond

Figure 2. Structure of a peptide bond.

BASIC BIOLOGY OF PEPTIDES

The opioid peptides—beta–endorphin, dynorphin and the enkephalins—are a class of peptides that display such opiate-like activity as analgesia and a decrease in gut smooth muscle contractions in a wide variety of species. During the early 1970s researchers found that there were receptors present in the central nervous system (CNS) that would bind exogenous opiate alkaloids such as morphine in a stereo-specific manner; yet, at that time, no endogenous ligand for these receptors had been identified (Pert et al, 1973; Simon et al, 1973; Terenius, 1973). In 1975, Hughes et al reported the isolation from brain extracts of two related pentapeptides that possessed opioid-like activity. These two peptides, leucine- and methionine-enkephalin, shared the same first four amino acids—tyrosine– glycine–glycine–phenylalanine—and differed only in the amino acid in their fifth position having either leucine or methionine. The amino acid sequence of try– gly–gly–phe–leu or –met is necessary for opioid activity, and is found repeatedly in the three opioid gene families shown in Figure 3.

The most thoroughly studied of the opioid peptides has been beta–endorphin, a 31 amino acid peptide. Beta–endorphin is cleaved from a larger peptide, beta– lipotropin, a 91 amino acid peptide found in the pituitary. The discovery that a biologically active peptide such as beta–endorphin was formed from a precursor protein was quite exciting, and introduced a new level of complexity into our appreciation of CNS functioning. Beta–lipotropin is also part of a larger precursor termed proopiomelanocortin (POMC), which gives rise to ACTH, beta–endorphin, beta–lipotropin and alpha–, beta–, and gamma–MSH as shown in Figure 3. The remainder of this section will focus on our current knowledge of POMC biosynthesis and processing as a model for other neuropeptides. (See Figure 3 caption for more information on all three opioid families).

The first evidence of a common precursor for ACTH and beta–endorphin was discovered in the mid 1970s. Mains et al (1977) reported that in a mouse pituitary tumor cell line, ACTH and beta–endorphin were both present in the same 31,000 dalton precursor protein. This was determined in a pulse-chase paradigm in which cultured pituitary cells were incubated in a medium containing a radioactive amino acid for short periods of time (that is, the "pulse") so that the proteins synthesized during this interval contained a radioactive amino acid: For example, ^{3}H phenylalanine. The cells were then "chased" with a medium containing no radioactive amino acids and an excess of nonradioactive amino acids. All proteins were extracted at different time points after the chase: Those containing ACTH or beta–endorphin were precipitated with specific antisera and separated by SDS polyacrylamide gel electrophoresis to determine molecular weights. Mains et al (1977) found that a labelled 31,000 dalton protein containing both ACTH and beta–endorphin immunoreactivity appeared after a short duration of labeling, and was gradually processed to smaller sized peptides as the time of the chase was increased. This indicated that both ACTH and beta– endorphin are synthesized as part of a larger precursor that was processed to the final products ACTH, beta–endorphin, beta–lipotropin, and so forth.

The evidence for a common precursor for ACTH and beta–endorphin was made even more compelling in 1979 when POMC messenger RNA was sequenced by Nakanishi et al (1979) through the use of recombinant DNA methodology

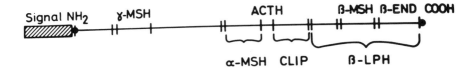

A: POMC

Signal NH₂   γ-MSH   ACTH   ß-MSH ß-END COOH

α-MSH   CLIP   ß-LPH

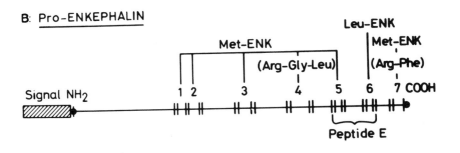

B: Pro-ENKEPHALIN

Leu-ENK

Met-ENK

Met-ENK

(Arg-Gly-Leu)

(Arg-Phe)

Signal NH₂   1 2   3   4   5   6   7 COOH

Peptide E

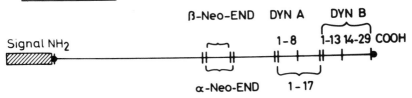

C: Pro-DYNORPHIN

ß-Neo-END   DYN A   DYN B

1-8   1-13 14-29 COOH

Signal NH₂

α-Neo-END   1-17

Figure 3. Diagrammatic representation of the three opioid peptide precursors: proopiomelanocortin (Nakanishi et al, 1979), proenkephalin (Noda et al, 1982) and prodynorphin (Kakidani et al, 1982). Sites of dibasic amino acid residues where cleavage occurs are marked by vertical lines. All three precursors have signal sequences at their amino terminus and, with the exception of gamma–MSH in POMC, the biologically active peptide products are located at the carboxy terminus. All three precursors contain multiple peptides, and repetitive nucleic acid sequences within precursors suggest gene duplication as the manner in which many of these sequences may have arisen (that is alpha, beta and gamma–MSH or met–enkephalin).

(see Figure 4 for information on cloning). By isolating the specific message (mRNA) from a tissue rich in POMC—that is, the intermediate lobe of the bovine pituitary—and cloning it into a bacterial plasmid (a small circular double stranded DNA molecule that infects bacteria, often conferring resistance to one or more antibiotics), it was possible to greatly amplify the number of copies of each mRNA (now present in plasmid DNA) simply by growing the host bacteria (E.

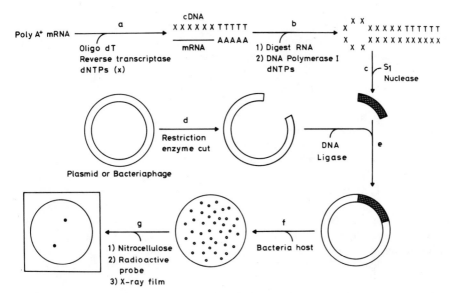

Figure 4. Cloning mRNA. This figure is a simplified illustration of mRNA coding for a specific protein. Poly A+ mRNA (see Figure 5 for addition of poly A tail to mRNA) from a tissue rich in the specific protein—that is, pituitary intermediate lobe for POMC—is isolated and mixed (a) with a synthetic nucleotide oligomer of poly dT, which will anneal to the poly A tail and form a double stranded primer for reverse transcriptase. Using deoxy nucleotide triphosphates (dNTPs), reverse transcriptase copies RNA into DNA; the double strand (with DNA represented as x's) is treated to remove the RNA (b); and the remaining DNA forms transient hairpins (loops) that serve as primers for the large frag- ment of DNA polymerase I, which lacks the exonuclease activity of the intact enzyme. S_1 nuclease (c), which cuts single stranded nucleic acids, removes the hairpin and produces a double stranded piece of DNA.

A restriction enzyme (restriction enzymes recognize specific nucleotide sequences 4–6 base pairs long) cuts (d) of plasmid or bacteriophage to open the circular DNA, allowing the foreign DNA (stippled box) to be inserted and joined to the vector with DNA ligase (e). Infection (f) of a bacterial host with subsequent plating in a culture dish forms bacterial colonies, some of which have the inserted DNA and some of which have simply religated vector. By binding the colonies to nitrocellulose paper (g), mixing with a radioactive probe (a synthetic DNA sequence 12–18 bases long that is derived from a portion of the protein's primary structure) and exposing the paper to X–ray film (h), the colonies containing plasmid with inserted DNA can be identified as dark spots on the film. By returning to the original plate, the correct colony can be grown in a culture to produce large quantities of a single species of DNA that represents the protein mRNA sequence. The entire amino acid sequence can then be determined, or the cloned DNA can be used for measuring levels of mRNA in tissue.

coli) and separating plasmid DNA from host DNA by density centrifugation. Since the amino acid sequence of part of the precursor was known, a synthetic oligonucleotide was constructed. The synthetic DNA sequence was comple- mentary to a portion of the POMC mRNA and used as a "probe" to detect clones that had POMC mRNA sequences as part of the plasmid DNA. (For a general review of cloning, see the September 1983 issue of *Trends in Neuroscience* and Figure 4.). Once the proper clones were selected and grown it was possible to sequence the POMC DNA (Maxam and Gilbert 1977), infer the mRNA sequence that would be transcribed from the DNA and, by using the triplet genetic code, deduce the amino acid sequence of the protein. This general strategy has been of great importance in furthering our understanding of neuropeptides in recent years.

Figure 3 illustrates the overall structure of three opioid peptide precursors—proopiomelanocortin, proenkephalin and prodynorphin—each of which was determined using a strategy similar to that described above. Figure 5 depicts major aspects of the cellular biology of peptide synthesis, starting at the level of the gene. All three precursors possess signal sequences: that is, 15–25 amino acids at the amino terminus of the precursor that are important for guiding the growing peptide chain into the rough endoplasmic reticulum (RER) (Blobel and Sabatini, 1971). Signal sequences are characteristic of secreted proteins. Upon entry of the signal sequence into the RER, it is cleaved by a signal peptidase. Further cleavage of the precursor into smaller products is generally considered to occur in the secretory granules that bud from the Golgi apparatus. Included in the secretory granules with the proprotein are all the enzymes necessary for site specific cleavage to form the final products. This site specific cleavage often occurs at pairs of basic amino acid residues, lysine or arginine, in all three precursors (Figure 3). A trypsin-like enzyme with a pH optimum of 5.0, identical to the internal pH of the granules, is thought to make the initial cut, and the remaining basic amino acid is removed by a carboxy peptidase-like enzyme.

Site specific cleavage is not always identical in all tissues. For example, the processing of POMC in the anterior lobe of the pituitary and in the cells of the arcuate nucleus of the hypothalamus differ in their processing, as shown in Figure 6. In the anterior lobe of the pituitary, POMC is proteolytically cleaved to form ACTH, beta–lipotropin (LPH) and some beta–endorphin. In contrast, ACTH is not found as an end product in brain POMC neurons, but is further processed to ACTH 1–13 amide or, even further, to alpha–MSH. Amino acids 15–18 of ACTH are –lys–lys–arg–arg–, which is easily recognized as sequence one would expect to find at a cleavage site. In addition, beta–endorphin is the major product derived from beta–lipotropin. These differences in processing are probably due to different enzyme specificities located within the secretory granules of each cell group. This type of cleavage can be seen in the other two opioid precursors. For example, in positions six and seven of beta–neoendorphin, dynorphin A and dynorphin B (all derived from prodynorphin) are the sequences arg–lys, arg–arg, and arg–arg respectively. These are potential cleavage sites and are possible indirect sources for leu–enkephalin. It is important to keep in mind that since processing is occurring in the secretory granules, exocytosis of the granule will release its total contents; that is, several fully processed peptides, peptide products that are not usually considered biologically active, and, possibly, enzymes involved in processing. Parallel release of peptide products has been demonstrated for ACTH and beta–endorphin in the anterior lobe of the pituitary, with equimolar concentrations of each peptide being released (Guillemin et al, 1977).

Cleavage of the larger prohormones occurs at dibasic amino acid residues. When combined with the deduced amino acid sequence of the precursors via recombinant DNA methods, this realization led to a clearer understanding of the processing of the prohormone into its daughter peptides. In the case of

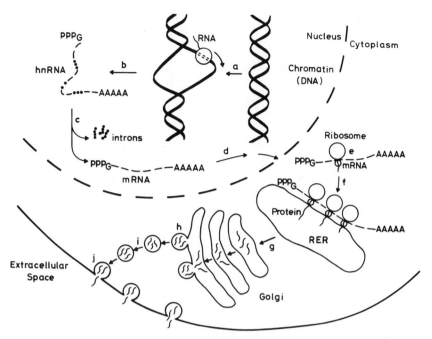

Figure 5. Protein processing. This figure summarizes events from transcription of a secretory protein gene (a) to its eventual exocytosis (j). Within the nucleus of the cell, the gene for a secretory protein is transcribed (a) into heteronuclear (hn) RNA (b) by RNA polymerase II after local unwinding of the chromatin. The hnRNA is "capped" with a guanosine triphosphate at the 5' end, and a poly A tail is added at the 3' end. Both modifications are important for stability of the RNA in the cytoplasm. HnRNA is a mixture of exons—pieces of RNA that will be present in the mature messenger RNA (mRNA)—and introns, which are noncoding and do not appear in mRNA. Introns, which served an unknown function, are excised from hnRNA (c) and degraded in the nucleus. The mRNA, which is the spliced exons (POMC, for example, has 3 exons and 2 introns), is transported (d) from the nucleus to the cytoplasm, associates with free ribosomes (e) and begins translation of the mRNA into a protein. After the signal peptide has emerged from the ribosome, translation is halted by the binding of a signal recognition particle (not shown). Upon association of the free ribosome, mRNA, signal peptide complex and the endoplasmic reticulum (f), translation starts again as the growing peptide is discharged into the rough endoplasmic reticulum (RER). The signal peptide is rapidly cleaved by a signal peptidase, and the proprotein is transported through the golgi apparatus (g). Any phosphorylation or glycosylation occurs in either the RER or golgi. Secretory vesicles "bud" (h) from the golgi and contain the proprotein; that is, uncleaved POMC, and the necessary processing enzymes. Proteolytic processing occurs as the secretory granules move toward the membrane (i), where they fuse (j) with the membrane and release their contents upon appropriate stimulation.

POMC and prodynorphin, it was also possible to identify two previously unreported potential peptide products. These were gamma–MSH in the amino terminal portion of POMC, which shows a high degree of homology with alpha– and beta–MSH; and dynorphin B, a 29 amino acid peptide with leu–enkephalin at its amino terminus, which is found at the carboxy terminus end of prodynorphin.

To summarize: All three opioid peptide families—beta–endorphin, leu– and

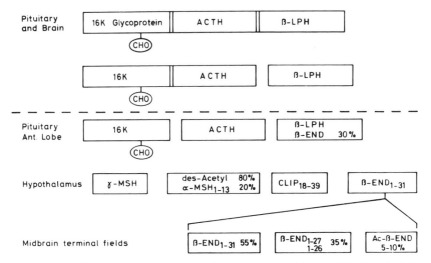

Figure 6. Differential processing of POMC in pituitary and brain. POMC in both brain and pituitary is a 31,000 dalton glycosylated (CHO) protein. The initial cleavage is at the junction of ACTH and beta–LPH followed by a separation of ACTH from the 16K glycoprotein. In the anterior lobe of the pituitary approximately 30 percent of beta–LPH is further processed to beta–end.

Processing of POMC in the arcuate nucleus of the hypothalamus occurs to a greater extent than in the anterior lobe of the pituitary. The 16K glycoprotein is cleaved to produce gamma–MSH, and ACTH is cleaved to alpha–MSH (20 percent) des–acetyl MSH (80 percent) and corticotropin-like intermediate lobe peptide (CLIP). In contrast to the pituitary, beta–LPH is completely processed to beta–endorphin. In the midbrain terminal fields of the arcuate nucleus, 35 percent of beta–endorphin is found as beta–endorphin 1–27, 1–26 and ten percent as N–acetylated–Beta–endorphin. Acetylation of beta–endorphin inactivates its opioid properties. This additional processing occurs in the secretory vesicles as they are transported down the axon.

met–enkephalin, and dynorphin—come from larger precursors that have been fully sequenced by cloning their respective mRNAs. In each precursor, the smaller end products are cleaved from the larger prohormone at dibasic amino acid residues. While this processing is highly specific, it is not identical in all cell groups (for example, the anterior lobe corticotrophs and the neurons of the arcuate lobe in the hypothalamus, in the case of POMC). Prodynorphin might also reveal differential processing with leu–enkephalin as a final product in some cell groups. Since this processing occurs in the secretory granules, exocytosis of the granules contents releases a mixture of peptide products and, probably, enzymes into the extracellular space. Finally, the principles of recombinant DNA technology are important tools for students of the nervous system, not only for sequence determination, but also as a more molecular probe for questions of regulation starting at the level of the genome.

CLINICAL RELEVANCE OF THE ACTH/BETA-ENDORPHIN FAMILY OF PEPTIDES IN AFFECTIVE DISEASE

The relevance of neuropeptides to psychiatric disorders in general and to affective disorders in particular has been the subject of much research over the past few years. We will now examine what is known about the role that POMC derivative peptides (that is, ACTH and beta–LPH/beta–endorphin) play in the pathophysiology of endogenous depression.

Hypothalamic–Pituitary–Adrenal (HPA) Dysfunction in Endogenous Depression

Studies by several investigators (Sachar et al, 1973; Carroll et al, 1976; Carroll et al, 1981) have demonstrated a faulty regulation of cortisol secretion in endogenously depressed patients. This dysfunction consists of: hypersecretion of cortisol with altered circadian rhythmicity; and failure to suppress cortisol secretion after the oral administration of 1 or 2 mg of dexamethasone. This latter abnormality has led to the development and standardization of the Dexamethasone Suppression Test (DST) (Carroll et al, 1981). Administration of the synthetic steroid dexamethasone will lead, in normal cases, to a blockade of ACTH release due to negative feedback (see Figure 7) and to a subsequent suppression of cortisol secretion by the adrenals. An abnormal DST is defined as a serum cortisol level of greater than 5 μg/dl at either 0800, 1600 and/or 2300 hrs after

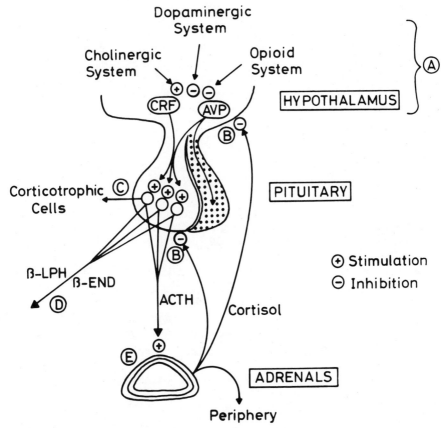

Figure 7. Schematic of the hypothalamo pituitary adrenal axis.

the administration of dexamethasone at 2300 hrs the night before. Such an abnormality is found in 30 to 60 percent of endogenously depressed patients (Carroll et al, 1976; Schlesser et al, 1980; Rush et al, 1982; Winokur et al, 1982), but is found in only about five percent of nonendogenously depressed patients and normal controls. Although the specificity of the test has recently been debated, there seems to be a disturbance in HPA regulation in a subtype of depressed individuals; and this defect disappears with normalization of the individual's mood (Greden et al, 1982; Greden et al, 1983; Albala et al, 1981).

Possible Sites of the HPA Defect

The secretion of cortisol by the adrenals is stimulated by the peptide ACTH as shown in Figure 7. ACTH is co-released with beta–LPH and beta–endorphin from the corticotrophic cells in the anterior lobe of the pituitary. The release of these peptides is, in turn, controlled by a variety of hypothalamic factors, including corticotropin releasing factor (CRF) (Vale et al, 1981) and vasopressin (Vale et al, 1968). Normally, peripheral cortisol inhibits the synthesis and release of ACTH and beta–LPH/beta–endorphin. This is done through negative feedback, both at the pituitary and hypothalamic levels.

There seem to be two types of negative feedback. One type is a "fast feedback" mechanism that is sensitive to the *rate of rise of cortisol levels* and blocks ACTH release within minutes of a sharp secretion—for example after acute stresss (Jones et al, 1974). The second type is a delayed feedback (Jones et al, 1974) that may regulate the transcription of the POMC gene and consequent synthesis of POMC, as well as regulate the processing of the precursor into ACTH and beta–LPH. This delayed feedback process takes more than ten hours to produce any change in the amount of POMC and its products.

One of the most widely held hypotheses concerning the location of the HPA defect in endogenously depressed patients proposes a disruption in a limbic monoaminergic system or its counterbalancing elements, such as the cholinergic system (Janowsky et al, 1980). This disturbance in a central neurotransmitter control of the hypothalamus could lead to a dysregulation of CRF, vasopressin or other factors controlling ACTH release. This, in turn, would lead to hypersecretion of ACTH and thus increased cortisol synthesis and release (Figure 7, site A). When the limbic system normalizes, either upon spontaneous remission or with antidepressant therapy, the faulty CRF control would be corrected and the remainder of the cascade of events returned to normal. Most studies of this model use the study of the HPA axis as a "window to the brain" to understand the underlying limbic defect.

There are certainly other possible explanations for the faulty HPA regulation. For example, there could be a defect in the corticosteroid receptors in the hypothalamus or pituitary (Figure 7, site B), with loss of the feedback inhibition necessary to suppress ACTH and/or CRF release. There could be a supersensitivity of the pituitary corticotrophic cells to CRF (Figure 7, site C), leading to increased release of the POMC peptides by the pituitary, despite normal CRF secretion. The defect could also lie in the biosynthetic or releasing mechanism for the POMC peptide (Figure 7, site D), which could lead to increased synthesis of particular peptides (that is, ACTH or gamma–MSH); or the defect could be caused by an abnormal ratio of peptides which, in turn, could promote exaggerated adrenal steriodogenesis. Finally, the defect could lie in the adrenal cortex itself (Figure 7, site E), which could be hyperresponsive to ACTH or to other POMC peptides (such as gamma–MSH) and produce hypercortisolemia.

There is, of course, the possibility—even the probability—that there are subgroups of patients with endogenous depression who manifest different regulatory disturbances in the HPA axis, or that there may be multiple disturbances operating at the same time.

POMC Peptides and Pituitary Disturbances

There have been a number of studies investigating ACTH levels in depression, both before and after dexamethasone challenge, in an attempt to discover evidence of pituitary involvement in the endocrine derangement found in depression.

There is some evidence that ACTH levels, both before and after dexamethasone, are higher in DST cortisol nonsuppressors than in suppressors (Reus et al, 1982; Kalin et al, 1982; Demiskah et al, 1983). This is consistent with the hypothesis of ACTH hypersecretion. However, other studies have found no such difference in ACTH levels (Fang et al, 1981; Yerevanian et al, 1983).

The disagreements among these studies may arise from the nature of ACTH secretion, which occurs in pulsatile bursts, with a half-life of approximately ten to 20 minutes. If ACTH sampling is done at only one time point, plasma values may represent either a peak or a valley in secretion and may not accurately reflect the mean ACTH values. Both of the negative studies used only one time point sample. Another explanation for the inconsistencies in these studies may be the *dissociation* between ACTH and cortisol responses. In an interesting study, Yerevanian et al (1983) measured ACTH levels both at the time of admission and after clinical recovery in depressed patients, all of whom were DST nonsuppressors. Half the patients reverted to normal cortisol suppression, while the other half did not. There was a significant reduction of ACTH levels in the cortisol "normalized" group, while ACTH levels remained high in the group that continued to be nonsuppressors. Thus, this study accounted for individual variation in ACTH sensitivity and was suggestive of an ACTH mediated mechanism in a DST nonsuppressor.

Another strategy for studying possible pituitary dysfunction is the measurement of the opioid peptide beta–endorphin. Since we know that beta–endorphin and ACTH are co-released by anterior pituitary corticotrophs, we would expect dysregulation of beta–endorphin, as well. A recent study from this laboratory (Matthews et al, 1982), using a well characterized beta–endorphin radio-immunoassay (RIA) (Cahill et al, 1983), found that 50 percent of endogenously despressed patients *did not decrease* their beta–endorphin levels after dexamethasone, as compared with only eight percent of nonendogenous psychiatric controls.

It is reasonable to conclude, then, that there is strong evidence for a disturbance in ACTH and beta–endorphin regulation in some endogenously depressed patients. This disturbance points to a pituitary dysfunction as a factor in the observed HPA abnormalities in this group of patients.

Abnormalities at Different Levels of the Axis

Is the group of patients who show abnormal cortisol suppression to dexamethasone the same group that shows abnormalities at the pituitary levels? The answer is "not necessarily." This question was asked by Fang et al (1981), who found no relationship between patients with abnormal cortisol DSTs and those with abnormal plasma ACTH levels after dexamethasone. In the study by Matthews and co-workers (Matthews et al, 1982), 33 percent of endogenous depressed patients had an abnormal cortisol response to DST, while 50 percent had an abnormal beta–endorphin response to DST; only a very small percentage (approximately 15 percent) had an abnormality in *both tests*. In other words, there is a high proportion of endogenously depressed patients who do not show abnormal cortisol secretion but who *do show* an abnormal regulation of their beta–endorphin secretion by the pituitary. The combination of both tests yielded an abnormality rate of 70 percent for endogenous depressed patients, versus eight percent for the psychiatric controls.

This result suggests that the cortisol–DST alone does not detect a group of patients who may have faulty pituitary peptide regulation; the idea that there is a one-to-one relationship between cortisol and pituitary hypersecretion is too simplistic. The evidence points to a multi-level HPA disturbance in depression.

There is also evidence that the HPA defect may lie above the pituitary level. In an attempt to address the role of the hypothalamus in affective disease, Risch et al (1982) showed that beta–endorphin levels, after physostigmine infusion, were significantly higher in depressed than in control subjects. These data are interpreted as indicating a *central* alteration in the HPA axis in depression and a possible role for the cholinergic system, possibly as a regulator of CRF neuronal activity.

Finally, at the other end of the HPA axis, there is some preliminary evidence (Amsterdam et al, 1983) that in some depressed patients, the adrenal itself is more sensitive to ACTH infusion than in controls, suggesting that the deficit is peripheral rather than central.

In summary, three conclusions can be drawn from the available evidence: First, there is an HPA disturbance in endogenous depression; second, the disturbances seem to occur at all three levels of the HPA; and third, a disturbance at one level does not necessarily reflect disturbances in the others.

CONCLUSION

The implication of these clinical endocrine data is that the multiple levels of control on the brain–HPA system are complex and interrelated, but capable of independent regulation. For example, within the corticotroph the defect could occur at several levels, starting with transcription and/or translation of the POMC gene; processing of precursor; or final release from the corticotroph, with modification both by the hypothalamic input and adrenal steroid feedback.

Even if we hypothesize a basic defect (for example, a limbic imbalance), the system will try to achieve homeostasis by using various mechanisms, entering its own loops of checks and balances at the hypothalamic neuronal level, the corticotroph or even the adrenal level. As we have seen, the use of only one test (that is, peripheral measurements of cortisol) may not be enough to detect other abnormalities higher in the system. In order to uncover patterns or profiles of HPA dysfunction, we must challenge the system by using such different methods as a CRF challenge, studying corticoid feedback modulation, or the nature of the peptides released by the pituitary. Nonetheless, the study of the HPA axis as a "window to the brain" has shown us that this is a "distorted window," because it can itself become disturbed. And even though we now know that there is a dysregulation of beta–endorphin and ACTH at the pituitary level, it may very well be that the defect lies higher in the HPA axis. Studies higher in the axis clearly deserve major investigation; the potential exists for real improvement in our knowledge of the role of neuropeptides in CNS and in psychiatry.

REFERENCES

Albala AA, Greden JF, Tarika J, et al: Changes in serial dexamethasone suppression tests among unipolar depressives receiving electro-convulsive treatment. Biol Psychiatry 16:551-560, 1981

Amsterdam JD, Winokur A, Abelman E, et al: Cosyntropin stimulation test in depressed patients and healthy subjects. Am J Psychiatry 140:907-908, 1983

Blobel G, Sabatini DD: In Biomembranes, vol. 2. Edited by Manson LA. New York, Plenum Press, 1971

Cahill C, Watson S, Knobloch, M, et al: POMC in rhesus anterior pituitary and plasma: Evidence of N–acetylated beta–endorphin and alpha–MSH. Life Sci 33:53-56, 1983

Carroll BJ, Curtis GC, Mendels J: Neuroendocrine regulation in depression: I. Limbic system–adrenocortical dysfunction. Arch Gen Psychiatry 33:1039-1044, 1976

Carroll BJ, Feinberg M, Greden JF, et al: A specific laboratory test for the diagnosis of melancholia. Arch Gen Psychiatry 38:15-22, 1981

Chang T, Loh YP: Characterization of proopiocortin converting activity in rat anterior pituitary secretory granules. Endocrinology 112:1832-1838, 1983

Demiskah K, Demisch L, Bochnick MS, et al: Comparison of the ACTH suppression test and dexamethasone suppression test in depressed patients. Am J Psychiatry 140:1511-1512, 1983

Fang VS, Tricou BJ, Robertson A, et al: Plasma ACTH and cortisol levels in depressed patients: relation to dexamethasone suppression test. Life Sci 29:931-938, 1981

Greden JF, de Vigne JP, Albala AA, et al: Serial dexamethasone suppression tests among rapidly cycling bipolar patients. Biol Psychiatry 17:455-462, 1982

Greden JF, Gardner R, King D, et al: Dexamethasone suppression tests in antidepressant treatment of melancholia. Arch Gen Psychiatry 40:493-500, 1983

Guillemin R, Vargo T, Rossier J, et al: Beta-endorphin and adrenocorticotropin are secreted concomitantly in the pituitary. Science 197:1367-1369, 1977

Hughes JU, Smith TW, Kosterlitz HW, et al: Identification of two related pentapeptides from the brain with potent opiate agonist activity. Nature 258:577-579, 1975

Janowsky DS, Risch SC, Parker D, et al: Increased vulnerability to cholinergic stimulation in affective disorder patients. Psychopharmacol Bull 16:29-31, 1980

Jones MT, Tiptaft EM, Brush FR, et al: Evidence for dual corticosteroid receptor mechanisms in the feedback control of ACTH secretion. J Endocrinol 60:223-233, 1974

Kakidani H, Furutani Y, Takahashi H, et al: Cloning and sequence analysis of cDNA for porcine beta–neo–endorphin/dynorphin precursor. Nature 298:245-248, 1982

Kalin NH, Weiler SJ, Shelten SE: Plasma ACTH and cortisol concentrations before and after dexamethasone. Psychiatry Res 7:87-92, 1983

Mains RE, Eipper BA, Ling N: Common precursor to corticotropins and endorphins. Proc Natl Acad Sci USA 74:3014-3018, 1977

Maxam AM, Gilbert W: A new method for sequencing DNA. Proc Natl Acad Sci USA 74:560-564, 1977

Matthews J, Akil H, Greden J, et al: Plasma measures of beta–endorphin-like immuno-reactivity in depressives and other psychiatric subjects. Life Sci 31:1867-1870, 1982

Nakanishi S, Inoue A, Kita T, et al: Nucleotide sequence of cloned cDNA for bovine corticotropin–beta–lipotropin precursor. Nature 278:423-427, 1979

Noda M, Furutani Y, Takahashi H, et al: Cloning and sequence analysis for bovine adrenal preproenkephalin. Nature 295:202-206, 1982

Pert CB, Pasternak GW, Snyder SH: Opiate agonists and antagonists discriminated by receptor binding in brain. Science 182:1359-1361, 1973

Reus VI, Joseph MS, Dallman ME: ACTH levels after the dexamethasone suppression test in depression. N Engl J Med 306:238-239, 1982

Risch SC: Beta–endorphin hypersecretion in depression: possible cholinergic mechanisms. Biol Psychiatry 17:1071-1079, 1982

Rush AJ, Giles DE, Roffmary HP, et al: Sleep EEG and dexamethasone suppression test findings in outpatients with unipolar major depressive disorders. Biol Psychiatry 17:327-341, 1982

Sachar EJ, Mellman L, Roffmary MP, et al: Disrupted 24 hour pattern of cortisol secretion in psychotic depression. Arch Gen Psychiatry 28:19-24, 1973

Schlesser MA, Winokur G, Sherman BM: Hypothalamic–pituitary–adrenal axis activity in depressive illness: its relationship to classification. Arch Gen Psychiatry 37:737-743, 1980

Simon EJ, Hiller JM, Edelman I: Stereospecific binding of the potent narcotic analgesic (^{3}H)etorphine to rat-brain homogenate. Proc Natl Acad Sci USA 70:1947-1949, 1973

Stryer, L: Biochemistry, 2nd ed. San Francisco, W H Freeman & Co, 1981

Terenius L: Characteristics of the "receptor" for narcotic analgesics in synaptic plasma membrane fraction from the rat brain. Acta Pharmacol Toxicol 33:377-384, 1973

Vale W, Fleischer N: Inhibition of vasopressin indirect ACTH release from the pituitary by glucocorticoids in vitro. Endocrinology 83:1232, 1968

Vale W, Speiss J, Rivier J, et al: Characterization of a 41 residue ovine hypothalamic peptide that stimulates secretions of corticotrophin and beta–endorphin. Science 213:1394-1397, 1981

Winokur A, Amsterdam J, Caroff S, et al: Variability of hormonal responses to a series of neuroendocrine challenges in depressed patients. Am J Psychiatry 139:39-44, 1982

Yerevanian BI, Woolf PD: Plasma ACTH levels in primary depression: relationship to the 24 hr dexamethasone suppression test. Psychiatry Res 9:319-327, 1983

Yerevanian BI, Woolf PD, Iker MP: Plasma ACTH levels in depression before and after recovery: relationship to the dexamethasone suppression test. Psychiatry Res 10:175-181, 1983

Afterword

by Joseph T. Coyle, M.D.

We must look to the future and consider the full impact of the advances in synaptic neurochemistry and molecular psychopharmacology that have been reviewed in the previous chapters. The following developments are in their embryonic stages, but are likely to affect clinical management in psychiatry over the next decade:

Ligand-binding methods to characterize neurotransmitter and drug receptors will be exploited by the pharmaceutical industry to develop much more potent and specific psychotropic drugs. As discussed in this section, current evidence suggests the existence of subtypes of benzodiazepine receptors and opiate receptors that are likely to lead to the development of anxiolytics and analgesics that are devoid of sedating or respiratory-depressing side effects.

The fusion of molecular biology with neurobiology alluded to in Chapter 6 by Watson and colleagues will lead to the mapping on the human chromosomes of the genetic coding for the neurotransmitter processes. This information will allow for more incisive and compelling studies of heritable factors that now appear, in results from clinical studies, to play a role in vulnerability to major psychiatric disorders.

Whole new classes of drugs, heretofore not considered, will be developed to manipulate specific brain transmitter systems. Current psychotropic drugs interact with only a small fraction of identified neurotransmitter systems in the brain. The brain neuropeptides, the most rapidly expanding group of neurotransmitters, hold particular promise for development of new classes of psychotropics.

The elucidation of the neuroanatomic organization and functional role of the specific neurotransmitter systems in the brain will set the stage for determination of their involvement in an expanding number of neurologic and psychiatric disorders. While much research will exploit post mortem synaptic neurochemical analysis of brain tissue from patients with specific diagnoses, the expansion of new technologies such as positron emission tomography will allow neurotransmitter specific probes to be studied in the living patient.

Ultimately, it is anticipated that these advances in neurobiology will lead to more specific, effective, and well-tolerated psychotropic medications. These advances should not erode the humanistic foundation of psychiatry, but, rather, should free the clinician to exploit psychotherapeutic interventions in a more confident manner, as the biological aspects of psychiatric disorders are clarified.

II

Neuropsychiatry

Contents

Section II
Neuropsychiatry
Introduction
by Stuart C. Yudofsky, M.D., Section Editor

Psychiatrists are intrigued as well as troubled by boundaries. We attempt to define the line between normal and abnormal behavior. We search to understand which symptomatologies stem from a patient's biology and which from his life experiences. We struggle to know what is mind and what is brain, what is psychiatry and what is neurology. A philosopher once asked his students the question, "What is the most important part of an oxcart?" Some of his students answered, "the ox"; others, "the cart"; and still others, "the driver." When one student responded that the wheel was the most important component, the philosopher acknowledged that this answer was closest to the "correct" one. For, to the philosopher, the most important part of an oxcart is the **concept** of an oxcart. Once the concept exists, almost anyone can then fashion a wheel, build a cart, join it to an ox and create an oxcart. Although concepts are not tangible—that is, do not "really" exist in the material world—they are manifestly useful. Neither psychiatry nor neurology "really" exists, but each is a conceptual tool, an invention of man. To take too seriously the boundary between psychiatry and neurology is, therefore, to take ourselves and our inventions too seriously. For instance, certain investigators have reported that specific subtypes of schizophrenia are associated with increased size of lateral ventricles as well as fibrillary gliosis in periventricular regions of the brain. Does this imply that schizophrenia, with all of the associated impairments in interpersonal relationships, mood, affect and cognition, should be considered a neurological illness? Consequently, the authors of this section intentionally do not focus upon the boundaries between psychiatry and neurology; but, rather, upon the interfaces between these disciplines. We have chosen the title "Neuropsychiatry" in order to emphasize the inevitable inseparability of these two specialties.

In Chapter 7, Drs. Taylor, Sierles and Abrams focus on the neuropsychiatric evaluation. They point out that ten to 15 percent of hospitalized acute medical or surgical patients suffer from delirium of varying degrees, and that an additional 25 percent of hospitalized medical patients suffer significant cognitive impairment. They also state that although 15 to 20 percent of acute psychiatric patients suffer from some behavioral neurologic disorder, psychiatrists are, as a rule, ill-equipped to evaluate the role of the patient's central nervous system (CNS) in his emotional, behavioral or cognitive impairment. For this reason, the authors provide the structure for a comprehensive neuropsychiatric evaluation. Special emphasis is placed upon the content and process of securing a neuropsychiatric mental status evaluation, as well as upon techniques for testing cognitive functions. Special emphasis is also placed upon evaluating language and memory function. Finally, the authors provide an approach to the evaluation of cortical functioning of the specific brain lobes and include a review of common syndromes that arise from discrete lesions in particular lobes of the brain.

In Chapter 8, "Psychiatric Aspects of Brain Injury: Trauma, Stroke and Tumor," Drs. Yudofsky and Silver underscore the common occurrence of severe brain injury. They report that the largest cause of death of people under 35 years of age in the United States is automobile accidents, 70 percent of which result from head trauma. An even higher number sustain nonfatal but neurologically disabling head trauma secondary to such accidents. The incidence of brain injury in the United States is approximately one-half the incidence of schizophrenia. In financial terms, motor vehicle accidents rank second, and stroke ranks fourth among the most costly illnesses in this country. The authors review the emotional and cognitive changes associated with brain injury, which include exacerbation of preexisting character or personality disorders, personality changes secondary to the injury, intellectual changes and psychotic changes.

Following cardiac disease and cancer, stroke ranks as the most common cause of death. Investigators find that the long-term psychiatric disability in stroke victims is far more severe than are the physical disabilities. Approximately one-third of those who suffer strokes are depressed six months following the acute event. Depression correlates significantly with stroke victims' failure to resume social activity. It is important to note that 60 percent of patients with left anterior stroke meet the criteria for major depressive disorders, while only 12 percent with left posterior region strokes meet these criteria. Drs. Yudofsky and Silver emphasize that explosive rage and violent behavior are commonly associated with both focal lesions and diffuse damage in the CNS. They outline the diagnostic criteria for organic aggressive syndrome (intermittent explosive disorder), and later review the most recent approaches to the management of this severely disabling condition.

Primary brain tumors constitute nearly ten percent of nontraumatic neurological disease, and metastatic cerebral neoplasms far outnumber primary tumors. Chapter Eight reviews the most commonly occurring psychiatric symptomatologies associated with various types of tumors in different locations in the brain. This chapter also discusses the psychological reactions of patients who are diagnosed as having brain tumors. In addition, this chapter emphasizes prevention, which includes the use of seat belts with upper torso restraints for the reduction of head injuries secondary to motor vehicle accidents, and the diagnosis and treatment of hypertension for the reduction of cerebral vascular accidents. Finally, the authors review the psychopharmacologic management of patients with brain injury, with special emphasis on increased sensitivity of the injured brain to side effects of specific agents.

Drs. Jeste, Grebb and Wyatt review psychiatric aspects of movement disorders and demyelinating disease in Chapter 9. The authors point out that the CNS must translate thoughts, feelings and drives into behavior which, most often, is expressed through motoric function. They emphasize that just as dance relates movement to emotion, the disorders affecting movement have major emotional components. They divide their topic into disorders that primarily affect the basal ganglia (Huntington's Disease, Parkinson's Disease, Sydenham's Chorea and Wilson's Disease); disorders that affect the cerebellum; drug-induced movement disorders (tardive dyskinesia); demyelinating diseases (multiple sclerosis); and miscellaneous movement disorders (Tourette's syndrome, Creutzfeldt-Jakob Disease). The authors thoroughly review the literature on behavioral and emotional concomitants of these illnesses. They point out that in Huntington's Disease, psychiatric diagnoses account for 46 percent of first admissions, and that suicide is often a major clinical concern in these patients. For Parkinson's Disease, the prevalence of dementia ranges from 30 to 80 percent, depending upon the study, and different studies have reported the prevalence of depression in the disorder to be from 60 to 90 percent. The authors underscore the fact that the medications used to treat Parkinson's disease have psychosis as a prominent side effect, and that those medications used to treat psychosis have, as prominent side effects, parkinsonian symptomatologies. The high percentage of patients (40 to 50 percent) with disorders of the cerebellum who also have psychotic symptoms is revealed. The authors extensively review the special problems related to tardive dyskinesia from a basic science as well as a clinical perspective. Prevention, diagnosis and treatment of tardive dyskinesia is emphasized. Finally, the authors review the extensive literature on psychiatric aspects of multiple sclerosis. The literature reports up to a 90 percent prevalence of emotional distress or affective symptoms in progressing MS, and a 40 percent prevalence in stable patients.

Drs. Bear, Friedman, Shiff and Greenberg address the subject of behavioral alterations in patients with temporal lobe epilepsy in Chapter 10. They emphasize that temporal lobe epilepsy is the most frequent form of epilepsy in adulthood. According to some estimates, 30 to 40 percent of patients with temporal lobe epilepsy experience persistent psychiatric symptoms, which can become the most incapacitating aspect of their illness. The authors discuss symptoms associated with temporal lobe epilepsy, which include alterations of physiological drives, changes in intellectual and personality qualities, and the emergence of paranoid symptoms and dissociative states. The neurological presentation of temporal lobe epilepsy is highlighted and the prominent changes on electroencephalogram (EEG) and other diagnostic tests are reviewed. Finally, theoretical and research questions related to interictal behavior syndromes are discussed in an effort to increase our understanding of normal brain function.

In Chapter 11, on dementia syndromes, Drs. Read, Small and Jarvik illustrate the magnitude of the problem of dementia by estimating that five percent of those 65 years or older suffer from dementia, and that the prevalence rises to 20 percent of those aged 80 and over. The authors believe that since these age groups are the fastest growing of any in our population, dementia of the Alzheimer type (DAT) can be appropriately termed "an approaching epidemic." They emphasize the syndromic nature of dementia, as opposed to the long-held belief that the disorder results from a unitary disease process. The earliest stages of dementia of the Alzheimer's type can be obscure, and there is a tendency among family and friends to underestimate the initial deficit. The authors focus on amnestic, aphasic, and visuospatial changes that are characteristic of the illness. They also review delirium (which is characterized by clouding of consciousness and may also include florid hallucinosis), agitation and other mental status changes. Abnormalities of the EEG are important diagnostic features, and usually consist of relative generalized slowing, as compared with the characteristically normal EEGs in the early stages of dementia. The authors caution that the failure to recognize delirium is a serious clinical error and may result in missed opportunities for significant therapeutic interventions. They review the relationship between depression and dementia. They present their view that the designation "pseudodementia" is misleading, because the dementia syndrome is as "real" when depression is the underlying etiology as it is when dementia results from any other dysfunction. A clinical approach for assessing and treating dementia associated with affective illness is provided. Finally the authors offer a clinical approach to the treatment of patients with dementia. They advocate accurate assessment through thorough medical and neuropsychological examinations, the treatment of any underlying disease process, psychosocial management and psychopharmacologic treatments.

Drs. Gold, Estroff and Pottash review substance-induced organic mental disorders in Chapter 12. They point out that psychiatric symptoms occur in approximately three percent of patients who take prescribed medication on a regular basis. The authors also review prominent psychiatric side effects and toxic effects of psychotropic agents, antihypertensive agents, antiarrhythmic drugs, anticonvulsant medications, and other prescribed medications. Specific emphasis is placed upon an anticholinergic toxicity which can result from the use of agents commonly prescribed in psychiatry, such as antidepressants, belladona alkaloids, antipsychotics, benztropine, and trihexyphenidyl. Antihypertensive agents, such as reserpine and alpha methyldopa, are well known to cause depression as a prominent side effect. In contrast, depression in patients who receive propranolol is relatively low, at less than one percent. The authors emphasize that illicit drug use should be a component of the differential diagnosis of almost every patient who presents to a psychiatrist. Chronic opiate administration is associated with high rates of major and minor depressions; and among the detoxification of patients with opiate addictions, one-third of this population exhibit depression. Alcohol is the most dangerous drug in our society, and the authors review the various psychiatric syndromes that can result from alcohol intoxication, dependence and withdrawal.

Robert Post introduces Chapter 13, on the future interfaces between psychiatry and neurology, with a discussion of the historical relationship between the two disciplines. He emphasizes that one of the first major somatic interventions for a psychiatric illness involved the initiation of a special neurologic state: electroconvulsive treatment (ECT)-induced seizures to treat depression. By pointing out that one of our newer somatic interventions in manic depressive illness paradoxically uses an anticonvulsant agent, Dr. Post underscores the complexity of the interface between neurology and psychiatry.

He focuses on seven areas of future interfaces between psychiatry and neurology. First, he outlines the complex interactions between psychiatric disturbances and seizure disorders and predicts that a better understanding of the fundamental mechanisms in seizure disorders will provide rewarding insights into the pathogenesis of many psychiatric disorders. Second, he reviews the relationship between endocrinology and the brain. The newly discovered cerebral peptides, as well as the earlier discovered neurotransmitters (such as dopamine, norepinephrine, epinephrine, serotonin and GABA) are involved in major psychiatric disorders as well as neurologic disorders (such as the epilepsies). To demonstrate the explosive impact in diagnosis and treatment that our increasing knowledge about brain endocrinology is likely to have, Dr. Post focuses upon a single neuropeptide, somatostatin, and emphasizes its implications in our understanding and treatment of diseases such as Alzheimer's dementia, depression, and Huntington's Chorea. In his discussion of the advances in neurobiology, he concludes that it is conceivable that certain psychoanalytic concepts and traditionally psychological states may ultimately have definable biochemical, physiologic, and perhaps anatomical substrates.

Dr. Post also speculates about the manipulation of peptides with recombinant DNA techniques. He discusses the techniques that have been used to isolate the gene involved in the production of Huntington's Chorea, and raises the possibility that alterations in gene function by direct recombinant DNA techniques may, in the future, alleviate neurological and behavioral diseases presently treated by the "juggling" of brain chemicals and relevant receptors.

In the area of diagnosis, Dr. Post discusses the dramatic impact that computerized axial tomography (CAT) scans have had on neurologic diagnosis, as well as its putative diagnostic value for such psychiatric illnesses as schizophrenia. He discusses the promise of other diagnostic techniques, such as nuclear magnetic resonance and positron emission tomography (PET) for diagnosis in psychiatry. Finally, Dr. Post speculates optimistically on new horizons for electrophysiologic and electromagnetic interventions for both psychiatric and neurologic dysfunctions. He draws a parallel between the use of electrical pacing of cardiac tissue and the use of electrical devices to regulate brain function.

In summary, the authors of all the chapters in this section emphasize the inherent indivisibility of neurology and psychiatry. Repeatedly, the authors demonstrate, using examples from the scientific literature, that all neurologic illness has prominent psychiatric components, and that most psychiatric illness has a prominent neurologic interface. Consistently, the authors stress that the emotional and behavioral disturbances of chronic neurologic illness are far more disabling than the sensory and motor dysfunctions. On the other hand, they reveal that neuroanatomical and neurophysiologic changes are most likely to be involved in all of the major psychiatric illnesses. The authors encourage both psychosocial and neurobiologic interventions for most patients with severe psychiatric or neurologic illness. They predict that future research will reveal an ever enlarging interface between psychiatry and neurology, and that this knowledge will be translated into more effective prevention, diagnosis and treatment.

Chapter 7

The Neuropsychiatric Evaluation

by Michael Alan Taylor, M.D., Frederick Sierles, M.D. and Richard Abrams, M.D.

The neuropsychiatric evaluation is not an esoteric exercise appropriate solely to the ivory tower academician. Studies (Taylor and Abrams, 1978; Sierles, 1982) indicate that ten to 15 percent of hospitalized acute medical or surgical patients suffer from deliria of varying severities; that an additional 25 percent of hospitalized medical patients have significant cognitive impairment that interferes with the management of their systemic illness; and that 15 to 20 percent of acute psychiatric patients suffer from "organic" mental disorders. The psychiatric practitioner is expected by members of his profession, by his colleagues in other branches of medicine and by society, to be expert in caring for such patients. The knowledge and skill required to provide this care are fundamental to the practice of modern psychiatry.

The neuropsychiatric examination conducted by a psychiatrist, and the subsequent laboratory assessment of the patient's central nervous system (CNS), may best be compared to the examination performed by other specialists (for example, a cardiologist's evaluation of the heart). The neuropsychiatric examination is more elaborate and more specialized than the examination performed by the average clinician, but it is still only a part of the complete physical examination, without which it has limited meaning. The goals of the neuropsychiatric examination are: to establish a reasonable doctor-patient relationship; to thoroughly evaluate the patient's present behavior and neurologic functioning; to form a diagnosis; and to develop, execute and monitor a treatment plan. The examination should not be haphazard. Some structuring is important, and questions and testing procedures should proceed in a logical pattern, while remaining responsive to the specific needs and behaviors of the patient. Open-ended questioning—during which the examiner is passive and nondirective, permitting the patient to control the topics of the interview—is rarely a useful strategy. The sequence of questions can vary and "lead-ins" to questions must be individualized, but a basic sequence of topics and a standardized tactical approach for each symptom area should characterize the examination.

Neuropsychiatry is increasingly merging with the relatively new field of behavioral neurology: the clinical discipline in which normal and abnormal behaviors are linked to functioning of specific areas or regional systems of the brain. For example, the ability to perform skilled fine motor tasks (such as typing) is associated with the frontal lobe of the dominant hemisphere; the loss of such abilities is usually associated with dominant frontal lobe dysfunction. The basic science of behavioral neurology is neuropsychology, which is concerned with understanding the relationships between cognitive functions, behavior and brain structure (Pincus and Tucker, 1978; Heilman and Valenstein, 1979).

In the traditional, "routine" evaluation of neurologic function, examiners focus almost exclusively upon such structures as the brainstem, cerebellum, basal ganglia, motor and sensory strips and the "long tracts." In contrast, the associational areas of the cortex and their related subcortical structures (areas primarily associated with behavior) are often given a cursory examination. This attitude is, in part, due to past unreliability of clinical testing procedures and the consequent difficulty in localizing lesions that result in defects of higher cortical functions. Testing of these higher cortical functions can, however, be reliable, valid and sensitive, often identifying a lesion before it is noted on a computerized axial tomography (CAT) scan or electroencephalogram (EEG) (Golden, 1978; Klove, 1974; Matarazzo et al, 1976; Matarazzo, 1972; Wheeler and Reitan, 1962; Folstein et al, 1975; Tsai and Tsuang, 1979). Whether the clinician relies on interpretations from standard assessment instruments, or performs his or her own neuropsychiatric examination, a knowledge of modern neuropsychological concepts is essential for a real understanding of the patient's disorder.

DOMINANT AND NONDOMINANT HEMISPHERES

The term "dominant hemisphere" refers to the cerebral hemisphere that is organized to express language. For 97 percent of the population, the dominant hemisphere is the left. For three percent, the dominant hemisphere is either the right, or dominance is mixed. Hemispheric dominance is not synonymous with hand preference, although there is a relationship. Ninety percent of the population is right-handed (dextral), and in 99 percent of those who are right-handed, the left hemisphere is dominant for language. Ten percent of the population is left-handed (sinistral). Among those who are left-handed, 60 percent have language organized in their left hemisphere (it is "dominant"); 40 percent have either mixed dominance for language, or language organized in their right hemisphere. Thus, the clinician should be alert to the possibility of mixed or right hemispheric dominance for language in sinistrals (Benson and Geschwind, 1968; Seamon, 1974; Geschwind, 1974; Pincus and Tucker, 1978; Golden, 1978; Heilman and Valenstein, 1979).

A patient's preferred hand for writing is a crude but clinically useful guide to determining which of his hemispheres is organized for language or is dominant (Beaumont, 1974). To confirm that the patient's hand preference for writing is a natural tendency, and not the product of having been required as a child to write with the nonpreferred hand, the patient should be asked to state his hand preference, and demonstrate with which hand he pours liquids, holds his knife to cut food, holds scissors, throws a ball, and holds a thread when threading a needle. Most individuals who write with their right hand will use their right hand for these purposes. Left-handed persons often give a mixed response.

There is considerable evidence that the two hemispheres process information differently and have different functional specializations. The dominant hemisphere—usually the left—appears to process information in a sequential, analytic, linear fashion and is particularly efficient at processing language and other symbolic information. The "nondominant" hemisphere—usually the right—appears to process information in a gestaltic, holistic, parallel fashion and is particularly efficient at processing visuo-spatial information (Benson and Geschwind, 1968; Seamon, 1974; Heilman and Valenstein, 1979). Anatomical

---

and biochemical asymmetries may underlie these functional differences (Geschwind, 1974).

INTERHEMISPHERIC CONNECTIONS

The corpus callosum and other structures deep within the hemispheres are responsible for transferring and integrating information between the two hemispheres. Although sensory and motor long tracts do not pass through the interhemispheric structures, messages from one associational cortical region to another in the opposite hemisphere do pass through them. For example: In a left-hemisphere dominant patient, the instruction, "With your left hand, show me how you would hit a nail with a hammer" is processed by the associational cortex for speech in the left hemisphere, and by the associational cortices of the left parietal and frontal lobes. A "message" is then transmitted to the right hemisphere to initiate the motor response in the left hand. The message from the right frontal lobe motor areas to the spinal cord and to the left hand does not pass through the corpus callosum (Geschwind, 1965) (See Figure 1).

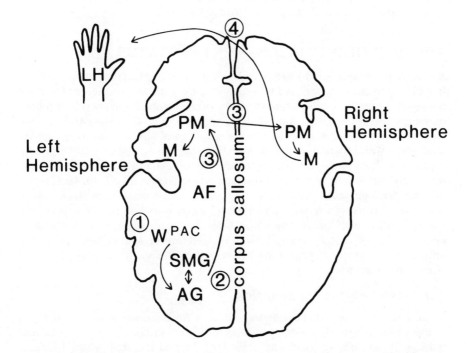

Figure 1. Interhemispheric Connections. LH, left hand; W–PAC, Wernicke's area—primary auditory cortex; SMG, supramarginal gyrus; AG, angular gyrus; AF, arcuate fasiculus; PM, premotor area; M, motor area; 1—patient decodes information "With your left hand, show me how you would use a hammer"; 2—control of ideokinetic praxis; 3—transmission of ideokinetic information from dominant parietal area to dominant frontal area and then across corpus callosum to nondominant frontal area; 4—transmission of motor sequencing (i.e., hammering) along pyramidal tract to spinal cord and then to left upper extremity.

THE NEUROPSYCHIATRIC EVALUATION

The neuropsychiatric evaluation includes: a complete assessment of systemic and neurologic functions; an examination for "soft" neurologic signs (palmomental reflexes, grasp reflex, snout reflex, adventitious motor overflow, double simultaneous discrimination); and a detailed mental status and cognitive assessment. In addition, it includes such ancillary clinical tests as: the "Minimental State"; the Aphasia Screening Test; Paired Associate Learning; Babcock Story Recall and Memory for Design; WAIS Non-Proverb Comprehension and Similarities Subtests; and Stanford-Binet Verbal and Pictorial Absurdities. Also included are such neurological laboratory tests as neuropsychological assessment; electrophysiologic studies (EEG, evoked response); CAT scan or Nuclear Magnetic Resonance (NMR) scan; spinal fluid studies; cerebral angiography; and skull X–ray. General systemic tests include chemistries (for example, SMA–6, SMA–12) and urinalysis. Such specific systemic tests as intermediate tuberculin purified protein derivative (PPD); Venereal Disease Research Laboratories (VDRL); electrocardiogram; chest X–ray; endocrine studies; and nutritional studies are also included. The clinician interested in further information about the systemic and neurologic examinations and related laboratory tests is referred to Wells and Duncan, 1980; Strub and Black, 1981; and Scheinberg, 1981.

THE NEUROPSYCHIATRIC MENTAL STATUS

A change in an individual's behavior is often the earliest sign of brain dysfunction. The person who, for the first time, exhibits inefficiency at work, a general feeling of lassitude, inattentiveness, slight circumstantiality in speech or moodiness, may be in the early stages of dementia. Although CAT scan and EEG are usually still within normal limits at this early stage of illness, a thorough behavioral history and mental status examination may reveal psychopathology and cognitive deficits suggesting coarse brain disease, even in the absence of more traditional neurologic indicators (Peterson, 1978; Fitzhugh-Bell, 1978). Clusters of abnormal behaviors may also be suggestive of regional brain dysfunction, and a well-structured mental status examination can thus be a sensitive and specific indicator of brain disease. A brief review of the mental status as a neuropsychiatric assessment technique is therefore presented here. Historical information, helpful in diagnosing behavioral neurologic disease, is presented elsewhere in the text.

The Mental Status Examination

Acquiring information that correlates with specific diagnoses is an essential goal of this examination. Whenever possible, the examiner should greet the patient outside the examining room and walk with him to the area selected for the interview. This initial pseudo-informal introductory period permits the examiner to observe the patient's general appearance and manner. Observations of the patient's behavior on the ward are also extremely helpful. The examiner should deliberately review the patient's age, sex, race/ethnic background, body type, nutrition, personal hygiene and state of consciousness. No detail should be overlooked: A short, stocky, hirsute "depressed" woman might have adrenal hyperplasia; an unkempt, dazed, ataxic man with urine-stained pants might have normal pressure hydrocephalus; a man with the left side of his face unshaven may have left spatial neglect caused by nondominant parietal lobe disease (Critchley, 1953).

Motor behavior is also observed upon meeting the patient and walking with him to the examining room. Observations of motor behavior should include a description of gait, abnormal movements, frequency of movement, rhythm, coordination and speed. The wide-based or ataxic gait of the alcoholic, the hesitant gait of the Huntington's patient, the stooped shuffle of the patient with frontal lobe disease, the manneristic hopping and tiptoe gaits of the catatonic are but a few of the unusual motor behaviors that can be observed at this time. Just as motor behavior is regulated by frontal lobe systems (Luria, 1973; Heilman and Valenstein, 1979), motor abnormalities—including the catatonic syndrome, severe hyperactivity, and stupor—may reflect coarse frontal lobe disease.

Affect is studied in this examination. Affect is the emotional tone underlying all behaviors; it can be understood quantitatively as having a range, intensity (quantity or amount), modulation and stability; and qualitatively as having appropriateness of mood, quality of mood and relatedness. Mood is the content of affect and refers to expressions of sadness, happiness, anger and anxiety.

In mental illness the quality of mood may be constant despite changes in the patient's immediate surroundings (Taylor, 1981). For example, patients with affective disorder express a constant mood of sadness, elation, irritability or dysphoria. Variability of emotional expression over time is the range of affect, and can be compared to the variations and modulation in music. A person with a constricted affect essentially expresses only one mood over a period of time, regardless of surrounding events.

In contrast, some patients have rapid mood shifts (Taylor, 1981), moving quickly from tears, to laughter, to angry outbursts. Often, these outbursts occur with minimal or no provoking stimuli. This instability of emotional expression is termed lability of affect. Constriction and lability of affect are opposite extremes of emotional expression.

Moods can vary in intensity as well as quality (Taylor, 1981). Intensity of mood refers to the degree or amplitude of emotional expression. Thus, anger is more intense than irritability, and euphoria is more intense than happiness. In many patients, affectivity can be intense while being constricted in range (restricted to a single quality of mood). The psychomotor epileptic, for example, can shout and rage with great force, never varying his mood until overcome by exhaustion. His range of affect is severely constricted, but the amplitude of his affect is great.

Mood appropriateness refers only to the patient's moods expressed during the mental status examination and is determined, in part, by the examiner's own mental state and empathic understanding of the patient's behavior ("What's appropriate for me is appropriate for the patient."). A patient's inappropriateness of mood (such as laughing in a sad situation) may be a pathognomonic sign of serious illness, but it may also reflect normal anxiety (for example, "gallows" humor).

The most difficult parameter of affect to evaluate is relatedness, or an individual's ability to express warmth, to interact emotionally and to establish rapport.

Schizophrenics are notoriously unable to respond in this manner and often appear cold and unfeeling. They are said to have emotional blunting. Emotional blunting has been considered a core sign of schizophrenia since the earliest descriptions of the syndrome. Recently, reliable measures for determining the presence of emotional blunting have been reported (Abrams and Taylor, 1978; Andreasen, 1979). Patients with emotional blunting have a paucity of emotional response.

Occasionally, patients with emotional blunting will make silly jokes and express a fatuous, shallow mood, incongruous to the situation. This is termed *Witzelsucht* and is associated with frontal lobe disease. Motor aprosodia, an expression of nondominant frontal lobe disease in which the patient is unable to express emotion in speech, may be mistaken for emotional blunting (Ross, 1981). Unlike the emotionally blunted patient, however, the patient with motor aprosodia has all the usual desires and feelings, but cannot express them. The aprosodias are discussed below.

The assessment of language has been given insufficient attention in most discussions of the mental status examination. Thought processes are inferred from a person's speech and use of language. The form of speech and language differs from thought content. The form of speech is characterized by its rate, pressure, rhythm, idiosyncrasy of work usage, grammar, syntax and associational linkage. The form of speech is process; what he is talking about is content. Content primarily reflects cultural and personal life experience rather than the disease process in question. Thought content is rarely of diagnostic importance. Exceptions to this rule are the thoughts of suicide, guilt and hopelessness often expressed by depressed patients; or the grandiose ideas of great wealth, power or high birth expressed by manics. These, however, can also be conceptualized as the content of a profound, unremitting sadness and dysphoria, which is the essential psychopathological form of major depressive illness; or, the content of an intense euphoric mood, a cardinal feature of mania. Strange or "bizarre" ideas are never diagnostic and can occur in many conditions (Taylor, 1981).

Delusional phenomena are characterized by false or arbitrary ideas developed without adequate proof. These phenomena, each of distinct psychopathological form, include: delusional mood and ideas of reference, delusional ideas (primary and secondary), autochthonous delusional ideas, and delusional perceptions (Taylor, 1981). Delusional phenomena are frequently observed in severely ill psychiatric patients. However, they are not pathognomonic of schizophrenia and are frequently found in patients with affective disorder and coarse brain disease (Taylor, 1981; Abrams and Taylor, 1983). The delusion that familiar people are impostors (Capgras syndrome) has been associated with nondominant hemisphere disease (Hayman and Abrams, 1977; Alexander et al, 1979).

Perceptual disturbances are very common among psychiatric patients. Hallucinations can occur in all sensory modalities; visual, auditory, olfactory, gustatory, tactile and visceral, and can occur in a variety of nonpathological conditions, such as fatigue, distractability, falling asleep and awakening. Nearly 50 percent of people without any mental disorder have hallucinated at some time (Taylor, 1981). Anyone who has heard his name paged when no sound came from the loudspeakers has hallucinated. Although no perceptual dysfunction is pathognomonic, the presence of any of the following strongly suggests coarse brain disease: dysmegalopsia, panoramic hallucinations, autoscopy, extracampine hallucinations, pervasive hypnagogic or hypnopompic hallucinations, vivid olfactory hallucinations, or any vivid hallucination which occurs in the absence of other significant psychopathology (Davidson and Bagley, 1969; Taylor, 1981; Benson and Blumer, 1982).

The late Kurt Schneider, the German psychiatrist who first systematically described clinical phenomena he termed "first-rank symptoms" (Schneider, 1959), wrote, "when any of these modes of experiences is undeniably present, and no basic somatic illness can be found, we may make the decisive clinical diagnosis of schizophrenia." Schneider regarded these symptoms as "first-rank" only in the diagnostic sense. They were correlative assumptions formed purely from clinical experience and were without relationship to any theoretical concept. Although his descriptions and definitions have generated great interest in the phenomenologic study of schizophrenia, investigations have demonstrated that, though first-rank symptoms occur in 60 to 75 percent of rigorously defined schizophrenics, they are also experienced by individuals with affective disease, particularly during manic episodes (Taylor, 1981; Abrams and Taylor, 1983).

Schneider listed 11 first-rank symptoms that can be conveniently categorized under five major headings: thought-broadcasting; experiences of influence; experiences of alienation; complete auditory hallucinations; and delusional perceptions. Although first-rank symptoms have never been associated with specific neurologic disease, experiences of alienation appear identical to denial of left-sided body parts in patients with right parietal lobe lesions (Critchley, 1953).

TECHNIQUES FOR TESTING OF COGNITIVE FUNCTIONS

Cognitive assessment must be performed thoroughly and systematically in order to be valid. Our preferred strategy is to test: motor behavior; language; frontal lobe functions; memory; dominant parietal lobe functions; nondominant parietal lobe functions; occipital lobe functions; and soft neurologic signs.

The various examination strategies can be cross-checked by using Table 1. For example, if motor testing reveals echopraxia and language testing reveals expressive aphasia, both abnormalities can be seen as manifestations of frontal lobe dysfunction.

Most tasks in the examination are designed to focus on specific higher cortical functions and associational cortical regions and systems. Nevertheless, functional intactness of the entire system (afferent and efferent) is required for the correct performance of a given task. Thus, when a patient makes an error, the examiner must put the error into the context of what has been gleaned about the patient from tasks already completed, and may need to perform other tasks to localize the dysfunction (Wheeler and Reitan, 1962; Klove, 1974; Matarazzo et al, 1976; Golden, 1978; Heilman and Valenstein, 1979). Other sources of error include the patient misunderstanding the instructions, being insufficiently fluent in the examiner's language, or being uncooperative or poorly motivated.

Table 1. Cortical Mapping

	Frontal	Dominant Temporo-Parietal	Dominant Parietal	Nondominant Parietal	Nondominant Temporo-Parietal	Occipital	Corpus Callosum
Normal Function							
Motor Behavior	• Motor persistence • Initiation and stopping • Rapid sequential movement • Resistance to stimulus binding • Learned complex motor behavior	• Writing	• Ideokinetic (ideomotor) praxis • Kinesthetic praxis	• Constructional praxis • Dressing praxis • Kinesthetic praxis			• Tying shoelaces with eyes closed • Ideokinetic praxis in hand ipsilateral to dominant hemisphere
Language	• Verbal fluency • Spontaneous prosody and gesturing* • Ability to repeat with prosodic affective variation*	• Comprehension of spoken language • Reading • Relevance and word usage • Naming • Writing • Letter gnosis • Number gnosis	• Symbolic categorization		• Auditory comprehension of affective components of prosody • Visual comprehension of affective components of prosody		• Writing • Reading
Memory	• Short-term memory store	• Rehearsed consolidated memory (30 sec–30 min)			• Rehearsed consolidated memory (30 sec–30 min) • Musical memory	• Visual memory	
Other	• Concentration • Global orientation • Judgment • Problem-solving • Abstracting ability • Right spatial recognition		• Finger gnosis • Calculation • Right-left orientation • East-West orientation • Stereognosis • Graphesthesia	• Stereognosis • Graphesthesia • Recognition of familiar faces and other things		• Visual pattern recognition (visual gnosis)	• Stereognosis • Graphesthesia

Table 1. Cortical Mapping—Continued

	Frontal	Dominant Temporo-Parietal	Dominant Parietal	Nondominant Parietal	Nondominant Temporo-Parietal	Occipital	Corpus Callosum
Brain Dysfunctions							
Motor Abnormalities	• Motor impersistence • Inertia • Impaired rapid sequential movements • Stimulus-bound behavior (e.g., echopraxia, gegenhalten)	• Dysgraphia	• Ideokinetic (ideomotor) dyspraxia • Kinesthetic dyspraxia	• Constructional dyspraxia • Dressing dyspraxia • Kinesthetic dyspraxia			• Inability to tie shoes with eyes closed • Ideokinetic dyspraxia in hand ipsilateral to dominant hemisphere • Constructional dyspraxia in hand contralateral to dominant hemisphere
Language Abnormalities	• Broca's aphasia • Transcortical aphasia • Motor aprosodia* • Verbigeration	• Wernicke's aphasia • Pure word deafness • Drivelling, word approximations, stock phrases, phonemic paraphasias, private use of words • Dysgraphia • Dyslexia • Dysnomia • Letter agnosia • Number agnosia • Sensory aprosodia					
Memory Abnormalities	• Impaired short-term memory store	• Impairment of rehearsed consolidated memory			• Impaired musical memory • Impaired comprehension of prosody and gesturing • Impaired rehearsed consolidated memory (30 sec-30 min)	• Impaired visual memory • Visual agnosia	
Other Abnormalities	• Impaired concentration • Global disorientation • Impaired judgment • Impaired problem solving • Impaired abstraction • Right spatial neglect		• Finger Agnosia • Dyscalculia • Right-left disorientation • East-west disorientation • Astereognosis • Graphanesthesia • Impaired symbolic categorization	• Astereognosis • Graphanesthesia • Anosognosia • Prosopagnosia • Paragnosia • Reduplicative paramnesia • Left spatial neglect			• Astereognosis of hand ipsilateral to dominant hemisphere • Graphanesthesia of hand ipsilateral to dominant hemisphere

*nondominant frontal lobe

OBSERVATION AND TESTING OF SPECIFIC FUNCTIONS

Motor Functions

The assessment of motor behavior is a prominent part of the traditional mental status examination. The examiner is expected to note the general level of motor activity, the gait, the presence of tremors, choreo-athetoid movements, intrusiveness, agitation and inertia. The behavioral neurologic examination requires further testing for motor regulation dysfunctions, such as motor impersistence, perseveration, stimulus-bound phenomena, catatonia, and a praxias.

The examiner tests motor persistence by noting whether the patient is able to sustain a motor action. He should ask the patient to perform at least four tasks, such as, "Hold out your arms"; "Make a fist with both of your hands"; "Stick out your tongue"; "Close your eyes tightly," and note whether the patient is able to continue each task for about 20 seconds. Inability to persist with eyes open may be due to frontal lobe dysfuction (that is, motor impersistence), or to motor weakness (Ben-Yishay et al, 1968; Heilman and Valenstein, 1979). To distinguish between the two, motor strength is tested as in the general neurologic examination. The patient with normal motor persistence and strength should then be asked to close his eyes and again hold out his arms for 20 seconds. If one arm drifts downward sooner than 20 seconds, the parietal lobe contralateral to the drifting hand may be affected (Critchley, 1953; Heilman and Valenstein, 1979).

The ability to start and stop motor actions is associated with frontal lobe function (Luria, 1973). One abnormality of this ability is termed perseveration, which is the unnecessary repetition or maintenance of an action. It can present itself or be elicited in a number of ways: The patient can be asked to copy or spontaneously draw a design or shape which "lends itself" to unnecessary repetition; the patient can be asked to perform a three-stage command such as, "Take this piece of paper in your right hand, fold it in half, and return it to me" (a common perseverated response is for the patient to fold the paper in fourths or eighths); the patient can be asked to perform a task such as "Place your left hand to your right ear," and despite precise instructions to lower his hand once the task is completed, he maintains the posture; occasionally a patient can be asked to perform a sequence of tasks. If, following a request to perform a new task, he continues to perform an action that had been requested earlier in the examination, he has perseverated (Luria, 1973; Quitkin et al, 1976).

Related to motor perseveration is the difficulty in initiating motor tasks. Some patients will be virtually immobile, moving extremely slowly and hesitantly. The combination of difficulty initiating motor tasks and difficulty stopping the task once started (perseveration) is termed motor inertia (Luria, 1973). In patients with dysfunctions such as perseveration, frontal lobe abnormalities often produce false positive findings on testing of functions of other brain regions (for example, perseverating a previous task response when requested to perform a new task) (Heilman and Valenstein, 1979; Taylor, 1981).

The ability to willfully control one's motor actions based on thinking or reasoning—despite the presence of visual, tactile or other stimuli that might lead one with brain dysfunction to lose control over those actions—is called stimulus-resistant motor behavior. It is principally a frontal lobe function (Luria, 1973;

Heilman and Valenstein, 1979). Abnormalities of stimulus-resistant motor regulation (termed stimulus-bound behavior) include echopraxia and *gegenhalten*, each a feature of catatonia (Abrams et al, 1979).

Echopraxia occurs when the patient imitates an action of the examiner after receiving specific instructions not to do so. Echopraxia is elicited by an instruction to the patient such as, "When I touch my nose, you touch your chin." The examiner then touches his nose; if the patient touches his nose, he has manifested echopraxia. Several trials may be needed to assess: first, whether the patient understood the request; and, second, the severity of the echopraxia.

The examiner might also ask the patient to extend his upper extremities in an anterior direction and then state, "I'd like you to do with your right hand what I do with my right hand." Once he is convinced that the patient understands the question, he places the fingers and palm of his right hand in various positions. If the patient copies these hand positions with his left hand (mirroring the examiner's right hand), he has demonstrated echopraxia. Another example of stimulus-bound motor dysregulation is elicited by instructing the patient, "Don't shake my hand," while the examiner extends his arm in a handshaking position. If the patient shakes the examiner's hand despite understanding the instruction, he has manifested stimulus-bound behavior.

Gegenhalten, or paratonia, refers to uneven resistance of the limbs to passive movement. To test for *gegenhalten* the examiner instructs the patient to relax his arms, then attempts to flex and extend the patient's hand, forearm or arm. If the patient's muscles give equal and opposite resistance to the examiner's maneuvers, the patient has manifested *gegenhalten*. Although *gegenhalten* is localized in the frontal lobe, it is considered a neurologic "soft sign" (Paulson and Gottlieb, 1968).

The *catatonic* patient may show echopraxia or *gegenhalten*, or any of the following signs of motor dysregulation: stupor with mutism; automatic obedience; catalepsy; mannerisms; stereotypies; *mitgehen*; and posturing. Catatonic behaviors are often seen in patients with frontal lobe dysfunction (Heilman and Valenstein, 1979; Abrams et al, 1979; Luria, 1973).

The examiner should test the patient's ability to perform rapid sequential fine movement by asking the patient to mimic his finger movements. With his hands in the prone position and his palms on a flat surface, the examiner proceeds to tap each finger, one at a time (little finger, ring finger, middle finger, forefinger, thumb), rapidly and in sequence. The patient without upper limb pathology should be able to mimic these rapid sequential finger movements; if he cannot, he may have contralateral frontal lobe dysfunction (Luria, 1973; Heilman and Valenstein, 1979). If, as the examiner tests one hand for sequential finger movements, the fingers of the other hand start to wiggle or tap, the patient has manifested adventitious motor overflow (choreiform movements is another example of adventitious motor overflow). Although this sign is sometimes localized in the frontal lobe, it is considered a neurologic "soft sign" (Quitkin et al, 1976; Paulson and Gottlieb, 1968).

Ideokinetic (ideomotor) praxis is the ability to perform an action from memory upon request without props or cues (Critchley, 1953; Geschwind, 1965; Luria, 1973; Geschwind, 1974; Golden, 1978; Heilman and Valenstein, 1979; Taylor, 1981). Primary motor and sensory function must be intact and the patient must fully understand the task. To rule out the effect of interhemispheric dysconnection, the nonpreferred hand is tested first, and the patient should not be allowed to cue himself by restating the instruction. The patient is asked to demonstrate the use of a key, comb and hammer, and to flip a coin first with the nonpreferred and then with the preferred hand. Common errors include: awkward performance of these actions, miming only with proximal movements (movements of the shoulder and arm) while distal movements (hand and wrist) are stiff or absent; use of the hand as the object itself, instead of as the bearer of the object (for example, combing the hair by running the hand through the hair, hitting the imaginary nail with the fist); and the inability to perform the task without verbalizing the action (verbal overflow) (Critchley, 1953; Geschwind, 1965; Luria, 1973; Geschwind, 1974; Heilman and Valenstein, 1979; Golden, 1978; Taylor, 1981). In patients with interhemispheric dysconnection, ideokinetic praxis may be normal in the hand (usually the right), contralateral to the dominant (usually the left) hemisphere, and abnormal in the other hand (Geschwind, 1965, 1974). In patients with dominant parietal lobe dysfunction, ideokinetic dyspraxia will be manifest with both hands (Critchley, 1953; Geschwind, 1965; Luria, 1973; Geschwind, 1974; Golden, 1978; Heilman and Valenstein, 1979; Taylor, 1981).

Kinesthetic praxis is usually tested by asking the patient to mimic hand, finger, and other limb positions presented to the patient by the examiner (Critchley, 1953; Luria, 1973; Heilman and Valenstein, 1979; Taylor, 1981). If the patient cannot reproduce these hand positions, he is manifesting kinesthetic dyspraxia, reflecting malfunction in the parietal lobe contralateral to the hand being tested (Critchley, 1953; Geschwind, 1965; Luria, 1973; Geschwind, 1974; Golden, 1978; Heilman and Valenstein, 1979).

Constructional ability is usually tested by asking the patient to copy the outline of a shape (for example, a square, a triangle, a Greek cross) (Wheeler and Reitan, 1962; Klove, 1974; Heilman and Valenstein, 1979). The patient is asked to copy only the outline of the drawing because accurate copying of the small details within the object's boundaries may require verbal reasoning (dominant hemisphere), as well as nondominant parietal lobe functioning (Gainotti et al, 1977). In order to eliminate facilitating cues (for example, straight lines) or distracting cues (for example, other drawings), each drawing should be done on a separate, blank, 8½" x 11" unlined sheet of paper. The examiner should instruct the patient to copy the *outline* of the shape, without taking his pencil off the paper. The copy should be the same size as the test shape and should be drawn in the center of the page. If the patient lifts the pen during the task, he should repeat the drawing. If the drawing is markedly inaccurate, or if the patient cannot complete the drawing unless he lifts his pen in mid-task, he may have constructional dyspraxia. He should repeat the drawing with his nonpreferred hand. If the preferred-hand drawing is worse than the nonpreferred hand drawing, the dysfunction is probably the product of interhemispheric dysconnection or dysfunction in dominant hemisphere structures (LeDoux et al, 1978). If both drawings are inaccurate, the dysfunction is probably in the nondominant parietal region (Wheeler and Reitan, 1962; Klove, 1974; Heilman and Valenstein, 1979).

Dressing praxis is the ability of the patient to dress and undress himself efficiently. When patients make errors, such as putting on clothes inside out, or putting their feet in their shirtsleeves, they probably have nondominant parietal dysfunction (Wheeler and Reitan, 1962; Klove, 1974; Heilman and Valenstein, 1979).

Language Functions

Assessment of language is an extension of the "thought processes and content" section of the mental status examination. Language functions include spontaneous speech, naming, reading and writing. Language functions are, by definition, primarily served by the dominant hemisphere; but the "affective components" of speech (called prosody) are served by the nondominant hemisphere (Benson, 1979; Ross, 1981).

The function of speech is localized primarily in the parasylvian areas of the frontal, temporal and parietal lobes of the dominant (for words and word usage) and nondominant (for the "affectivity" of speech) hemispheres. In the dominant hemisphere, this includes: Broca's area; the frontal cortex deep to Broca's area; the supplementary motor cortex; the arcuate fasciculus connecting Broca's to Wernicke's area; Wernicke's area and adjacent temporal lobe structures; and the supramarginal gyrus of the parietal lobe (Geschwind, 1965, 1974; Golden, 1978; Benson, 1979; Heilman and Valenstein, 1979).

Fluency of speech is a function of Broca's area, the frontal cortex deep to it, and the supplementary motor cortex. Speech fluency can be grossly estimated by simply listening to the extent, continuity and fluidity of the patient's utterances. A standardized, sensitive test of general verbal fluency should be administered by asking the patient to name as many animals as he can (or words beginning with a specific letter) as fast as he can. If expressive language function is normal, the patient can name 20 to 30 animals (or 20 to 30 alliterated words) in 60 seconds (Pincus and Tucker, 1978; Golden, 1978; Heilman and Valenstein, 1979; Benson, 1979). Abnormalities of speech fluency include Broca's aphasia, transcortical motor aphasia and mixed aphasias (Geschwind, 1974; Golden, 1978; Benson, 1979).

Broca's (motor) aphasia results from damage to the left posterior inferior region of the left frontal lobe (Broca's area). Although they may have some comprehension and thinking deficits, patients with Broca's aphasia often understand spoken language reasonably well. Characteristically, however, they are unable to express themselves fluently and are occasionally totally mute. Most can speak, but struggle to "get the words out." Their speech is often dysarthric, with labored utterances or mispronounced syllables (for example, "Messodist Episcopal" for "Methodist Episcopal"). Their sentences are most commonly missing small words such as "the," or "to," or "a." Without these articles of speech, language resembles telegrams("don't write, send money"), and is hence termed "telegraphic."

Because of the extent of brain tissue damage associated with most diseases producing Broca's aphasia, abnormalities not directly related to spoken language often accompany it (Wheeler and Reitan, 1962; Geschwind, 1974; Benson, 1979). These abnormalities include: ideokinetic dyspraxia of the ipsilateral hand; buccolingual dyspraxia (the patient may have trouble puffing out his cheeks, whistling, or blowing out a match); weakness or paralysis of the contralateral extremity, and dysgraphia of the ipsilateral (and sometimes the contralateral) hand.

Transcortical motor aphasia results from damage to the frontal lobe deep to Broca's area. In this type of aphasia, the patient manifests a paucity of speech. Speech, as in Broca's aphasia, is labored; however, it is not telegraphic. Comprehension and thinking may be affected.

Sometimes, a mild motor aphasia is not immediately recognized by the examiner, who should routinely test for it in all patients by having the patient repeat sentences or phrases containing small words (such as, "The Polish Pope now lives in the Vatican," "No ifs, ands, or buts") or phrases that are difficult to pronounce (such as "Methodist Episcopal," "Massachusetts Avenue"). Repetitive language also involves decoding and phonemic expression; therefore, dysfunction in posterior language areas must be ruled out if a patient has difficulty repeating sentences.

Auditory comprehension and linkage of words to visual images are associated with the posterior two-thirds of the superior temporal gyrus, encompassing the transverse auditory gyrus of Heschl (the medial third of the superior temporal gyrus), Wernicke's area (the posterior third); and the angular gyrus. Dysfunctions in either these regions, or in tracts such as the arcuate fasciculus connecting Wernicke's area to Broca's area, can produce Wernicke's aphasia, impaired auditory comprehension, dysnomia and conduction aphasia. (See Figure 1.)

Wernicke's (receptive) aphasia is the product of a lesion in or near Wernicke's area and is characterized by fluent jargon-filled speech (drivelling), paraphasic utterances, loss of word complexity, phonemic problems and impaired comprehension of the speech of others. Syntax appears intact but the content is often meaningless. Writing is usually aphasic.

The poor auditory comprehension of a Wernicke's aphasia patient may be immediately apparent in his lack of appropriate response to simple requests. Evidence of poor auditory comprehension may have to be elicited, however, by presenting the patient with requests of gradually increasing complexity. Sometimes a patient who can respond properly to a simple request (such as, "Would you sit down, please?") will be unable to respond to a more complex one (such as, "Show me all the pictures that contain white, black or red"). On occasion, a lesion of the middle third of the superior temporal gyrus will produce a solitary defect of auditory comprehension. Here the patient's speech is fluent, clear and understandable, but the patient has grossly impaired comprehension of the speech of others.

The patient with dysnomia (or anomia) has difficulty naming objects. The examiner first asks the patient to name a series of common objects (such as a pen, a wristwatch, a tie, a lightswitch and a thermostat) commensurate with the patient's level of education. The examiner also asks the patient to point to various items that the examiner names (for example, "Point to your belt," "Show me a button"). Dysnomia can be the product of a dominant temporal or a dominant parietal lesion.

A recent study (Faber et al, 1983) demonstrated that patients with schizophrenia and formal thought disorder, and neurologic patients with posterior aphasia, exhibited elements of aphasic speech with equal frequency. Both groups had fluent speech and speech with reduced content or meaning (fewer nouns and more pronouns). The schizophrenics, however, were able to use multisyllabic words (for example, "military industrial complex"); the posterior aphasics did not use such words and, in addition, tended to exhibit auditory comprehension deficits.

Reading and writing are, in addition to speech, language functions associated with the dominant temporoparietal region (Critchley, 1953; Luria, 1973; Geschwind, 1974; Seamon, 1974; Benson, 1979; Heilman and Valenstein, 1979). To test reading, the patient is asked to read several words and sentences. He should also be asked to demonstrate reading comprehension by reading a sentence, then doing what it says (for example, "Touch your left hand to your right ear"). Impaired reading ability is called dyslexia; when the disability is profound, it is called alexia.

Writing is tested by first asking the patient to write one or several words from memory and then to write a sentence. The patient should be instructed to use cursive writing ("Write in script," "Use your handwriting") rather than printing, because testing of cursive writing permits detection of subtle dysgraphia that would be unnoticed in printing. If the patient cannot write cursively—which itself represents dysgraphia or agraphia—he can print. The examiner also evaluates what is written for letter construction, syntax and word usage.

Recent studies of regional blood flow during spontaneous speech have revealed changes in the parasylvian regions of the nondominant hemisphere. During speech, activity in these regions "mirrors" changes in homologous regions of the dominant hemisphere, serving the functions of prosody and emotional gesturing: the "affective components" of language (Seamon, 1974; Heilman and Valenstein, 1979; Benson, 1979; Ross, 1981). Patients with normal dominant hemispheric functioning and lesions in the nondominant hemisphere manifest normal spontaneity, clarity and comprehension of speech. But they may have impairments of range, modulation and melody of voice, of gesturing with speech, or of comprehension of the emotional tone of the speech of others. These abnormalities are analogous to aphasic disturbances due to dominant hemisphere dysfunction. For example, in an anterior (frontal) prosodic disturbance, there is impaired spontaneous emotionality and gesturing with speech; in posterior (temporal) prosodic disturbance, there is impaired comprehension of the prosody and gesturing of others. The assessment of language-related functions of the nondominant hemisphere include: observations of the patient's range, modulation, and melody of voice, the spontaneity of his gestures and their ability to convey the feeling associated with what he is saying; the patient's ability to repeat a sentence with the same affective quality as the examiner (the examiner presents statements using a happy, sad, tearful, disinterested, angry, or surprised voice, and the patient is requested to repeat these statements in the same way); the patient's ability to comprehend (rather than simply mimic) the emotions of others, which is analogous to the assessment of the comprehension of speech (to test this, the examiner stands behind the patient, and presents the patient with sentences devoid of emotionally laden words, with varying affective tones; the patient is then asked to state whether the sentence was spoken with an "angry, sad, happy, indifferent, surprised or fearful tone"); and the patient's ability to comprehend emotional gesturing. The examiner faces the patient and mimes a facial expression to convey one of the above-mentioned moods. The patient is then asked to describe the mood portrayed. If he is unable to do this, he is given the choices and asked to choose the correct one.

Sometimes, dysprosodia can be distinguished from emotional blunting by the patient's stating that he experiences moods normally, but is unable to convey them, and is troubled by this problem. Emotional blunting is, by definition, associated with other affective incompetence; dysprosodia can be, and often is, a solitary affective dysfunction.

Memory

Memory assessment is rarely performed adequately during the mental status examination. This is unfortunate because there are many tests of memory function available to the clinician. Memory assessment should include an evaluation of immediate retention span learning and retrieval of recently learned and long-stored information. Specific verbal and visual memory testing should be done.

Questioning patients about their past and about the sequence of events and details surrounding their recent illness can provide an impression of their memory function (Barbizet, 1970). A standardized clinical assessment of memory should also be done. The extent of this evaluation will obviously be determined by the individual clinical situation. Long-term memory can be tested by asking the patient to recite information learned by rote in early childhood (such as the alphabet, number series, simple multiplication tables, days of the week and months of the year, the Pledge of Allegiance, childhood rhymes and prayers). Any error or inability to start or to complete these verbal automatisms suggests significant impairment.

Short-term learning can be tested by having the patient learn a list of ten word pairs (six simple pairs and four difficult pairs), such as those presented in the well-known Paired Associate Learning test from the Wechsler Memory Scale. The patient is instructed to listen carefully as the examiner reads a list of word pairs aloud (for example: come–go; lead–pencil; in–although). After a five second pause, the examiner reads one word aloud from each pair (in random order) and the patient tries to recall each co-word. The patient is given three trials to learn the ten word pairs. This paired associate learning task has the advantage of being standardized and (unlike the usual task of asking the patient to remember three or four words) this test has been administered to thousands of normal subjects of various age groups so that it may be scored. Scoring entails dividing by two the sum of all the correct responses (over three trials) for the simple words, plus the sum of all the correct responses (over three trials) for the difficult words. A perfect score is 21. If a patient is alert and attentive, severe impairment is indicated by scores equal to or less than: 13 (ages 20–39); 10 (ages 40–54); 7 (ages 55–69); 6 (70 or older).

Immediate retention can be tested by either having the patient learn a series of eight or nine digits (up to 12 trials are allowed and two consecutive correct repetitions is the goal), or by having the patient listen to a standardized 21 unit story paragraph (Table 2) that he is asked to immediately recall (one point is earned for each unit recalled and the score is adjusted by adding four, giving a maximum score of 25; a score equal to or less than 11 indicates severe dysfunction) (Lezak, 1983). The advantage of story recall over serial digit learning is that the paragraph can be used to test short-term retrieval by reading it a second

Table 2.   Story Recall Test

December 6./ Last week/ a river/ overflowed/ in a small town/ ten miles/ from Albany./ Water covered the streets/ and entered the houses./ Fourteen persons/ were drowned/ and 600 persons/ caught cold/ because of the dampness/ and cold weather./ In saving/ a boy/ who was caught/ under a bridge,/ a man/ cut his hands.

---

time, then asking the patient to recall it after 20 minutes (the maximum score is 21 and a score equal to or less than 11 indicates severe dysfunction).

Visual memory can be tested in a variety of ways. One method is to present the patient with a series of geometric designs, such as those included in the Memory-for-Designs Test, each presented for five seconds. The patient immediately tries to reproduce each design. Rotations and reversals, missed major elements or loss of configuration each indicates dysfunction. When 15 designs are presented, a standard scoring system can be used (that is, one point for two or more errors with gestalt of design preserved; two points with configuration lost or a major element missing; three points for rotations and reversals or failure to draw anything), with scores of 0–4 within the normal range, 5–11 a borderline performance and scores of 12 or greater suggestive of brain damage (Lezak, 1983; Benton et al, 1983).

Temporal Lobes

Language and memory assessment tests, in part, temporal lobe function. Temporal lobe dysfunction can be expressed as a variety of psychomotor states; the presence of psychomotor symptoms should suggest a temporal lobe lesion (although discharges in other areas of the brain, such as the frontal lobe or the parietal lobe, can also produce psychomotor features).

Some patients without temporal lobe epilepsy will, nevertheless, have temporal lobe lesions. Patients with stroke, head injury, viral disease (particularly herpes), vascular malformations and degenerative disease involving the temporal lobes can present with delusions, hallucinations (particularly auditory and panoramic visual) and mood disturbances. Patients with posterior (temporoparietal) aphasia and patients with formal thought disorder share many of the same elements of language dysfunction. There is a strong association between temporal lobe dysfunction and psychopathology. In the absence of a classical epileptic picture and course, a temporal lobe etiology in the differential diagnosis of a psychotic patient must be considered (Davidson and Bagley, 1969; Hayman and Abrams, 1977; Pincus and Tucker, 1978; Heilman and Valenstein, 1979; Taylor, 1981; Benson and Blumer, 1982; Koella and Trimble, 1982).

Disturbances in language and memory are most commonly observed in psychiatric patients with temporal lobe dysfunction. Bilateral involvement is typically associated with dementia. When the dysfunction is in the dominant temporal lobe, euphoria, auditory hallucinations (often "complete" voices), formal thought disorder and primary delusional ideas are the likely psychopathology. These clinical phenomena are associated with such cognitive deficits as decreased learning and retention of verbal material (read or heard), and poor speech and reading comprehension. When the dysfunction is in the nondominant temporal lobe, dysphoria, irritability, depression, and inappropriate emotional expression (aprosodia) are the likely psychopathologies. These clinical phenomena are associated with such cognitive deficits as decreased recognition and recall of visual and environmental sounds, amusia (loss of ability to repeat musical sounds), poor visual memory, decreased auditory discrimination and comprehension of tonal patterns, and decreased ability to learn and recognize nonsense figures and geometric shapes (Pincus and Tucker, 1978; Golden, 1978; Heilman and Valenstein, 1979; Cummings, 1982).

Frontal Lobe Functions

The frontal lobes comprise 25 percent of adult brain weight. The portion of the frontal lobes rostral to the motor areas has control over other cortical areas, and is considered by many to be the association cortex for the limbic system. Frontal lobe dysfunction (either intrinsic or secondary to limbic system dysfunction) adversely affects performance on tasks designed to test other cortical areas; the clinician must be especially careful in trying to diagnose the locus of a lesion in the presence of frontal lobe dysfunction (Luria, 1973; Golden, 1978; Pincus and Tucker, 1978; Heilman and Valenstein, 1979).

Motor behavior and expressive language are regulated by frontal lobe systems. Additional frontal lobe functions should be assessed, beginning with an evaluation of the patient's ability to concentrate on or attend to a task. This is reliably and readily done by asking the patient to subtract sevens serially from 100. Another useful test of concentration is to have the patient spell a five letter word (such as earth, world or money) backwards. (Spear and Green, 1966; Luria, 1973; Folstein et al, 1975; Golden, 1978).

Reasoning and thinking abilities should be assessed as part of the evaluation of frontal lobe, as well as other dominant hemisphere, functioning. Proverb or adage interpretation is the most widely used mental status tool for assessing thinking. Unfortunately, responses to proverbs do not correlate well with deficits in abstract thinking (Andreasen, 1977); fewer than 22 percent of non-brain-damaged adults fully understand them (Matarazzo, 1972). Because thinking is not a monolithic function, no single test spans all the cognitive processes subsumed under that rubric. A clinical assessment of "thinking," however, can be obtained by specifically assessing a patient's comprehension, concept formation and reasoning; the extent of this assessment is determined by the individual clinical situation.

Some of the nonproverb items from the comprehension subtest of the WAIS (Matarazzo, 1972; Lezak, 1983) can be used to clinically assess a patient's comprehension. Three of the test questions are: Why do we wash clothes? Why does a train have an engine? Why should we keep away from bad company?

Encouraging and asking the patient to elaborate his answer may be needed to obtain the patient's best performance. However, the examiner should terminate the test after three consecutive failures. As these items are extracted from the WAIS, normative data are not specifically available for them. However, if one scores each response as 0–poor, 1–fair, or 2–full comprehension, a score of 8 or less suggests significant impairment.

The similarities subtest of the Wechsler Adult Intelligence Scale (WAIS) is a good test of verbal concept formation (Matarazzo, 1972; Lezak, 1983, pp. 265-266). The examiner should introduce each item by saying, "In what way are "A" and "B" alike?" For item one (orange and banana), if the subject replies "they are both fruit," the examiner simply proceeds with item two. If the subject's response to item one is inadequate, the examiner should state, "They are alike in that they are both fruit" and proceed with item two, but offer no help on this or on succeeding items. After three consecutive failures, the test should be terminated. As with the WAIS comprehension, each item may be scored 0, 1, 2, with a score of 10 or less suggesting serious dysfunction. Three examples from a subtest of the WAIS are: 1) Orange. . . .Banana; 2) Coat. . . .Dress; 3) Axe. . . .Saw.

A good test of reasoning can be adopted from the verbal and pictorial absurdities sections of the Stanford-Binet (Lezak, 1983). (The Stanford-Binet Third Revision (form L-M) discussed here is published by the Riverside Publishing Company, copyright 1973. The Fourth Edition carries a 1986 copyright). To test verbal reasoning, the patient is asked to listen to a statement and then tell the examiner what is "foolish" about the statement. Some examples of test statements are:

1. A man had flu twice. The first time it killed him, but the second time he got well quickly.
2. In the year 1980, many more women than men got married in the United States.
3. A man wished to dig a hole in which to bury some rubbish, but could not decide what to do with the dirt from the hole. A friend suggested that he dig the hole large enough to hold the dirt, too.
4. They began the meeting late, but they set the hands of the clock back so that the meeting might surely close before sunset.
5. When there is a collision, the last car of the train is usually damaged most. So they decided that it will be best if the last car is always taken off before the train starts.

Visual reasoning is tested in a similar way, by showing the patient several pictures. After examining each picture, he must tell the examiner what is "foolish" about it. Verbal and visual reasoning can be scored similarly, with 0–poor, 1–fair, and 2–good response. In a five item reasoning test, a score of less than five suggests significant impairment.

Other tests of frontal lobe function include orientation to time, place and person (Luria, 1973; Golden, 1978); assessing the patient's ability to recognize the right side of space or the right side of his body (Damasio et al, 1980); and testing for active perception (Luria, 1973; Ratcliff, 1979). Orientation is tested in the manner familiar to those experienced in the mental status examination. If the patient reads only the left side of printed material (for example, if he reads "MGW" as "MG"), if he doesn't shave the right side of his face, or if he bumps only into objects to his right (Damasio et al 1980), he does not recognize the right side of space. Active perception—that is, the ability to "mentally" rotate an item in one's visual field—is a nondominant hemisphere function and is tested by asking the patient to identify a picture of an object (such as a baby or a hat) presented in a sideways or upside-down position. The patient should be able to identify the rotated object without tilting his head.

Frontal lobe dysfunction can also be expressed in behavioral change. Two major frontal lobe syndromes have been described: the convexity syndrome and the medial-orbital syndrome (Luria, 1969, 1973, Hecaen and Albert, 1975; Heilman and Valenstein, 1979). The convexity syndrome, related to lesions within or near the lateral surface of the frontal lobes, is characterized by "negative symptoms." Patients with convexity syndrome are apathetic, indifferent to their surroundings and emotionally unresponsive. They appear to have lost all drive and ambition. Loss of social graces is common and they frequently appear disheveled and dirty. Their movements are slow and reduced in frequency (motor inertia). Occasionally, they may remain in positions for prolonged periods (catalepsy) and may posture. A slight flexion at the waist, knees and elbows is a typical body position of these patients. They occasionally move with a floppy shuffling gait, progressively picking up steam, only to gradually slow down to a stop (glissando/deglissando gait). Unlike patients with Parkinson's disease, muscle tone is decreased and "pill rolling" is not present. These patients have difficulty attending to tasks but do respond to irrelevant, particularly intense stimuli. They tend to walk next to walls (just touching them) rather than walk in the middle of the hallway; they may even follow architectural contours rather than take a direct route across open space.

If the convexity syndrome is due to dominant hemisphere pathology, it is also associated with a deficit in language and verbal thinking. Impoverished thinking (vague and without detail) is almost always present; verbal fluency is significantly impaired; speech is often stereotyped with perseverative and verbigerated utterances; Broca's or transcortical aphasia may be present. Most frontal lobe cognitive and soft neurologic signs can be observed in these patients, who may also be dyspraxic (gait, bucco–linguo–facial, or ideomotor dyspraxias) and incontinent of urine.

A second frontal lobe syndrome is associated with dysfunction in the medial-orbital areas of the frontal lobes and is termed orbitomedial syndrome. Some patients may be asthenic and easily fatigued, bland, akinetic, aphonic, withdrawn and fearful. They may have diminished wakefulness, or may be in an oneiroid (dream-like, clouded) or even stuporous state. Other patients may have an intense affect, expressing euphoria, irritability or extreme lability of affect, with rapid mood shifts and mixed and cycling mood states. *Witzelsucht* is common. These affectively intense patients are hyperactive and overresponsive to stimuli. They rapidly terminate one incomplete goal-directed behavior only to start another, and may appear frenetic as they run from one activity to another, never completing a task. These patients lose their inhibitions and become reckless. They are impulsive and may engage in buying sprees or other high risk behaviors. They lack foresight, cannot make decisions, are unable to persevere and have uncontrollable associations. They are strongly stimulus bound, distractable, intrusive and importunate. They will interrupt conversations and will mimic the examiner's movements and comments. These are the patients who, despite repeated injunctions, will continually enter a room in which a group of people are in conference; or will pull fire alarms; or will change channels continually on television sets, simply because they see the dial. These patients may have uncontrollable, often fantastic confabulations, and when prevented from doing as they please, may have violent outbursts.

The obvious similarity in behaviors between patients with orbitomedial syndrome and patients with bipolar affective disorder requires particularly careful diagnostic evaluation. Neurologic (particularly soft) signs, shallowness of affect, a prolonged and insidious onset, a chronic nonepisodic course, a negative family history for affective disorder, and localized CAT scan and EEG abnormalities would suggest coarse brain disease.

The Parietal Lobes

Touch, pain and temperature senses are represented in the primary cortex in the posterior central gyrus, located in the anterior portion of the parietal lobe opposite (contralateral) to the side of the body where the sensation is being tested. Proprioception, stereognosis and graphesthesis are functions represented in the secondary cortex in the contralateral parietal lobe, just caudal to the posterior central gyrus (Critchley, 1953; Luria, 1973).

The largest part of each parietal lobe is tertiary cortex. The nondominant parietal lobe coordinates motor, sensory and spatial perception. Its functions include: the awareness of one's body in space; the recognition of faces; and the ability to copy the outline of simple objects (Critchley, 1953; Luria, 1973; Golden, 1978; Heilman and Valenstein, 1979).

The dominant parietal lobe coordinates visual and language functions, which include reading (lexic function), writing (graphic function) and parietal lobe language functions. Two other parietal lobe functions, kinesthetic praxis and ideokinetic (ideomotor) praxis, have also been discussed (Critchley, 1953; Luria, 1973; Golden, 1978; Heilman and Valenstein, 1979). Others include finger gnosis, calculation, right-left orientation, symbolic categorization, graphesthesis, and stereoagnosis.

The examiner tests finger gnosis (Neilsen, 1938; Critchley, 1953) by pointing to each of the patient's fingers without touching them, and asking the patient to name them. Inability to do this suggests finger agnosia or dysnomia. The examiner may then assign a number to all ten fingers. When the patient has learned the numbering system, he should be instructed to interlock his fingers (as if in prayer) and to rotate his wrists so that the interlocking fingers face the patient. If the patient is then able to identify his fingers by number, finger gnosis is intact.

The patient's ability to compute simple mathematical problems is assessed by asking him to perform, on paper, several calculations in which he is asked to "carry" one or two digits (Critchley, 1953; Luria, 1973; Golden, 1978; Pincus and Tucker, 1978; Heilman and Valenstein, 1979). The way the patient writes the problem on paper may reveal dysfunctions other than dominant parietal dysfunction. For example, if the patient miscalculates and also transcribes the numbers in a rotated alignment, he is making an error of visual-motor coordination revealing parietal dysfunction. If, however, he perseverates numbers rather than miscalculating, his dysfunction is likely to be frontal. Single digit computations (such as $4+4$, 5×3) should not be used, because they may have become overlearned, rote responses.

Right-left orientation (Neilsen, 1938; Critchley, 1953; Luria, 1973) is tested by asking the patient to perform several tasks, each of which requires that he distinguish between left and right while crossing his body midline. For example, he is told, "Touch your left hand to your right ear"; "Touch your right hand to your left elbow"; "Touch your right hand to your right knee."

Another dominant parietal lobe function is symbolic categorization (Critchley, 1953; Luria, 1973), which can be tested by asking the patient to identify relationships between members of a family. For example, the patient can be asked: "What would be the relationship to you of your brother's father?" (or father's brother, or son's daughter). Symbolic categorization requires that the patient make a "mental diagram" in order to answer the question correctly.

As in the assessment of kinesthetic praxis, the evaluation of graphesthesia and stereognosis tests the parietal lobe contralateral to the hand being tested, and the connections between the two hemispheres (Critchley, 1953; Luria, 1973; Golden, 1978; Pincus and Tucker, 1978; Heilman and Valenstein, 1979). The examiner tests graphesthesia by tracing letters, one at a time, on the palms of the patient's hands while the patient's eyes are closed. After each letter, the examiner asks the patient to name it. If the patient experiences difficulty, the examiner should test for letter gnosis as previously mentioned. If letter gnosis is intact, the error is called graphanesthesia: It could be due either to dysfunction of the contralateral parietal lobe, or to dysfunction of the interhemispheric connections such as the corpus callosum. Figure 1 illustrates the reason for this. Following the test for graphesthesia on the hand ipsilateral to the patient's dominant hemisphere, graphesthesia should be tested for on the other hand. If the patient manifests graphanesthesia on that hand, the abnormality is probably in the contralateral parietal lobe.

The examiner tests stereognosis by placing several objects (such as a key, several coins of different sizes, a button, a paper clip—all items that don't make noise when palpated), one at a time, in the palms of the patient's hand while the patient's eyes are closed. After each placement, the patient is asked to "feel it with your fingers and then name it." If the patient experiences difficulty, and if his naming ability as previously tested was intact, the patient is manifesting astereognosis. It could be due to dysfunction of the contralateral parietal lobe, or to dysfunction of the interhemispheric connections such as the corpus callosum, if errors are primarily lateralized to the nonpreferred hand.

We have discussed functions of the nondominant parietal lobe, including constructional praxis, dressing praxis, kinesthetic praxis (of the contralateral hand), graphesthesia (of the contralateral hand) and stereognosis (of the contralateral hand) (Critchley, 1953; Luria, 1973; Golden, 1978; Pincus and Tucker, 1978; Heilman and Valenstein, 1979). Additional functions can be characterized as the abilities "to recognize," "to be familiar with," or "to be aware of" people and things. Abnormalities include nonrecognition of: serious medical disability (anosognosia); the left side of one's body or of objects in the left visual field (left spatial nonrecognition); and familiar people and faces (prosopagnosia). These abnormalities, when present, are often so obvious that the examiner's questions are usually required only to reaffirm and elaborate upon his impression of the existence of such a disability.

Anosognosia (Critchley, 1953; Weinstein and Kahn, 1955; Luria, 1973; Golden, 1978; Pincus and Tucker, 1978; Heilman and Valenstein, 1979) is nonrecognition of a serious medical disability. For example, in Babinski's agnosia, a patient with hemiparalysis will attempt to get out of bed and walk, despite evidence of paralysis from repeated failures to walk, and despite instructions from staff and visitors not to walk. It is possible that other phenomena routinely described as "denial" are actually the product of posterior nondominant hemisphere dysfunction.

Some patients with intact left-right orientation pay no attention to the left side of their body or to objects in their left visual field. This left spatial nonrecognition (a product of nondominant parietal lobe dysfunction (Critchley, 1953; Weinstein and Kahn, 1955; Luria, 1973; Golden, 1978; Pincus and Tucker, 1978; Heilman and Valenstein, 1979) may reveal itself in a number of ways, including not shaving the left side of the face, bumping into objects on the left, or reading only the right side of printed materials. East-west orientation (Critchley, 1953; Luria, 1973) is also a "spatial" orientation function of the nondominant parietal lobe. The examiner assesses this function by drawing two crossed arrows to represent the directions on an imaginary map, then asking the patient to identify which portions of the map would be north, south, east and west.

Occasionally, a patient with normal global orientation (who will select the correct answer when given a series of choices about his location) is unable to spontaneously state where he is. When asked to do so, he will make a series of wild guesses. For example, a patient on a psychiatric ward is unable to correctly answer the question, "Where are we now?" Instead, he answers in rapid succession, "At the McDonald's"; "At the railway station"; "In a highrise building." This wild guessing is called paragnosia, and is often associated with lesions in the nondominant parietal lobe (Critchley, 1953; Luria, 1973).

Prosopagnosia (Critchley, 1953; Luria, 1973; Meadows, 1974) is nonrecognition of faces that should be familiar. It is sometimes diagnosed when the patient accuses one or more familiar persons, usually a family member, of being an impostor (that is, Capgras' syndrome) (Hayman and Abrams, 1977; Alexander et al, 1979). Some recent evidence suggests that prosopagnosia extends to the nonrecognition of other nonfacial visual phenomena and that lesions are often bilateral.

A related phenomenon is called the Fregoli syndrome (Christodoulou, 1976). In this syndrome, the patient mistakenly thinks other persons not well known to him are very familiar (for example, he thinks the other person is a friend, relative or famous person), despite the fact that there is no resemblance. For example, a patient in a psychiatric ward was convinced that Charlton Heston and Marilyn Monroe had been admitted to his ward.

Another, related phenomenon is reduplicative paramnesia (doppelganger phenomenon) (Critchley, 1953; Weinstein and Kahn, 1955; Luria, 1973), in which a patient with nondominant parietal dysfunction manifests a delusion that a duplicate of a person or place exists elsewhere. For example, a white woman on a psychiatric service had the delusion that she had a twin sister, and that this twin sister was a black woman. This patient also manifested Capgras' syndrome, thinking that her husband was an impostor sent to spy on her.

Parietal lobe dysfunction can be associated with significant psychopathology (such as delusional ideas, experiences of alienation), which can lead to misdiagnoses and inappropriate treatment for "functional" disorders (Critchley, 1953;

Luria, 1973; Heilman and Valenstein, 1979). Two general patterns of symptoms have been observed. Lesions of the dominant parietal lobe are usually associated with: disorders of language (dyslexia, word finding problems, conduction aphasia); problems of calculation; dyspraxias (ideomotor, kinesthetic); difficulties in spatially related abstraction; and contralateral sensory (graphanasthesia, astereognosis) and motor (hypotonia, posturing, paucity of movement) deficits. The best known dominant parietal syndrome is the controversial Gerstmann's syndrome (dysgraphia, dyscalculia, right-left disorientation, finger agnosia) (Neilsen, 1938), putatively involving a lesion in the posterior-inferior aspect (angular gyrus) of the dominant parietal lobe. Although the validity of the syndrome has been questioned by some authors, it has been reported in over 20 percent of chronic psychiatric patients (Birkett, 1967).

Lesions of the nondominant parietal lobe are associated with profound (occasionally delusional) denial of illness (anosognosia), left sided spatial neglect, constructional difficulties, dressing dyspraxia, and contralateral sensory and motor deficits. Capgras' syndrome (delusional ideas that close friends or relatives are impostors) and the first-rank symptom of experience of alienation (body parts or thoughts not belonging to one) have been described in patients with nondominant parietal lesions. One patient, observing his own left arm, thought there was another person in bed with him. He complained to his relatives about this, who in turn complained to the chief of the department of neurology, that "overcrowding at this hospital has gone too far." These patients may also have difficulty orienting themselves to their environment. They complain that "things look confused" or "jumbled." They say they cannot find their way along previously familiar routes and that they can no longer drive a car because they lose track of the other vehicles around them. They may complain that their body is somehow different; that an arm or leg feels heavy, bigger than usual; or that they are not always sure of the location of an arm or leg.

The Occipital Lobe

We can test primary occipital cortical functions, such as visual fields or color vision; otherwise, it is difficult to test separately for right and left hemispheric occipital lobe functioning. Thus, errors on tests for associational occipital cortical functioning cannot readily be lateralized (Pincus and Tucker, 1978; Golden, 1978; Heilman and Valenstein, 1979). A gross test of occipital lobe associational cortex functioning requires the patient to identify a visual pattern in the presence of a distracting background (Luria, 1973). The patient is shown a drawing and asked to name it. If he cannot do so, and his capacity to name objects is intact, he may have occipital lobe dysfunction.

"Soft" Neurological Signs

These are clinical features that indicate brain dysfunction but which cannot routinely be localized within the brain, despite their association by some neurologists with frontal lobe dysfunction. When present, these signs are well correlated with psychiatric illnesses and other behavior disorders (Ben-Yishay et al, 1968; Pincus and Tucker, 1978; Cox and Ludwig, 1979; Taylor, 1981; Nasrallah et al, 1983).

The examiner tests the palmar-mental reflex by repeatedly scratching the base of the patient's thumb. If the lower lip and jaw move slightly downward, and if this response does not extinguish, the patient has manifested a palmar-mental reflex (50 percent of the population exhibits this feature, but it will quickly extinguish with repeated stimulation). The examiner tests the grasp reflex by pressing his fingers into the palm of one or both of the patient's hands. If the patient's hand grasps the examiner's fingers, the examination has revealed a grasp reflex. The snout (rooting) reflex is tested when the examiner strokes the corner of the subject's mouth. If the patient's lips purse and the lips or head move towards the stroking, the patient has a snout reflex. Adventitious motor overflow is tested by asking the patient to tap rapidly and repetitively with one hand on his knee or on a table. If he also begins to tap or move the other hand, he has shown adventitious motor overflow. Each hand should be tested separately.

Double simultaneous discrimination is tested with the patient's eyes closed. The examiner simultaneously brushes one of his fingers against one of the patient's cheeks and another finger against one of the patients hands. He asks the patient where he feels the touch. When a patient has impaired double simultaneous discrimination, the touch on the hands is usually not perceived. Occasionally, only stimuli on one side of the body are extinguished, which suggests contralateral dysfunction. Some patients with large parietal lobe lesions (usually the right) locate the stimuli outside their body parts. The phenomena of motor impersistence and *gegenhalten* are also thought by some to be soft neurologic signs.

THE NEUROLOGIC HISTORY

The neurologic history and examination (of the spinal cord, peripheral nerves and primary cortex) is part of a complete neuropsychiatric evaluation. In practice, it usually precedes the cognitive and behavioral examinations. A careful review of systems, of the patient's nutritional status, exposure to toxins and substances of abuse, history of surgical procedures, trauma, hospitalizations, seizures, antenatal and perinatal difficulties, may each provide the necessary clue to the etiology of the patient's present symptoms.

Some common symptoms of nervous system dysfunction include: headache; spinal pain; pain in the extremities; disorders of memory and thinking; loss of interest, drive and energy; clumsiness or weakness of the extremities; tremors and involuntary movements; change in speech and difficulty in swallowing; loss of balance and vertigo; loss of hearing and tinnitus; blurring or dimness of vision; diplopia; sensory distortions (paresthesias); sensory loss; difficulty urinating; and signs and symptoms of convulsive disorder. Despite the association of the above symptoms with neurologic disease, a large body of data has accumulated in the past two decades that makes discrimination of "neurologic" from "psychiatric" disorder difficult, if the traditional neurologic vs. nonneurologic variables are used without qualification.

Important Historical Antecedents of
Coarse Brain (Neurologic) Disease

Although virtually any neurologic disease that affects brain functioning can lead to behavioral changes, head trauma is the most common historical antecedent of brain syndromes. To be of sufficient magnitude to result in subsequent behavioral changes, a closed head injury will likely be associated with a skull fracture, unconsciousness of 30 minutes or longer, anterograde amnesia of several hours or longer, focal neurologic signs (even if transient) or blood in the spinal fluid. "Bumps on the head," even when suturing is required, do not correlate highly with most brain syndromes (Luria, 1969; Sisler, 1978). Mild to moderate trauma is, however, a typical antecedent of the postconcussion syndrome (Rowe and Carlson, 1980). A documented history of epilepsy is also commonly associated with behavioral syndromes (Davidson and Bagley, 1969; Benson and Blumer, 1982; Koella and Trimble, 1982), as is a history of major systemic disease (Hall, 1980).

Physical Signs of Coarse Brain Disease

Physical examination findings consistent with coarse neurologic disease include focal neurologic features (such as abnormal cranial nerve signs, pathological reflexes, paralysis) and sufficient signs of a systemic illness known to produce behavioral change (Peterson, 1978; Hall, 1980). Soft neurologic signs have been reported in 40 to 70 percent of "functional" psychotics and are not useful in discriminating neurologic from psychiatric conditions (Quitkin et al, 1976; Cox and Ludwig, 1979; Nasrallah et al, 1983).

LABORATORY STUDIES

The use of laboratory studies to distinguish neurologic from psychiatric disorders has been complicated by recent work, which demonstrates that schizophrenics and patients with affective disorder have abnormalities on a variety of laboratory measures. Nevertheless, there are specific differences in the laboratory findings of psychiatric patients and patients with coarse brain disease, which can be diagnostically useful.

Many computer enhanced tomographic studies (Weinberger et al, 1982) have found that, compared to normal controls, schizophrenics have enlarged lateral ventricles, reduced cortical thickness, decreased gray matter density, greater or reversed cerebral asymmetry and reduced cerebellar mass. Several investigators have reported similar findings in patients with affective disorder (Nasrallah et al, 1982) and psychiatrically ill children (Reiss et al, 1983), while others have failed to confirm differences between patients and controls (Benes et al, 1982). Although theoretically interesting, these findings are primarily based on group mean comparisons, and few individual subjects have CAT scan images that would be clinically reported as abnormal. An individual scan characterized as clinically abnormal (for example, circumscribed lesion, significant cortical atrophy) is consistent with the diagnosis of neurologic coarse brain disease (Peterson, 1978; Cummings, 1982).

Similarly, many studies have reported that from 40 to 50 percent of schizophrenics have clinically abnormal resting EEG findings, usually nonspecific slowing (Abrams and Taylor, 1979). None of these studies, however, has been able to demonstrate a characteristic schizophrenic EEG pattern. Although less numerous, EEG studies in affective disorder (Abrams and Taylor, 1979) and other psychiatric conditions (Kiloh et al, 1974) have also failed to identify specific abnormalities. A resting EEG with a specific clinical abnormality (for example, spike and low wave complexes, paroxysmal bursts of slow waves, circumscribed abnormalities) is inconsistent with a "functional" psychiatric diagnosis, and indicates the patient may have coarse brain disease. Power/spectral studies (Flor-Henry, 1976) and evoked response studies (Rockstroh et al, 1982), each suggesting differences between psychotic patients and normal controls, have not yet proven diagnostically useful. Evoked response studies, however, can be helpful in determining the presence of demyelinating disease (Green and Walcoff, 1982).

Neuropsychological testing of affective disorder patients and schizophrenics has captured the imagination of many investigators. Despite a common notion that schizophrenics exhibit dominant hemisphere dysfunction, while those patients with affective disorder exhibit nondominant hemisphere dysfunction, the data overwhelmingly demonstrate that most schizophrenics have bilateral and diffuse cognitive impairment (perhaps more profound in the anterior dominant regions); and a smaller proportion of patients with affective disorder show evidence of bilateral anterior impairment and general nondominant hemisphere dysfunction (Silverstein, 1983; Taylor and Abrams, 1984). A circumscribed neuropsychological deficit is inconsistent with the major functional psychoses and suggests the patient has coarse brain disease (Golden, 1978; Fitzhugh-Bell, 1978; Heilman and Valenstein, 1979). There are only a few neuropsychological studies of other functional disorders (such as Briquet's syndrome, psychopathy, obsessive-compulsive disorder), and clear-cut patterns of dysfunction have not been reported. None of these disorders, however, appears to be associated with severe or focal cognitive impairment (Marin and Tucker, 1981).

Any cerebrospinal fluid (CSF) abnormality, any abnormal blood finding associated with causes of dementia (for example, low serum B12, low serum T3) or other laboratory findings consistent with a systemic illness known to produce behavioral change (such as X–ray evidence of pneumonia, EKG evidence of a recent myocardial infarct) should strongly influence the clinician toward a diagnosis of coarse brain disease, as these abnormalities are rarely reported in the primary functional states (Peterson, 1978). In some samples of psychotic patients (Hall, 1980) nearly 40 percent had systemic illness that appeared to be the most likely cause of the behavioral syndrome. Investigative techniques, such as brain electrical area mapping (BEAM) (Morihisa et al, 1983) and cerebral blood flow studies (Mathew et al, 1982; Uytdenhoef et al, 1983), show promise as discriminating measures of various behavioral syndromes. Many more patients, however, will have to be studied by these techniques before consistent and clear-cut differences emerge.

ANCILLARY CLINICAL TESTS

Neuropsychological tests used primarily for identification and localization of coarse brain disease, and the assessment of cognitive dysfunction, include two screening tests and two test batteries. The screening tests are the Reitan-Indiana Aphasia Screening Test (Wheeler and Reitan, 1962) and the Minimental State Examination of Folstein, Folstein and McHugh (Folstein et al, 1975; Tsai and Tsuang, 1979); the test batteries are the Luria-Nebraska Battery (Golden, 1978) and the Halstead-Reitan Battery (Klove, 1974; Matarazzo et al, 1976). Other ancillary clinical tests have been discussed above.

The Reitan-Indiana Aphasia Screening Test and the Minimental State Examination are easily administered, brief (five to 20 minutes), noninvasive tests designed to identify, localize, and lateralize brain dysfunction. Comparing the results of Aphasia Screening Tests with the results of neurosurgical procedures performed on the tested patients, Wheeler and Reitan (1962) demonstrated the concurrent validity of the Aphasia Screening Test in terms of its capacity to lateralize lesions.

Comparing the results of Minimental State Examinations with clinical diagnoses and WAIS results on the same patients, Folstein, Folstein and McHugh (1975) demonstrated the concurrent validity of the Minimental State Examination in terms of its capacity to distinguish diffuse cortical dysfunction from normal cortical function or from focal cortical dysfunction. Tsai and Tsuang (1979) demonstrated concurrent validity of this test by comparing its results to computerized tomographic scan results. Folstein, Folstein and McHugh have also demonstrated the high reliability of the Minimental State Examination. The maximum score on the Minimental State is 30. The range of scores for normals is 26–30. A score of 23 or less suggests diffuse cognitive impairment consistent with a diagnosis of dementia or delirium. Elderly patients with endogenous depression and associated cognitive impairment (sometimes called pseudodementia) score in the range of 13–27. Patients with psychiatric syndromes other than dementia, delirium or pseudodementia usually perform in the 26–30 range. Table 3 shows the Minimental State Examination.

The Luria Battery

This battery was developed by Alexander Luria (1973) and a formal scoring system was developed by Golden and associates (Golden, 1978; Golden et al 1978). The battery consists of tests of a wide variety of cognitive functions. The concurrent validity of the Luria battery is good. Golden and co-workers (1978) compared 50 hospitalized control patients with 50 matched neurological patients having a clinical diagnosis of coarse brain disease, and were able to separate the groups with 100 percent accuracy.

The Halstead-Reitan Battery

This battery is a modification, by Reitan, of an examination developed by Halstead for the investigation of behavior in brain-damaged and normal persons. It takes longer to administer than does the Luria battery (six to eight hours), but more psychologists are currently able to administer this battery. It contains ten subtests, including the MMPI (a self report personality inventory), the WAIS, and the Reitan-Indiana Aphasia Screening Test. In addition to identifying and localizing brain dysfunction, it is useful in providing feedback for vocational rehabilitation and other rehabilitation programs (Wheeler and Reitan, 1962; Matarazzo, 1972; Klove, 1974; Matarazzo et al, 1976). Matarazzo et al (1976) demonstrated high test-retest reliability for this battery; the validity of the Halstead-Reitan battery is also high.

Table 3. The Minimental State Examination of Folstein, Folstein and McHugh

Specific Test	Function Tested	Points Score
1. What is the year/season/day/date/month?	Orientation	5
2. What is the state/county/town/hospital/floor?	Orientation	5
3. Repeat three items.	Registration	3
4. Serial subtraction of sevens or spell "world" backwards.	Concentration	5
5. Name wristwatch and pen.	Naming	2
6. Say "No ifs, ands, or buts."	Expressive speech	1
7. Take this paper in your right hand, fold it in half, and put it on the table.	Three-stage command	3
8. Read "close your eyes" and do it.	Reading	1
9. Remember the three items from part three.	Short-term memory	3
10. Write a sentence.	Writing	1
11. Copy intersecting pentagons.	"Construction"	1

Reprinted with permission from the *Journal of Psychiatric Research*, Vol. 12, Folstein, Folstein and McHugh, "Minimental State: A Practical Method for Grading the Cognitive State of Patients for the Clinician." Copyright © 1975, Pergamon Press, Ltd.

SUMMARY

In our presentation of the neuropsychiatric evaluation, we have described an approach to behavioral assessment that emphasizes the increasing value and relevance of the interface between neurology and psychiatry. In this interface, specific behaviors and mental events—both functional and dysfunctional—are linked to specific structural systems in the brain. It is our belief that technological advances in the neurosciences and neuropsychological assessment will generate a wealth of new data that will enhance our present understanding of the relationships between regional brain dysfunction and emotional and behavioral abnormalities. The neuropsychiatric evaluation also provides a useful structure for eliciting, assessing and organizing clinical data encompassing psychopathology, neurological and cognitive deficits, and brain function and structure. It is hoped that the mastery of this evaluation by clinicians will translate into more comprehensive assessment and specificity of treatment of patients who suffer from psychiatric disorders.

REFERENCES

Abrams R, Taylor MA: A rating scale for emotional blunting. Am J Psychiatry 135:225-229, 1978

Abrams R, Taylor MA: Differential EEG patterns in affective disorder and schizophrenia. Arch Gen Psychiatry 36:1355-1358, 1979

Abrams R, Taylor MA: The importance of schizophrenic symptoms in the diagnosis of mania. Am J Psychiatry 138:658-661, 1983

Abrams R, Taylor MA, Stolrow KAC: Catatonia and mania: patterns of cerebral dysfunction. Biol Psychiatry 14:111-117, 1979

Alexander MP, Struss DT, Benson DF: Capgras' syndrome: a reduplicative phenomena. Neurology 29:334-339, 1979

Andreasen NC: Reliability and validity of proverb interpretation to assess mental status. Compr Psychiatry 18:465-472, 1977

Andreasen N: Affective flattening and the criteria for schizophrenia. Am J Psychiatry 136:944-947, 1979

Barbizet J: Human Memory and its Pathology. Translated by Jardine DK. San Francisco, W.H. Freeman and Co., 1970

Beaumont JG: Handedness and Hemisphere Function, in Hemisphere Function in the Human Brain. Edited by Dimond SJ, Beaumont JG. New York, Halstead Press, 1974

Benes F, Sunderland P, Jones BD, et al: Normal ventricles in young schizophrenics. Br J Psychiatry 141:90-93, 1982

Benson DF: Aphasia, Alexia and Agraphia: Clinical Neurology and Neurosurgery Monographs. Edinburgh, Churchill Livingstone, 1979

Benson DF, Blumer D: Psychiatric Manifestations of Epilepsy, in Psychiatric Aspects of Neurologic Disease, vol. II. Edited by Benson DF, Blumer D. New York, Grune and Stratton, 1982

Benson F, Geschwind N: Cerebral dominance and its disturbances. Pediatr Clin North Am 15:759-769, 1968

Benton AL, Hamsher K des, Varney NR, et al: Contributions to Neuropsychological Assessment: A Clinical Manual. New York, Oxford University Press, 1983

Ben-Yishay Y, Diller L, Gerstman L, et al: The relationship between impersistence, intellectual function and outcome of rehabilitation in patients with left hemiplegia. Neurology 18:852-861, 1968

Birkett DP: Gerstmann's syndrome. Br J Psychiatry 113:801, 1967

Christodoulou GN: Delusional hyper-identifications of the Fregoli type: organic pathogenetic contributors. Acta Psychiatr Scand. 54:305-314, 1976

Cox SM, Ludwig AM: Neurological soft signs and psychopathology; I: findings in schizophrenia. J Nerv Ment Dis 167:161-165, 1979

Critchley M: The Parietal Lobes. New York, Hafner Press, 1953

Cummings JL: Cortical Dementias, in Psychiatric Aspects of Neurologic Disease, vol. 2. Edited by Benson DF, Blumer D. New York, Grune and Stratton, 1982

Damasio AR, Damasio H, Chui HC: Neglect following damage to frontal lobe or basal ganglia. Neuropsychologia 18:123-132, 1980

Davidson K, Bagley CR: Schizophrenia-like psychoses associated with organic disorders of the central nervous system: a review of the literature, in Current Problems in Neuropsychiatry. Br J Psychiatry Special Publication 4:113-184, 1969

Faber R, Abrams R, Taylor MA, et al: Formal thought disorder and aphasia: comparison of schizophrenic patients with formal thought disorder, and neurologically impaired patients with aphasia. Am J Psychiatry 140:1348-1351, 1983

Fitzhugh-Bell KB: Neuropsychological evaluation in the management of brain disorders, in Brain Disorders: Clinical Diagnosis and Management. The Psychiatric Clinics of North America, vol. 1. Edited by Hendric HC. Philadelphia, W.B. Saunders, 1978

Flor-Henry P: Lateralized temporal-limbic dysfunction and pathology. Ann NY Acad Sci 280:777-797, 1976

Folstein MF, Folstein SW, McHugh PR: "Mini-Mental State": a practical method of grading the cognitive state of patients for the clinician. J Psychiatr Res 12:189-198, 1975

Gainotti G, Miceli G, Caltagirone C: Constructional apraxia in left brain-damaged patients: a planning disorder? Cortex 13:109-118, 1977

Geschwind N: Disconnection syndromes in animals and man. Part I: Brain 88:237-294, 1965; Part II: Brain 88:585-644, 1965

Geschwind N: The anatomical basis of hemisphere differentiation, in Hemisphere Function in the Human Brain. Edited by Dimond SJ, Beaumont JG. New York, Halstead Press, 1974a

Geschwind N: Selected Papers on Language and the Brain. Boston, Reidel, 1974b

Golden CJ: Diagnosis and Rehabilitation in Clinical Neuropsychology. Springfield, Illinois, Charles C Thomas, 1978.

Golden C, Hammeke T, Purisch A: Diagnostic validity of a standardized neuropsychological battery from Luria's neuropsychological tests. J Consult Clin Psychol 48:1258-1265, 1978

Green JB, Walcoff MR: Evoked potentials in multiple sclerosis. Arch Neurol 39:696-697, 1982

Hall RCW: Psychiatric Presentations of Medical Illness: Somatopsychic Disorders. New York, SP Medical and Scientific Books, 1980

Hayman M, Abrams R: Capgras' syndrome and cerebral dysfunction. Br J Psychiatry 130:68-71, 1977

Hecaen H, Albert ML: Disorders of mental functioning related to frontal lobe pathology, in Psychiatric Aspects of Neurologic Disease, vol 1. Edited by Benson DF, Blumer D. New York, Grune and Stratton, 1975

Heilman KM, Valenstein E: Clinical Neuropsychology. New York, Oxford University Press, 1979

Kiloh LG, McComas AJ, Osselton JW: Clinical Electroencephalography, 2nd edition. London, Butterworths, 1974

Klove H: Validation studies in adult neuropsychology, in Clinical Neuropsychology: Current Status and Applications. Edited by Reitan R, Davidson L. Washington, DC, V.H. Winston, 1974

Koella WP, Trimble MR: Temporal Lobe Epilepsy, Mania and Schizophrenia and the Limbic System: Advances in Biological Psychiatry, vol 8. Basel, S. Kruger, 1982

LeDoux JE, Wilson DH, Gazzaniga MS: Block design performance following callosal sectioning: observations on functional recovery. Arch Neurol 35:506-508, 1978

Lezak MD: Neuropsychological Assessment, 3rd edition. New York, Oxford University Press, 1983

Luria AR: Frontal lobe syndromes, in Handbook of Clinical Neurology, vol. II: Localization in Clinical Neurology. Edited by Vinken PJ, Bruyn GW. New York, Elsevier-North Holland, 1969

Luria AR: The Working Brain: An Introduction to Neuropsychology. Translated by Hough B. New York, Basic Books, 1973

Marin RS, Tucker GJ: Psychopathology and hemispheric dysfunction: a review. J Nerv Ment Dis 169:546-557, 1981

Matarazzo J: Wechsler's Measurement and Appraisal of Adult Intelligence. New York, Oxford University Press, 1972

Matarazzo JD, Matarazzo RG, Wiens AM, et al: Retest reliability of the Halstead Impairment Index in normals, schizophrenics and two samples of organic patients. J Clin Psychol 32:338-354, 1976

Mathew RJ, Duncan GC, Weinman ML, et al: Regional cerebral blood flow in schizophrenia. Arch Gen Psychiatry 39:1121-1124, 1982

Meadows J: The anatomical basis of prosopagnosia. J Neurol Neurosurg Psychiatry 37:489-501, 1974

Morihisa JM, Duffy FH, Wyatt RJ: Brain electrical activity mapping (BEAM) in schizophrenic patients. Arch Gen Psychiatry 40:719-728, 1983

Nasrallah HA, McCalley-Whitters M, Jacoby CG: Cerebral ventricular enlargement in young manic males: a controlled CT study. J Affective Disord 4:15-19, 1982

Nasrallah HA, Tippin J, McCalley-Whitters M: Neuropsychological soft signs in manic patients, a comparison with schizophrenics and control groups. J Affective Disord 5:45-50, 1983

Neilsen J: Gerstmann's syndrome: finger agnosia, agraphia, comparison of right and left and acalculia. Archives of Neurology and Psychopathology 39:536-560, 1983

Paulson G, Gottlieb G: Development reflexes: the reappearance of foetal and neonatal reflexes in aged patients. Brain 91:37-52, 1968

Peterson GC: Organic brain syndrome, differential diagnosis and investigative procedures in adults, in Brain Disorders: Clinical Diagnosis and Management. The Psychiatric Clinics of North America, vol. 1. Edited by Hendrie HC. Philadelphia, W.B. Saunders, 1978

Pincus JH, Tucker GJ: Behavioral Neurology, 2nd edition. Oxford University Press, New York, 1978

Quitkin F, Rifkin A, Klein DF: Neurologic soft signs in schizophrenia and character disorders, organicity in schizophrenia with premorbid associality and emotionally unstable character disorders. Arch Gen Psychiatry 33:845-853, 1976

Ratcliff G: Spatial thought, mental rotation and the right cerebral hemisphere. Neuropsychologia 17:49-54, 1979

Reiss D, Feinstein C, Weinberger DR, et al: Ventricular enlargement in child psychiatric patients: a controlled study with planimetric measurements. Am J Psychiatry 140:453-456, 1983

Rockstroh B, Elbert T, Berbaumer N, et al: Slow Brain Potentials and Behavior. Baltimore, 1982

Ross ED: The aprosodias: functional anatomic organization of the affective components of language in the right hemisphere. Arch Neurol 38:561-569, 1981

Rowe MJ, Carlson C: Brain stem auditory evoked potentials in post-concussional dizziness. Arch Neurol 37:679-683, 1980

Scheinberg P: Modern Practical Neurology: An Introduction to Diagnosis and Management of Common Neurologic Disorders. 2nd edition. New York, Raven Press, 1981

Schneider K: Clinical Psychopathology. Translated by Hamilton MW. New York, Grune and Stratton, 1959

Seamon JG: Coding and Retrieval Processes and the Hemispheres of the Brain, in Hemisphere Function in the Human Brain. Edited by Dimond SJ, Beaumont JG. New York, Halstead Press, 1974

Sierles F: Behavioral medicine, in Clinical Behavioral Science. Edited by Sierles F. New York, SP Medical and Scientific Books, 1982

Silverstein M: Neuropsychological dysfunction in the major psychoses, in Laterality and Psychopathology. Edited by Flor-Henry F, Gruzelier J. Amsterdam, Elsevier-North Holland, 1983

Sisler GC: Psychiatric Disorder Associated with Head Injury, in The Psychiatric Clinics of North America: Brain Disorders, Clinical Diagnosis and Management, vol. I. Edited by Hendrie HC. Philadelphia, W.B. Saunders, 1978

Spear FG, Green R: Inability to concentrate. Br J Psychiatry 112:913-915, 1966

Strub RL, Black, FW: Organic Brain Syndromes: An Introduction to Neurobehavioral Disorders. Philadelphia, F.A. Davis Co., 1981

Taylor MA: The Neuropsychiatric Mental Status Examination. New York, SP Medical and Scientific Books, 1981

Taylor MA, Abrams R: The prevalence of schizophrenia: A reassessment using modern diagnostic criteria. Am J Psychiatry 135:945-948, 1978

Taylor MA, Abrams R: Cognitive impairment in schizophrenia. Am J Psychiatry 141:196-201, 1984

Tsai L, Tsuang MT: The "Mini-Mental State" and computerized tomography. Am J Psychiatry 136:436-439, 1979

Uytdenhoef P, Portelange P, Jacquy J, et al: Regional cerebral blood flow and lateralized hemispheric dysfunction in depression. Br J Psychiatry 143:128-132, 1983

Weinberger DR, DeLisi LE, Perman GP, et al: Computed tomography in schizophreniform disorder and other acute psychiatric disorders. Arch Gen Psychiatry 39:778-783, 1982

Weinstein EA, Kahn RL: Denial of Illness: Symbolic and Physiological Aspects. Springfield, Illinois, Charles C Thomas, 1955

Wells CE, Duncan GW: Neurology for Psychiatrists. Philadelphia, F.A. Davis Co., 1980

Wheeler L, Reitan RM: Presence and laterality of brain damage predicted from responses to a short aphasia screening test. Perceptual Motor Skills 15:783-799, 1962

Chapter 8

Psychiatric Aspects of Brain Injury: Trauma, Stroke and Tumor

by Stuart C. Yudofsky, M.D. and Jonathan M. Silver, M.D.

Each year in the United States over one million people suffer severe brain injury. A far larger number are afflicted with chronic sequelae of such injuries. This chapter will focus upon the three most common sources of brain injury: trauma, stroke and tumor. The role of the psychiatrist in the prevention, diagnosis and treatment of the cognitive, behavioral and emotional aspects of brain injury will be reviewed.

TRAUMATIC BRAIN INJURY

It is commonly taught to medical students in introductory psychiatric courses that suicide is the second most common cause of death in persons under 35 years of age. What is less emphasized is that the number one cause of death in this population is automobile accidents. In the United States in 1982 there were 46,000 automobile-related deaths (National Safety Council, 1983). Approximately 70 percent of automobile-related deaths result from head trauma (Poleck, 1967). An even higher number of persons sustain nonfatal, but disabling head trauma secondary to traffic accidents. From an epidemiologic survey conducted in San Diego County in which the incidence, causes, and destructiveness of brain damage were studied, it was calculated that there are 410,000 brain injuries that occur each year in the United States, and 180,000 of these injuries are secondary to motor vehicle accidents. In addition, it was found that 21 percent of brain injuries occur from falls, 12 percent of brain injuries result from assaults, ten percent from sports, and six percent from firearms. Five to 10 percent of these cases have residual neurological damage (Kraus et al, 1984). The incidence of brain injuries in the United States of 180 per 100,000 population is approximately one-half the incidence of schizophrenia. Hartunian and associates (1980) compared the economic costs of various illnesses and found that the total economic cost per year for cancer is 23.1 billion dollars; for motor vehicle injuries 14.4 billion dollars; for heart disease 13.7 billion dollars; and for stroke 6.5 billion dollars. Children are highly vulnerable in accidents as passengers and as pedestrians, to falls, to impacts from moving objects such as rocks or baseballs and to sports injuries (Hendrick et al, 1965). The authors belabor these statistics for two purposes: first, to sensitize the clinician to the common occurrence of disabling head injuries; and, second, to propose that all practitioners in their roles as advisors and authority figures encourage preventative measures. As will later be delineated, brain injuries are potentially preventable, as opposed to many other common neurologic and psychiatric disorders. To focus solely upon the accurate diagnosis and state of the art treatment of head injury is short sighted and incomplete.

Emotional and Cognitive Changes Associated With Brain Injury

Although brain injury subsequent to serious automobile, occupational, or sports accidents may not result in diagnostic enigmas for the psychiatrist, less severe trauma may first present as relatively subtle behavioral or affective change. Prototypic examples of brain damage in which the patient, while providing a history, may fail to associate with the traumatic event include: the alcoholic who is amnestic for a fall which occurred while inebriated; the ten-year-old whose head was hit while falling from his bicycle, but who fails to so inform his parents; or the housewife who was beaten by her husband, but who is either fearful or ashamed to report her injury to her family physician. Such trauma may be associated with confusion, intellectual changes, affective lability, and/or psychosis; and the patient may first present to the psychiatrist for evaluation and treatment. The following changes secondary to brain injury are among the most frequently seen by psychiatrists:

EXACERBATION OF PREEXISTING CHARACTER OR PERSONALITY DISORDERS. Prominent behavioral traits such as disorderliness, suspiciousness, argumentativeness, isolativeness, disruptiveness, anxiousness, and so forth, become more pronounced with brain injury (Fordyce et al, 1983; Weddell et al, 1980; Thomsen, 1984). Also, symptomatologies associated with personality disorders or major psychiatric illness occur after brain injury. For example, the affective lability of the borderline patient may intensify to the point that previous feelings of sadness and depression become life-threatening suicidal or self-mutilative behaviors. Nonpsychiatric physicians may dismiss these behaviors as "crazy and intolerable"; however, the alert psychiatrist will detect from a careful history and mental status examination that an exacerbation of preexisting psychopathology has occurred that is not fully explained by social or psychological events. As always, when discrete mental changes cannot be traced to specific stressors, an organic etiology must be suspected and explored.

PERSONALITY CHANGES. Because of the vulnerability of the prefrontal and frontal regions of the cortex to injury, specific changes in personality known as frontal lobe syndrome are not uncommon. In the prototypic patient with frontal lobe syndrome, the cognitive functions of the patient are preserved while personality changes abound. These changes include decreased motivation, impaired social judgment and labile affect. A patient may display uncharacteristic lewdness, inability to appreciate the effects of his/her behavior or remarks on others, a loss of social graces (such as eating manners), a lack of attention to personal appearance and hygiene, and boisterousness. In addition, impaired judgment may also be prominent and take the form of diminished concern for the future, an increase in risk taking, unrestrained drinking of alcoholic beverages, and indiscriminate selection of food. The patient may appear shallow, indifferent or apathetic, with a global lack of concern for the consequences of his or her behavior.

INTELLECTUAL CHANGES. Problems with intellectual functioning may be among the most subtle manifestations of brain injury. Changes may occur in the capacity to concentrate, to use language, to abstract, to calculate, to reason, to remember and to process information (Rimel et al, 1981, Brooks and Aughton, 1979). An example of a change in intellectual functioning as the first symptom of brain injury is that of the 36-year-old corporate attorney who was self referred to a psychiatrist. The attorney sought help for what he felt were motivational problems related to his job. Specifically, he complained of being unable to concentrate upon or to synthesize data related to the complex contracts and negotiations of his profession. A friend advised him that his decreased capacities to concentrate and to work were likely symptoms of depression, a premise for which he sought treatment from a psychiatrist. The careful history secured by the psychiatrist revealed that the patient had been suffering from recurrent nausea and from headaches that were ameliorated by aspirin. Upon a careful neurologic workup, a left parietal-temporal subdural hematoma was discovered from a computerized axial tomography (CAT) scan. At that point, the patient recalled having been struck on the head by a friend's elbow during a basketball game. When discrete changes in intellectual functioning antedate affective change, the clinician should suspect an organic etiology.

AFFECTIVE CHANGES. Preexisting affective illness is aggravated by brain injury. Head trauma, like other stresses, is well known to precipitate manic or depressive states in patients with bipolar illness. Others may develop major depressive episodes *de novo* subsequent to the brain damage. (Robinson and Szetela, 1981). A condition known as episodic dyscontrol or intermittent explosive disorder commonly follows brain trauma, and is associated with pronounced rage and other affective changes. Episodic dyscontrol will be considered in a separate section within this chapter, because it is common and involves behavioral as well as affective changes. Patients whose affective illness fails to respond to aggressive psychiatric treatment, and patients who exhibit side effects at relatively low doses of psychotropic medications or other drugs that affect the brain, may have central nervous system (CNS) lesions.

PSYCHOTIC CHANGES. Posttraumatic psychoses can occur either immediately following brain injury, or after a latency of many months of normal functioning. The psychiatrist is often consulted as the brain injured patient is emerging from coma. At that time, the patient may be restless, agitated, confused, disoriented, delusional and/or hallucinatory. Although the psychiatrist is usually summoned to manage the behavior of the patient, he or she should be aware that the patient's agitation and psychosis may be secondary to etiologies other than the trauma that initiated the coma. Included among the etiologies of psychoses in patients emerging from coma are: fluid and electrolyte imbalance; side effects of medications; environmental factors, such as sensory monotony or decreased oxygen levels; infections; disorders of blood, blood volume or blood viscosity; and withdrawal from drugs that were being administered prior to the traumatic event. Psychosis that occurs after a span of time subsequent to trauma may be more difficult to diagnose and to treat. Such psychosis may be associated with posttraumatic seizures that develop in five percent of closed head injuries, and in approximately 50 percent of injuries in which the dura mater has been penetrated (Adams and Victor, 1981). It must be noted that depressed skull fractures and intracranial hematomas are associated with a high incidence of late onset seizures. Psychosis and other psychological changes related to seizure disorders are covered more fully in Chapter Ten of this volume, by Dr. David Bear and colleagues. Hillbom (1960) surveyed a large number of patients whose head injuries occurred during war. He found that left-sided injuries were more often associated with psychiatric illness in general and with psychosis in particular. Lishman (1978) reported that patients with schizophrenic-like symptoms subsequent to brain injury may be "indistinguishable" from symptoms of the "naturally occurring" disorder. Reviews of the literature reveal one to 15 percent of schizophrenic inpatients have histories of head injury (Davison and Bagley, 1969). It must be recalled that *DSM-III* criteria for schizophrenia exclude those cases for which there is a known traumatic etiology. The correct *DSM-III* diagnosis in such cases would be organic delusional syndrome or organic hallucinosis.

CEREBROVASCULAR DISEASE

As a result of significant physical, emotional, social, and occupational disruptions, victims of stroke and their families frequently seek assistance from psychiatry. Over 500,000 people in the United States are "new" stroke victims each year (Wolf et al, 1977). Stroke ranks third as the highest overall cause of death after cardiac disease and cancer; cerebrovascular accidents account for 200,000 deaths per year (Wolf et al, 1977). Brain damage and disability are significant among those who do not die from their strokes. In the Framingham study that examined the status of long-term survivors of strokes over a seven-year period, investigators found that 15 percent required institutionalization; 63 percent exhibited decreased vocational functioning; 59 percent demonstrated decreased social functioning outside of the home; and 47 percent showed decreased avocational interest in hobbies and reading. In this study, the most frequent disability that resulted from stroke was psychosocial rather than physical (Greshman et al, 1979). In another study of psychosocial disability in long-term stroke survivors with restored physical deficits, Labi, Phillips and Greshman (1980) found that a significant proportion of survivors manifested psychological and social disability despite complete physical restoration. In a three-year follow-up study of the quality of life after stroke, Lawrence and Christi (1979) found that "it was evident that stroke had devastated many people's lives; they ceased to work prematurely, their interpersonal relations had deteriorated, and over 70 percent viewed their future with uncertainty and gloom. Physical disability in itself was less important than the people's response to their disability. . . . " It must be noted that the risk of incurring a stroke by age 70 is 5 percent, and that 20 percent of strokes occur in people under 65 years of age (Wolf et al, 1977). From these data we learn that, as with brain injury, cerebrovascular accidents are common and result in significant psychosocial disability.

Emotional and Cognitive Changes Associated With Cerebrovascular Disease

AFFECTIVE CHANGES. Many studies document the high incidence of major affective change following stroke. Robinson and Price (1982) followed 103 patients attending a stroke clinic to assess poststroke depressive disorders over a 12-month period. They found almost one-third of the patients were depressed at the time of the initial assessment, and two-thirds of these remained depressed when reevaluated after seven to eight months. In 91 stroke patients, Feibel and Springer (1982) found a 26 percent incidence of depression six months following the stroke. Depression correlated significantly with failure to resume social activities; depressed patients lost a mean of 67 percent of previous activities while nondepressed patients lost a mean of 43 percent of such activities. Mania secondary to stroke has also been reported with lesions in either the dominant or nondominant hemisphere (Jampala and Abrams, 1983). This condition, however, as judged from the paucity of published case reports in the scientific literature, is extremely rare. As with brain trauma, the question is raised as to whether the depression subsequent to stroke is related to the significant disability engendered by stroke, whether it is related to organic changes secondary to brain damage, or whether it is related to a combination of both. Folstein and co-workers (1977) compared mood disorder in patients following strokes with mood disorder in patients with significant orthopedic injury. They found that 45 percent of stroke patients were depressed, as opposed to ten percent of patients with orthopedic injuries. They concluded that the mood disorder was a specific complication of brain damage related to stroke, rather than a reaction to physical disability. When Robinson and co-workers (1983) measured the incidence of affective change subsequent to right vs left cerebral hemispheric lesions, depression with vegetative symptomatologies was significantly higher in patients with left hemispheric cerebrovascular accidents. They also found that 60 percent of those patients with left anterior strokes met criteria for major depressive disorder, while only 12 percent with left posterior lesions did. One interesting finding was that five out of six patients in Robinson's study with right anterior (frontoparietal) lesions subsequent to stroke showed undue cheerfulness. Finally, dexamethasone suppression testing of patients subsequent to stroke showed an abnormal dexamethasone suppression test (failed to suppress) in 52 percent of patients (Finkelstein et al, 1982).

INTELLECTUAL AND PERCEPTUAL CHANGES. The nature and extent of intellectual changes following stroke are directly related to the location of the lesion. Multiple infarct dementia has recently received considerable attention. The signs and symptoms of this disorder will be discussed in greater detail in Chapter 11 of this volume. Strokes in and around Broca's area are particularly disabling and frustrating, because comprehension is preserved while expression and communication are impaired. Investigators find that impairments of expression and communication are far more disabling from social and vocational standpoints than are the concomitant physical disabilities. All too often, rehabilitative efforts are placed upon motoric aspects of a person's recovery from stroke rather than on the cognitive, volitional and communicative problems resulting from the lesion. Brain damage related to strokes in temporal regions of the brain can give rise to hallucinatory phenomena (auditory, visual, olfactory), as well as to dissociative disorders; and, in rare cases, strokes in occipital regions may lead to visual hallucinatory experiences. Such conditions do not often create diagnostic difficulties for the clinician; however, management of mood disorders and life adjustment related to the poststroke disabilities are common and important challenges for the psychiatrist. Irritability, which is found in approximately 70 percent of patients with right hemispheric lesions (Folstein et al, 1977), and dyscontrol of rage and violent behavior secondary to strokes in various regions of the brain, will be considered in the next section.

ORGANIC AGGRESSIVE SYNDROME (INTERMITTENT EXPLOSIVE DISORDER)

Pathology and Definition

Explosive rage and violent behavior have long been associated with focal lesions as well as with diffuse damage to the CNS. Various investigators and nosological systems have labeled and described this condition in different ways. *DSM-III* calls the condition Intermittent Explosive Disorder, and places the category under "disorders of impulse control not elsewhere classified" (American Psychiatric Association, 1980). *DSM-III* diagnostic criteria for intermittent explosive disorder are as follows:

a). Several discrete episodes of loss of control of aggressive impulses resulting in serious assault or destruction of property.
b). Behavior that is grossly out of proportion to any precipitating psychosocial stressor.
c). Absence of signs from generalized impulsivity or aggressiveness between episodes.
d). Not due to schizophrenia, antisocial personality disorder or to conduct disorder.

Other names for the syndrome include episodic dyscontrol syndrome, disinhibition syndrome, and explosive personality disorder. It is our feeling that the existing diagnostic labels, including that found in *DSM-III*, can be confusing. Since organic etiologies for the condition are, in our experience, quite common, we do not agree with the statement under "differential diagnosis" in *DSM-III* that purports "an underlying physical disorder, such as brain tumor or epilepsy, may in rare cases cause this syndrome" (American Psychiatric Association, 1980). Elliott (1982) studied 286 patients with recurrent attacks of intermittent rage, and found 94 percent of this population had evidence of either developmental or acquired brain deficit. He further points out that 30 percent of the population have complex partial seizures. We agree with *DSM-III* that "any toxic agents such as alcohol, that may lower the threshold for violent outbursts, and conditions conducive to brain dysfunction such as perinatal trauma, infantile seizures, head trauma, and encephalitis may predispose to this disorder." We therefore submit that the condition should be reclassified as an organic mental disorder and be called organic aggressive syndrome with the following criteria:

a). Persistent or recurrent aggressive outbursts, either of a verbal or a physical nature.
b). The outbursts are out of proportion to the precipitating stress or provocation.
c). Evidence from the history, physical examination, or laboratory tests of a specific organic factor that is judged to be etiologically related to the disturbance.

d). The outbursts are *not* primarily related to personality features or disorders such as paranoia, manic disorder, antisocial or narcissistic personality disorder, borderline disorder, or conduct disorder.

Note that the *DSM-III* designation, "organic affective syndrome" is primarily a disturbance in mood "resembling either a manic episode or a major depressive episode," which is due to a specific organic factor. Clearly, the rage and violent outbursts associated with brain lesions are highly distinct from disturbances of mood, and distinct even from those depressions or manias related to organic illness of the CNS.

BRAIN TUMORS

Primary brain tumors constitute nearly ten percent of nontraumatic neurological disease, and metastatic cerebral neoplasms far outnumber primary tumors. Metastatic tumors arise most commonly from the lung, breast, stomach, thyroid or kidney. Secondary cerebral tumors often invade multiple areas of the brain and are characterized by rapid growth. Among the primary tumors, gliomas are the most common form of intracranial neoplasm. These tumors derive from cells that form the glia, or the supporting tissue of the nervous system. Among the gliomas are: astrocytomas, which can occur at any age in both cerebral and cerebellar regions, and which may be relatively benign; the glioblastoma multiforme, which is highly malignant, occurs in middle age, and is almost exclusive to the cerebral hemispheres; and the medulloblastoma, which is frequently found in children, often located in the cerebellum, and which grows rapidly. Oligodendrogliomas and ependymomas are rare, slowly growing tumors. The meningiomas are extracerebral tumors that arise from arachnoid cells, and tend to invade the overlying bone of the skull with characteristic hyperostotic changes visible on X–ray. These cells can be found along intracranial venous sinuses, particularly the superior sagittal sinus. They therefore remain clinically silent until they become large. Tumors may arise from cerebral blood vessels (angioblastomas and angiomas); from the pituitary (chromophobe adenoma, chromophil adenoma, and craniopharyngioma); from the pineal gland, and from the choroid plexus of the third ventricle (colloid cysts); and from cranial nerves (acoustic neuromas). Such tumors tend to be more benign, and their destructiveness is related to their location and size. Seizures are the most common presenting sign of brain tumor. Focal neurologic deficits (such as visual field cuts and sensory and motor changes), as well as symptoms related to raised intracranial pressure (such as headaches or blurred vision) are also common presentations. When mental disturbance is the most prominent feature of brain tumor, the patient may first seek the help of a psychiatrist and run the risk of a delayed or even totally missed diagnosis. Lishman (1978) reviewed the problem of misdiagnosing tumors as a primary psychiatric illness. He found that although the incidence of brain tumor among psychiatric patients may be relatively low (less than five percent on autopsy), a significant percentage of these would have been treatable with early diagnosis.

Emotional and Cognitive Changes Associated With Tumors

Impaired level of consciousness is the most common psychiatric change associated with brain tumor. This disability may take the form of diminished ability to focus and to concentrate, loss of energy, impaired memory and, later, drowsiness and stupor. Intellectual changes also commonly occur with tumor, and may at first be subtle alterations in the capacity to abstract or to perform highly technical tasks related to employment. As with other lesions of the CNS, depression and irritability are among the early manifestations of brain tumors. As the tumor becomes larger, the previously mentioned symptomatologies become more pronounced, with increased confusion, apathy, seizures, and even coma. As has been stated previously, perceptual changes in patients with tumors depend largely upon the location of the lesion. Temporal lobe tumors can be associated with complex visual, auditory, olfactory and/or gustatory hallucinations, while occipital tumors may give rise to less complex visual hallucinations such as a geometric figure. Tactile and kinesthetic hallucinations may be secondary to parietal lobe tumors. Finally, it is important to note that frontal lobe tumors may give rise to significant differential diagnostic problems: apathy, intellectual changes and impaired judgment may occur without the presence of obvious neurologic signs.

Psychiatric management of patients in whom brain tumors are diagnosed is important and complex. First, the psychological impact on a person who is told that either he, she, or a member of his or her immediate family has a brain tumor, cannot be underestimated. Even if a patient who is diagnosed to have a brain tumor is "fortunate" enough to have a benign tumor and "fortunate" enough to not have neurological sequelae from consequent brain surgery, the psychological significance of the entire episode is far-reaching. It is common for a patient who survives a neurosurgical procedure with a positive prognosis to be expected by his surgeons and his family to feel overjoyed and grateful at the propitious outcome. He is told, "Be thankful that the tumor was detected so soon, before it could cause much damage." We, as psychiatrists, should be aware that the psychological damage to the patient begins with the diagnosis or, upon occasion, with the misdiagnosis of a brain tumor.

It is crucial for the psychiatrist to be involved from the earliest phases of medical treatment once a brain tumor has been detected. The psychiatrist can assess the patient's ability to withstand the idea of having a tumor within the brain, the patient's capacity to undergo potentially frightening diagnostic procedures, and the patient's capacity to deal with the disfigurements and physical, cognitive and sensory disabilities that so commonly are associated with this illness. It must be remembered that disabilities may be more severe after the surgery than they were at the time of presentation. The psychiatrist must assess the extent to which a patient's family or support group can care for the patient's physical and psychological needs during convalescence. As with trauma and stroke, the incidence of affective illness in patients with brain tumors is high. A major clinical consideration involves the use of electroconvulsive therapy (ECT) in the presence of brain tumor. One study has reviewed the clinical basis for the long established contraindication of ECT in the presence of brain tumor (Maltbie et al, 1980). Based on clinical data from 35 cases, there was a 74 percent overall morbidity and 28 percent one month mortality rate for patients with brain tumors who received ECT.

PREVENTION OF BRAIN INJURY

Brain Trauma

MOTOR VEHICLE ACCIDENTS. According to all responsible sources, the proper use of seat belts with upper torso restraints is a highly effective but little used (less than ten percent) measure for the prevention of head injury (Haddon and Baker, 1981). The proper use of safety belts is 50 to 65 percent effective in the prevention of fatalities and injuries, and this would translate to 12,000 to 16,000 lives saved per year (National Safety Council, 1983). It is also calculated that the installation of "air bag" safety devices in automobiles would save from 6,000 to 9,000 lives per year (National Safety Council, 1983).

Psychiatrists recognize that alcoholism per se is a highly prevalent and destructive illness. In addition, alcohol abuse is a common concomitant of affective and characterologic disorders. In the United States, it is estimated by the National Safety Council that alcohol ingestion is implicated in over 50 percent of all automobile related fatalities (Haddon and Baker, 1981). Therefore, in all psychiatric and other medical histories, a detailed inquiry about alcohol use, driving patterns (accident records, violations, driving while intoxicated, speeding patterns, car maintenance, presence of distractions such as children and animals, hazardous driving conditions, and so forth), as well as seat belt use, is essential. Clearly, the use of motorcycles—with or without helmets—and bicycles for commuting purposes are strongly associated with head injury, even when safety precautions are taken and driving regulations are observed.

Once the practitioner identifies the patient to be at high risk for head trauma, preventive measures must be undertaken. Among such interventions are the proper use of psychotropic medications, of psychological interventions, of family and peer support, and of specialized treatment groups such as Alcoholics Anonymous. In addition, the psychiatrist must counsel patients to use seat belts, not to drive after drinking, and to drive safely in a safe automobile.

BRAIN INJURY IN CHILDREN. Beyond nurturance, children rely on their parents or guardians for guidance and protection. Each year in the United States over 1,400 children under 13 years of age die as motor vehicle passengers, and over 90 percent of these were not using car seat restraints (Insurance Institute for Highway Safety, 1983). Child seats have been found to be 80 to 90 percent effective in the prevention of deaths and severe injuries to children (National Safety Council, 1983). Unfortunately, it is not uncommon for head trauma to result from more overt child abuse on the part of parents, other adults and peers. The clinician must always be alert to the possibility that his patients may be neglectful, may utilize poor judgment, and may even be directly violent in their treatment of children. Often, psychiatrists feel it is a violation of their patient's trust and confidentiality to intervene directly in cases of child abuse. Not only is such intervention ethically appropriate but, in most states, it is mandated by law. We encourage directive counselling of patients who do not consistently use infant and child car seats for their children.

RISK TAKING. Psychiatric patients with affective illness, with problems of substance abuse, with impulse disorders, and with characterologic disorders (such as antisocial, borderline and narcissistic personality disorders) are prone to the taking of risks. Representative examples include: the suicidally depressed patient who drives at high speeds under the influence of alcohol; the irritable manic patient who provokes a fight in a bar; and the construction worker with narcissistic personality disorder who takes unnecessary risks and refuses to wear protective gear in order to capture the attention and admiration of his co-workers. Sports such as boxing, football, rugby, ice hockey, sky diving, mountain climbing, hang gliding, and professions such as the military, law enforcement, fire fighting and above ground construction, not only attract risk takers but also result in a disproportionately high incidence of head trauma. The psychiatrist should be aware that self-destructive behavior may be camouflaged by the violence, contact and other dangers inherent in such activities.

Guns and war give rise to a significant amount of serious head trauma. Fifty percent of reported suicides in males and 25 percent of reported suicides in females in the United States are from gunshot wounds. Homicides and assaults in the United States involve guns in an exponentially higher number of cases than in countries where handguns are strictly prohibited. The psychiatrist is often reluctant to inquire about the ownership of or access to weapons—especially by the violent, paranoid, or impulsive patient. These patients, as well as others with diagnoses of affective illness, substance abuse disorders or antisocial personalities, should be encouraged by the psychiatrist to dispose of their weapons prior to a crisis. This may prove to be a life-saving intervention.

Stroke

As with brain damage secondary to trauma, the preventive measures for cerebrovascular disease should not be ignored by the psychiatrist. Among the treatable risk factors for stroke are: hypertension, heart disease, diabetes, elevated blood lipid levels, cigarette smoking, alcoholism and obesity. Among this group, hypertension is the most significant potentially reversible risk factor. Stroke incidence increases sixfold in patients with hypertension; and 50 percent of the cerebrovascular accidents occur in the 20 percent of adults who have hypertension (Wolf and Kannel, 1982). In a large, five-year cooperative study of the effects of hypertension detection and treatment, it was found that the death rate from cerebrovascular disease decreased in the treated hypertensive population to a level approaching that of the general U.S. population (Hypertension Detection and Follow-up Program Cooperative Group, 1982). Finnish investigators have reported that even occasional ethanol intoxication increases the risk of ischemic brain infarction and subarachnoid hemmorhage in both adolescents and adults. They reported that ethanol intoxication preceding strokes was over three times as common as ethanol intoxication in the general Finnish population of the same age and sex (Hillbom and Kaste, 1981a and 1981b).

Investigators have related recent stressful life events as well as "type A" personality factors to the severity of disability following cerebrovascular accidents (Carasso et al, 1981). A psychiatrist may aid in the prevention of strokes by encouraging all adult patients to have regular physical examinations, by carefully monitoring the blood pressure of his or her patients at highest risk, by treating alcoholism and cigarette smoking, and by helping a patient with his or her reduction of life stress. Special attention must be paid by the psychiatrist to those psychiatric medications and treatments that effect blood pressure. Monoamine oxidase inhibitors, in combination with food substances containing tyramine, can result in dramatic and life-threatening increases in blood pressure. The psychiatrist should also be aware that psychotropic medications that lower blood pressure—such as antidepressants and antipsychotic agents—may adversely affect cerebral vascular perfusion, particularly in elderly patients with histories of high systolic or diastolic blood pressures. Even with excellent anesthetic modification of motoric activity, blood pressure increases during ECT. These increases are aggravated by the presence of medications such as steriods, mono-amine oxidase inhibiting agents and beta blocking agents. The psychiatrist must pay special attention to the preECT blood pressures in these patients, as well as employ continuous intratreatment monitoring.

TREATMENT

The safe use of automobiles and automobile safety devices, judgment in the use of alcohol, reduction of violence and the availability of hand guns, appropriate prescription of medications and the treatment of hypertension are effective measures for the prevention of most brain injuries. For the large number of people who are brain injured, there are many useful therapeutic approaches available.

Psychopharmacologic Treatment of Brain Injury

Psychopharmacologic treatments of brain injury are directed toward associated symptomatologies. An important general principle is that patients with brain injury of any type are far more likely to be sensitive to the effects and side effects of medication than the nonbrain-injured population. For example, dis-abling sedative and anticholinergic side effects from thioridazine (Mellaril), when used to treat psychosis in a poststroke patient, may occur at doses lower than 50 mg per day; side effects of such severity are rarely encountered in the nonbrain-injured patient at doses lower than 500 mg per day.

AFFECTIVE ILLNESS. Affective disorder related to brain damage is, as we have pointed out, common, and is destructive to a patient's rehabilitation and socialization. The published literature is sparse regarding the effects of antide-pressant agents in the treatment of patients with brain damage. However, one study, a hospital treatment survey of depression after stroke, suggested that antidepressant medications are underutilized in this population (Lim and Ebra-him, 1983). As a rule, it is best to use antidepressants with the fewest sedative, hypotensive and anticholinergic side effects. In a double blind study, Lipsey and associates (1984) examined the efficacy of nortriptyline in poststroke depres-sions. They found that patients on nortriptyline had a significantly greater response than placebo-treated controls. An important finding was that therapeutic blood levels of drug were achieved in oral doses from 50 to 100 mgs. We prefer desipramine, (10 mg three times a day) and nortriptyline, with initial doses of 10 mg per day and the careful monitoring of plasma levels of the parent compound and its metabolites. Should the patient become sedated, confused, or severly hypotensive, the dosage of these drugs may be reduced to as low as 5 mg twice a day, with the possibility of antidepressant efficacy. Depending upon the sever-ity and nature of the brain injury, approximately 33 percent to 50 percent of the standard treatment dose is adequate in most cases for an antidepressant benefit.

Blood levels of nortriptyline are also important because of the therapeutic window in which plasma levels above 150 nanograms per milliliter can reverse the therapeutic benefit. Except for those patients with increased intracranial pressure and brain tumors, ECT remains a highly effective and underutilized modality for the treatment of patients with both depression and brain damage. In our experience, nondominant unilateral ECT, using pulsatile currents, increased spacing of treatments (2 to 3 days between each treatment), and fewer treatments in an entire course (4 to 6), results in amelioration of depressive symptomatology without major memory deficits as side effects. Lithium has been reported to aggravate confusion in patients with brain damage (Schiff et al, 1982), as well as to induce nausea, manual tremor, ataxia, and lethargy. We limit the use of lithium to those patients with mania, and to patients with recurrent depressive illness that preceded brain damage. Carbamazepine (Tegretol) is effective in the treatment of patients with bipolar illness; however, the use of this medication to treat mania in patients with brain damage has yet to be examined.

PSYCHOSIS. In treating patients with psychosis resulting from brain injury, principles similar to those detailed for antidepressants should be followed. In addition to problems of hypotension, sedation and confusion, psychotic patients with brain injury are also subject to severe dystonias, akathisias, and Parkinsonian side effects when even relatively low doses of antipsychotic medications are used. If patients show agitation with psychosis, aliphatic phenothiazines such as chlorpromazine, in doses beginning at 5 mg three times a day, might be attempted. In this instance, therapeutic use is made of the sedative side effect of chlorpromazine in order to treat the agitation. In less agitated patients, piperazine phenothiazines such as fluphenazine (Prolixin) (0.5mg twice a day) or butyrophenones, haloperidol (Haldol) (beginning at 0.5 mg orally twice a day) may be tried. We have had difficulty maintaining brain damaged patients on haloperidol in doses above 5 mg orally per day because of akathesias and dystonias. Such motoric side effects often require two to three months to resolve following the discontinuation of haloperidol. A general principle to remember in treating brain injured patients with psychotropics is that all medications must be raised and lowered in very small increments over protracted periods of time to avoid seizures.

ANXIETY. Panic and anxiety are common symptoms in patients with brain injury. Nonpsychiatric clinicians tend to overutilize minor tranquilizers, sedatives and hypnotics. We prefer to treat the anxiety of brain injured patients with supportive psychotherapy and social interventions. When the symptoms are so severe that they require pharmacologic intervention, we prefer such short-acting benzodiazepines as oxazepam and lorazepam, so that sedative and confusional side effects are less likely to occur. Sleep patterns of patients with brain damage are often impaired; therefore, barbiturates, alcohol and long-acting minor tranquilizers such as flurazepam (Dalmane) must be avoided because of their interference with REM and stage 4 sleep patterns. The clinician should advise brain injured patients against using over the counter preparations for sleep and colds because of the prominent anticholinergic side effects of these remedies.

ORGANIC AGGRESSIVE SYNDROME. Patients with organic dyscontrol of rage and violent behavior are most often treated with major tranquilizers. In essence, clinicians make use of the sedative side effects of antipsychotics in order to control agitation and aggression. This clinical approach is often unsuccessful because of side effects (akathisias, dyskinesias, dystonias, and lethargy). With the lowering of seizure threshold inherent in most antipsychotic agents, organic dyscontrol may intensify. Recently, investigators have reported that propranolol is specifically effective in treating the rage and violent behavior of patients with brain damage. This approach has been reported to be effective in patients with brain trauma, seizure disorders, Alzheimer's Disease, Korsakoff's Syndrome, mental retardation, and other brain disorders in both adults and children (Yudofsky et al, 1981, 1984; Williams et al, 1982; Ratey et al, 1983; Mansheim, 1981; Petrie and Ban, 1981; Schreier, 1979; Elliot, 1977). Neither cardiovascular side effects such as hypotension and bradycardia, nor psychological side effects such as emotional blunting, depression, or confusion, preclude safe treatment of this population. In the adult patient, we initiate propranolol at an oral dose of 10 mg three times a day, and monitor the patient's pulse rate and blood pressure. After several days of stable vital signs, we increase the dose by 20 mg per day, every other day, until either disabling side effects (blood pressure, heart rate, ataxia), or therapeutic effects, emerge. In our experience, in the prototypic male receiving 70 kg, cardiovascular side effects such as hypotension and bradycardia stabilize at doses below 400 mg per day. Occasionally, patients must be raised to doses over 1 gram per day. A latency period of six to eight weeks after the patient has achieved a high dose of propranolol may be required before results are achieved. Many so-called "treatment failures" occur because subtherapeutic doses have been utilized over too brief a time period. Those patients who have chronic obstructive pulmonary disease, asthma, brittle diabetes, congestive heart failure, or recent myocardial infarctions may not be treated in this fashion. Anticonvulsants such as carbamazepine have also been suggested for the treatment of organic aggressive syndrome (Luchins, 1983; Neppe, 1982; Folks et al, 1982; Hakoloa and Laulumaa, 1982; Tunks and Demer, 1977).

Psychological Interventions

In the broadest terms, psychological issues involving patients who incur brain injury revolve around four major themes: psychopathology that preceded the injury; psychological response to the traumatic event; psychological reactions to deficits of brain injury; and psychological issues related to potential recurrence of brain injury. In our experience, preexisting psychiatric illness is intensified by brain injury. Therefore, for example, the paranoid patient often becomes more suspicious and guarded after stroke, and the patient suffering from depression often shows more prominent affective symptomatology with brain trauma. Because attention, concentration, and intellectual functions are often diminished with brain injury, the usefulness of psychological and psychotherapeutic approaches is also diminished. It is true that certain patients who had perviously shown improvement with interpretive psychodynamic treatment may be unable to respond to this approach. Nevertheless, clinicians frequently underestimate the capacities of the brain injured patient to respond to traditional psychological interventions. For every patient suffering from brain injury, we recommend an assessment of the capacity to benefit from psychologic treatments.

The events surrounding brain injury often have far-reaching experiential and symbolic significance for the patient. Such issues as guilt, punishment, magical wishes and fears crystallize about the nidus of the brain injury. For example, a patient with oedipal conflicts revolving around a seductive mother and an exploitive and aggressive father may view the diagnosis of brain tumor as "the deserved punishment." In such a case, mere reassurance and homilies about his lack of responsibility for his illness will be less productive than psychological exploration. After successful medical intervention, a patient may retain complex psychological responses to his brain injury. Unless the psychological issues are addressed, such symptoms as anxiety, insomnia, affective changes, and poor interpersonal relations may emerge. The psychiatrist should not neglect the psychological responses of the patient's family, who also experience the shock of and adjustment to the brain injury of a loved one. Oddy and co-workers (1978) evaluated 54 relatives of patients with brain injury within one, six and 12 months of the traumatic event. Their study revealed that approximately 40 percent of the relatives showed depressive symptomatologies within one month of the event, and 25 percent of the relatives showed significant physical or psychological illness within six and 12 months of the brain damage. By treating the psychological responses of relatives of a patient with brain injury, the clinician can foster a supportive and therapeutic atmosphere for his patient. A patient's reactions to being disabled secondary to brain damage also have concrete as well as symbolic significance. When intense effort is required for a patient to form a word or to move a limb, frustration may be expressed as anger, depression, anxiety or fear. Particularly in cases in which brain injury results in permanent impairment, a psychiatrist may experience countertransferential discomfort resulting in failure to directly discuss the patient's disabilities and limitations. Gratuitous optimism, collaboration with denial of the patient, and facile solutions to complex problems are rarely effective and can erode ongoing treatment. By gently and persistently directing the patient's attention to the reality of his disabilities, the psychiatrist may help the patient to begin the process of acceptance and adjustment to his impairment. Clinical judgment should guide the psychiatrist in deciding whether explorations of the symbolic significance of the patient's brain injury should be pursued. The persistence of anxiety, guilt and fear beyond normative stages of adjustment and rehabilitation may indicate that psychodynamic approaches are required.

It is a distressing fact that many of the most severe types of brain injury recur. Strokes, brain tumors and even trauma from accidents occur more commonly in patients who have already suffered from such events than in those who have not. Therefore, patients' fears and anxieties about recurrence of brain injury are more than just efforts at magical control over terrifying situations. Therapeutic emphasis should be placed upon those actions and activities that will aid in preventing recurrence. A patient will feel less impotent and passive when working toward reducing blood pressure, diminishing life stress, and correcting deleterious habits that may have led to the initial event.

Invariably, brain injury leads to emotional damage in the patient and his family. In this chapter, we have reviewed the most frequently occurring types of brain injury and the resulting psychiatric symptomatologies. We have emphasized how the informed psychiatrist is not only effective but also essential in the prevention of brain injury and in the treatment of its sequelae.

REFERENCES

Adams RD, Victor M: Principles of Neurology. New York, McGraw-Hill Company, 1981

American Psychiatric Association, Diagonostic and Statistical Manual of Mental Disorders, 3rd edition. Washington, DC, American Psychiatric Association, 1980

Brooks DN, Aughton ME: Psychological consequences of blunt head injury. Int Rehabil Med 1:160-165, 1979

Carasso R, Yehuda S, Ben-Uriah Y: Personality type, life events and sudden cerebrovascular attack. Int J Neurosci 14:223-225, 1981

Cooper PR: Head Injury. Baltimore, Williams and Wilkins, 1982

Davison K, Bagley CR: Schizophrenic-like psychoses associated with organic disorders of the central nervous system: a review of the literature, in Current Problems in Neuropsychiatry; Schizophrenia, Epilepsy, the Temporal Lobe. Edited by Herrington RN. Br J Psychiatry, spec pub No 4, 1969

Elliott FA: Propanolol for the control of belligerent behavior following acute brain damage. Ann Neurol 1:489-491, 1977

Elliott FA: Neurological findings in adult minimal brain dysfunction and the dyscontrol syndrome. J Nerv Ment Dis 170:680-687, 1982

Feibel JH, Springer CJ: Depression and failure to resume social activities after stroke. Arch Phys Med Rehabil 63:276-277, 1982

Finkelstein S, Benowitz LI, Baldessarini RJ, et al: Mood, vegetative disturbance and dexamethasone depression test after stroke. Ann Neurol 12:463-468, 1982

Folks, DG, King LD, Dowdy SB, et al: Carbamazepine treatment of selective affectively disordered inpatients. Am J Psychiatry 139:115-117, 1982

Folstein MF, Maiberger R, McHugh PR: Mood disorder as a specific complication of stroke. J Neurol Neurosurg Psychiatry 40:1018-1020, 1977

Fordyce DJ, Roueche JR, Prigatano GP: Enhanced emotional reactions in chronic head trauma patients. J. Neurol Neurosurg Psychiatry 46:620-624, 1983

Gresham GE, Phillips TF, Wolf PA, et al: Epidemiologic profile of long-term stroke disability: the Framingham Study. Arch Phys Med Rehabil 60:487-491, 1979

Haddon JW, Baker SP: Injury control, in Preventive and Community Medicine. Edited by Clark D, McMahn B. Boston, Little Brown Co., 1981

Hakoloa HP, Laulumaa VA: Carbamazepine in treatment of violent schizophrenics (letter). Lancet 1:1358, 1982

Hartunian NS, Smart CN, Thomas MS: The incidence and economic cost of cancer, motor vehicle injuries, coronary heart disease and stroke: a comparative analysis. Am J Pub Health 70:1249-1260, 1980

Hendrick EB, Harwood-Hash DCF, Hudson AR: Head injuries in children: A survey of 4465 consecutive cases at the Hospial for Sick Children, Toronto, Canada. Clin Neurosurg 11:46-65, 1965

Hillbom E: After-effects of brain injuries. Acta Psychiatrica et Neurologica Scandinavica Supplement 142:1-195, 1960

Hillbom M, Kaste M: Does alcohol intoxication precipitate aneurysmal subarachnoid hemorrhage? J Neurol Neurosurg Psychiatry 44:523-526, 1981a

Hillbom M, Kaste M: Ethanol intoxication: a risk factor for ischemic brain infarction in adolescents and young adults. Stroke 12:422-425, 1981b

Hypertension Detection and Follow-up Program Cooperative Group. Five-year findings of the hypertension detection and follow-up program. III. Reduction in stroke incidence among persons with high blood pressure. JAMA 247:633-638, 1982.

Insurance Institute for Highway Safety: Children in crashes. Washington, DC, Insurance Inst for Highway Safety, May 1983

Jampala VC, Abrams R: Mania secondary to left and right hemisphere damage. Am J Psychiatry 140:1197-1199, 1983

Kraus JF, Black MA, Hessol N, et al: The incidence of acute brain injury and serious impairment in a defined population. Am J Epidemiol 119:186-201, 1984

Labi ML, Phillips TF, Gresham GE: Psychosocial disability in physically restored long-term stroke survivors. Arch Phys Med Rehabil 61:561-565, 1980

Lawrence L, Christie D: Quality of life after stroke: a three-year follow-up. Age Ageing 8:167-172, 1979

Lim ML, Ebrahim SB: Depression after stroke: hospital treatment survey. Postgrad Med J 59:489-491, 1983

Lipsey JR, Robinson RG, Pearlson, GD, et al: Nortriptyline treatment of post-stroke depression: a double-blind study. Lancet 1:297-300, 1984

Lishman WA: Organic of Psychiatry: the psychological consequences of cerebral disorder. London, Blackwell Scientific Pub, 1978

Luchins DJ: Carbamazepine for the violent psychiatric patient. Lancet 2:766, 1983

Maltbie AA, Wingfield MS, Volow MR, et al: Electroconvulsive therapy in the presence of brain tumor: case reports and an evaluation of risk. J Nerv Ment Dis 168:400-405, 1980

Mansheim P: Treatment with propranolol of the behavioral sequelae of brain damage. J Clin Psychiatry 42:132, 1981

National Safety Council. Accident Facts. Chicago, National Safety Council, 1983

Neppe VM: Carbamazepine in the psychiatric patient. Lancet 2:334, 1982

Oddy M, Humphrey M, Uttley D: Stresses upon the relatives of head-injured patients. Br J Psychiatry 133:507-513, 1978

Petrie WM, Ban TA: Propranolol in organic agitation. Lancet 1:324, 1981

Poleck DG: The body: what happens to it in a crash. Traffic Safety Magazine, April, 1967

Ratey JS, Morrill R, Oxenkrug G: Use of propranolol for provoked and unprovoked episodes of rage. Am J Psychiatry 140:1356-1357, 1983

Rimel RW, Giordano B, Barth JT, et al: Disability caused by minor head injury. Neurosurgery 9:221-228, 1981

Robinson RG, Price TR: Post-stroke depressive disorders: a follow-up study of 103 patients. Stroke 13:635-641, 1982

Robinson RG, Szetela B: Mood change following left hemisphere brain injury. Ann Neurol 9:447-453, 1981

Robinson RG, Kubos KL, Starr LB, et al: Mood changes in stroke patients: relationship to lesion location. Compr Psychiatry 6:555-566, 1983

Robinson, RG, Starr LB, Price TR: A two year longitudinal study of mood disorders following stroke: prevalence and duration at six months follow-up. Br J Psychiatry 144:256-262, 1984

Schiff HB, Sabin TD, Geller A, et al: Lithium in aggressive behavior. Am J Psychiatry 139:1346-1348, 1982

Schreier HA: Use of propranolol in the treatment of postencephalitic psychosis. Am J Psychiatry 136:840-841, 1979

Thomsen IV: Late outcome of very severe blunt head trauma: a 10-15 year second follow-up. J Neurol Neurosurg Psychiatry 47:260-268, 1984

Tunks ER, Dever SW: Carbamazepine in the dyscontrol syndrome associated with limbic dysfunction. J. Nerv Ment Dis 164:56-63, 1977

Weddell R, Oddy M, Jenkins D: Social adjustment after rehabilitation: a two year follow-up of patients with severe head injury. Psychol Med 10:257-263, 1980

Williams DT, Mehl R, Yudofsky S, et al: The effect of propranolol on uncontrolled rage outbursts in children and adolescents with organic brain dysfunction. J Am Acad Child Psychiatry 21:129-135, 1982

Wolf P, Kannel W: Controllable risk factors for stroke: preventive implications of trends in stroke mortality, in Diagnosis and Management of Stroke and TIA's. Edited by Meyer JS, Shaw T. Menlo Park, California, Addison-Wesley Pub Co., 1982

Wolf PA, Dawber TR, Thomas HE, et al: Epidemiology of stroke. Adv Neurol 16:5-19, 1977

Yudofsky SC, Williams D, Gorman J: Propranolol in the treatment of rage and violent behavior in patients with chronic brain syndromes. Am J Psychiatry 138:218-220, 1981

Yudofsky SC, Stevens L, Silver J, et al: Propranolol in the treatment of rage and violent behavior associated with Korsakoff's psychosis. Am J Psychiatry 141:114-115, 1984

Chapter 9

Psychiatric Aspects of Movement Disorders and Demyelinating Diseases

by Dilip V. Jeste, M.D., Jack A. Grebb, M.D. and Richard Jed Wyatt, M.D.

Important functions of the central nervous system (CNS) include translation of thoughts, feelings and drives into behavior which, practically speaking, is virtually synonymous with movement. Indeed, the movements of dance bespeak a relationship between movement and emotion. Therefore, it is not surprising that many of the disorders affecting movement also have major psychiatric symptoms.

The major CNS structures involved in movement include the cerebral cortex, basal ganglia, thalamus, cerebellum, red nucleus, brainstem and spinal cord. The complex interactions of these structures have recently been reviewed by Humphrey (1983). The physiology of these systems continues to be explored using new techniques such as regional cerebral blood flow (Roland et al, 1982) and positron emission tomography (PET) scanning (Bustany et al, 1983; Hawkins et al, 1983; Kahl et al, 1981). The neurotransmitters utilized within these structures include dopamine (DA), norepinephrine (NE), acetylcholine (ACh), serotonin (5–HT), gamma–aminobutyric acid (GABA) and glutamate, as well as many of the peptide neurotransmitters (Buck and Yamamura, 1982). Again, new techniques such as visualization of dopamine receptors in living man (Garnett et al, 1983) promise further appreciation of the functioning of neurotransmitter systems.

Table 1 lists specific motor abnormalities. There are variations in the literature regarding the definitions of these terms. Two recent reviews offer some clinical guidelines for the assessment of abnormal involuntary movements (Jeste and Wyatt, 1982; Yung, 1983a). Yung (1983b) has also published a flow chart to help in the differential diagnosis of movement disorders.

This chapter will emphasize the neuropsychiatric aspects of the major movement disorders. Adams and Victor (1977) provide further clinical information on these disorders, and Heimer (1983) offers an elegant guide to neuroanatomy. When considering the neuropsychiatric symptoms of movement disorders, it is important to realize that they could be: secondary to the lesion that also caused the movement disorder; a psychologic response to the movement disorder; secondary to the social ramifications of the primary disorder; or secondary to the medical treatment of the primary disorder. Furthermore, in any single case, it is possible that two independent disorders—one motor and one psychiatric—coexist by chance alone.

Table 1. Different Types of Motor Abnormalities

Akathisia—subjective sense of inner "tension" often evidenced by motor restlessness

Akinesia—an extreme form of bradykinesia (see below)

Astasia–abasia—inability to stand or walk, in the absence of any organic lesion affecting leg movements

Asterixis—"flapping" or "wing beating" tremor of outstretched arms, seen in various metabolic encephalopathies

Ataxia—loss of muscle coordination

Athetosis—slow, writhing, purposeless movements

Ballismus—sudden, rapid, violent extensions of limbs (hemibalismus affects one side)

Bradykinesia—abnormal slowness of movement not related to paralysis or apraxia

Chorea—rapid, jerky, quasi-purposeful, nonrhythmic movements (hemichorea affects one side of the body)

Choreoathetosis—combination of chorea and athetosis

Compulsion—irresistible, sometimes complex, motor act or behavior occurring despite a conscious effort to avoid it

Dyskinesia—generic term for involuntary, abnormal movements

Dystonia—slow, sustained, muscular contraction or spasm that can result in an involuntary movement

Hyperkinesia—general term for increased motor activity

Hypokinesia—general term for decreased motor activity (a milder form of bradykinesia)

Mannerism—irregularly repetitive, somewhat purposeful movement or discrete behavior that is often peculiar to an individual

Myoclonus—abrupt, irregular contraction of muscles sometimes producing sudden, jerky movements

Paralysis—loss of ability to move certain muscles

Paresis—weakness of certain muscles

Rabbit syndrome—fine, rapid tremor of lips, seen after neuroleptic treatment

Rigidity—stiffness of muscles typically seen in extrapyramidal disorders

Spasticity—hypertonia, usually with hyperreflexia, characteristic of corticospinal tract lesions

Stereotypy—repetitive, uniform, purposeless movements or discrete behaviors

Tics—brief, sudden, recurrent contractions of related muscles producing apparently purposeful movements

Tremors—rhythmic, regular, oscillatory movements, varying in speed from 3 to 20 per second

Intention Tremor—tremor present when a limb approaches a target; for example, intention tremor of cerebellar disorders

Static or Rest Tremor—tremor present when a limb is at rest or in a certain position; for example, "pill rolling" tremor of Parkinson's disease

DISORDERS PRIMARILY AFFECTING THE BASAL GANGLIA

The four best-known movement disorders affecting the basal ganglia are Huntington's disease, Parkinson's disease, Sydenham's chorea, and Wilson's disease. Although other CNS structures are also affected in these disorders, the basal ganglia are considered to be the major site of pathology. All four of these conditions, as well as Fahr's Syndrome and Hallervorden–Spatz disease, have major neuropsychiatric symptoms that are discussed below and summarized in Table 2.

Anatomy and Physiology of the Basal Ganglia

As with the motor system as a whole, the basal ganglia are proving to be more complex in their interconnections than previously supposed (Mehler, 1981; Marsden, 1982a, 1982b; Barnes, 1983). There is no agreement on which structures are considered to comprise the "basal ganglia," and various texts include either more or fewer anatomic structures in that category. Moreover, the concept of "basal ganglia" is misleading, inasmuch as it implies that these structures work together as a single unit for a single purpose; this is most unlikely to be the case. The components of the basal ganglia are summarized in Table 3.

Basal Ganglia and Higher Mental Functions

One of the reigning oversimplifications regarding the brain is that the cerebral cortex is concerned with "higher mental functions," such as thinking and planning, and that the basal ganglia are concerned with "motor" functions. Yet there are grounds for believing that the basal ganglia may have a more extensive action upon the functions of the cerebrum (Jeste et al, 1984a,b; Marsden, 1982b). The basal ganglia receive input from almost all areas of the neocortex (Graybiel and Ragsdale, 1979), and could affect the workings of most parts of the brain. Four recent reviews further consider this question (Nauta, 1982; Chozick, 1983; Stern, 1983; Vicedomini et al, 1984).

Related to the role of the basal ganglia is the concept of the so-called "subcortical dementia" (Benson, 1983; Mayeaux et al, 1983). Dementia was previously thought to be a pathognomonic sign of damage to the cerebral cortex. As will be pointed out in the discussions of individual movement disorders, there are neuropsychiatric disorders with sparing of the cerebral cortex that are, nonetheless, characterized by dementia. The clinical characteristics of such subcortical dementias are thought to include: abnormal involuntary movements; psychomotor retardation; forgetfulness without inability to learn new material; situation-dependent apathy; and absence of cortical signs such as aphasia or aparaxia (Benson, 1983).

Also related to the role of the basal ganglia in higher mental functions is their possible role in schizophrenia (Lidsky et al, 1979). In an interesting review by Bowman and Lewis (1980), the authors tabulated the subcortical sites of damage in 22 neurological diseases with symptoms resembling schizophrenia, and found that basal ganglia were the most often involved structures in these conditions.

Huntington's Disease

Huntington's disease is an autosomal dominant (with complete penetrance), degenerative disease of the CNS. The physiologic mechanisms controlled by

Table 2. Summary of Movement Disorders Involving the Basal Ganglia

	Huntington's Disease	Parkinson's Disease	Striatonigral Degeneration	Sydenham's Chorea	Wilson's Disease	Fahr's Syndrome	Hallervorden-Spatz Disease
Average Age of Onset	30–50	50–60	50–65	5–15	20–30	20–60	10–15
Characteristic Motor Abnormalities	Chorea	Bradykinesia Rigidity Tremor (Pill Rolling) Postural Instability	Bradykinesia Rigidity	Chorea	Bradykinesia Rigidity Tremor (Wing Beating)	Similar to Parkinson's	Rigidity Dystonia Choreoathetosis Spasticity
Common Neuropsychiatric Associations							
• Dementia	Yes	Yes	Yes	No	Yes	Yes	Yes
• Affective Disorders	Yes	Yes	Yes	Rare	Yes	Yes	?
• Psychoses	Yes	Uncommon (Except drug-induced)	?	Schizophrenia?	Yes	Yes	?
Major Sites of Pathology in Basal Ganglia	Striatum	Substantia nigra	Striatum, Substantia nigra	Caudate? Subthalamic Nuclei?	Globus pallidus Putamen	Generalized	Substantia nigra Globus pallidus Red nucleus
Major Neurotransmitters Implicated	GABA Somatostatin?	Dopamine Norepinephrine	Dopamine	?	?	?	?
Genetics	Autosomal dominant	*	*	*	Usually autosomal recessive	Hereditary	Autosomal recessive
Other Characteristics	Rigidity in Westphal variant (early onset)	Sometimes secondary to other etiologies	Nonresponsive to L-dopa	Post-Group A streptococcal infection	Kayser Fleisher rings in cornea Hepatic failure Low serum ceruloplasmin	Calcified Basal Ganglia	Iron deposition in basal ganglia

*No identified genetic basis; however, familial cases have been reported.

Table 3. Components of the Basal Ganglia

Corpus Striatum
Substantia Nigra
Subthalamic Nucleus of Luys
Other Structures*
Amygdala
Cerebellum
Locus Coeruleus
Red Nucleus
Thalamus

*Different authors vary as to which of these other structures, if any, are included in the "basal ganglia."

this gene are unknown; however, the first step in unravelling this mystery has been taken by locating the restriction enzyme marker of the involved gene (Gusella et al, 1983). The disease is characterized by a progressive movement disorder and mental changes, with onset in the third to fifth decades, and an incidence of 5/100,000. The movement disorder can begin as seemingly minor restless movements, but then progresses to chorea involving the entire body. One laboratory test that is of some diagnostic use is computerized tomography (CT) scan showing atrophy of the caudate in some cases. A dopamine challenge test with dopaminergic drugs such as L–dopa to bring out a movement disorder in asymptomatic but at-risk family members is not currently being used because of practical and ethical issues. The disease usually takes a relentless course of physical and mental decline resulting in death approximately 15 years after onset of symptoms. A thorough compilation of information on this disease can be found in the book edited by Chase et al (1979).

The disease process involves degeneration of normally developed neurons in the basal ganglia, especially in the striatum. Layers three, five and six of the frontal and parietal cortex are also atrophied. The cerebellum has been reported to be involved in some cases (Jeste et al, 1984a). It is interesting to note that a study of Huntington's disease patients with PET showed decreased glucose metabolism (indicative of decreased neuronal activity), in spite of normal CT scans (Kahl et al, 1981).

Neurochemically, GABA (McGeer and McGeer, 1976), methionine–enkephalin (Emson et al, 1980a), cholecystokinin (Emson et al, 1980b), acetylcholine (McGeer and McGeer, 1976), and substance P (Aronin et al, 1983) have all been reported to have reduced activities in these patients. The dopaminergic and noradrenergic systems are relatively spared, although there may be a net over-activity of dopamine (Marsden, 1982a, 1982b) because of the reduction in other neurotransmitter systems. A recent report (Aronin et al, 1983) found concentrations of somatostatin increased three- to fivefold in the caudate and globus pallidus. Pharmacologically, neuroleptics have been used to decrease the movements, but other approaches involving GABA-ergic or cholinergic agents have not been particularly successful.

DEMENTIA. Table 4 is a summary of ten studies on neuropsychiatric syndromes in Huntington's disease reviewed by Jeste et al (1984b). Dementia was a prodromal symptom in ten percent, and a reason for first admission in eight percent of these patients. Fisher et al (1983) studied 30 Huntington's disease patients, nine Parkinson's disease patients, and 19 controls. Huntington's patients had deficits in memory, sequencing and organizational skills with sparing of language and factual information, a profile consistent with the concept of the so-called subcortical dementia. This study also found increasing intellectual decline with advancing disease, and in comparison with the Parkinson's disease patients, the dementia of Huntington's disease was a more significant source of disability early in the course of the illness.

PSYCHIATRIC SYMPTOMS. Table 4 summarizes the psychiatric syndromes of Huntington's disease. Psychiatric diagnoses account for 46 percent of the first admissions in these studies. Suicide is often a major clinical concern with these patients. A recent study (Caine and Shoulson, 1983) of 30 Huntington's patients followed for two to six years found the following numbers of patients with *DSM-III* syndromes: no psychiatric syndrome (six); dysthymic (six); major depressive (five); schizophrenia (three); atypical psychotic (two); anxiety (two); intermittent explosive (two); paranoid (one); other disturbances not conforming to *DSM-III* (seven). The relatively high prevalence of neuropsychiatric symptoms in Huntington's argues against this coexistence being due solely to chance. Furthermore, since onset of the neuropsychiatric symptoms often precedes the appearance of the movement disorder, viewing these symptoms as secondary phenomena does not seem to be the most logical explanation. There is a possibility that the neuropsychiatric symptoms might be manifestations of the primary structural lesion.

Parkinson's Disease

Cardinal symptoms of Parkinson's disease are bradykinesia, rigidity, "resting" tremor, stooped posture, and a festinating gait, with an age of onset usually in the fifth or sixth decade. Parkinson's disease is pathologically characterized by degeneration of pigmented neurons, most markedly in the zona compacta of the substantia nigra, ventral tegmental area, and the locus coeruleus. The degree

Table 4. Huntington's Disease and Psychiatric Symptoms: A Summary of 10 Studies*

Patients With:	Overall Prevalence (Percentage)
Psychiatric Symptoms	91
Dementia	89
Affective Disorders	42
Schizophrenia-Like Psychoses	18
Neuroses and Personality Disorders	23
Other	9

*Adapted from Jeste et al, 1984b.
Some patients have multiple symptoms.

of decreased dopamine in the striatum and substantia nigra is correlated with the severity of the motor symptoms (Marsden, 1982a, 1982b). Decreased dopamine concentrations in the limbic system (Hornykiewicz, 1981) and decreased turnover of 5–HT and norepinephrine (Olsson and Roos, 1968; Puite et al, 1973) have also been reported. The most common form is idiopathic; however, the syndrome can also follow encephalitis, carbon monoxide or manganese poisoning, head injury, and ingestion of 1–methyl–4–phenyl–1,2,5,6–tetrahydropyridine (MPTP), a derivative of meperidine that has been sold illicitly (Langston et al, 1983). It has also been suggested that Parkinson's disease might have an infectious or toxic etiology (Calne and Langston, 1983). The use of regional cerebral blood flow (Globus et al, 1983; Leenders et al, 1983) and PET (Bustany et al, 1983) should help further our understanding of this disorder. The work on brain transplants of substantia nigra (Freed, 1983) offers futuristic promise.

DEMENTIA. An excellent recent review of the studies of dementia in Parkinson's disease is by Mayeux and Stern (1983). The authors report estimated prevalence of dementia in Parkinson's disease to range from 30 percent to 80 percent; however, they conclude that some degree of intellectual impairment could be expected in nearly every patient with Parkinson's disease, and that "clinically, the point at which intellectual difficulties progress to dementia may be less than clear-cut." The degree of intellectual impairment has been related to age of onset of the disease (Lieberman et al, 1979b). Clinical, radiographic, and neuropathological evidence has been reported to suggest a similarity between the dementia of Parkinson's disease and that of Alzheimer's disease (Hakim and Mathieson, 1978; Boller et al, 1980; Sroka et al, 1981). Moreover, 40 out of 65 Alzheimer patients in one study were reported to have extrapyramidal symptoms (Pearce, 1974). Not all demented patients with Parkinson's disease have Alzheimer-type neuropathology, however; a proportion of Parkinson's patients have dementia resembling that seen in Huntington's disease.

PSYCHIATRIC SYMPTOMS. Depression is a major psychiatric consideration in Parkinson's disease, but its assessment is particularly difficult because of the similar appearances of the masked facies and psychomotor retardation in both conditions (Serby, 1980). Different studies have reported prevalence of depression in Parkinson's disease to be 56 percent in females and 71 percent in males (Warburton, 1967), 65 percent in females (Mindham, 1970) and 90 percent in males (Lieberman et al, 1979a). Two studies used control groups of similarly disabled neurological controls, and found depression to be more prevalent in the parkinsonian groups (Horn, 1974; Robins, 1976), which suggests that depression may have a specific relationship to the parkinsonian disease process. Lieberman et al (1979a) reported equal degrees of depression in 520 demented and nondemented patients, indicating that these two neuropsychiatric syndromes may be independent.

Using a genetic approach to the question of depression, Duvoisin et al (1981) studied 12 monozygotic twin pairs discordant for Parkinson's disease. The investigators found personality differences dating back to adolescence in seven of the 12 pairs. The affected twins were described as having been "nervous, quieter, more introverted, and more serious." Three of the patients and none of the siblings had been under psychiatric care for depression. In support of genetic predisposition to depressive illness in parkinsonian patients, Stern et al (1977) reported a 24 percent prevalence of depression in first-degree relatives of patients; however, Winokur et al (1978) were not able to replicate this finding.

Pharmacologically, it is interesting that a reduction of dopaminergic and noradrenergic activities has been implicated in both Parkinson's disease and depression (Willner, 1983). Furthermore, levodopa, the mainstay of treatment for parkinsonism, has been reported to elevate mood in depressed, non-parkinsonian patients (Goodwin et al, 1970). Celesia and Wanamaker (1972) reported a decrease in the number of parkinsonian patients with depression from 37 percent to 24 percent after 1–2 years of levodopa treatment; however, Marsh and Markham (1973) reported no change in depressive symptoms despite improved motor status after one year of treatment. It is also noteworthy that desipramine, a tricyclic antidepressant, has been reported to benefit the movement disorder in parkinsonism (Laitinen, 1968).

There is an interesting theoretical relationship between Parkinson's disease and schizophrenia, inasmuch as Parkinson's disease is a hypo-dopaminergic state, and schizophrenia has been hypothesized to be a hyper-dopaminergic state. The oversimplicity of such hypotheses is suggested by reports of Parkinson's disease and schizophrenia coexisting in the same patient (Hollister and Glazener, 1961; Crow et al, 1976).

Levodopa treatment can often complicate the psychiatric presentation of patients with Parkinson's disease. Psychosis has been reported in up to 60 percent of parkinsonian patients after six years of treatment (Sweet et al, 1976), an observation for which Moskovitz et al (1978) have hypothesized a kindling model. Levodopa can also cause affective symptoms and confusion. The movement disorders induced by levodopa are discussed in the section on drug-related movement disorders.

Striatonigral Degeneration

Related to Parkinson's disease is striatonigral degeneration that has a similar age of onset of the classical parkinsonian symptoms, but is distinguished from Parkinson's disease by having less tremor, poor response to levodopa, greater morbidity, and a shorter course until death (Adams and Victor, 1977; Kan, 1978). Although there is loss of neurons in the substantia nigra as there is in Parkinson's disease, there is an even more striking loss of neurons in the putamen, caudate, and globus pallidus. Some of the reports have observed no changes in mental status; others have, however, noted dementia (Kosada et al, 1981; Nakamura, 1982).

Sydenham's Chorea

Sydenham's chorea (chorea minor) is a movement disorder affecting children and early adolescents (Schwartzman et al, 1948; Thiebaut, 1968; Nausieda et al, 1980). It is considered to be a delayed complication of infection with group A streptococcus; however, evidence supporting this prior infection (for example, increased antibody titers, coexisting rheumatic heart disease) is present in only one-half to two-thirds of these patients (Stollerman, 1983). Nevertheless, a strong argument for a rheumatic origin of most cases has been made (Taranta and Stollerman, 1956; Taranta, 1959). The disease has been hypothesized to be an antibody-mediated condition (Waksman, 1983), and antibodies specifically reacting with the cytoplasm of subthalamic and caudate nuclei have been reported (Husby et al, 1976; Husby et al, 1977). The neuropathologic descriptions have included "rheumatic" changes in cerebral blood vessels (Breutsch, 1940; 1944), inflammatory and degenerative changes (Grinber and Sahs, 1966), and edema, congestion and degeneration of neurons (Brain and Walton, 1969).

NONSCHIZOPHRENIC PSYCHIATRIC SYMPTOMS AND SEQUELAE.   In a review of 175 cases of Syndenham's chorea, Schwartzman (1959) found that the most common behavioral changes were shyness and introversion, and a tendency to cry easily. If rheumatic infection did commonly affect the brain, one would expect to find a higher incidence of abnormal mental status in patients who had either rheumatic fever or Sydenham's chorea. Five follow-up studies with an emphasis on psychological adjustment have been published. The largest study, involving 2,687 patients (Wertheimer, 1963) found that patients who had contracted rheumatic fever at puberty were four times more likely to have subsequent "functional" psychiatric illnesses than control populations. Two other controlled studies supported this general finding (Keeler and Bender, 1952; Freeman et al, 1965). Freeman and colleagues (1965) interviewed 40 patients, 30 years after their acute illness, and found that 33 of the 40 patients (83 percent) suffered from either a personality disorder or a psychoneurosis as compared with only 25 percent of controls. The two remaining studies did not support this finding; however, one observed only ten patients who had recovered from chorea (Sacks et al, 1962) and the other used the Minnesota Multiphasic Personality Inventory (MMPI) as its only assessment tool (Stehbens and Macqueen, 1972). Bird et al (1976) compared 26 patients convalescing from Sydenham's chorea with siblings and matched rheumatic fever controls. Using clinical examination, neuropsychological testing and EEGs, this group concluded that "uncomplicated Sydenham's chorea is not necessarily a benign self-limited affliction of the central nervous system and that some patients are left with a definite, albeit minimal, neurologic residual."

HYPOTHESIZED LINK TO SCHIZOPHRENIA.   In 1961, Wertheimer published a paper entitled "Rheumatic Schizophrenia," which described an epidemiologic study involving over 2,500 schizophrenic patients. The results supported the author's hypothesis that "a large portion of schizophrenics, including many who present a typical course and symptomatology with no outstanding organic symptoms and no traditional signs of rheumatic fever, may nonetheless have psychoses resulting from rheumatic disease." Many earlier reports, some reviewed by Lewis and Minski (1935), had hypothesized a relationship between rheumatic disease and schizophrenia. Wertheimer (1961) developed the hypothesis that, depending upon the age of the affected individual when first infected, a syndrome varying in the relative proportion of movement disorder to mental symptoms would evolve: The later a patient was infected, the more prominent the mental symptoms would be. Wertheimer further hypothesized that a patient could present with only mental symptoms, and no other stigmata of rheumatic infection. In her first paper, Wertheimer (1957) reported a prevalence of 8.2 percent for rheumatic histories in 147 college-educated schizophrenic patients, as compared to 2.4 percent in 420 normal college freshmen.

Neuropathologic evidence for a link between schizophrenia and rheumatic infection was provided by Bruetsch (1940, 1944), who reported 100 consecutive autopsies on schizophrenic patients and found a prevalence of nine percent for histories of previous rheumatic infection, a figure well above that for nonschizophrenic populations from the same period. Guttman (1936) reported similar findings twice as often in schizophrenics as in manic-depressive patients, although diagnostic questions regarding specificity can be raised.

Wilson's Disease (Hepatolenticular Degeneration)

Wilson's disease is usually transmitted as an autosomal recessive trait associated with a deficiency of the copper-binding enzyme ceruloplasmin, thereby causing copper to be deposited in various tissues, especially the liver and CNS, most notably the basal ganglia. Clinical manifestations include jaundice, Kayser-Fleischer rings in the cornea, "blue moons" on the fingernails and "wing-beating" tremor; and other CNS symptoms including rigidity, dysarthria, dysphagia and emotional disturbances. Dobyns et al (1979) reported the findings in 58 patients with Wilson's disease. Ten patients had presented with hepatic symptoms, 19 with CNS symptoms, and 24 with both. Five of the 19 patients with CNS involvement presented with psychiatric illness. Kendall et al (1981) studied CT scans of 12 patients with Wilson's disease. Seven patients had CT evidence of either low density or atrophy of basal ganglia, and all of these patients had signs of intellectual deterioration. There was only a moderate correlation between cerebral atrophy and the degree of dementia. Another CT study (Williams and Walshe, 1981) examined CT scans of 60 patients with Wilson's disease. Ventricular dilatation was present in 73 percent, cortical atrophy in 55 percent, and hypodense basal ganglia in 45 percent. Fourteen of the 19 patients were rescanned after treatment with a copper chelating agent, and showed moderate to marked improvement in the hypodensity of the basal ganglia that correlated with clinical improvement. Most recently, PET with F^{18}–fluorodeoxyglucose in four patients with Wilson's disease demonstrated globally reduced metabolism as compared to controls (Hawkins et al, 1983).

Fahr's Syndrome

Fahr's syndrome, also called idiopathic calcification of the basal ganglia, is a rare, hereditary disorder and is diagnosed on the basis of a clinical triad consisting of a movement disorder, neuropsychiatric symptoms, and abnormal calcification of the basal ganglia. The calcification is concentrated in the walls of arterioles and capillaries, and in the perivascular areas (especially in the basal ganglia, dentate nucleus of the cerebellum and, more generally, in white matter). The differential diagnosis for calcification of the basal ganglia includes parathyroid disorders, infectious conditions, toxic disorders, and other hereditary conditions (Cummings et al, 1983). The motor symptoms include a Parkinson-like syndrome, choreoathetosis, cerebellar ataxia and paralysis. Neuropsychiatric symptoms include dementia, schizophrenia-like psychoses and depression (Cummings et al, 1983; Francis, 1979; Konig and Haller, 1982). There may be two subtypes of this syndrome: one having an onset at approximately the age of 30 and presenting with psychosis; the other having a later onset at approximately the age of 50, presenting with dementia (Cummings et al, 1983). All patients eventually develop dementia (Francis, 1979).

Hallervorden–Spatz Disease

Hallervorden–Spatz disease is a rare, hereditary (autosomal recessive) condition involving the pathological deposition of iron pigment in the globus pallidus, pars reticulata of the substantia nigra, and the red nucleus (Adams and Victor, 1977; Dooling et al, 1974). Approximately 60 cases had been reported in the literature as of 1974 (Dooling et al, 1974). The disease symptoms usually begin at age ten to 15, and the early signs are both extrapyramidal (rigidity, dystonia, choreoathetosis), and corticospinal (spasticity, hyperreflexia). Ataxia and myoclonus have also been reported. There is a gradual and relentless dementia, and the movement disorder progresses steadily over approximately a 20-year period, at which time death usually occurs. There is no known diagnostic test; however, there is one case report suggesting that CT scans might be of some value (Dooling et al, 1980). There is no known treatment.

DISORDERS OF THE CEREBELLUM

The cerebellum includes vermis, cortex and nuclei (dentate, emboliform, globose and fastigial). The cerebellum has reciprocal innervations with the cerebral cortex, limbic system, brainstem, and spinal cord. The efferent loop to the cortex is by way of the thalamus. Traditionally the cerebellum has been thought to have as its principal function the coordination of motor activity. Lesions of the cerebellum produce ataxia, muscle incoordination, irregular, broad-based gait, intention tremor (for example, finger oscillating more as it nears its target on the finger-to-nose test), jerky conjugate eye movements and irregular, slurred speech. It is increasingly clear that the cerebellum also coordinates the autonomic, limbic, cortical, visual, auditory and tactile information that it receives through its connections with the cerebral cortex, limbic system, and special sensory systems (Dow, 1974; Snider and Maiti, 1976; Watson, 1978). A recent finding was that lesions of the dentate nucleus in rabbits abolished the classically conditioned eyelid response. This response was not abolished with lesions of the hippocampus or neocortex, suggesting a very direct role for the cerebellum in learning and production of classically conditioned responses (McCormick and Thompson, 1984).

Psychiatric Symptoms

Psychiatric symptoms have been reported in patients with cerebellar lesions. In 1979, Heath and colleagues reported neuropathologic changes in the cerebellar vermis in 40 percent of patients with a diagnosis of functional psychosis. In a subsequent paper (Heath et al, 1982), this group reported the visual and computer-analyzed readings of 1,700 CT scans; 50 percent of patients with functional psychosis and 38 percent of patients with seizures had vermal atrophy, as compared with 0.5–3.7 percent for other disorders. About one-half of the psychotic group were schizophrenics; therefore, the authors concluded that the findings did not have diagnostic significance, but might point to a behavioral syndrome of emotional dyscontrol and anhedonia. Vermal atrophy has also been reported in bipolar patients (Nasrallah et al, 1981; Lippman et al, 1982). Mental deficiency has been reported as a result of bilateral cerebellar agenesis (Dow and Moruzzi,

1958), and dyslexia might be related to cerebellar-vestibular dysfunction (Levinson, 1980). Hamilton et al (1983) reported on three cases that had been diagnosed for approximately two to three years as having functional psychiatric disorders, until more careful neurological assessment led to diagnoses of cerebellar lesions. Weinberger and co-workers (1979) noted that schizophrenics had a higher incidence of vermal atrophy on CT scans when compared to controls. In another study, Dewan and colleagues (1983) found similar results, but only in a subgroup of schizophrenic patients.

On the other hand, several groups of investigators have failed to find evidence of cerebellar lesions in schizophrenic and other psychiatric patients (for example, Coffman et al, 1981; Nasrallah et al, 1981a, 1981b). In a recent study, Jeste and colleagues (1984a) found no significant difference in cerebellar Purkinje cell density among schizophrenic patients, patients with other psychiatric disorders and age-matched normal controls.

DRUG–INDUCED MOVEMENT DISORDERS

Neuroleptic–Related Movement Disorders

The most serious movement disorder induced by neuroleptics is tardive dyskinesia. The prevalence of tardive dyskinesia among patients on long-term neuroleptic treatment is about 25 percent (Jeste and Wyatt, 1982). In nearly two-thirds of these patients, symptoms persist for months or years after neuroleptics have been discontinued. As the prevalence of spontaneous dyskinesia is about six percent, the risk of *neuroleptic-induced* persistent tardive dyskinesia is approximately 13 percent.

While a number of drugs induce dyskinesia, only neuroleptic use has been associated with persistent tardive dyskinesia. No definite data exist on the neuropathology of tardive dyskinesia. Contrary to popular belief, postsynaptic dopamine receptor supersensitivity in the nigrostriatal system may not be the only crucial pathogenic disturbance. Noradrenergic hyperactivity, GABA-ergic underactivity and other mechanisms may be more important in subgroups of patients.

In view of the heterogeneity of diagnostic criteria for tardive dyskinesia used by different investigators, we have developed a set of criteria that may be useful for diagnosing tardive dyskinesia, at least for research purposes (Jeste and Wyatt, 1982).

Phenomenology of Movement Disorder
- Choreoathetoid or rhythmic abnormal involuntary movements, reduced by voluntary movements of affected body parts and increased by those of unaffected areas.
- Involvement of one or more of these areas: tongue, jaw and extremities.

Onset and Duration of Abnormal Movements
- Onset after at least three continuous months of neuroleptic treatment, with dyskinesia appearing either during a course of drug treatment or within a few weeks of neuroleptic withdrawal.
- Duration: At least three weeks.

Pharmacologic Response
- Temporary suppression by increasing neuroleptic dose and, at least temporarily, aggravation by dose reduction or discontinuation.
- Nonresponse to or worsening by anticholinergic drugs (possible exception: certain tardive dystonias).

Differential Diagnosis of Movement Disorder
- Rule out tremors, acute dystonias, myoclonus, mannerisms, and compulsions.
- Exclude other causes of dyskinesia such as Huntington's disease, Wilson's disease, ill-fitting dentures, and so forth.

Severity (for Research Purposes)
- Mean global rating of at least two on the 0–to–4 Abnormal Involuntary Movement Scale (AIMS).

TARDIVE DYSKINESIA AND PSYCHOPATHOLOGY. Several groups of investigators have reported a relatively high prevalence of tardive dyskinesia in patients with major affective disorders, especially depression (see Kane et al, 1984). It is, however, uncertain whether this increased prevalence is due to a direct association between dyskinesia and depression, or due to certain treatment related variables such as high-dose intermittent neuroleptic use in patients with affective disorders (see Jeste and Wyatt, 1982). Cutler et al (1982) noted that the severity of dyskinesia in two or three bipolar patients was related to the intensity of depression. Glazer et al (1984) reported an inverse correlation between intensity of depression and that of dyskinesia in their schizophrenic patients.

Degkwitz (1969) and Hippius and Lange (1970) found a positive relationship between severity of psychosis and that of dyskinesia. Chouinard and Jones (1980) proposed that some dyskinetic patients have a "supersensitivity psychosis" characterized predominantly by positive symptoms of schizophrenia (such as delusions, hallucinations), attributed to supersensitivity of mesolimbic dopamine receptors. It is, however, unclear whether such a condition exists with any noticeable frequency.

We recently studied 47 schizophrenic inpatients, including eight with persistent tardive dyskinesia, nine with intermittent tardive dyskinesia and 30 without tardive dyskinesia (Jeste et al, 1984b). Patients were regularly rated on a number of rating scales. Our study found an association of tardive dyskinesia (especially persistent tardive dyskinesia) with negative symptoms (which included emotional withdrawal, motor retardation and blunted affect). It is interesting to relate our findings to the controversial concept of the "subcortical dementia" reported in certain conditions such as Huntington's disease, Wilson's disease and progressive supranuclear palsy. In these disorders, abnormal involuntary movements are frequently associated with psychomotor retardation, apathy and slow retrieval of learned material without true amnesia (Benson, 1983). Our patients with tardive dyskinesia (especially persistent tardive dyskinesia) had abnormal movements, motor retardation and apathy. Their memory difficulty, if any, remains to be tested with the help of neuropsychological testing. The apparent similarity between our findings and the reported subcortical dementias raises a possibility that subcortical (for example, basal ganglia) damage might be related to certain major clinical manifestations of our persistent tardive dyskinesia patients. A number of alternative explanations are also possible (see Jeste et al, 1984b).

Elsewhere, we have reviewed treatment strategies against tardive dyskinesia (Jeste and Wyatt, 1982). Suffice it to say here that prevention is better than the currently available methods of management. Judicious use of neuroleptics is warranted.

Other Drug–Related Movement Disorders

Levo–dopa (L–dopa) is the most successful therapeutic agent for the treatment of Parkinson's disease; however, it can produce akathisia, choreoathetosis, myoclonus, tremor, dyskinesia and dystonia (Jeste and Wyatt, 1982; Weiner and Bergun, 1977). The prevalence of L–dopa induced movement disorders is 40 to 80 percent, and this effect is related primarily to the dosage of the drug. The onset usually occurs after three to 12 months of treatment, and has only been reported to occur in parkinsonian patients or patients with other extrapyramidal diseases or CNS structural lesions. Often the clinician and the patient are faced with the dilemma of choosing between too high a dose (causing dyskinesia) and too low a dose (poorly controlling Parkinson's disease). Sometimes the patient must be willing to tolerate some dyskinesia in order for L–dopa to control the symptoms of Parkinson's disease.

Tricyclic antidepressants and lithium can also cause movement disorders, as can several other agents. These are summarized in Table 5.

MISCELLANEOUS MOVEMENT DISORDERS

Gilles de la Tourette's Syndrome

Tics ("habit spasms") appear transiently in 10 to 20 percent of normal children from ages five to ten. Tourette's syndrome is, however, a chronic condition characterized by multiple, transient motor tics, vocalizations (clicks, yelps, sniffs, and so forth), behavioral tics (sometimes of a sexual nature), and echophenomena (repeating the words or actions of others). Coprolalia, the involuntary utterance of curse words, is present in about 60 percent of patients. The cause and the pathophysiology of Tourette's syndrome are unknown. The cingulate gyrus (Bonnet, 1982), association cortex (Sutherland et al, 1982) and midbrain (Devinsky, 1983) have been implicated; nevertheless, no definitive conclusion regarding the neuropathology can be made (Richardson, 1982). Neuroleptics, especially haloperidol, trifluoperazine and pimozide, and α-receptor agonist, clonidine, are the most useful agents for controlling the tics. Cholinergic, serotonergic, and GABA-ergic agents have been tried with little success (Messiha and Carlson, 1983). A comprehensive review of Tourette's syndrome can be found in Cohen (1984).

Although some texts have referred to an absence of pathology other than tics, abnormal EEGs are found in 25 to 60 percent of Tourette's syndrome patients (Shapiro, 1978); "soft" neurologic signs (for example, motor asymmetries, clumsiness) are also present in many patients (Sweet et al, 1973). Neuropsychological testing has demonstrated a large discrepancy between verbal and performance IQs, abnormal performance on the Bender-Gestalt test (Shapiro, 1978); decreased

Table 5. Some Drug–Related Movement Disorders*

Movement Disorder	Tricyclic Antidepressants	Lithium	Other Chemicals
Akathisia	—	—	Benzodiazepine withdrawal
Ataxia	Acute intoxication	Acute intoxication	Alcohol, phenytoin, and many other drugs in toxic doses
Choreoathetosis	Rare	Rare	Amphetamine Anticholinergics Antihistamines Benzhexol Caffeine Methyldopa Oral Contraceptives Phenytoin
Myoclonus	Rare	Rare	Heavy metals Strychnine
Tics	—	—	Amphetamines Methylphenidate
Tremor	Uncommon	Yes	Alcohol Caffeine
Acute Dyskinesia	Rare	—	Amantadine Amphetamine Antihistamines Benzodiazepines Estrogens Fenfluramine Monoamine Oxidase Inhibitors Phenytoin
Dystonia	—	—	Metoclopramide
Tardive Dyskinesia	Rare	—	Metoclopramide

*See text for movement disorders related to neuroleptics and levodopa.

nonconstructional visuopractic abilities (Incagnoli and Kane, 1981); and deficits in memory (Sutherland et al, 1982). However, one intensive, prospective study of three patients did not demonstrate any singular pattern on neuropsychologic testing (Joschko and Rourke, 1982).

Psychologically, the heterogeneity and variability of symptoms in Tourette's syndrome should be recognized (Caine et al, 1982). Nee et al (1980) reported that 68 percent of their patients had obsessive-compulsive illness, and 32 percent had disturbed sexual behavior. Wilson et al (1982) reported that behavior disturbances in Tourette's syndrome patients exceeded those in normal children; there was, however, no difference between treated and untreated patients. The severity of the movement disorder was predictive of the degree of behavioral abnormality, but the pattern of behavioral problems was still quite variable.

With regard to the prevalence of obsessive-compulsive symptoms, Fernando (1976) reported a 31 percent, Morphew (1969) a 35 percent, and Kelman (1965) an 11.4 percent rate of occurrence. Montgomery's (1982) recent study found obsessive-compulsive illness in 66 percent of the patients, and in 30 out of 53 relatives. He also found a wide range of other psychiatric disorders in the patients' relatives, including anxiety, depression, and substance abuse.

Obsessive-Compulsive Disorder (OCD)

DSM-III requires the presence of either obsessions or compulsions for the diagnosis of obsessive-compulsive disorder. When compulsions are present, OCD could be considered a movement disorder inasmuch as the behavior (movement) is often under minimal voluntary control. The differentiation between complex "tics" in Tourette's syndrome and compulsions in OCD is frequently unclear. OCD has been the subject of several recent reviews (Insel and Murphy, 1981; Salzman and Thaler, 1981; Jenike, 1983). The cause of OCD is unknown. Insel et al (1982a) reported that some patients with OCD had EEG abnormalities, and neuropsychological testing was suggestive of an organic lesion. A possible link with depressive disorders has been suggested by abnormal dexamethasone suppression test (Insel et al, 1982b) and sleep EEG patterns (with less stage 4 sleep and shortened REM latency in OCD patients (Insel et al, 1983a). Clomipramine, a serotonergic tricyclic antidepressant, has been the most effective pharmacologic agent tried so far (Insel et al, 1983b); but monoamine oxidase inhibitors (Jenike et al, 1983), clonidine (Knesevich, 1982), and naloxone, an opiate antagonist (Insel and Pikar, 1983) have also been reported to be of possible benefit.

Although it may seem to be stretching the point to include OCD as a movement disorder, its inclusion makes the point that differentiation between more classic movement disorders with psychiatric symptoms, and classical psychiatric syndromes with abnormal movements, is not always clear.

Creutzfeldt-Jakob Disease (CJD)

Creutzfeldt-Jakob Disease (CJD) is a rare (one case per million population) disorder that appears to be caused by a transmissible virus with an incubation period of approximately two years. There is a strong inheritance pattern in approximately ten percent of the cases; this may, however, represent a genetic susceptibility to infection. The first symptoms are usually nervousness, memory loss and confusion, which progress to profound dementia and sometimes psychosis. The progressive motor symptoms include myoclonus and rigidity. The course runs an average of nine months (range one month to six years) until death. The EEG sometimes shows characteristic high voltage bursts of biphasic and triphasic slow waves; definitive diagnosis can, however, be made only upon examination of brain tissue. The cerebellum, basal ganglia and pyramidal systems are most affected, but the thalamus has also been reported to be involved (Martin, 1968). There are two relatively recent reviews of CJD (Kirschbaum, 1968; Traub, 1983).

It is important for the clinician to know that CJD could explain the symptoms of a patient who presents with mild neuropsychiatric manifestations. Although it is a very rare condition, it is worthwhile for the busy clinician to be careful with needles and lumbar punctures on patients because of the transmissable nature of this devastating malady.

Progressive Supranuclear Palsy

Progressive supranuclear palsy (Steele, 1964) has its onset in the fifth to seventh decade with a gradual progression of symptoms, including supranuclear opthalmoplegia, pseudobulbar palsy, axial dystonia, neck extension, and neuropsychiatric symptoms. The cause is unknown and there is no successful treatment. The dementia is characterized by forgetfulness, slowing of thought processes and impaired ability to manipulate acquired knowledge (Albert et al, 1974). Psychiatric symptoms tend to fall into two categories: indifference, apathy, depression, and progressive irritability, and/or euphoria (Albert et al, 1974).

Dystonia Musculorum Deformans

Dystonia musculorum deformans usually has its onset in childhood (six to 14 years of age) as an intermittent dystonic movement that may seem to be merely a nervous tic; however, as the disease progresses, there is a development of major dystonic movements in almost all muscle groups (Eldridge, 1970). There are two different inheritance patterns and subtypes of this disease. One subtype is inherited in an autosomal recessive pattern, and affects children (aged six to 14), predominantly Ashkenazi Jews. This form has a relatively fast progression, leaving the patients in almost continuous, uncontrollable movement. This subtype has been associated with superior intelligence (Riklan et al, 1976). The second type is autosomal dominant in inheritance, with an average age of onset of 28 (range 18 to 59) and no predilection for any ethnic group. The progression is slower, and does not necessarily lead to complete disability. Although first thought to be a manifestation of hysteria, neither form has been associated with psychopathology or dementia.

Meige Syndrome

This syndrome is characterized by dystonia involving the orofacial muscles. Usually the onset is after 50 years of age. Three recent studies (Marsden, 1976; Tolosa, 1981; Jankovic and Ford, 1983) have reported that approximately one-fourth to one-half of the patients were depressed before or during the onset of the movement disorder. Diagnosis in these studies was done retrospectively; however, the possible association between Meige syndrome and depression is of interest.

Spontaneous Movement Disorders in Psychiatric Patients

Both Kraepelin (1919) and Bleuler (1950) described stereotypy and mannerisms in their schizophrenic patients. Chorea, athetosis, and dystonia had not been reported in nonmedicated schizophrenic patients (Bleuler, 1950), although Kraepelin referred to one irregular movement of some patients as "athetoid ataxia." It is possible that some of the elderly patients diagnosed as having schizophrenia had disorders now clearly recognized as neurologic disorders—a realization which may well pertain to our patients in the future. Mettler and Crandell (1959), reported a prevalence of only 0.5 percent of chorea and athetosis in state hospital patients in the preneuroleptic era. Morrison (1973) reported a prevalence of 24 percent for stereotypies and 14 percent for mannerisms in untreated patients. Besides the movement disorders of schizophrenics, the bradykinesia and masked facies of depression can often cause a diagnostic confusion with Parkinson's disease. Early neurologists felt that focal pathology would account for the movement disorders of psychiatric patients, and later psychiatrists developed symbolic meanings for these movements. We are now perhaps returning to the earlier view, although the environment may indeed contribute to some of the specific abnormal movements. For instance, the effects of institutionalization have been studied, and the isolation of nonhuman primates has produced an increase in stereotyped behavior patterns (Berkson et al, 1963). The subject of spontaneous movement disorders in psychiatric patients is more completely reviewed by Casey (1984).

Conversion Disorders

Conversion disorders can sometimes present as movement disorders, and it is incorrect to automatically associate their presence with hysterical personality disorder (Lazare, 1981). Virtually any movement disorder may be imitated by a conversion disorder; but a very careful neurological examination and close observation for inconsistencies in the movement when the patient thinks he is unobserved might point toward the correct diagnosis. The fluctuation of the symptoms with levels of stress does not separate conversion disorder from neurologic movement disorders. The high incidence of conversion symptoms in patients with a history of head injury and other organic mental syndromes (Lazare, 1981), and the finding of EEG abnormalities in hysteria (Flor-Henry, 1981) suggest that there may be a neurological or biological basis for some aspects of conversion and hysterical personality disorders.

DEMYELINATING DISEASES

Multiple Sclerosis (MS)

The cardinal features of multiple sclerosis (MS) are the presence of symptoms of more than one lesion at more than one time, and a course of remissions and exacerbations (Adams and Victor, 1977; McFarlin and McFarland, 1983). Neuropathologically, there are macroscopic areas of demyelination scattered throughout the white matter of the CNS. Biological markers suggestive of MS in the cerebrospinal fluid (CSF) are a mild increase in protein and/or lymphocytes, an increase in IgG in 70 percent of patients, the presence of oligoclonal bands in 90 percent of patients, and occasional elevations of IgM or IgA. The etiology is unknown, but both infectious and autoimmune mechanisms have been suggested.

There is a large body of literature on psychiatric aspects of MS (see Trimble and Grant, 1982). One of the complicating issues regarding the etiology of these psychiatric symptoms is that treatment of MS exacerbations with prednisone and adrenocorticotropin (ACTH) can cause euphoria, irritability, depression or psychosis. It is of clinical interest that Flak et al (1979) found that lithium was successful in prophylactically reducing psychiatric side effects of prednisone and ACTH treatment in neurologic patients (Goggans et al, 1983).

INTELLECTUAL IMPAIRMENT.   Virtually every study of neuropsychological testing in MS patients has indicated some impairment (Trimble and Grant, 1982). The deficits have most often involved decreased performance scores on intelligence tests, decreased performance on timed and problem-solving motor tasks, and decreased abstracting abilities. In a majority of studies, the cognitive deficits were positively correlated with duration and severity of the disease (Pratt, 1951; Canter, 1951; Surridge, 1969; Invik, 1978a, 1978b; Staples and Lincoln, 1979), although one recent study (Bertrando et al, 1983) did not find a correlation between cognitive impairment and patient's age at onset of MS, duration, or degree of disability. Canter's study (1951) found that neuropsychological test scores declined in patients with MS over a six-month period, whereas scores for normals increased because of the effect of "practising" the test. Ross and Reitan (1955) also made an important contribution by using two control groups, matched for age, education and IQ—one with intracranial mass lesions or trauma, and one mixed group of psychiatric and neurologic patients. The MS group performed less well than the nonbrain-damaged control group, thereby reducing the possibility that the finding was related to depression, anxiety or cooperation with testing. Of particular interest to clinicians are reports of MS patients with dementia as the primary or presenting symptom (Bergin, 1957; Koenig, 1968; Young, 1976). Another group of investigators has further suggested that the neuropsychological profiles were related to specific neurologic symptoms (Peyser et al, 1980a), and that neuropsychological testing could possibly be used to subtype MS patients (Peyser et al, 1980b).

AFFECTIVE SYMPTOMS.   Early reports and uncontrolled studies reported depression, euphoria, and disregard for physical disabilities in MS patients. Braceland and Griffin (1950) conducted a large uncontrolled study of 75 patients, and reported depression in 75 percent, euphoria in 10 percent, emotional lability in 18 percent, and irritability in 12 percent. This study also found an increase in euphoria, with increasing intellectual deterioration and neurologic disability. Two studies using neurologically disabled controls have reported conflicting evidence regarding depression. Surridge (1969) examined 108 patients with MS and 39 controls with muscular dystrophy, finding a nonsignificant difference with depression being present in 18 percent of MS patients and 13 percent of controls. Whitlock and Siskind (1980) studied 30 MS patients and 30 neurologically disabled controls using the Beck Depressive Mood Inventory, and found more depression in MS patients both before and after the onset of neurological symptoms. The degree of depression was not related to the duration of illness. A recent prospective, controlled study (Dalos et al, 1983) used the General Health Questionnaire as a nonspecific measure of emotional distress, and found that the degree of emotional disturbance was associated with the course of disease activity. The prevalence of emotional distress was 90 percent in progressing MS, and 39 percent in stable patients. The test scores were not related to age, gender, duration or severity of neurologic symptoms. To further address the question of whether the depression was a result of the physical disability or a symptom of the disease process itself, Schiffer et al (1983) compared 15 MS patients with primarily cerebral involvement with a group of 15 patients with cerebellar and spinal cord involvement, matched for age, duration and disability. This was a retrospective study of neuropsychiatric test results. There was more major depression and more depressed mood in the group with primary cerebral involvement. The authors interpreted this to mean that depression in MS may be related to subcortical cerebral demyelination itself. In further support of this concept, there have been at least four reports of patients who had severe depression before the onset of neurologic symptoms (O'Malley, 1966; Mur et al, 1966; Young et al, 1976; Goodstein and Farrell, 1977). Furthermore, the depression reported by Whitlock and Siskind (1980) had other "classic" symptoms of depression, such as guilt, suicidal thoughts, diurnal mood changes and vegetative symptoms. A major complication of depression in MS is the potential for suicide; a rate 14 times higher than that for the general population was reported in one large study from South Africa (Kahana et al, 1971).

Surridge (1969) confirmed the earlier reports of increased euphoria in MS in a study of 108 patients. The euphoria was associated with more disability and incontinence. There have been at least three case reports of MS associated with mania (Cremieux et al, 1959; Mapelli and Ramelli, 1981; Peselow et al, 1981).

It is possible that CNS lesions in varying locations could give rise to different psychiatric presentations. Moreover, it is at least hypothetically possible that psychiatric syndromes, even when they appear without neurological symptoms, could represent exacerbations of the underlying disease process.

OTHER PSYCHIATRIC SYMPTOMS. Davison and Bagley (1969) provided a comprehensive review of psychosis in patients with MS. They summarized 39 reports by 26 authors, and concluded that the coexistence of schizophrenia-like psychoses and MS was no greater than that due to chance alone. This seems to be in agreement with Surridge (1969), who reported only one case with schizophrenia-like symptoms in his 108 patients.

The other major psychiatric question regarding MS is whether a certain personality type is more prone to develop the disease. This relates to the concept of "personality bias," namely, patients develop specific diseases relating to their premorbid personality. Langworthy (1948) held that poor premorbid adjustment led to multiple sclerosis. Most of the studies addressing this issue have used the MMPI as a measurement tool, but at least two authors have warned against interpreting MMPI data in nonpsychiatric patients (Wilson et al, 1982a; Marsh et al, 1982). Warren et al (1982) conducted a controlled study of 100 MS patients and found no difference between MS patients and controls in happiness in childhood or premorbid reactions to life's problems. Interestingly, the investigators did find a greater number of stressful life events in the MS patients in the two years prior to onset. It is certainly hypothetically possible that stress immunologically precipitates an exacerbation of the disease process.

Leukodystrophies

The leukodystrophies are a group of heritable, progressive degenerations of cerebral white matter. Metachromatic leukodystrophy (MLD) is a metabolic disorder caused by a deficiency of the enzyme arylsulfatase A, resulting in an accumulation of sulfatide in myelin and a degeneration of the affected areas. There is demyelination and axonal loss in the basal ganglia and cerebellum, as well as in the cerebral hemispheres, brainstem and spinal cord. In Sweden the incidence is 1/40,000 births (MacFaul et al, 1982). There is no treatment, and the diagnosis is made on the basis of metachromasia in the urine, increased urinary excretion of sulfatide, and low levels of the enzyme itself in urine or leukocyte cultures. A peripheral nerve biopsy is the most definitive confirmation of the diagnosis which may be suspected on clinical grounds, abnormal evoked potentials, and/or white matter destruction on CT (Scully et al, 1984).

MLD has at least three forms: infantile, juvenile, and adult. A recent review of the juvenile form (Haltia et al, 1980) described an onset from five to 20 years of age with motor and intellectual dysfunction. Clumsiness, tremor and speech dysfunction were early manifestations, followed by progressive motor and intellectual impairment. A recent survey of 18 state hospital patients who had not responded to neuroleptics revealed three patients (17 percent) with increased urinary sulfatide excretion and decreased leukocyte arylsulfatase A (Mahon-Haft et al, 1981). This study suggests that MLD might be more common than recognized in psychiatric patients, and that the diagnosis particularly should be considered in patients with a family history suggestive of the disorder.

Two other forms of leukodystrophy are adrenoleukodystrophy and Krabbe's disease. Adrenoleukodystrophy (Schilder's or Schaumberg's disease) is an enzymatic disorder of myelin that presents with Addison's disease (adrenal insufficiency), dementia and motor symptoms. Krabbe's disease is primarily confined to infancy and is caused by a decreased amount of galactosylceramidase. An interesting report (Christomanou et al, 1981) demonstrated lower full scale IQs in heterozygous, nonaffected carriers of Krabbe's disease than in seven noncarriers from the same family.

IMPLICATIONS FOR PSYCHIATRY

Clinical Implications

There are several clinical implications that derive from this consideration of movement disorders:

1). Many of the movement disorders considered here may present with psychiatric manifestations either alone or as the primary symptoms; it is, therefore, necessary for psychiatrists to consider these disorders in their differential diagnoses.
2). When consulting on a patient with a movement disorder, it is not always correct to assume that psychiatric symptoms are a "normal reaction" to the primary illness or treatment. The psychiatric symptoms may be as much a result of the primary lesion as the movement disorder, and deserving of specific treatment.
3). Treatment planning for movement disorder patients should include careful assessment of their intellectual functioning, because directly addressing organic intellectual impairments may well facilitate rehabilitation (Hamilton et al, 1983).
4). The clinician should bear in mind the possibility that pharmacotherapy for a movement disorder might aggravate psychiatric symptoms (for example,

L–dopa induced psychosis), or vice versa (for example, neuroleptic induced dyskinesia).

5). Finally, a study of neuropsychiatric aspects of movement disorders and demyelinating diseases illustrates the fallacy of body-mind dichotomy. We cannot but agree heartily with Charles Burr: "It is incorrect to divide off insanity arbitrarily as a thing to be studied apart from other diseases. There is no doubt that if we studied the mental conditions of physically ill persons with the same care as we study their physical symptoms, much would be learned which would throw light on psychiatry" (Burr, 1908).

Further Understanding of Psychiatric Disorders

Study of movement disorders may help improve our understanding of the pathophysiology of certain psychiatric illnesses. Wertheimer (1957) expressed this view in her paper on "rheumatic" schizophrenia:

> It should be emphasized that there is no reason to believe, from the present data, that rheumatic fever is related to all, or even to a large portion of all, the cases diagnosed as schizophrenia. However, if rheumatic fever can be validly implicated in even a portion of cases, it does suggest new directions for therapy and prevention. Perhaps equally important, if any group within the present "wastebasket" category of schizophrenia can be legitimately separated out on the basis of etiology, such separation would simplify the study of the remaining cases.

"LOCALIZATION" OF CEREBRAL FUNCTIONS. Traditionally, the concept has been that the cerebral cortex is the site of "the higher mental functions," and that the basal ganglia, cerebellum, and other "subcortical" structures have to do with motor control. This view is overly simplistic. With the explosion of information in the basic and clinical neurosciences, the scientist and the philosopher of the mind should be willing to let go of even the most "generally accepted" conceptual models of how the brain works.

PSYCHIATRIC DIAGNOSIS. The study by Caine et al (1983), which demonstrated almost the complete range of *DSM-III* diagnoses in patients with Huntington's disease—a disease with a *single* etiology—should provide psychiatric diagnosticians with some food for thought. This is not a new lesson, since neurosyphilis has long been called the "great imitator." Moreover, Parkinson's disease is an example of a single syndrome with multiple etiologies. The classic concept of one cause–one disease does not apply to a number of neuropsychiatric disorders. Symptoms or even symptom clusters may not necessarily suggest a specific etiology. The term "diagnosis" literally means "seeing through." Psychiatric manifestations alone may not be enough to make a diagnosis in the sense of seeing through the etiopathology of that disorder. One possible alternative would be further studies using biological markers as the independent variable for psychiatric syndrome classification.

REFERENCES

Adams RD, Victor M: Principles of Neurology. New York, McGraw-Hill, 1977

Albert ML, Feldman RG, Willis AL: The 'subcortical dementia' of progressive supranuclear palsy. J Neurol Neurosurg Psychiatry 37:121-130, 1974

Aronin N, Cooper PE, Lorenz LJ, et al: Somatostatin is increased in the basal ganglia in Huntington's disease. Ann Neurol 13:519-526, 1983

Barnes CD: The basal ganglion in extrapyramidal dysfunction. Brain Res Bull 11:271-275, 1983

Benson DF: Subcortical dementia: a clinical approach, in The Dementias. Edited by Mayeux R, Rosen WG. New York, Raven Press, 1983

Bergin JD: Rapidly progressing dementia in disseminated sclerosis. J Neurol Neurosurg Psychiatry 20:285-292, 1957

Berkson G, Mason WA, Saxon SV: Situation and stimulus effects on sterotyped behaviors of chimpanzees. J Comp Psychol 56:786, 1963

Bertrando P, Maffei C, Ghezzi A: A study of neuropsychological alterations on multiple sclerosis. Acta Psychiatry Belg 83:13-21, 1983

Bleuler EP: Textbook of Psychiatry. New York, Dover, 1950

Bird MT, Palkes H, Prensky AL: A follow-up study of Sydenham's chorea. Neurology 26:601-606, 1976

Boller F, Mizutani T, Roessmann U, et al: Parkinson disease, dementia, and Alzheimer disease: clinicopathological correlations. Ann Neurol 7:329-335, 1980

Bonnet KA: Neurobiological dissection of Tourette Syndrome: a neurochemical focus on a human neuroanatomical model, in Advances in Neurology, vol. 35, Gilles de la Tourette Syndrome. Edited by Friedhoff AJ, Chase TN. New York, Raven Press, 1982

Bowman M, Lewis MS: Sites of subcortical damage in diseases which resemble schizophrenia. Neuropsychologia 18:597-601, 1980

Braceland FJ, Griffin ME: The mental changes associated with multiple sclerosis. Research Association for Research in Nervous and Mental Disease 28:450-455, 1980

Brain L, Walton JN: Brain's Diseases of the Nervous System, 7th ed. New York, Oxford University Press, 1969

Bruetsch WL: Chronic rheumatic brain disease as a possible factor in the causation of some cases of dementia praecox. Am J Psychiatry 97:276-296, 1940

Bruetsch WL: Late cerebral sequelae of rheumatic fever. Arch Intern Med 73:472-476, 1944

Buck SH, Yamamura HI: Neuropeptides in normal and pathological basal ganglia, in Advances in Neurology, vol. 35, Gilles de la Tourette Syndrome. Edited by Friedhoff AJ, Chase TN. New York, Raven Pess, 1982

Burr CW: The mental state in chorea and choreiform affections. J Nerv Ment Dis 35:353-364, 1908

Bustany P, Henry JF, de Rotrov J: Local cerebral metabolite rate of ^{11}C–L–Methionine in early stages of dementia, schizophrenia, Parkinson's disease. Journal of Cerebral Blood Flow and Metabolism 3 (Suppl 1):S492-S493, 1983

Caine ED, Schoulson I: Psychiatric syndromes in Huntington's disease. Am J Psychiatry 140:728-733, 1983

Caine ED, Polinsky RJ, Ludlon CL, et al: Heterogeneity and variability in Tourette syndrome, in Advances in Neurology, vol. 35, Gilles de la Tourette Syndrome. Edited by Friedhoff AJ, Chase TN. New York, Raven Press, 1982

Calne DB, Langston JW: Aetiology of Parkinson's disease. Lancet 2:1457-1459, 1983

Canter AH: Direct and indirect measures of psychological deficit in multiple sclerosis. J Gen Psychol 44:3-50, 1951

Casey D: Spontaneous dyskinesias, in Neuropsychiatric Movement Disorders. Edited by Jeste DV and Wyatt RJ. Washington, D.C., American Psychiatric Press, 1984

Celesia GC, Wanamaker WM: Psychiatric disturbances in Parkinson's disease. Diseases of the Nervous System 33:577-583, 1972

Chase TN, Wexler NS, Barbeau A (Eds): Advances in Neurology, vol. 23, Huntington's Disease. New York, Raven Press, 1979

Chouinard G, Jones BD: Neuroleptic-induced supersensitivity psychosis: clinical and pharmacologic characteristics. Am J Psychiatry 137:16-21, 1980

Chozick BS: The behavioral effects of lesions of the corpus striatum: a review. Int J Neurosci 19:143-160, 1983

Christomanou H, Jaffe S, Martinus J, et al: Biochemical, genetic, psychometric, and neuropsychological studies in heterozygotes of family with globoid cell leukodystrophy (Krabbe's Disease). Hum Genet 58:179-183, 1981

Coffman JA, Mefferd J, Golden CJ, et al: Cerebellar atrophy in chronic schizophrenia (Letter to editor). Lancet 1:666, 1981

Cohen D: Gilles de la Tourette's syndrome, in Neuropsychiatric Movement Disorders. Edited by Jeste DV and Wyatt RJ. Washington, D.C., American Psychiatric Press, 1984

Crow TJ: Is schizophrenia an infectious disease? Lancet 1:173-175, 1983

Crow TJ, Johnstone EC, McClelland HA: The coincidence of schizophrenia and parkinsonism: some neurochemical implications. Psychol Med 6:227-233, 1976

Cremieux A, Alliez J, Tonga M, et al: Sclerose en plaques debut par troubles mentaux: etude anatomo-clinique. Rev Neurol (Paris) 101:45-51, 1959

Cummings JL, Gosenfeld LF, Houlihan JP, et al: Neuropsychiatric disturbance associated with idiopathic calcification of the basal ganglia. Biol Psychiatry 18:591-601, 1983

Cutler NR, Post RM: State-related cyclical dyskinesia in manic-depressive illness. J Clin Psychopharmacol 2:350-354, 1982

Dalos NP, Rabins PV, Brooks BR, et al: Disease activity and emotional state in multiple sclerosis. Ann Neurol 13:573-577, 1983

Davison K, Bagley CR: Schizophrenia-like psychoses associated with organic disorders of the central nervous system: review of the literature, in Current Problems in Neuropsychiatry. Edited by Herrington RN. Kent, England, Headley Brothers, 1969

Degkwitz R: Extrapyramidal motor disorders following long-term treatment with neuroleptic drugs, in Psychotropic Drugs and Dysfunctions of the Basal Ganglia (US Public Health Service Publication No. 1938). Edited by Crane GE, Gardner JR Jr. Washington, U.S. Government Printing Office, 1969

Devinsky O: Nemoanatomy of Gilles de la Tourette's syndrome. Arch Neurol 40:508-514, 1983

Dewan MJ, Pandurangi AK, Lee SH: Cerebellar morphology in chronic schizophrenic patients: a controlled computed tomographic study. Psychiatry Res 10:97-103, 1983

Dobyns WB, Goldstein NP, Gordon H: Clinical spectrum of Wilson's disease (hepatolenticular degeneration). Mayo Clin Proc 54:35-42, 1979

Dooling EC, Schoene WC, Richardson EP: Hallervorden-Spatz syndrome. Arch Neurol 30:70-83, 1974

Dooling EC, Richardson EP, Davis KR: Computed tomography in Hallervorden-Spatz disease. Neurology 30:1128-1130, 1980

Dow RS: Some novel concepts of cerebellar pathology. Mt Sinai J Med (NY) 41:103-119, 1974

Dow RS, Moruzzi G: The Physiology and Pathology of the Cerebellum. Minneapolis, University of Minnesota Press, 1958

Duvoisin R, Eldridge R, Williams A, et al: Twin study of Parkinson disease. Neurology 31:77-80, 1981

Eldridge, R: The torsion dystonias: literature review and genetic and clinical studies. Neurology 20:1, 1970

Emson PC, Arregui A, Clement-Jones V, et al: Regional distribution of methionine enkephalin and substance P-like immunoreactivity in normal human brain and in Huntington's disease. Brain Res 199:147-160, 1980a

Emson PC, Rehfield JF, Langevin H, et al: Reduction in cholecystokinin-like immunoreactivity in the basal ganglia in Huntington's disease. Brain Res 198:497-500, 1980b

Feinberg I: Schizophrenia: caused by a fault in programmed synaptic elimination during adolescence? J Psychiat Res 17:319-334, 1982/83

Fernando SJM: Six cases of Gilles de la Tourette's syndrome. Br J Psychiatry 128:436-441, 1976

Fisher JM, Kennedy JL, Caine ED, et al: Dementia in Huntington's disease, in Advances in Neurology, vol. 38, The Dementias. Edited by Mayeux R, Rosen WG. New York, Raven Press, 1983

Flak WE, Mahnke MD, Paskanzer MD: Lithium prophylaxis of corticotrophin induced psychosis. JAMA 241:1011-1012, 1979

Flor-Henry P, Fromm-Auch D, Tapper M, et al: A neuropsychological study of the stable syndrome of hysteria. Biol Psychiatry 16:601-626, 1981

Francis FA: Familial basal ganglia calcification and schizophreniform psychosis. Br J Psychiatry 135:360-362, 1979

Freed WJ: Functional brain tissue transplantation: reversal of lesion-induced rotation by intraventricular substantia nigra and adrenal medulla grafts, with a note on intracranial retinal grafts. Biol Psychiatry 18:1205-1267, 1983

Freeman JM, Aron AM, Colland JE, et al: The emotional correlates of Sydenham's chorea. Pediatrics 35:42-49, 1965

Friedhoff AJ, Chase TN: Advances in Neurology, vol. 35, Gilles de la Tourette Syndrome. New York, Raven Press, 1982

Garnett ES, Firnau G, Nahmias C: Dopamine visualized in the basal ganglia of living man. Nature 305:137-138, 1983

Glazer WM, Moore DC, Schooler NR, et al: Tardive dyskinesia: a discontinuation study. Arch Gen Psychiatry 41:623-627, 1984

Globus M, Mildorf B, Melamed E: rCBF changes in Parkinson's disease: correlation with dementia. Journal of Cerebral Blood Flow and Metabolism 3(Suppl. 1):S508-S509, 1983

Goggans FC, Weisberg LJ, Koran LM: Lithium prophylaxis of predonisone psychosis. J Clin Psychiatry 44:111-112, 1983

Goodstein RK, Farrell RB: Multiple sclerosis presenting as a depressive illness. Diseases of the Nervous System 38:127-131, 1977

Goodwin FK, Murphy DL, Brodie HKH, et al: L-DOPA, catecholamines, and behavior: a clinical and biochemical study in depressed patients. Biol Psychiatry 2:341-366, 1970

Graybiel AM, Ragsdale CW Jr: Fiber connections of the basal ganglia. Prog Brain Res 51:239-283, 1979

Grinber RR, Sahs AL: Neurology, 6th ed. Springfield, Illinois, Charles C Thomas, 1966

Gusella JF, Wexler NS, Conneally PM, et al: A polymorphic DNA marker genetically linked to Huntington's disease. Nature 306:234-239, 1983

Guttman E: On some constitutional aspects of chorea and on its sequelae. Journal of Neurology and Psychopathology 17:16, 1936

Hakim AM, Mathieson G: Basis of dementia in Parkinson's disease. Lancet 2:729, 1978

Haltia T, Palo J, Haltia M, et al: Juvenile metachromatic leukodystrophy: clinical biochemical, and neuropathologic studies in nine new cases. Arch Neurol 37:42-46, 1980

Hamilton NG, Frick RB, Takahashi T, et al: Psychiatric symptoms and cerebellar pathology. Am J Psychiatry 140:1322-1326, 1983

Hawkins RA, Phelps ME, Mazziotta JC, et al: A study of Wilson's disease with F-18 FDG and positron tomography. Journal of Cerebral Blood Flow Metab 3 (Suppl 1):S498-S499, 1983

Heath RG, Franklin DE, Shraberg D: Gross pathology of the cerebellum in patients diagnosed and treated as functional psychiatric disorders. J Nerv Ment Dis 167:585-592, 1979

Heath RG, Franklin DE, Walker CF, et al: Cerebellar vermal atrophy in psychiatric patients. Biol Psychiatry 17:569-583, 1982

Heimer L: The Human Brain and Spinal Cord. New York, Springer-Verlag, 1983

Hippius M, Lange J: Zur problematik der spaten extrapyramidalen hyperkinesen nach Langfristiger neuroleptischer Therapie. Arzneimittel-Forschung 20:888-890, 1970

Hollister LE, Glazener FS: Concurrent paralysis agitans and schizophrenia. Dis Nerv Syst 22:188-189,1961

Horn S: Some psychological factors in parkinsonism. J Neurol Neurosurg Psychiatry 37:27-31,1974

Hornykiewicz O: Biochemical determinants of Parkinson's disease, in Handbook of Biological Psychiatry, Part IV. Edited by Van Praag H. New York, Marcel Dekker, 1981

Humphrey DR: Cortocospinal systems and their control by premotor cortex, basal ganglia, and cerebellum, in The Clinical Neurosciences, Neurobiology. Edited by Rosenberg RN, Willis WD. New York, Churchill Livingston, 1983

Husby G, Van de Rign I, Zabriskie JB, et al: Antibodies reacting with cytoplasm of subthalamic and caudate nuclei neurons in chorea and acute rheumatic fever. J Exper Med 144:1094-1110, 1976

Husby G, Van de Rign I, Zabriskie JB, et al: Antineuronal antibody in Sydenham's chorea. Lancel 1:1028, 1977

Incagnoli T, Kane R: Neuropsychological functioning in Gilles de la Tourette's syndrome. J Clin Neuropsychol 3:165-169, 1981

Insel TR, Murphy DL: The psychopharmacological treatment of obsessive-compulsive disorder: a review. J Clin Psychopharmacol 1:304-311, 1981

Insel TR, Pickar D: Naloxone administration in obsessive-compulsive disorders: report of two cases. Am J Psychiatry 140:1219-1220, 1983

Insel TR, Gillin JC, Moore A, et al: The sleep of patients with obsessive-compulsive disorder. Arch Gen Psychiatry 39:1372-1377, 1982a

Insel, TR, Kalin NH, Guttmacher LB, et al: The dexamethasone suppression test in patients with primary obsessive-compulsive disorder. Psychiatry Res 6:153-160, 1982b

Insel TR, Donnelly EF, Lalakea ML: Neurological and neuropsychological studies of patients with obsessive-compulsive disorder. Biol Psychiatry 18:741-751, 1983a

Insel TR, Murphy DL, Cohen RM, et al: Obsessive-compulsive disorder: a double-blind trial of clomipramine and clorgyline. Arch Gen Psychiatry 40:605-612, 1983b

Invnik RJ: Neuropsychological stability in multiple sclerosis. J Consult Clin Psychol 46:913-923, 1978a

Invnik RJ: Neuropsychological test performance as a function of duration of multiple sclerosis-related symptomatology. J Clin Psychol 39:304-307, 311-331, 1978b

Jankovic J, Ford J: Blepharospasm and orofacial-cervical dystonia: clinical and pharmacological findings in 100 patients. Ann Neurol 13:402-411, 1983

Jenike MA: Obsessive compulsive disorder. Compr Psychiatry 24:94-115, 1983

Jenike MA, Surman OS, Cassem NH, et al: Monoamine oxidase inhibitors in obsessive-compulsive disorder. J Clin Psychiatry 44:131-132, 1983

Jeste DV, Wyatt, RJ: Understanding and Treating Tardive Dyskinesia. New York, The Guilford Press, 1982

Jeste DV, Barban L, Parisi J: Reduced cerebellar Purkinje cell density in Huntington's disease. Exp Neurol 85:78-86, 1984a

Jeste DV, Karson CN, Wyatt RJ: Movement disorders and psychopathology, in Neuropsychiatric Movement Disorders. Edited by Jeste DV, Wyatt RJ, Washington, American Psychiatric Press, 1984b

Joschko M, Rourke BP: Neuropsychological dimensions of Tourette syndrome: test-retest stability and implications for intervention, in Advances in Neurology, vol. 35, Gilles de la Tourette Syndrome. Edited by Friedhoff AJ, Chase TN. New York, Raven Press, 1982

Kahana E, Liebowitz U, Alter M: Cerebral multiple sclerosis. Neurology 21:1170-1176, 1971

Kahl D, Phelps M, Mankham C, et al: Local cerebral glucose metabolism in Huntington's disease determined by emission computed tomography of 18F-fluorodeoxyglucose. Journal of Cerebral Blood Flow and Metabolism 1:S459, 1981

Kan AE: Striatonigral degeneration. Pathology 10:45-52, 1978

Kane JM: Tardive dyskinesia, in Neuropsychiatric Movement Disorders. Edited by Jeste DV, Wyatt RJ. Washington, American Psychiatric Press, 1984

Keeler WR, Bender L: A follow-up study of children with behavior disorder and Sydenham's chorea. Am J Psychiatry 109:421-428, 1952

Kelman DH: Gilles de la Tourette's disease in children: a review of the literature. J Child Psychol 6:219-226, 1965

Kendall BE, Pollock SS, Bass NM, et al: Wilson's disease—clinical correlation with cranial computed tomography. Neuroradiology 22:1-5, 1981

Kirschbaum WR: Jakob-Creutzfeldt Disease. New York, American Elsevier Publishing Company, Inc, 1968

Knesevich JW: Successful treatment of obsessive-compulsive disorder with clonidine hydrochloride. Am J Psychiatry 139:364-365, 1982

Koenig H: Dementia associated with multiple sclerosis. Trans Am Neurol Assoc 93:227-228, 1968

Konig P, Haller R: Initial psychopathological alterations in Fahr's syndrome: a preliminary report. Biol Psychiatry 17:449-453, 1982

Kosaka K, Iizuka R, Mizutani Y, et al: Striatonigral degeneration combined with Alzheimer's disease. Acta Neuropathol (Berl) 54:253-256, 1981

Kraepelin E: Dementia Praecox and Paraphrenia. Edinburgh, Livingstone, 1919

Laitinen L: Desipramine in treatment of Parkinson's Disease, Third Symposium on Parkinson's Disease 1968

Langston JW, Ballard P, Tetrud JW, et al: Chronic parkinsonism in humans due to a product of meperidine-analog synthesis. Science 219:974-980, 1983

Langworthy OR: Relation of personality problems to onset and progress of multiple sclerosis. Arch Neurol Psychiatry 59:13-28, 1948

Lazare A: Conversion symptoms. N Engl J Med 305:745-748, 1981

Leenders K, Wolfson L, Gibbs J: Regional cerebral blood flow and oxygen metabolism in Parkinson's disease and their response to L-Dopa. Journal of Cerebral Blood Flow and Metabolism 3 (Suppl 1):S488-S489, 1983

Levinson HN: A Solution to the Riddle Dyslexia. New York, Springer-Verlag, 1980

Lewis A, Minski L: Chorea and psychosis. Lancet 1:536-538, 1935

Lidsky TI, Weinhold PM, Levine FM: Implications of basal ganglionic dysfunction for schizophrenia. Biol Psychiatry 14:3-12, 1979

Lieberman A, Dziatolowski M, Kupersmith M, et al: Dementia in Parkinson's disease. Ann Neurol 6:355-359, 1979a

Lieberman A, Dziatolowski M, Neophytides A, et al: Dementias of Huntington's and Parkinson's disease, in Advances in Neurology, vol. 23. Edited by Chase TN, Wexler NS, Barbeau A. New York, Raven Press, 1979b

Lippman S, Manshadi M, Baldwin H, et al: Cerebellar vermis dimensions on computerized tomographic scans of schizophrenic and bipolar patients. Am J Psychiatry 139:667-668, 1982

Mahon-Haft H, Stone RK, Johnson R, et al: Biochemical abnormalities of metachromatic leukodystrophy in an adult psychiatric population. Am J Psychiatry 138:1372-1374, 1981

Mapelli G, Ramelli E: Manic syndrome associated with multiple sclerosis: secondary mania? Acta Psychiatr Belg 81:337-349, 1981

Marsden CD: Basal ganglia disease. Lancel 2:1141-1146, 1982a

Marsden CD: The mysterious motor function of the basal ganglia: the Robert Wartenberg lecture. Neurology 32:514-539, 1982b

Marsden CO: Blepharospasm-oromandibular dystonia syndrome (Brueghel's syndrome): a variant of adult-onset torsion dystonia? J Neurol Neurosurg Psychiatry 39:1204, 1976

Marsh GG, Markham CH: Does levodopa alter depression and psychopathology in parkinsonism patients? J Neurol Neurosurg Psychiatry 36:925-935, 1973

Marsh GG, Hirsch SH, Leung G: Use or Misuse of the MMPI in multiple sclerosis. Psychol Rep 51:1127-1134, 1982

Martin JJ: Thalamic syndromes, in Handbook of Clinical Neurology, vol. 2. Edited by Vinken PJ, Bruyn GW. Amsterdam, North Holland, 1968

Mayeux R, Stern Y: Intellectual dysfunction and dementia in Parkinson's disease, in The Dementias. Edited by Mayeux R, Rosen WG. New York, Raven Press, 1983

Mayeux R, Stern Y, Rosen J, et al: Is "subcortical dementia" a recognizable clinical entity? Ann Neurol 14:278-283, 1983

Mehler WR: The basal ganglia–circa 1982: a review and commentary. Appl Neurophysiol 44:261-290, 1981

Mettler FA, Grandell A: Neurologic disorders in psychiatric institutions. J Nerv Ment Dis 128:148-154, 1959

Messiha FS, Carlson JC: Behavioral and clinical profiles of Tourette's disease: a comprehensive review. Brain Res Bull 11:195-204, 1983

McCormick DA, Thompson RF: Cerebellum: essential involvement in the classically conditioned eyelid response. Science 223:296-299, 1984

McFarlin DE, McFarland HF: Multiple sclerosis (First of two parts). N Engl J Med 307:1183-1188, 1983

McFaul R, Cavanagh N, Lake BD, et al: Metachromatic leukodystrophy: review of 28 cases. Archives of Disease in Childhood 57:168-175, 1982

McGeer PL, McGeer EG: Enzymes associated with the metabolism of catecholamines, acetylcholine and GABA in human controls and patients with Parkinson's disease and Huntington's chorea. J Neurochem 26:65-76, 1976

Mindham R: Psychiatric symptoms in Parkinsonism. J Neurol Neurosurg Psychiatry 33:188-191, 1970

Montgomery MA, Clayton PJ, Friedhoff AJ: Psychiatric illness in Tourette's syndrome patients and first-degree relatives, in Advances in Neurology, vol. 35, Gilles de la Tourette syndrome. Edited by Friedhoff AJ, Chase TN. New York, Raven Press, 1982

Morphew JA, Sim A: Gilles de la Tourette's syndrome: a clinical and psychopathological study. Br J Med Psychol 42:293-301, 1969

Morrison JR: Catatonia: retarded and excited types. Arch Gen Psychiatry 28:39-41, 1973

Moskovitz C, Moses H, Klawans HL: Levodopa-induced psychosis: a kindling phenomenon. Am J Psychiatry 135:669-675, 1978

Mur J, Kumpel G, Dostal S: An anergic phase of disseminated sclerosis with psychiatric course. Cofinia Neurologica 28:37-49, 1966

Nakamura Y: Familial neuroaxonal dystrophy with principal lesions of nigropallido-subthalamic degeneration. Folia Psychiatrica et Neurologia 36:151-162, 1982

Nasrallah HA, Jacoby CG, McCalley-Whittle M: Cerebellar atrophy in schizophrenia and mania (letter to editor). Lancet 1:1102, 1981

Nausieda PA, Grossman BJ, Koller WC, et al: Syndenham's chorea: an update. Neurology 30:331-334, 1980

Nauta WJH: Limbic innervation of the striatum, in Advances in Neurology, vol. 35, Gilles de la Tourette's Syndrome. Edited by Friedhoff AJ, Chase TN. New York, Raven Press, 1982

Nee LE, Caine ED, Polinsky RJ, et al: Gilles de la Tourette syndrome: clinical and family study of 50 cases. Ann Neurol 7:41-49, 1980

Olsson R, Roos BE: Concentration of 5-hydroxyindoleacetic acid and homovanillic acid in the cerebrospinal fluid after treatment with probenecid in patients with Parkinson's disease. Nature 219:502-503, 1968

O'Malley PP: Severe mental symptoms in disseminated sclerosis: a neuropathological study. J Irish Med Assoc 55:115-127, 1966

Pearce J: The extrapyramidal disorder of Alzheimer's disease. Eur Neurol 12:94-103, 1974

Peselow ED, Deutsch SI, Fieve RR, et al: Coexistant manic symptoms and multiple sclerosis. Psychosomatics 22:824-825, 1981

Peyser JM, Edwards KR, Poser CM: Psychological profiles in patients with multiple sclerosis. Arch Neurol 37:437-440, 1980a

Peyser JM, Edwards KR, Poser CM, et al: Cognitive function in patients with multiple sclerosis. Arch Neurol 37:577-579, 1980b

Pratt RTC: An investigation of the psychiatric aspects of disseminated sclerosis. J Neurol Neurosurg Psychiatry 14:326-335, 1951

Puite JK, Schut T, Van Praag HM, et al: Monoamine metabolism and depression in Parkinson's patients. Psychiatria, Neurologia, Neurochirurgia 76:61-70, 1973

Richardson EP: Neuropsychological studies of Tourette's syndrome in Advances of Neurology, vol. 35, Gilles de la Tourette's Syndrome. New York, Raven Press, 1982

Riklan M, Cullinan T, Cooper IS; Psychological studies in dystonia musculorum deformans, in Advances in Neurology, vol. 14. Edited by Eldridge R, Fahn S. New York, Raven Press, 1976

Robins AM: Depression in patients with parkinsonism. Br J Psychiatry 128:141-145, 1976

Roland PE, Meyer E, Shibasaki T, et al: Regional cerebral blood flow changes in cortex and basal ganglia during voluntary movements in normal human volunteers. J Neurophysiol 48:467-480, 1982

Ross AT, Reitan RM: Intellectual and affective functions in multiple sclerosis. Arch neurol Psychiatry 73:663-677, 1955

Sacks L, Feinstein AR, Taranta A: A controlled psychologic study of Sydenham's chorea. J Pediatrics 61:714-722, 1962

Salzman L, Thaler FH: Obsessive-compulsive disorders: a review of the literature. Am J Psychiatry 138:286-296, 1981

Schiffer RB, Caine ED, Bamford KA, et al: Depressive episodes in patients with multiple sclerosis. Am J Psychiatry 140:1498-1500, 1983

Schwartzman J: Chorea minor: review of 175 cases with reference to etiology, treatment and sequelae. Rheumatism, 1950

Schwartzman J, MacDonald DM, Perillo L: Sydenham's chorea. Archives of Pediatrics 65:6-24, 1948

Scully RE, Monk EJ, McNeely BU: Case records of the Massachusetts General Hospital. N Engl J Med 310:445-455, 1984

Serby M: Psychiatric issues in Parkinson's disease. Compr Psychiatry 21:317-322, 1980

Shapiro AM, Shapiro E, Brunn R, et al: Gilles de la Tourette's Syndrome. New York, Raven Press, 1978

Snider RS, Maiti A: Cerebellar contributions to the Papez circuit. J Neurosci Res 2:133-146, 1976

Speedie LJ, Heilman KM: Anterograde memory deficits for visuospatial material after infarction of the right thalamus. Arch Neurol 40:183-186, 1983

Sroka H, Elizan TS, Yahr MD, et al: Organic mental syndrome and confusional states in Parkinson's disease. Arch Neurol 38:339-342, 1981

Staples D, Lincoln NB: Impairment in multiple sclerosis and its relation to functional abilities. Rheumatic Rehabil 18:153-160, 1979

Steele JC, Richardson JC, Olszewski J: Progressive supranuclear palsy. Arch Neurol 10:333-359, 1964

Stehbens JA, Macqueen JC: The psychological adjustment of rheumatic fever patients with and without chorea. Clin Pediatr 11:638-640, 1972

Stern SL, Hurtig HI, Mendels J, et al: Psychiatric illness in relatives of patients with Parkinson's disease: a preliminary report. Am J Psychiatry 134:443-444, 1977

Stern Y: Behavior and the basal ganglia, in The Dementias. Edited by Mayeux R, Rosen WG. New York, Raven Press, 1983

Stollerman GH: Rheumatic fever, in Principles of Internal Medicine. Edited by Petersdorf RG, Adams AD, Brauwald E, et al. New York, McGraw-Hill, 1983

Surridge D: An investigation into some psychiatric aspects of multiple sclerosis. Br J Psychiatry 155:749-764, 1969

Sutherland RJ, Kolb B, Schoel WM: Neuropsychological assessment of children and adults with Tourette's syndrome: a comparison with learning disabilities and schizophrenia, in Advances in Neurology, vol. 35, Gilles de la Tourette's Syndrome. Edited by Friedhoff AJ, Chase TN. New York, Raven Press, 1982

Sweet RD, Solomon GF, Wayne HL: Neurological features of Gilles de la Tourette's Syndrome. J Neurol Neurosurg Psychiatry 36:1-9, 1973

Sweet RD, McDowell FH, Fergenson JS, et al: Mental symptoms in Parkinson's disease during chronic treatment with levodopa. Neurology 26:305-310, 1976

Taranta A: Relation of isolated recurrences of Sydenham's chorea to preceding streptococcal infections. N Engl J Med 260:1204-1210, 1959

Taranta A, Stollerman GH: The relationship of Sydenham's chorea to infection with group A streptococci. Am J Med 20:170-175, 1956

Thiebaut F: Sydenham's chorea, in Handbook of Neurology, vol. 6. Edited by Vinken PJ, Bruyn GW. New York, American Elsevier, 1968

Tolosa ES: Clinical features of Meige's disease (idiopathic orofacial dystonia): a report of 17 cases. Arch Neurol 38:147-151, 1981

Traub RD: Recent data and hypotheses on Creutzfeld-Jakob Disease, in Advances in Neurology, vol. 38, The Dementias. Edited by Mayeux R, Rosen WG. New York, Raven Press, 1983

Trimble MR, Grant I: Psychiatric aspects of multiple sclerosis, in Psychiatric Aspects of Neurologic Disease, vol. 2. Edited by Benson DF, Blumer D. New York, Grune and Stratton, 1982

Vicedomini JP, Isaac WL, Nonneman AJ: Role of the caudate nucleus in recovery from neonatal mediofrontal cortex lesion in the rat. Dev Psychobiol 17:51-65, 1984

Waksman BH: Immunity and the nervous system: basic tenets. Ann Neurol 13:587-591, 1983

Wallesch CW, Kornhuber HH, Kunz T, et al: Neuropsychological deficits associated with small unilateral thalamic lesions. Brain 106:141-152, 1983

Warburton JW: Depressive symptoms in Parkinson's patients referred for thalomotomy. J Neurol Neurosurg Psychiatry 30:368-370, 1967

Warren S, Greenhill S, Warren KG: Emotional stress and the development of multiple sclerosis; case-control evidence of a relationship. J Chronic Dis 35:821-831, 1982

Watson PJ: Non-motor functions of the cerebellum. Psychol Bull 85:944-967, 1978

Weinberger DR, Torrey EF, Wyatt RJ: Cerebellar atrophy in chronic schizophrenia. Lancet 1:718-719, 1979

Weiner WJ, Bergun D: Prevention and management of the side effects of levodopa, in Clinical Neuropharmacology, vol. 2. Edited by Klawans HL. New York, Raven Press, 1977

Wertheimer NM: The differential incidence of rheumatic fever in the histories of paranoid and non-paranoid schizophrenics. J Nerv Ment Dis 125:637-641, 1957

Wertheimer NM: "Rheumatic" schizophrenia. Arch Gen Psychiatry 4:579-596, 1961

Wertheimer NM: A psychiatric follow-up of children with rheumatic fever and other chronic diseases. J Chronic Dis 16:223-237, 1963

Whitlock FA, Siskind MM: Depression as a major symptom of multiple sclerosis. J Neurol Neurosurg Psychiatry 43:861-865, 1980

Williams FJB, Walshe JM: Wilson's disease: an analysis of the cranial computerized tomographic appearances found in 60 patients and the changes in response to treatment with chelating agents. Brain 104:735-752, 1981

Willner P: Dopamine and depression: a review of recent evidence. Brain Res Rev 6:211-224, 1983

Wilson H, Olson WH, Gascon GG, et al: Personality characteristics and multiple sclerosis. Psychol Rep 51:791-806, 1982

Wilson RS, Garron DC, Tanner CM, et al: Behavior disturbance in children with Tourette's syndrome, in Advances in Neurology, vol. 35, Gilles de la Tourette's Syndrome. Edited by Friedhoff AJ, Chase TN. New York, Raven Press, 1982

Winokur A, Dugan J, Mendels J, et al: Psychiatric illness in relatives of patients with Parkinson's disease: an expanded survey. Am J Psychiatry 135:854-855, 1978

Young AC, Saunders J, Ponsford JR: Mental change as an early feature of multiple sclerosis. J Neurol Neurosurg Psychiatry 39:1008-1013, 1976

Yung CY: Clinical features of movement disorders. Brain Res Bull 11:167-171, 1983a

Yung CY: Evaluation and differential diagnosis of movement disorders: a flow chart approach. Brain Res Bull 11:149-152, 1983b

This chapter was written by the authors in their private capacities. No official support or endorsement by NIMH is intended or should be inferred.

Chapter 10

Interictal Behavioral Changes in Patients With Temporal Lobe Epilepsy

by David Bear, M.D., Roy Freeman, M.D., David Schiff, B.A. and Mark Greenberg, Ph.D.

The issue of behavioral changes in patients with temporal lobe epilepsy is important for several reasons. Temporal lobe epilepsy is a common illness—the most frequent form of epilepsy in adults—with a prevalence of roughly three per 1,000. According to some estimates, 30 to 40 percent of patients experience persistent psychiatric symptoms, which often become the most incapacitating aspect of the illness (Blumer and Benson, 1982; Lishman, 1978). Moreover, temporal lobe epilepsy may serve as a valuable model illness in neuropsychiatry by allowing a direct correlation between localized, electrical dysfunction within the limbic structures of the temporal lobe and specific features of human emotion, cognition, and personality (Bear, 1979d).

It would be an error to dismiss the careful documentation of behavioral symptoms in many patients with temporal lobe epilepsy. In fact, much apparent controversy has no bearing on the reality of behavioral changes per se, but on independent, secondary, and often confused issues: the frequency of such changes among temporal lobe epileptics; the specificity of these behavioral changes to this neurological illness; or the differentiation of particular behavioral features from those of idiopathic psychiatric syndromes.

Some confusion regarding behavioral observations centers upon a failure to distinguish ictal (seizure-like) from interictal events. For example, it has sometimes been assumed that, if behavior were affected by a limbic epileptic focus, the alterations would take the form of brief, episodic, paroxysmal activation of basic biological drives such as sex or aggression; following these ictal perturbations in behavior, the patient would revert to an unremarkable interictal personality. However, the facts show that this is not the case. During the ictal period, the limbic functions of drive activation and memory are most commonly *inhibited*, as suggested by the terms absence, automatism, or psychoparesis (Bear, 1979c). In contrast, the interictal emotional state is generally characterized by an *intensification* of affective responses. This intensification forms the basis of the majority of behavioral features to be described (Bear, 1979c), (Bear and Fedio, 1977), Waxman and Geschwind, 1975).

The deepening of affect may lead to characteristic features of interictal behavior, but many of these traits—such as an interest in cosmic issues or a tendency to write extensively—need not constitute psychopathology as defined by *DSM-III*. Many commentaries on "interictal psychopathology" in temporal lobe epilepsy erroneously equate specific behavior patterns with psychopathology, as measured by psychological tests or reflected in admission to psychiatric hospitals.

In this chapter, through the use of case examples, we attempt to provide a picture of interictal behavioral changes without the attribution of pathological diagnostic labels. These behavioral observations include: changes in physiological drives such as sexuality and aggression; changes in emotional and intellectual behavior, including circumstantiality, religious or philosophical interests, interpersonal viscosity, and hypergraphia; psychosis (Davidson and Bagley, 1969; Slater and Beard, 1963); and the rarer phenomena of prolonged dissociative states or multiple personality (Bear, 1979c; Davidson and Bagley, 1969; Lishman, 1978; Waxman and Geschwind, 1975). We will then summarize the neurological approach to the evaluation of the suspected temporal lobe epileptic. Following the presentation of these clinical features, we will consider unresolved issues related to the frequency, specificity, neural mechanism, and treatment of temporal lobe seizures.

INTERICTAL CHANGES IN PHYSIOLOGICAL DRIVES

Sexuality

The importance of the temporal lobes in mediating sexual behavior has been demonstrated by numerous investigations in humans and animals through stimulation and ablation studies (Kluver and Bucy, 1937; McLean, 1957). A wide range of sexual behaviors has been described during the ictal, interictal, and postictal periods in patients with temporal lobe epilepsy. Gastaut and Colomb (1954) drew attention to global hyposexuality occurring interictally in some temporal lobe epileptics. Their observations have been repeatedly confirmed in case reports and retrospective studies and include: lack of sexual interest and curiosity; absence of sexual dreams and fantasies; loss of libido; inability to experience orgasm; and dimunition in frequency of sexual intercourse or masturbation (Blumer and Walker, 1967; Ellison, 1982; Jensen and Larsen, 1979a; Kolersky et al, 1967; Shukula et al, 1979; Taylor, 1969).

Other authors have drawn attention to the occurrence of impotence in temporal lobe epilepsy, although most patients have developed normal secondary sexual characteristics and remain capable of complete sexual arousal (Hierons and Saunders, 1966; Johnsen, 1965). An inverse relationship between temporal lobe epileptic activity and sexual behavior is suggested by the return of normal sexual behavior following control of seizures by medication or surgery (Ellison, 1982). This observation contradicts the view that hyposexuality in epileptic patients is an adverse effect of seizures medication. This inverse relationship is further supported by the occasional development of hypersexuality in the months following a temporal lobectomy and the return of hyposexuality if seizures recur (Blumer, 1970). The frequency of changes in sexual behavior may be underestimated because hyposexuality in the temporal lobe epileptic is often perceived as ego-syntonic (Blumer and Walker, 1967; Ellison, 1982). This is particularly likely when the epileptic focus has been present prior to development of secondary sexual characteristics.

Temporal lobe epilepsy has also been associated with sexual deviations and paraphillias in numerous case studies. Transvestism, transexualism, voyeurism, exhibitionism, fetishism, sadism, masochism, heterosexual and homosexual pederasty, and genital self-mutilation have all been reported (Ellison, 1982; Epstein, 1961; Hierons and Saunders, 1966; Hoerig and Kenna, 1979; Kolersy et al, 1967; Taylor, 1969). In an unselected sample, 11 of 49 male temporal lobe epileptic patients showed deviant sexual behavior. Many of these patients had suffered temporal lobe damage prior to one year of age (Kolersky et al, 1967).

Case 1: *Hyposexuality followed by sexual preference conflict with deepened emotions, circumstantiality, and hypergraphia.*

A 34–year–old man suffered febrile convulsions early in childhood. He was aware of interruptions of consciousness during elementary school, but these were attributed to daydreaming and never evaluated medically. As a college freshman he suffered his first generalized tonic-clonic convulsion. An electroencephalogram (EEG) revealed a right temporal lobe spike focus. While taking anticonvulsants, he continued to experience complex partial seizures, heralded by an aura of dread, followed by rotation of the head to the left and lip smacking.

This man was a professional writer whose productions were marked by endless recitation of seemingly peripheral details. For his initial medical evaluation, he prepared a 20-page "essay" summarizing childhood experiences for the physician; no detail was left unexamined.

Of particular note was his sexual development. He had acquired secondary sexual characteristics early in adolescence. Yet he had "absolutely no" interest in sexual matters and virtually no knowledge of sexual anatomy until his freshman year in college. This hyposexuality was not a matter of concern, for he "preferred platonic relationships" with both men and women throughout high school. The phenomenon of dating had been a curiosity to him.

Classmates in college ridiculed him for his sexual naivete. He thereupon commenced a "crash course" in sexuality, proposing liaisons with both women and men through advertisements in a local newspaper. He first consummated a relationship with a female prostitute but subsequently had multiple sexual relations with men. Eventually, he entered a continuing sexual and deeply emotional relationship with a woman 40 years his elder. Privately, he also experimented with cross-dressing followed by masturbation in front of his mirror. His mannerisms and vocal habits became effeminate.

On rare occasions the ictus itself may include complex motor automatisms such as masturbatory activity, pelvic thrusting, or exhibitionism, for which the patient is usually amnesic (Currier et al, 1971; Freeman and Mavis, 1969; Hooshmand and Bravley, 1969; Sperber et al, 1983). Somatosensory genital sensations as well as sexual arousal, erotic thoughts or orgasm are infrequent ictal experiences (Hooshmand and Bravley, 1969; Sperber et al, 1983).

In the immediate postictal period, inappropriate sexual behavior such as exhibitionism or unseemly sexual advances may occur, perhaps due to lack of inhibition and judgment occurring in a setting of confusion and amnesia. Blumer has also drawn attention to appropriate postictal sexual arousal in some patients, usually expressed with a receptive partner or through masturbation in a private environment without associated confusion or amnesia (Blumer, 1970).

Anger and Aggression

The temporal lobe epileptic frequently experiences intensified feelings of anger or irritability. Occurring in conjunction with humorlessness and a moralistic sense of right and wrong, this personality alteration often results in sanctimonious or self-righteous behavior.

Few issues are more emotionally and legally charged than the association of aggression with epilepsy. Complicating the subject is the fact that epidemiological studies of overt aggression among temporal lobe epileptics in the general population are hampered by semantic, reporting and recognition difficulties. Studies of selected groups with a high incidence of violence (such as incarcerated prisoners) must control for other factors, such as head trauma and malnutrition, which may coincidentally increase the incidence of epilepsy.

The issue has been confused still further by the failure to distinguish among three clearly different patterns of aggression that may occur in the epileptic patient: ictal, postictal, and interictal aggression (Devinsky and Bear, 1984). In a recently reported study, a panel of experts reviewed the histories of 5,400 patients and then examined videotapes of 33 epileptic attacks in 19 patients thought to display ictal violence. Using strict criteria, only 13 were felt to have incontestable epilepsy; of these, only seven were felt to demonstrate unequivocal violence as defined by the "directed exertion of extreme and aggressive physical force which, if unrestrained, would result in injury, destruction, or abuse." (Delgado-Escuetta et al, 1981) The aggressive actions included spitting, shouting, swearing, scratching, karate blows and the destruction of property, and all lasted less than one minute. In five cases the aggression was accompanied by an angry mood; the other two patients appeared frightened and confused. In all cases there was amnesia for the event. However, while emphasizing the rarity of ictal violence, this study failed to address postictal or interictal aggression (Devinsky and Bear, 1984).

Postictal irritability is a well-described clinical event; in fact, in the above-mentioned study (Delgado-Escuetta et al, 1981), two patients demonstrated this phenomenon, screaming wildly as they were restrained three to four minutes postictally. This behavior may resemble the agitation of the confused or concussed patient who mistakes attempts at medical assistance for threats.

In contrast, directed aggression during the interictal period is a frequent and serious problem. In this situation, a patient might undertake an aggressive act for a clear motive, often following considerable planning in response to an objectively minor provocation. These acts often stem from moral concerns or a sense of outrage. The perpetrator does not generally claim amnesia for the event and may recall his actions with much regret (Devinsky and Bear, 1984).

Aggressive behavior is often associated with other features of the interictal behavior syndrome. In a recent study conducted in a psychiatric hospital, temporal lobe epileptics who demonstrated significant aggression were distinguished from patients with aggressive character disorders by the additional presence of religiosity, interpersonal clinging, circumstantiality, bizarre humor and philosophical interests. Contrary to prevailing clinical views, temporal lobe patients were more inclined to accept responsibility for angry outbursts and less inclined to claim amnesia or blame uncontrollable impulses for actions (Bear et al, 1982).

Case 2: *Aggression with deepened emotions, moralism, interpersonal clinging.*

A 38-year-old man experienced recurrent, paroxysmal attacks of flushing, tachycardia, diaphoresis, and feelings of fear or rage beginning in his 20s. Approximately one year subsequent to the onset of these spells, there was a dramatic decline in academic performance and conduct ratings pertaining to his military duties. During extensive medical, psychiatric, and neurologic examination, spike discharges were recorded bilaterally over the right and left temporal lobes on repeated EEGs. Pneumoencephalography revealed dilation of the left temporal horn. In the presence of a limbic spike focus, it seems likely that the episodes of autonomic discharge and dysphoric emotion represented complex partial seizures. The patient had suffered high fevers early in childhood but was unaware of associated febrile convulsion; no alternative etiology for the neurologic abnormalities was established.

His service records documented the onset of severe and bizarre forms of aggressivity approximately 18 months after the onset of the autonomic and emotional spells. Once he furiously punched a door, injuring the knuckles of his right hand. Involved in fights with fellow servicemen, he was confined to a stockade for several days. During the imprisonment he pulverized the plumbing fixtures in his cell, throwing the pieces through a metal barricade. When his sentence was thereby extended, he threatened to murder the magistrate. Only the identification of neurologic abnormality terminated this imprisonment.

When first questioned about his temper, the patient furiously responded that "I have more of a problem with anger than anyone I have ever met in my life." He described a constant struggle to contain vengeful feelings. During his hospitalization, he experienced paranoid distortions that technicians were laughing at him, which "almost made me throw one out of the (seventh story) window." His sense of indignation and rage was continual, and was in no sense limited to the paroxysmal sweating attacks.

Other aspects of the patient's personality were consistent with an interictal behavior syndrome: intense emotion with frequent tearfulness; moralistic concern with the plight of other patients, leading him to change linen and clean bedpans; extensive writing of personal reflections on good and evil, love overcoming anger, God vanquishing the Devil; a preoccupation with many details of his more than 500 pages of accumulated medical records; and an inappropriate interpersonal clinging to fellow patients and caretakers (stickiness, viscosity) (Devinsky and Bear, 1984).

Interictal aggressive behavior should be contrasted with the aggression occurring in frontal lobe disease, in which trivial stimuli elicit brief, aggressive outbursts that are usually unplanned, unsustained, ineffectual, and soon forgotten. The shallow mood and affect of the frontal lobe patient stand in sharp contrast to the deepened emotionality of temporal lobe epilepsy patients with the interictal behavior syndrome (Devinsky and Bear, 1984).

Epilepsy has been invoked as a defense in violent crimes with increasing frequency. For example, epilepsy was cited as a defense in five cases of murder in 1979 (Beresford, 1980). Defense attorneys most typically claim that violence occurred during a seizure. Because of the rarity of directed ictal aggression, we suspect that this defense is seldom justified.

INTERICTAL CHANGES IN EMOTIONAL AND INTELLECTUAL BEHAVIOR

In addition to biological drives such as sexuality and aggression, interictal behavior changes described in temporal lobe epilepsy include a cluster of emotional and intellectual characteristics. Underlying this behavioral pattern is a heightened intensity and attribution of significance to feelings and ideas.

In the affective sphere, this intensification may be present in the form of deepened emotions and emotional lability. Extremes of mood such as depression, elation or euphoria, and fear-related experiences such as anxiety, panic attacks, phobias or paranoia are common (Bear, 1979c; Bear and Fedio, 1977; Blumer and Benson, 1982; Waxman and Geschwind, 1975).

Interpersonal viscosity or "clinging" is a trait familiar to many physicians caring for the temporal lobe epileptic. Many such patients have an inability to terminate a conversation appropriately, and manifest an insensitivity to the temporal and spatial cues regarding social interaction. These patients may follow prolonged clinical interviews with frequent attempts to reestablish contact through phone calls, letters, notes, or messages (Bear, 1979c; Bear et al, 1982; Blumer and Benson, 1982). This excessive social cohesion is often associated with circumstantiality: a style of speaking or writing characterized by the incorporation of multiple, often peripheral details and containing an overabundance of clarifications, qualifications, and circumlocutions (Bear, 1979c; Bear and Fedio, 1977; Bear et al, 1982; Blumer and Benson, 1982; Waxman and Geschwind, 1975).

Waxman and Geschwind (1980) first documented the occurrence of hypergraphia, a tendency towards extensive and compulsive writing, in patients with temporal lobe epilepsy. The contents of these writings often reflect other aspects of the interictal behavior syndrome, such as verbosity, meticulous attention to details and frequent religious and metaphysical allusions. This behavior may be exhibited in the writing of notes, diaries, novels, poems, hymns, autobiographies; or letters to physicians, clergymen and politicians. The form of writing often incorporates idiosyncratic stylistic devices for emphasis: parentheses, underlining, use of different colored inks or the rewriting of numerals in arabic form. Some such patients also draw copiously.

Case 3: *Hypergraphia with emotional deepening, religious preoccupations, pansexuality and aggressivity.*

This 55-year-old black woman suffered seizures from early childhood. Originally she experienced interruptions of consciousness. She subsequently developed a prolonged aura consisting of foul odor, followed by focal movements of the left face and arm, which sometimes progressed to a generalized seizure. The EEG revealed a spike focus over the right temporal lobe; spike bursts were later recorded from the right amygdala with indwelling electrodes. A stereotactic radio frequency lesion within the right amygdala at age 42 produced no apparent change in seizure pattern or interictal behavior.

This patient initially presented her physician with more than 20 spiral notebooks filled with somber personal reflections, religious exegeses and angry diatribes against former physicians, police and politicians. She filled one 70-page notebook with writing each week for several months. Her efforts were all the more remarkable because she suffered painful and deforming rheumatoid arthritis which forced her to write with hand supports.

With her permission we include a sample page from these diaries.

She also carried satchels filled with audio cassettes of her own sermons on biblical themes. Despite her unmistakable religious and moral fervor, she reported sexual activity from age six with bisexual preference beginning in adolescence.

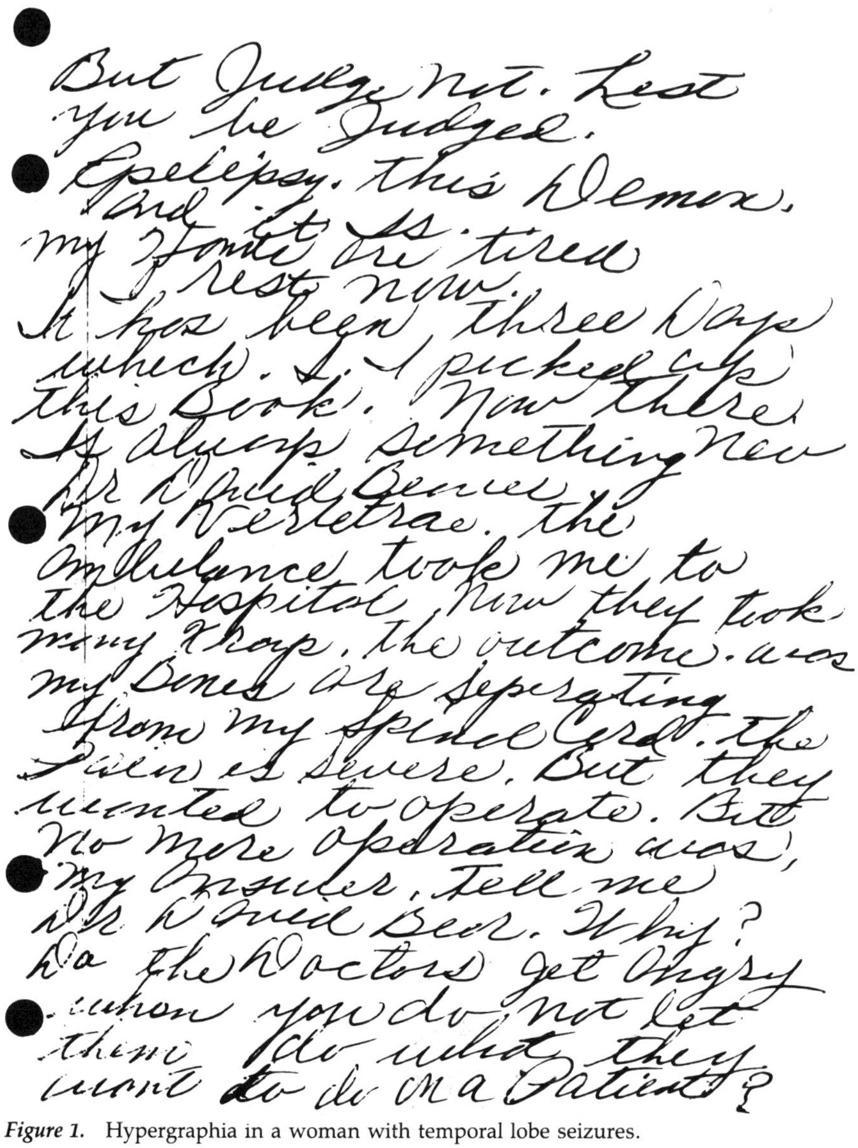
But Judge not. Lest
you be Judged.
Epilepsy. this Demon.
And it is. my Joints are tired
I rest now.
It has been three Days
which. I. I picked up
this Book. Now there.
Is always something New
Dr David Bear
My Vertebrae. the
ambulance took me to
the Hospital, Now they took
many Xrays, the outcome. was
my Bones are seperating
from my Spinal Cord. the
Pain is Severe. But they
wanted to operate. But
No more Operation was,
my Answer. Tell me
Dr David Bear. Why?
Do the Doctors get Angry
when you do not let
them do what they
want to do on a Patient?

Figure 1. Hypergraphia in a woman with temporal lobe seizures.

Yet another aspect of her intense emotionality was striking. She had been prosecuted for multiple aggravated assaults, including an attempt to castrate an unsatisfactory sexual partner and the beating of a policeman into unconsciousness.

Case 4: *Hypergraphia—poetry and paintings—with deepened emotions, philosophical interests, irritability, and sexual conflict.*

A 29-year-old single woman experienced the onset of spells eight years previously, during which "everything appeared wavy and faces looked like caricatures." These recurrent episodes included rushing thoughts and voices, and a sense of imminent disaster. At these times, she was aware of people talking to her but gave inappropriate responses to their questions. The EEG revealed bilateral midtemporal sharp waves on two occasions; neurological examination and cranial tomography (CT) scan were normal. The patient developed deepening emotions with a marked, self-reported tendency to become angry about trivial events. In the last two years, sounds of even normal volume led to violent outbursts in which she smashed furniture or struck her cat.

This highly intelligent woman composed music, wrote poems and frequently combined poetic texts with elaborately detailed or vividly colored illustrations. Philosophical reflections and moral aphorisms were frequently depicted, as exemplified by Figure 2.

Other features of the interictal behavior syndrome were present: readily elicitable sadness with recurrent suicidal depressions; religious preoccupation leading to enrollment in a divinity school; and continuing conflict regarding sexual preference (Devinsky and Bear, 1984).

The mechanisms of hypergraphia remains unresolved, although Waxman and Geschwind (1980) and Bear and Fedio (1977) have suggested that hypergraphia reflects intellectualized expression of intensified emotions. In a recent retrospective review, Roberts and colleagues (1982) noted the association of hypergraphia with right sided or predominantly right sided foci and emphasized the possible contribution of the intact language-dominant hemisphere. However, other studies have not confirmed this lateralization (Bear and Fedio, 1977; Seidman, 1978).

INTERICTAL PSYCHOSIS

Early investigators claimed an inverse relationship between seizure frequency and psychosis among epileptics (Gibbs, 1951; Glans, 1931), an observation which may have led von Meduna to introduce electroconvulsive therapy (ECT) as a treatment for schizophrenia. A more questionable concept of "antagonism" was based on the observation of early epidemiologists that the combination of schizophrenia and epilepsy occurred less frequently than predicted by chance. On the other hand, Slater and Beard (1963) believed that the association of epilepsy with psychosis occurred with a frequency far greater than predicted by chance. They described 69 such patients referred to two London hospitals over two years, arguing that this number was over ten times greater than would be predicted for the entire London area. The psychosis occurred on the average of 14.1 years after the onset of seizures, with a mean age of onset of 29.8 years. In over 70 percent of their patients, a temporal epileptic focus was located.

Such symptoms as delusions and hallucinations (in clear consciousness), paranoid behavior and, more rarely, thought-blocking, neologisms and catatonia were described in the interictal period of temporal lobe epilepsy. Slater and Beard (1963) emphasized that all the cardinal symptoms of schizophrenia were manifested at some time in their patients. However, they confirmed the observation of Pond (1957) that, in contrast to idiopathic schizophrenics, these patients usually had warm, appropriate affects and did not suffer the clinical deterioration of schizophrenia. This has led to the use of the term "schizophreniform

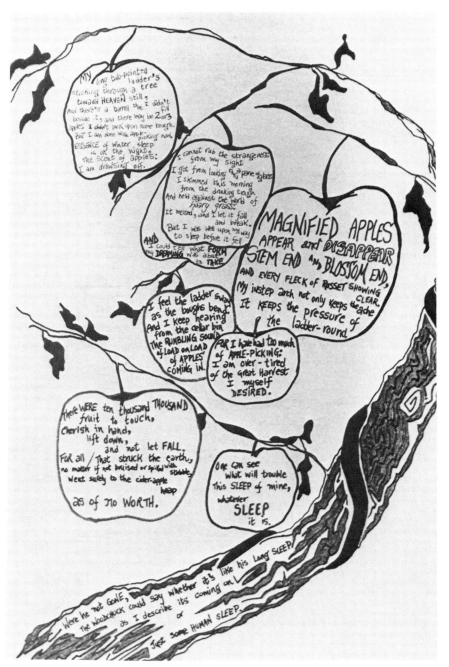

Figure 2. Philosophical reflections and moral aphorisms in a woman with temporal lobe epilepsy. Reprinted from D. Bear et al, "Behavioral Alterations in Patients with Temporal Lobe Epilepsy," in Psychiatric Aspects of Epilepsy. Edited by D. Blumer. Copyright © 1984 by Dietrich Blumer. Reprinted by permission.

psychosis of temporal lobe epilepsy" (Slater and Beard, 1963), which is *not* synonymous with the "Schizophreniform Disorder" defined in *DSM-III*.

Case 5: *Schizophreniform Psychosis with Somatic and Sexual Preoccupations, Hypergraphia, and Paranoid Delusions*

A 41-year-old man experienced seizures since the age of 4. These were characterized by lipsmacking, unpleasant abdominal sensation on some occasions followed by tonic-clonic movements affecting his right side, and deviation of the head and the eyes to the left. Numerous EEGs showed spike and sharp wave discharges emanating from the left temporal lobe. The patient was the product of a toxemic pregnancy with complicated delivery.

Because the seizures proved refractory to anticonvulsant treatment, he underwent a left temporal lobectomy in his early 30s; pathological examination identified a hamartoma. There was significant postoperative improvement in seizure control.

Nonetheless, his current behavior is characterized by somatic preoccupations concerning cleanliness, leading him to shave all the hair off his body. He has developed psychotic delusions regarding his bowels, reflected in the use of laxatives, idiosyncratic enemas, and the insertion of foreign bodies into the rectum. He has achieved sexual satisfaction from these pursuits while insisting that they have helped in controlling his seizures.

He is a frequent letter writer, usually sending a letter per week to his physician. These are remarkable for third person self-references and excessive inclusion of identification numbers: date, time, social security, telephone and post office box numbers. He usually follows the arabic numeral with its spelling.

Paranoid tendencies have resulted in litigation against employers, the owner of a restaurant in which he experienced a seizure, his landlord, former physicians, and the United States Post Office for failure to deliver his letters.

The development of psychosis in temporal lobe epilepsy has been connected to specific anatomic and clinical features. Taylor (1975) noted the association of hamartomas (congenital dysplasias) with psychosis in temporal lobe epilepsy. Specific types of auras have also been associated with the development of psychosis. Jensen and Larson (1979b) noted that psychosis occurred more commonly in patients with ictal hallucinations or complex motor automatisms than in patients with visceral auras. Hermann et al (1982), described the development of psychosis in patients with ictal fear.

INTERICTAL DISSOCIATIVE STATES

Several authors have drawn attention to the occurrence of dissociative states in temporal lobe epileptics (Mesulam, 1981; Schenk and Bear, 1981). Such behavior may encompass the classical multiple personality syndrome, in which two or more personalities take on an independent existence with amnesic barriers between them. In a less dramatic form of dissociative disorder, the patient, usually female, describes herself as having more than one side to her personality, attributing different thoughts and behaviors to alternative aspects of the self. Other patients have credited their actions, thoughts and emotions to benevolent or malevolent powers or spiritual entities.

Case 6: *Dissociative state (multiple personalities) with aggression, altered sexual orientation, self-destructive behavior*

This 21-year-old, right-handed woman reported absence attacks since age 14, as well as frequent déjà vu experiences. Within the last year, she has also suffered generalized (grand mal) convulsions. For years she has been troubled by auditory hallucinations, either of church bells or voices telling her to look out or to harm people. On one occasion, she had a visual hallucination of a car about to run her over.

The patient also gave a history of throbbing headaches with no prodrome. There was no family history of seizure disorder. While the etiology of her spells remains unclear, at four years of age she had a severe ear infection and at ten years of age lost consciousness following a skating accident. Repeated EEGs have been abnormal, showing bilateral temporal lobe spiking, more prominant on the right. Detailed neurological examination and CAT were within normal limits.

"Rebecca" displayed the deepened affects characteristic of the interictal behavior syndrome of temporal lobe epilepsy. She was angry and overtly aggressive. She wrote poetry, long letters, and a journal; she was also extremely interested in philosophy. She underwent a change in sexual preference, shifting from heterosexuality to homosexuality at age 17.

At age 15, while living with a foster family, Rebecca suddenly found herself in another state with strangers who referred to her as "Chris." Apparently she had stolen the foster family's car and driven off three weeks earlier; she denied any recollection of this three-week period. Following this experience, Rebecca underwent repeated psychiatric hospitalizations during which she experienced numerous episodes of "losing time."

Her roommate described the emergence of two distinct personalities during Rebecca's amnesic periods. One, who called herself Chris, was "like a teenage punk, angry, tough, threatening in her manner;" the other personality was a "childlike little girl," sweet, shy, cooperative and withdrawn.

Rebecca often behaved aggressively during her dissociative episodes. On one occasion she found herself lying on a grassy knoll with a bloody stick in her hand, next to the unconscious body of an unfamiliar man. She felt frightened and guilty, believing she had killed the man. On another occasion, she held a knife to her psychiatrist's throat for three hours. While claiming total amnesia for this episode, she later presented the therapist with a vial of her own blood by way of apology (Schenk and Bear, 1981).

In most reported cases, the dissociative states occur as interictal events in patients who are alert, attentive and capable of responding appropriately to their environments. It has been suggested that intensified, dysphoric affects that may develop as features of the interictal behavior syndrome predispose some individuals to dissociative reactions (Schenk and Bear, 1981). These phenomena should be distinguished from simple automatisms or fugue states that may occur as ictal or peri-ictal events.

NEUROLOGICAL PRESENTATION

This chapter has highlighted some long-term interictal behavioral changes associated with limbic epileptic foci. Most frequently such a focus declares itself in the form of the "complex partial" seizure. This type of seizure is defined as an alteration in consciousness preceding or following focal motor or sensory symptomatology; these events may secondarily generalize, eventuating in a grand mal convulsion. Ictal events (including the aura) rarely last more than two minutes, and are usually followed by a short period of postictal confusion.

The nature of the aura reflects the location and the discharge pattern of the seizure focus. Autonomic auras include epigastric sensations—"butterflies" or fullness—and, less frequently, cardiac arrhythmias, respiratory alterations, blushing, pallor, diaphoresis, or urinary incontinence. These commonly imply a seizure focus in the anterotemporal area, perhaps more frequently in the right hemisphere. Cognitive states such as déjà vu, jamais vu, forced thinking, and "dreamy states" are common clinical manifestations of temporal lobe seizures, as are such affective auras as fear, panic, depression and, occasionally, elation. Other typical auras are olfactory, gustatory, visual (simple and complex hallucinations, and illusions such as macropsia or micropsia), vertigo and somatosensory phenomena. The patient frequently has difficulty describing these idiosyncratic experiences (Guptaak et al, 1983).

Automatisms represent another category of ictal event. These may be simple behavioral patterns such as chewing, grimacing, blinking, head turning; foot, leg, arm, or hand movements; or complex behavioral patterns such as walking, picking at food, or other fragments of behavior in progress at the onset of a seizure. More unusual ictal phenomena include compulsive water drinking (Remillard et al, 1981), sexual seizures, prolonged confusional episodes or fugue states.

A lapse in consciousness or "absence" may accompany these phenomena and may be the only overt manifestation of temporal lobe seizures. This should be differentiated from petit mal epilepsy, a childhood disorder in which the seizure has no aura, no truncal movements, is of much shorter duration (approximately 10 seconds), and lacks postictal confusion.

The neurological examination in idiopathic temporal lobe epilepsy is frequently normal. A mild central facial weakness, particularly on spontaneous emotional smiling, may be present (Remillard et al, 1977). More rarely, upper quadrant visual field disorders may be uncovered. Neuropsychological testing may reveal subtle disorders of language or memory.

The EEG is the major laboratory tool in the evaluation of a patient with suspected temporal lobe epilepsy. Unfortunately, the usual scalp electrodes fail to detect a deep-lying limbic focus in up to 50 percent of patients. The sensitivity of the EEG may be increased by sleep deprivation or through specialized electrodes (sphenoidal or nasopharyngeal) more suitable for examination of the medial temporal lobe structures. Experimental techniques measuring local cerebral metabolism, such as the positron emission tomography (PET) scan and (SPEC) scan, may prove to be of additional value (Kuhl et al, 1980).

It must be remembered that an epileptic focus is the electrical manifestation of underlying abnormality in the brain. Therefore, its etiology should be carefully investigated. The most frequent pathologies identified during surgical treatment of temporal lobe epilepsy have been hamartomas and mesial temporal (hippocampal) sclerosis. The leading theories about the cause of the latter implicate injuries in utero or prolonged febrile convulsion in childhood. Moreover, because the orbital temporal poles are near the base of the skull, contusion of

Table 1. Ictal Versus Nonictal Aspects Of Temporal Lobe Epilepsy

Pre-ictal:	Irritability; fatigue; ataxia; dizziness; anomic aphasia; forgetfulness.
Aura:	Olfactory (often foul odor); gustatory (often a metallic taste); complex auditory or visual impression (for example, hearing bells, micropsia, macropsia, formed visual images); vertiginous, visceral sensations; emotions; localized paresthesias; distortions of time sense or familiarity (déjà vu, jamais vu).
Ictus:	Focal motor movements, often simple behavioral patterns such as chewing, swallowing, grimacing, fumbling with hands; more complex automatic sequences such as making a bed, walking or running to an unintended destination; fugue states; rarely water drinking, sexually aggressive behavior; these "complex partial" seizures may be followed by secondarily generalized (grand mal) seizures with or without incontinence.
Postictal Period:	Prolonged period of confusion regarding time and place; anterograde amnesia; aphasia (particularly anomia); occasionally a feeling of well-being or happiness; fatigue.
Interictal Period:	Alterations of emotional association—see text for discussion of interictal behavior syndrome.

this area is common; thus, head trauma is a frequent cause of temporal lobe epilepsy. Nonetheless, the possibility of brain tumor, encephalitis, granuloma, abscess, vasculitis, arteriovenous malformation, or stroke must be considered with the onset of seizures, even when clinical examination and neuropsychological tests are normal. We recommend that all such patients receive a lumbar puncture and a head CT scan.

The clinician is often required to separate psychogenic or pseudoseizures from genuine temporal lobe epilepsy. Pseudoseizures tend to be less stereotyped and are of longer duration than true seizures (Desai et al, 1982). They may terminate abruptly without postictal confusion or amnesia. Pseudoseizure frequency is often unrelated to drug levels. The differentiation of these two entities is made difficult by the frequent occurrence of pseudoseizures in patients with a legitimate seizure disorder (Class, 1975; King and Marsan, 1977; Theodore et al, 1983).

UNRESOLVED ISSUES

Measurement of Interictal Behavioral Changes

Standardized psychological tests designed to segregate patients into idiopathic psychiatric diagnostic categories are likely to be insensitive to the presence or severity of interictal behavioral changes. In the previously cited study of Bear and Fedio (1977), an inventory in which specific features ascribed to the interictal

Table 2. Differentiating Seizures From Pseudoseizures

	Complex Partial Seizures	Petit Mal Seizure	Pseudoseizure
Aura:	Frequently present — See Table 1	None	Often bizarre, atypical or unusual, frequently changing with each spell
Automatism:	Simple or elaborate movements of face, limbs and trunk	Simple stereotyped movement of face and eyes only	Often dramatic, unpredictable, with purposeful bilateral movements, often pelvic thrusting or other sexually suggestive movements; bilateral movements without loss of consciousness
Postictal Confusion:	Present—typically lasting several minutes	Absent	Frequently absent
Duration of Ictus:	Typically 15 seconds to 90 seconds	Typically 10 seconds	Often of longer duration
Serum Prolactin Level:	May be increased, particularly if there is generalization to whole body, tonic–clonic movement	Unchanged	Unchanged
Most typical EEG finding:	Focal spikes or slow waves	3 per second; generalized spike and wave	Normal
Amnesia for Ictus:	Frequently present	Present	Often Absent

behavioral syndrome—for example, writing interests, religious concerns, changes in sexual preference—clearly separated temporal lobe epileptics from normal controls, as well as from patients with other neurological disease. To our knowledge, in every study using this inventory, temporal lobe epileptics have obtained higher scores than normal subjects (Bear and Fedio, 1977; Mungas, 1982; Seidman, 1978; Wilson et al, 1982). The diagnostic power of such self-report instruments may be improved by future descriptions of previously unrecognized features of the interictal behavior syndrome.

In addition, indices of biological features underlying the interictal behavior syndrome may add objectivity and precision to the clinical picture. For example, alterations in neuroendocrine regulation of gonadotropins may be related to changes in sexual functioning (Herzog et al, 1982). Enhanced autonomic responses to neutral visual stimuli may provide direct evidence of increased emotionality (Bear and Schenk, 1981).

In the absence of satisfactory measures of behavioral change, its actual frequency remains unknown. Few observers doubt an elevated incidence of psychiatric illness, suicide attempts, aggressive disturbances, or sexual dysfunction among temporal lobe epileptics (Bear, 1979c; Blumer and Walker, 1967; Davidson and Bagley, 1969; Devinsky and Bear, 1984; Ellison, 1982; Lishman, 1978; Slater and Beard, 1963). However, these overt indications of psychopathology or maladaptive behavior may substantially underestimate the number of patients with more subtle features of an interictal behavior syndrome. For example, in a small sample of consecutively tested temporal lobe epileptics attending outpatient neurology clinics, one-third had attempted suicide and 40 percent had been admitted to psychiatric hospitals. Yet, based on questionnaire data sampling traits of the interictal behavior syndrome, more than 90 percent of the temporal lobe epilepsy patients could be distinguished from normal controls, as well as from other neurological patients, by a discriminant function analysis (Bear and Fedio, 1977). These results by no means constitute an estimate of the true frequency of behavioral changes, but indicate a high prevalence of such alterations in temporal lobe epilepsy.

Neurological Specificity

The observation of an "interictal behavior syndrome" associated with temporal lobe epilepsy implies that multiple features of behavior—such as deepened emotions, altered sexual behavior, and hypergraphia—appear in some patients with this disorder. We wish to emphasize the syndromic clustering of multiple aspects of behavior in individual patients (Bear, 1979c; Bear and Fedio, 1977; Bear et al, 1982; Waxman and Geschwind, 1975).

Such a behavioral syndrome has not been reported in response to the stress of general medical illnesses such as myocardial infarction, diabetes mellitus, or asthma (Bear, 1979c; Bear and Fedio, 1977). Furthermore, patients with life-threatening or disfiguring neurologic illness did not exhibit interictal features to a greater extent than normal controls (Bear and Fedio, 1977). Patients with multiple sclerosis or rheumatoid arthritis exhibited behavioral profiles differing from those of temporal lobe epileptics (Wilson et al, 1982).

The interictal behavior syndrome is also distinguished from behavioral syndromes resulting from other localized neurological lesions. For example, the intensification of affect contrasts with the flattened, transient emotions of patients following prefrontal lobe injury, the apathy of patients with Korsakoff amnesic syndrome, or the indifference reaction following right parietal lobe infarction (Bear, 1979b). Perhaps the most cogent argument for the neurological specificity of the interictal behavior syndrome is its behavioral antithesis, the Kluver-Bucy syndrome, resulting from structural, nonepileptogenic lesions of limbic structures in the medial temporal lobes (Kluver and Bucy, 1937). In this reproducible, anatomically specific behavior syndrome, aggression is reduced, sexual behavior is increased, social cohesion is diminished and exploratory behavior is promoted (Bear, 1979c; Blumer and Benson, 1982; Kluver and Bucy, 1937). Thus, it is difficult to attribute the interictal behavior syndrome to "nonspecific" effects of structural damage within the temporal lobe; indeed, beneficial behavorial consequences of temporal lobectomy may result from the effects of the destructive lesion on the *changes* produced by epilepsy (Falconer, 1973).

The observations frequently cited to dispute the neurological specificity of the interictal behavior syndrome are comparisons among patients with differing forms of epilepsy. Most commonly, patients with an electrographically documented temporal lobe focus have been contrasted with "grand mal" or "generalized" epileptics; both groups may show changes in behavior, with the differences between them failing to reach statistical significance. The results are summarized as a failure to observe specific behavioral changes in temporal lobe epilepsy (Migone et al, 1970; Small et al, 1962).

We believe that this type of comparison causes confusion. First, the fact that a patient has generalized seizures does not preclude the possibility that the epileptic focus lies within or activates the limbic system. Medially placed temporal lobe foci may escape EEG detection while secondary cortical dysrhythmias are observed (Bear, 1979c; Devinsky and Bear, 1984). Second, it has been repeatedly shown that kindling—the creation of new or secondary epileptic foci following repeated electrical stimulation (Goddard et al, 1969)—occurs most readily in limbic structures such as the amygdala. There is evidence from studies of experimental epilepsy in animals, as well as from clinical observations in man, that epileptogenic lesions outside the temporal limbic structures may induce daughter foci within the limbic system, resulting in the behavioral changes associated with limbic foci (Bear, 1979a; Bear, 1979c; Stamm and Warren, 1961).

In our view, these anatomical and physiological realities render behavioral comparisons between temporal lobe and generalized epileptics uninterpretable. The more appropriate but clinically difficult comparisons would be with other focal epilepsies or with patients having infrequent generalized seizures of metabolic origin, in which the probability of limbic kindling is low. In fact, there is evidence that patients with nontemporal focal epilepsy do not show these characteristic behavioral changes (Bear, 1979c; Dongier, 1959). Moreover, in the study of Sachdev and Waxman (1981), patients suffering only generalized withdrawal seizures were differentiated blindly from temporal lobe epileptics by the absence of hypergraphia and other features of interictal behavior within samples of their writing.

In summary, we believe that the interictal behavior syndrome is a frequent and specific consequence of limbic epileptic discharge. However, the recognition that the interictal behavior syndrome is specific does not imply that whenever the behavioral changes are observed, a temporal lobe focus must be present. There may well be analogous organic syndromes, such as those resulting from hallucinogens, which chemically affect or even "kindle" limbic structures (Bear, 1979a; Bear, 1979c). Furthermore, through genetic variation or environmental reinforcement, some fraction of nonepileptic individuals might exhibit a similar behavioral phenotype.

Psychiatric Specificity

The last controversial issue concerns the behavioral specificity or psychiatric "distinctiveness" of the interictal behavior changes. Are such features a potpourri of random psychiatric symptoms, indistinguishable from those found in the "typical psychiatric patient"? (Mungas, 1982).

Individual behavioral characteristics such as aggression, sexual dysfunction, and deepened mood occur frequently in psychiatric syndromes. However, the basis of most reports on behavior in temporal lobe epilepsy is precisely the distinctive syndromatic quality of the clinical picture: for example, the tendency to write at length coupled with philosophic or moralistic concerns, preoccupation with details, and aggressivity (Bear and Fedio, 1977; Waxman and Geschwind, 1975); or the combination of paranoid ideation with warm emotions and a tendency to maintain close social relations (Bear et al, 1982; Blumer and Benson, 1982; Slater and Beard, 1963). The interictal behavior syndrome is a *cluster* of behavioral features not typically seen together in other patients. In all likelihood, individual behavioral features such as aggression may occur more frequently or more intensely in syndromes other than temporal lobe epilepsy. Furthermore, because many of the traits sampled by the questionnaire of Bear and Fedio are closely correlated (for example, temper and overt aggression; circumstantiality, obsessiveness and viscosity; emotionality and altered mood), patients with other syndromes may present with multiple associated traits. The critical observation, both clinically and statistically, is the simultaneous occurrence of generally uncorrelated behavioral characteristics among temporal lobe epileptics. The existence of this cluster is not contradicted by the observation that one could obtain an "average" profile that includes many of the interictal behavior traits from a mixed group of psychiatric patients. This average profile of "nonspecific psychopathology" would not describe any particular patient. Indeed, it would be meaningless to try to interpret the statistical composite of, for example, a depressed patient, a schizophrenic, and a sociopath (Mungus, 1982).

In addition to the tendency of these behaviors to cluster in the temporal lobe epileptic, the *quality* of individual behaviors is often distinctive. For example, the morally justified aggressive acts with subsequent remorse, commonly seen in temporal lobe epilepsy, are quite rare in both idiopathic sociopathy and frontal lobe disease. In a recent study employing structured interviews to examine these and other distinctions among behavioral symptoms, observers blind to diagnosis found highly significant differences among profiles of patients with aggressive character disorder, affective disorder, or idiopathic schizophrenia compared to temporal lobe epileptics (Bear et al, 1982).

TREATMENT

The explanation of fundamental mechanisms and development of effective treatments are critical tasks for the future. It has been suggested that an increased tendency to associate drive-related (emotional) responses to many external stimuli may underlie the panoply of interictal behavior changes (Bear, 1979a; Bear, 1979c; Bear and Fedio, 1977). The finding that autonomic responses to visual stimuli appear to be enhanced during the interictal period in temporal lobe epileptics supports this hypothesis (Bear and Schenk, 1981).

Drawing on anatomical and physiological observations that limbic structures within the temporal lobe (such as the amygdala) link sensory association cortices with drive-controlling centers within the hypothalamus, researchers have suggested that an epileptic focus may lower the threshold for creation of sensory-limbic connections, facilitating fortuitous emotional associations (Bear, 1979c). The kindling phenomenon, readily demonstrated within the amygdala complex, provides a possible physiological model for this effect (Goddard et al, 1969).

The formation of such interictal "hyperconnections" (Bear, 1979c) may be a process independent of or even antagonistic to the ictal synchronization of neuronal firing which results in overt seizures. Thus, the observation that anticonvulsants such as phenytoin do not reverse interictal behavior changes (Blumer and Benson, 1982) and that seizure frequency may even correlate inversely with severity of interictal behavior (Landolt, 1969; Pond, 1957) are consistent with this view.

Several approaches to the control of interictal behavior are suggested by this model. Medications reducing the intensity of affect might be expected to reduce the frequency or severity of the associations; such agents include lithium carbonate (which may have anticonvulsant effects in a low therapeutic dose range), propranolol, or clonidine. Transmitter-active medications shown to inhibit the kindling effect in animals are worth testing: for example, cholinergic blockers, adrenergic agonists, or dopamine agonists. Carbamazepine may be an especially effective psychotropic agent because it combines anticonvulsant, antiimpulsive, and antikindling effects (Bear, 1979a).

Some patients suffer psychotic symptoms, usually within the setting of other interictal behavior changes. These individuals often require antipsychotic agents. Medicines producing the least increase in limbic excitability, such as the dihydroindolone, molindone, may be preferable (Oliver et al, 1982).

If the mechanisms sketched above are correct, prompt surgical removal of the epileptic focus—preventing paroxysmal seizures as well as halting the development of interictal change in limbic excitability—might be effective therapy (Falconer, 1973). Secondary surgical lesions within the limbic system involving the amygdala or the prefrontal cortex, or within the lateral hypothalamus, appear to improve particular behaviors, principally aggression (Kiloh et al, 1974; Vaernet and Madsen, 1970).

There is also a role for directive psychotherapy, which might be conceptualized as bringing altered emotional susceptibilities to the attention of intact, higher order association cortices within the brain. In our experience, group therapy meetings with temporal lobe epileptics manifesting interictal behavior changes have been especially efficacious, providing consensual validation of otherwise bizarre experiences and intense emotions, and serving as a forum for the development of innovative coping strategies.

In summary, the existence of distinct changes in physiological drive-related behavior, ideation, and emotion in a significant number of patients with temporal lobe epilepsy has been firmly established. Only further investigations will enable us to refine the clinical presentation and its variants, document its incidence and prevalence, and ameliorate its disabling consequences.

REFERENCES

Bear DM: Interictal behavior in temporal lobe epilepsy: possible anatomic and physiologic basis, in Epilepsy: Neurotransmitter, Behavior, and Pregnancy. Edited by Vancouver WJ, Joint Publication of Canadian League Against Epilepsy and Western Institute on Epilepsy, 1979a

Bear DM: Organic alterations in personality, in Outpatient Psychiatry: Diagnosis and Treatment. Edited by Lazare A. Baltimore, Williams and Wilkins Co., 1979b

Bear DM: Temporal lobe epilepsy: a syndrome of sensory-limbic hyper-connection. Cortex 15:357-384, 1979c

Bear DM: The temporal lobes: an approach to the study of organic behavioral changes, in Handbook of Behavioral Neurology, vol. 2. Edited by Gazzaniga M. London, Plenum Press, 1979d

Bear DM, Fedio P: Quantitative analysis of interictal behavior in temporal lobe epilepsy. Arch Neurol 34:454-467, 1977

Bear DM, Schenk L: Increased autonomic responses to neutral and emotional stimuli in patients with temporal lobe epilepsy. Am J Psychiatry 138:843-845, 1981

Bear DM, Levin K, Blumer D: Interictal behavior in hospitalized temporal lobe epileptics: relationship to idiopathic psychiatric syndromes. J Neurol Neurosurg Psychiatry 45:481-488, 1982

Bear DM, Freeman R, Greenberg M: Behavioral alterations in patients with temporal lobe epilepsy, in Psychiatric Aspects of Epilepsy. Edited by Blumer D. Washington, DC, American Psychiatric Press, 1984

Beresford HR: Letters to the editor, Neurology 30:1134-1140, 1980

Blumer D: Hypersexual episodes in temporal lobe epilepsy. Am J Psychiatry 126:1099-1106, 1970

Blumer D, Benson DF: Psychiatric manifestations of epilepsy, in Psychiatric Aspects of Neurologic Disease, vol 2. Edited by Blumer D and Benson DF. New York, Grune and Stratton, 1982: 25-48

Blumer D, Walker AE: Sexual behavior in temporal lobe epilepsy. Arch Neurol 16:37-43, 1967

Class D: Electroencephalographic manifestations of complex partial seizures. Adv Neurol 11:113-140, 1975

Currier FD, Little SC, Suess JF, et al: Sexual seizures. Arch Neurol 25:260-264, 1971

Davidson K, Bagley C: Schizophrenia-like psychoses associated with organic disorders of the central nervous system—review of literature. Br J Psychiatry 4:113-184, 1969

Delgado-Escuetta AV, Mattson RH, King L, et al: The nature of aggression during epileptic seizures. N Engl J Med 305:711-716, 1981

Desai BT, Porter RJ, Penry KJ: Psychogenic seizures: a study of 42 attacks in 6 patients with intensive monitoring. Arch Neurol 39:202-209, 1982

Devinsky O, Bear DM: Varieties of aggressive behavior in patients with temporal lobe epilepsy. Am J Psychiatry 141:651-655, 1984

Dongier S: Statistical study of clinical and EEG manifestations of 546 psychotic episodes occurring in 516 epileptics between clinical seizures. Epilepsia 1:117-142, 1959

Ellison J: Alterations of sexual behavior in temporal lobe epilepsy. Psychosomatics 23:499-500, 505-509, 1982

Epstein AV: Relationship of fetishism and transvestitism to brain and particularly to temporal lobe dysfunction. J Nerv Ment Dis 133:247-253, 1961

Falconer MA: Reversibility by temporal lobe resection of the behavioral abnormalities of temporal lobe epilepsy. N Engl J Med 289:451-455, 1973

Freeman FR, Mavis AH: Temporal lobe sexual seizures. Neurology 19:87-90, 1969

Gastaut H, Collomb H: Etude du comportement sexuel chez les epileptiques psychomoterus. Ann Med Psychol 112:657-696, 1954

Gibbs FA: Ictal and non-ictal psychiatric disorder in temporal lobe epilepsy. J Nerv Ment Dis 113:522-528, 1951

Glans A: Ueber kominationim von schizophrenie und epilepsie zum ges. Neurol Psychiatry 135:450-500, 1931

Goddard G, McIntyre D, Leech C: A permanent change in brain function resulting from daily electrical stimulation. Exp Neurol 25:295-330, 1969

Guptaak J, Jeavons PM, Hughes RC, et al: Aura in temporal lobe epilepsy: clinical and electroencephalographic correlations. J Neurol Neurosurg Psychiatry 46:1079-1083, 1983

Hermann B, Dikmen S, Schwartz M, et al: Interictal psychopathology in patients with ictal fear: a quantitative investigation. Neurology 32:7-11, 1982

Herzog AG, et al: Neuroendocrine dysfunction in temporal lobe epilepsy. Arch Neurol 39:133-135, 1982

Hierons R, Saunders N: Impotence in patients with temporal lobe lesions. Lancet 2:761-764, 1966

Hoerig J, Kenna JC: EEG abnormalities in transexualism. Br J Psychiatry 134:293-300, 1979

Hooshmand H, Bravley BW: Temporal lobe seizures and exhibitionism. Neurology 19:1119-1124, 1969

Jensen I, Larsen JK: Marital aspects of temporal lobe epilepsy. J Neurol Neurosurg Psychiatry 42:256-265, 1979a

Jensen I, Larsen JK: Psychoses in drug resistant temporal lobe epilepsy. J Neurol Neurosurg Psychiatry 42:948-954, 1979b

Johnsen J: Sexual impotence and the limbic system. Br J Psychiatry 3:300-303, 1965

Kiloh LG, Gye RS, Rushworth RG, et al: Stereotactic amygdalotomy for aggressive behavior. J Neurol Neurosurg Psychiatry 37:437-444, 1974

King DW, Marsan C: Clinical features and ictal patterns in epileptic patients with EEG temporal lobe foci. Ann Neurol 2:138-147, 1977

Kluver H, Bucy PC: "Psychic blindness" and other symptoms following bilateral temporal lobectomy in Rhesus monkeys. Am J Physiol 119:352-353, 1937

Kolersky A, Freuid K, Machak H, et al: Male sexual deviation—association with early temporal lobe damage. Arch Gen Psychiatry 17:735-743, 1967

Kuhl D, Engel J Jr., Phelps ME, Selin C: Epileptic patterns of localized cerebral metabolism and perfusion in humans determined by emission computed tomography of ^{18}FDG and ^{13}NH$_3$. Ann Neurol 8:348-360, 1980

Landolt H: Die Temporallappenepilepsie und ihre psychopathologie. Bibl Psychiatr Neurol 112:1-112, 1969

Lishman AW: Temporal Lobe Epilepsy in Organic Psychiatry. Oxford, Blackwell Scientific Publications, 1978

MacLean PD: Chemical and electrical stimulation of small hippocampus in unrestrained animals, Part II—Behavioral Findings. Arch Neurol Psychiatry 78:128-212, 1957

Mesulam MM: Dissociative states with abnormal temporal lobe EEG. Arch Neurol 38:176-181, 1981

Migone RJ, Donnelly EF, Sadowsky D: Psychological and neurological comparisons of psychomotor and nonpsychomotor epileptic patients. Epilepsia 11:345-349, 1970

Mungas D: Interictal behavior abnormality in temporal lobe epilepsy. Arch Gen Psychiatry 39:108-111, 1982

Oliver AP, Luchins DJ, Wyatt R: Neuroleptic-induced seizures. Arch Gen Psychiatry 39:206-209, 1982

Pond DA: Psychiatric aspects of epilepsy. J Indian Med Prof 3:1441-1451, 1957

Remillard GM, Andermann F, Rhi-Sausi A, et al: Facial asymmetry in patients with temporal lobe epilepsy. Neurology 27:109-114, 1977

Remillard GM, Anderman F, Gloor P, et al: Waterdrinking as ictal behavior in complex partial seizures. Neurology 31:117-124, 1981

Roberts JK, Robertson MM, Trimble MR: The lateralizing significance of hypergraphia in temporal lobe epilepsy. J Neurol Neurosurg Psychiatry 45:131-138, 1982

Sachdev HS, Waxman SG: Frequency of hypergraphia in temporal lobe epilepsy: an index of interictal behavior syndrome. J Neurol Neurosurg Psychiatry 44:358-360, 1981

Schenk L, Bear DM: Multiple personality and related dissociative phenomena in patients with temporal lobe epilepsy. Am J Psychiatry 138:1311-1326, 1981

Seidman L: Emotional and cognitive changes in temporal lobe epilepsy. Unpublished doctoral dissertation, Boston University, 1978

Shukula GD, Srivastava DN, Katiyar BC: Sexual disturbances in temporal lobe epilepsy: a controlled study. Br J Psychiatry 134:288-292, 1979

Slater E, Beard AW: Schizophrenia-like psychoses of epilepsy. Br J Psychiatry 109:95-150, 1963

Small JG, Milstein V, Stevens JR: Are psychomotor epileptics different? Arch Neurol 1:187-194, 1962

Sperber S, Sperber D, Williamson P, et al: Sexual automatism in complex partial seizures. Neurology 33:527-533, 1983

Stamm JS, Warren A: Learning and retention by monkeys with epileptogenic implants in posterior parietal cortex. Epilepsia 2:229-242, 1961

Taylor DC: Sexual behavior in temporal lobe epilepsy. Arch Neurol 21:510-516, 1969

Taylor DC: Factors influencing the occurrence of schizophrenia-like psychoses in patients with temporal lobe epilepsy. Psychol Med 5:249-254, 1975

Theodore WH, Porter RJ, Penry KJ: Complex partial seizures: clinical characteristics in differential diagnosis. Neurology 33:115-121, 1983

Vaernet K, Madsen A: Stereotaxic amygdalatomy and basofrontal tractotomy in psychotics with aggressive behavior. J Neurol Neurosurg Psychiatry 33:858-863, 1970

Waxman SA, Geschwind N: The interictal behavior syndrome of temporal lobe epilepsy. Arch Gen Psychiatry 32:1580-1586, 1975

Waxman SA, Geschwind N: Hypergraphia in temporal lobe epilepsy. Neurology 30:314-317, 1980

Chapter 11

Dementia Syndrome

by Stephen L. Read, M.D., Gary W. Small, M.D. and
Lissy F. Jarvik, M.D., Ph.D.

From CBS to OBS to OMS, the changing nomenclature reflects psychiatry's efforts to grapple with the complexities of the dementia syndrome. As the emphasis shifts from chronic to organic brain syndromes, and from organic brain syndromes to organic mental syndromes, our attempts at semantic clarification have been no more successful than have been our search for diagnostic markers. Our search for diagnostic markers, however, has barely begun. Indeed, it has only recently been recognized that dementia deserves both major biomedical research efforts and attention in health care policies. The magnitude of the problem is illustrated by the fact that an estimated five percent of those aged 65 years or older have dementia; the frequency rises to 20 percent for persons aged 80 and over (Mortimer and Schuman, 1981; Jarvik et al, 1980; Gurland and Cross, 1982). Since these are also the fastest growing age groups in the population, dementia of the Alzheimer type (DAT)—the most common form of primary degenerative dementia (PDD) and the most frequent cause of dementia in old age—has been termed "an approaching epidemic" (Plum, 1979).

RECOGNITION OF DEMENTIA IN THE ELDERLY

The consequences of impaired thinking vary, depending not only upon the particular social and occupational circumstances of the patient, but also upon the effect of a disease process on each patient's personality. One patient may seek medical attention after getting lost on the way to the market; another may be brought in by a distraught and angry spouse after receiving a foreclosure notice because the mortgage was not paid. The family may have known that the patient has been disoriented for some time, unable to balance the checkbook, and incapable of remembering the names of friends for months, if not years. Alternatively, they may insist that confusion is a reaction to a recent event or illness. Often the full panoply of symptoms must be elicited by careful questioning of family and friends. It may only be then that informants begin to realize how much they have been doing to compensate for the patient's deficits. This tendency to ignore deficits in memory is due, at least in part, to the fact that some memory decline is expected as an accompaniment of advancing age after maturity.

One of the hallmarks of aging—impaired memory, or forgetfulness—usually does *not* progress to the devastating deficits characteristic of dementia. In his

The opinions expressed are those of the authors and not necessarily those of the Veterans Administration. Supported in part by the Veterans Administration, NIMH Research Grant MH36205, Academic Award K08AG00200-02 from the National Institute on Aging (Dr. Small) and the Kaiser Foundation (Dr. Read).

retrospective analysis, Kral (1978) introduced the term "benign senescent forget-fulness" to differentiate certain age-related memory loss from the malignant global deterioration characteristic of dementia. In benign senescent forgetful-ness, the patient has transiently impaired recall of relatively unimportant aspects of a remote experience (such as a place, date or name) but can remember and relate the essence of the experience. Although Kral's specific criteria for discrim-ination have been criticized (La Rue, 1982), the concept is useful in distinguish-ing different patterns of memory loss in the aged.

Although many elderly persons maintain intellectual skills well into the ninth decade, some loss of psychomotor skills and decrements in performing serial learning tasks may be the rule (Jarvik et al, 1973). A caveat must therefore be directed toward the misclassification of elderly persons as brain damaged based on neuropsychological test norms developed for populations aged 16 to 64 years (Albert, 1981). Such misclassification becomes even more likely in the old who are physically ill (Steuer and Jarvik, 1981). Chronic illness increases in prevalence with increasing age, although data on cognitive impairment in the physically ill elderly are scant. Among the few data available are those on the effect of blood pressure on cognitive functioning (Wilkie and Eisdorfer, 1973) and, more recently, on the detrimental effects of even small increases in blood sugar (U'Ren and Lezak, University of Oregon, personal communication). Drug treatment is thought to cause some cognitive decrement but, again, data are generally absent. Sensory deprivation may impair perception and produce secondary withdrawal and loss of attention (Ernst et al, 1978). Nutritional and motivational factors, as well as cohort effects, are difficult to control (Goodwin et al, 1983). While awaiting further data, we caution against ascribing any decrement in cognitive function-ing to the aging process itself, and against assuming that all cognitive loss heralds a progressive or irreversible course.

DEFINITION OF DEMENTIA SYNDROME

The literature on dementia reflects a longstanding belief that the disorder results from a unitary disease process. Yet the truism that mental symptoms are nonspe-cific applies as much to cognitive dysfunction as to depression or psychosis. From the outset, then, we will emphasize the syndromic nature of dementia, which can result from many medical, psychiatric, and neurologic illnesses (Wells, 1977; Task Force, NIA, 1980; Small and Jarvik, 1982; Cummings and Benson, 1983). This transition to syndromic diagnosis is substantially, but not completely, reflected in the change from the second to the third edition of the Diagnostic and Statistical Manual of the American Psychiatric Association (1968, 1980). *DSM-II* devoted a total of two paragraphs to "Psychoses associated with organic brain syndromes"; *DSM-III* includes four pages discussing dementia. For clinical purposes, we use the *DSM-III* criteria for dementia, omitting the necessity of proving or presuming an organic cause (Table 1).

CLINICAL SYNDROMES AND DIFFERENTIAL DIAGNOSIS

Although Primary Degenerative Dementia (PDD) and Multi-Infarct Dementia (MID) are coded on Axis I in *DSM-III*, the differential diagnosis of dementia is

Table 1. Diagnostic Criteria for the Dementia Syndrome

A. A loss of intellectual abilities of sufficient severity to interfere with social or occupational functioning
B. Memory impairment
C. At least one of the following:
    (1) impairment of abstract thinking
    (2) impaired judgment
    (3) other disturbances of higher cortical function, such as aphasia, apraxia, or constructional difficulty
    (4) personality change
D. State of consciousness not clouded (that is, not delirium)

---

more consistently thought of as occurring on Axis III. From a long list of described causes (see Table 2), we focused on those marked by an asterisk because of their prevalence and interest to clinicians. A fuller treatment of this complex subject must be sought elsewhere (Wells, 1977; Cummings and Benson, 1983).

Dementia of the Alzheimer Type (DAT)

The initial identification of dementia as a syndrome came only in the nineteenth century with the work of Esquirol in France and Prichard in England. Among subsequent pathological studies appeared Alzheimer's case of a woman who died at age 51 after several years of progressive difficulty with memory, orientation, language, and the late development of poor motor function (reviewed in Cohen, 1983). Subsequent studies (Blessed et al, 1968; Tomlinson et al, 1970) have shown Alzheimer-type neuropathological changes to be the most frequent finding in progressive dementia, whether of senile or presenile onset. In these and subsequent autopsy studies, DAT accounted for about half the cases. The balance typically included multi-infarct dementia and a variety of other disorders; a few percent had no identifiable brain abnormality.

The earliest stages of DAT are obscure. By the time patients and their families consult a physician, amnesia, word-finding difficulties, and disorientation for place and time are often present. These patients typically show bland, untroubled responses and retain superficial social skills, which lead family, friends, and co-workers to underestimate their deficits. Attempts to define the beginning of the dementia syndrome may produce widely varying accounts; early episodes of confusion have often been attributed to plausibly extenuating circumstances. In cases where more abrupt onset is described (for example, after a spouse's death, a febrile illness, or a brain injury), gradually progressive impairment may have gone unrecognized. Personality changes, or other psychiatric symptoms, such as paranoid ideation, may at times be the earliest symptoms retrospectively attributable to DAT.

The diagnosis of Alzheimer's disease carries a grim prognosis and should not be made lightly. Clinical and neurological documentation of decline should, whenever possible, supplement history of progressive deterioration. The patient with DAT generally remains free of motor or sensory abnormality until late in the course of the disease. Findings on mental status examination include rather normal conversational style with:

Table 2. Differential Diagnosis of Dementia Syndrome

- Benign senescent forgetfulness and normal aging*
- Mental retardation and developmental disorders
- Focal Syndromes
  aphasia
  amnesia*
- Dementia of the Alzheimer Type (DAT)*
- Multi-Infarct Dementia*
- Pick Disease
- Unrecognized Disorders
- Depression*
- Conversion
- Anxiety Disorders
- Paranoia
- Drugs and Toxins*
  Antidepressants
  Lithium carbonate
  Atropine and related compounds
  Alcohol
  Benzodiazepines
  Barbiturates
  Bromides
  Phenytoin
  Propranolol
  Methyldopa
  Clonidine
  Mercury
  Arsenic
  Lead
  Organophosphates
  Carbon monoxide
- Major Organ Failure
  cardiac
  hematologic
  respiratory
  hepatic
  renal
- Metabolic Disorders
  volume depletion
  vitamin deficiency
  porphyria
  hyperlipidemia
  electrolyte imbalance
- Endocrine
  Hypoglycemia
  Hyperglycemia
  Hypothyroidism
  Hyperthyroidism
  Cushing syndrome
  Hypopituitarism
  Hypoparathyroidism
  Hyperparathyroidism
  Addison disease
- Inflammatory
  Systematic lupus erythematosus
  Temporal arteritis
  Sarcoidosis
  Behcet syndrome
- Infection
- Cardiac Arrhythmia
- Movement Disorders
  Parkinson disease
  Huntington disease
  Progressive supranuclear palsy*
  Wilson disease
  Cerebellar disorders
- Mass Lesions*
  Tumor
  Abscess
  Hematoma
  Hemorrhage
- Hydrocephalus
- Infections
  Meningitis
  Encephalitis
  Syphilis*
  Creutzfeldt-Jakob Disease*

*Discussed in the text
(Adapted from Small et al, 1981)

1). Amnesia—both verbal and visual, with an inability to use cues or to develop compensatory strategies. Memory impairment is a key factor in DAT, as it is in all dementias. According to clinical experience, the recall of recent events is impaired earlier and more severely than that of more remote events.

2). Aphasia—inability to generate items in a given category, followed by word finding difficulties; then, increasing comprehension difficulties, with relative preservation of the mechanics of repetition and reading aloud (Appell et al, 1982; Cummings et al, 1984a).

3). Visual-spatial difficulties—early loss of three-dimensional quality to reproduced drawings is followed by difficulty with even simple figures.

If any of the above features is atypical, the diagnosis must remain tentative.

Multi-Infarct Dementia (MID)

Cerebral infarctions rank second only to DAT as a cause of dementia. Hachinski and co-workers (1974) proposed this condition be called Multi-Infarct Dementia (MID). Although widely adopted, the concept has been criticized because of doubts about its frequency (Fisher, 1982), as well as concerns about current methods of antemortem and postmortem diagnosis (Liston and La Rue, 1983a, 1983b). In addition, other consequences of cardiovascular disease, such as hypoperfusion (due, for example, to ventricular fibrillation or brady-arrhythmia [Cummings et al, 1984b]), can lead to a dementia syndrome, although they are often not considered in the diagnosis (Read and Jarvik, 1984).

MID may be distinguished in life from DAT and other primary dementias by historical and clinical features. Diagnosis allows not only the possibility of arresting progression, but carries different implications for heritability and prognosis. In its course MID is differentiated from DAT by its sudden onset, frequent association with hypertension or other cardiovascular disorders, and stepwise decline in intellectual functioning (for example, a patient one day becomes apraxic; two months later he is confused and cannot recognize his wife). Depression, somatic complaints or emotional incontinence (for example, a patient having an angry outburst when confronted with a frustrating task) may be noted. Neurologic examination may reveal asymmetric reflexes or other residua of stroke. Although CT scan evidence of multiple infarcts is more common in clinically diagnosed multi-infarct dementia than in primary degenerative dementia, 50 percent or more of suspected cases of multi-infarct dementia do not have confirmatory CT findings.

In 1975, Hachinski and co-workers (1975) introduced an Ischemic Score (IS) based, in part, on the original clinical descriptions of vascular dementia by Sir Martin Roth (1955), based on cerebral blood flow studies. It has become a favored research tool. Several investigators (such as Rosen et al, 1980; Loeb and Gandolfo, 1983) have attempted to validate and modify the original IS. Methodological shortcomings, particularly the paucity of autopsy-verified studies, however, still raise questions about the applicability of these studies to the clinical situation (Liston and La Rue, 1983a, 1983b; Small, 1984).

Depression

As many as one-third of patients diagnosed as having early onset of organic dementia may be improved at follow-up (Nott and Fleminger, 1975; Ron et al,

1979). Presumably, these patients with remitting disorders suffered from other unrecognized psychiatric conditions. Depression appears to be the most common, and is the most extensively studied psychiatric illness to mimic dementia, a presentation often referred to as "pseudodementia" (McAllister, 1983). As we have remarked elsewhere (Small and Jarvik, 1982), this term is unfortunate—the cognitive dysfunction of depression is no less real than that of thyroid dysfunction, or DAT; it does, however, remit when mood improves. Caine (1981) pointed out that confusion in the discussion of "pseudodementia" may also stem from the comparison of studies of depressed patients with studies of patients suffering from a variety of other psychiatric disorders, including conversion, anxiety, manic and schizophreniform disorders.

The diagnostic differentiation of depression from dementia is confounded by the frequent presence of faulty memory, long recognized as a common complaint in depressed patients. Sternberg and Jarvik (1976) showed that memory impairment was typical of depressed younger adults (with or without subjective complaints) and that it improved early in the course of treatment with imipramine. This memory impairment is associated with changes in attention, encoding, recall and reaction time (see review by Weingartner and Silberman, 1982). Responses to proverbs and similarities tend to be concrete. Qualitative differences in response may also exist—there may be selective remote recall of dysphoric experiences, and a predominance of morbid or self-deprecatory themes. The impression of dementia may be transiently broken in the face of briefly improved affect (Lloyd and Lishman, 1975).

Changes in personality and judgment may be most striking. The depressed patient, then, often satisfies the phenomenological criteria for dementia. Important to note in this syndrome, which Folstein and McHugh (1978) proposed to call the "dementia syndrome of depression," is the absence of defects in higher cortical function. Aphasia, apraxia, agnosia and constructional difficulty are not characteristic of depression. Relatively sudden onset, personal or family history of affective disorder and the association of the onset of illness with psychological stress increase the suspicion of underlying affective disorder (Wells, 1979). History of affective disorder, however, does not offer absolute protection against the development of dementia.

Further work is needed to clarify the relationship of depression and dementia in the elderly. The clinical signs and symptoms presumably reflect dysfunction of specific neuroanatomical and neurochemical systems. Widely known is the evidence for neuroendocrine and central nervous system (CNS) catecholamine dysfunction in affective disorders (reviewed in Sachar, 1982; and Zis and Goodwin, 1982). The depression that accompanies neurologic disease is just beginning to draw attention. Thus, patients with multiple sclerosis (MS) whose disease affects the cerebrum may be more prone to depression than patients with a similar degree of functional disability whose disease affects primarily the spinal cord (Schifler et al, 1983); strokes in particular areas may be more likely to cause depression than strokes in other areas (Robinson, 1983). Although the lack of cortisol suppression to dexamethasone has been a disappointing marker (Raskind et al, 1982; Spar and Gerner, 1982; and Shapiro et al, 1983), more accurate distinction of neuropsychological and biological discriminators of depression from other causes of dementia may be anticipated.

Delirium and Medical Disorders

Clouding of consciousness is the key symptom of the confusional state termed Delirium in *DSM-III* (Liston, 1982; Lipowski, 1983). Although florid hallucinosis and agitation are often considered characteristic, the associated clinical findings may be variable, as recognized long ago in Bonhoeffer's seminal work (1909). Delirium usually has a relatively acute onset and fluctuates over hours and days, but the slowly developing confusion of a quiet patient is easily mistaken for a primary degenerative dementia. The hallmark deficits in attention and concentration can be documented by poor performance on such tests as digits forward (Wechsler, 1955) or the "A Test" (Rosvold et al, 1956). Agraphia may be a particularly sensitive sign (Chedru and Geschwind, 1972). The electroencephalogram (EEG) characteristically shows generalized slowing (Engel and Romano, 1959), whereas the EEG is normal in the early stages of many dementias. Serial EEGs may be especially useful because a single normal EEG is insufficient to rule out delirium (Pro and Wells, 1977).

Failure to recognize delirium is a grave clinical error; and it may be the only presentation of serious systemic illness, especially in the elderly (Liston, 1982). Thorough medical and laboratory evaluation on an urgent basis are the keys to correct diagnosis and successful treatment (Libow 1973, 1977). Despite this well known clinical caveat, data to substantiate the frequency and course of delirium are limited (for example, De Vaul, 1976; Arie, 1978).

Neurologic Disorders

Many neurologic disorders are associated with changes in perception or cognition. Unique characteristics of the cognitive dysfunction may reveal the diagnosis, but it often requires the recognition of associated neurological signs and symptoms. The study of these disorders may help to clarify the neuroanatomical basis of brain function and provide clues to etiology and physiology.

Movement disorders are discussed at greater length in Chapter Nine of this volume. These derive from conditions predominantly affecting structures from the midbrain to the basal ganglia. In patients with progressive supranuclear palsy, Albert and colleagues (1974) identified a syndrome of "subcortical dementia" consisting of forgetfulness, slowed thought processes, impaired ability to manipulate acquired knowledge and personality change (consisting of prominent apathy and depression) in the absence of amnesia, aphasia, agnosia or apraxia. Although dementia is also associated with Huntington's, Parkinson's and Wilson's diseases (as well as other disorders of the basal ganglia), there is controversy over the existence of a coherent "subcortical" syndrome and its anatomic specificity (Albert, 1978; Cummings and Benson, 1983).

Mass lesions (including tumor, abscess and subdural hematoma) typically present with a focal syndrome; but a gradually enlarging lesion in a relatively silent area of the brain may imitate dementia. The detection of such lesions is one of the major justifications for obtaining computerized tomographic (CT) scans of the head in the evaluation of patients with the dementia syndrome. Other intracranial conditions, such as hydrocephalus, hemorrhage, infarction and brain edema may also be visualized on CT scans. By contrast, evidence of cortical atrophy relates more to age than to degree of dementia (Wilson et al, 1982).

Intracranial infections, of course, usually have a more fulminant course than does dementia, but the indolent encephalitis or meningitis, particularly fungal, must be kept in mind in these patients. A gradual dementing process is the most common mental symptom of tertiary neurosyphilis. Peripheral signs may or may not be present, history of infection is typically unobtainable and routine serology is often nonreactive. Even specific serological tests are nonreactive in a percentage of patients. Examination of cerebrospinal fluid (CSF) is thus indicated when lues is a serious consideration (Hooshmand et al, 1972).

Creutzfeldt-Jakob disease is an uncommon disorder that produces dementia accompanied by motor signs, particularly myoclonus, early in the course of the disease. The progression is typically rapid, leading to death in eight months to two years. It is of heuristic significance because transmissibility has been shown by intracranial inoculation in primates and, suggestively, in humans. There is no evidence for transmission by normal human contact (Roos, 1981). The syndrome is referred to as a "slow virus" infection because it typically appears after a latent period of years.

CLINICAL APPROACH TO PATIENTS WITH DEMENTIA

Case Study

Dementia is not an acute remitting condition. Diagnosis and management, while conceptually separate, actually develop and interact over time. The following case study illustrates the interplay of principles to be discussed.

> Mr. A, a 64-year-old, right-handed man was brought to the Geropsychiatry Inpatient Service by his daughter, because he had become "unmanageable." During the previous two weeks at the nursing home he had at times been quite agitated, had slept little, and had mistaken his image in the mirror for an intruder. More remote history was patchy, but Mr. A had been a vigorous man, with a history of hypertension and prodigious drinking. Eighteen months prior to admission he was noted to have fluent, but essentially meaningless, conversation, although he continued to function socially. Six weeks prior to admission—shortly after separating from his wife—he had undergone alcohol detoxification complicated by alcoholic hepatitis. When his mental state failed to clear, Alzheimer's disease was diagnosed. He was placed in a nursing home and received haloperidol, but his agitation had worsened.

> Mr. A was ruddy and looked 50 rather than 64 years old. He had marked rigidity, slow movement, delayed response time, and a resting tremor. He was attentive, but did not identify his nose on written or oral command. He could neither write his name legibly nor produce any drawings. He was not dysarthric, his verbal output was fluent, but paraphasia was the rule and he erred particularly in naming. He was unable to name any President, but did manage to say "movie" for Mr. Reagan. When asked for earlier presidents, he said that the wife of one had just had a "stroke" as had, in fact, been reported by the media during the week before his admission. Mr. A conveyed a feeling of sadness and abandonment. His blood pressure was 160/100 mm Hg; physical and neurological examinations were otherwise unremarkable.

> His laboratory results showed mild macrocytosis with an occasional hypersegmented neutrophil. Serum B_{12} level was low normal, and a Schilling test suggested

impaired absorption. EEG was diffusely abnormal, and CT scan showed diffuse atrophy.

Mr. A's dementia most likely represented a combination of insults. The CT scan, history of hypertension, and persistent Wernicke-type aphasia suggested a previous stroke, with the possibility of other smaller lesions and multi-infarct dementia. Depression, fluctuating course, nocturnal confusion and stepwise progression were consonant with that diagnosis; focal neurological signs would be expected but were absent except for a localizing aphasia. Alcohol, hypertension and B_{12} deficiency may have been contributory.

Intermittent confusion and irritability were evident during his early hospital stay. Haloperidol seemed to worsen both symptoms, while occasional doses of oxazepam alleviated them. Propranolol (20 mg, three times a day) was prescribed for hypertension and seemed to reduce the need for tranquilizers. In response to the major defect in comprehension a particular nurse was assigned to Mr. A at each shift and gave him instructions in a very simplified form: For example, "It's time for dinner" became "Let's stand up," then "Let's go to the table," then "Let's sit down," and then "Let's eat."

Three months after administration of cyancobalamin, 1000 mg intramuscularly (IM), cognitive function seemed noticeably improved. At five months a dense, fluent (Wernicke-type) aphasia remained. Although unable to give the date, Mr. A accurately estimated the duration of his hospitalization and was well oriented to family members, staff, patients, and the ward topography, but he was intermittently confused, especially at night. He again became depressed and more confused when one of his favorite daughters chose to marry and live in Europe. Increased attention to Mr. A at this time, as well as extensive support of various family members and legal intervention, was necessary to resolve this crisis and arrange a suitable disposition.

Diagnosis

The course of dementia can provide critical diagnostic clues. The physician must obtain reliable collateral information from someone who knows the patient well. Of special importance, given the profound effect that medications can have on the mental status of geriatric patients, is an inventory of both prescription and over-the-counter drugs. A thorough physical examination and careful assessment of neurological status will help to identify underlying medical and neurological conditions.

Performing a full mental status examination, paying special attention to delineating the patient's cognitive function, is obviously crucial. To do this while maintaining rapport and preserving a patient's potentially threatened sense of dignity is the heart of the clinical task. Formal short tests, such as the Mental Status Questionnaire (Kahn et al, 1960) or the Mini-Mental State (Folstein et al, 1975), are useful for screening and for following severity over time; but diagnostic questions require more complete attention to various features, including: attention and concentration; language capability; both immediate recall and long-term memory; visuospatial skills; abstractions; mood; personality; motor behavior; and judgment. This approach (see, for example, Strub and Black, 1977) provides the best opportunity to identify a delirium, or one of the many focal syndromes that may be mistaken for dementia. An example of the latter is the angular gyrus syndrome misdiagnosed as Alzheimer's Disease (Benson et al, 1982).

Use of the laboratory is somewhat controversial. Unless the results of physical and mental status testing point to a clearcut diagnosis, we recommend a baseline battery (Table 3) somewhat more extensive than that of the National Institute on Aging Task Force (1980). Further investigations, such as cardiovascular evaluation, lumbar puncture, heavy metal screens and cisternography must be chosen on a case-by-case basis. New techniques such as nuclear magnetic resonance and evoked potentials may prove to be valuable, but their role is undefined at this time. Neuropsychological testing is useful for establishing a baseline to follow, especially in patients with early symptoms whose course remains to be established, and for delineating more fully abnormalities found in the clinical exam, including the role of personality traits, psychosis, stressors, and mood in cognitive dysfunction.

Management

The initial steps in management involve accurate diagnosis and treatment of specific identified disorder. In most cases this does not completely reverse the cognitive deficits; but it may arrest the dementing process and alleviate associated symptoms.

There are no specific treatments for Alzheimer-type or multi-infarct dementia—the most prevalent forms of dementia—but symptomatic treatments can maximize patient comfort and improve daily functioning (Small et al, 1981; Winograd and Jarvik, in press). Useful pharmacological agents include chloral hydrate or short-acting benzodiazepines for insomnia (for example, 0.5 mg lorazepam several hours before bedtime), high potency neuroleptics for agitation or paranoid symptoms (for example, 0.25–2.0 mg haloperidol daily) and antidepressants for concurrent depression (for example, 25 mg trazodone daily). The elderly with dementia often require reduced initial dosages in line with age-related changes in body function and pharmacokinetics. Dosages should be increased slowly and in small increments. Diphenhydramine and related compounds (often used as mild sedatives) should be avoided because of a tendency to cause anticholinergic toxicity in patients with cognitive deficits. Benzodiazepines may cause confusion, instability or ataxia, particularly undesirable side effects in the elderly.

Table 3. Screening Tests for Evaluating Dementia

1. Complete blood count
2. Urinalysis
3. Serum urea nitrogen and glucose; serum electrolytes (sodium, potassium, carbon dioxide content, chloride, calcium, phosphorus); bilirubin; serum vitamin B_{12}, folic acid, LDH, alkaline phosphatase, SGOT
4. T_4 (T_3 and TSH in appropriate situations)
5. Serological test for syphilis
6. Chest X–ray
7. Electrocardiogram
8. Electroencephalogram
9. Computerized tomography (CT scan) of the brain

Environmental management is also important. Patients with dementia do best with daily routines in familiar, constant surroundings. Prominently displayed clocks, calendars, nightlights, checklists, and diaries all aid the patient's orientation.

Psychological support for the patient may help maximize remaining abilities and adaptive skills, while psychotherapy for caregiving persons may lighten their emotional burden. Patients often need help in grieving cognitive losses and most, if not all, patients remain aware of such losses until the last stages of illness.

The importance of relatives in the care of the demented patient cannot be overemphasized. The great majority of patients with dementia reside in the community for the major period of their disability. Caregivers are most often family members, and their collaboration is essential for optimal management. Patients with progressive dementia will suffer if restrictions are imposed too early on the use of automobiles, stoves, and access to the street. Certain aids, such as identification bracelets, may increase the chances that patients will be able to get home. Legal transfer of authority should be considered early in the course of the disease so patients may be able to participate in the decision as to who should assume responsibilities for their property and person. Respite care (in day hospitals or nursing homes) and visiting nurses may sustain an overtaxed support system. Lay organizations, such as the Alzheimer's Disease and Related Disorder Association (ADRDA), provide invaluable support as well as information. The psychiatrist must be aware of and sensitive to the stresses inherent in caring for and watching a loved one deteriorate. Common issues among caregivers include dependency, guilt, anticipatory grief, and fears of their own mortality or mental failing.

FUTURE RESEARCH

The identification of effective treatments and preventive measures is, of course, the ultimate goal of physicians and scientists. Somatic treatments based on plausible hypotheses deserve careful clinical trials (Crook and Gershon, 1981; Greenwald and Davis, 1983). Methodology to ensure that responses are assessed accurately is necessary so that useful interventions are not mistakenly discarded and resources are not committed to approaches that have little promise. Historically, treatments have appeared before the cause of a given mental disease was understood; they have, at times, resulted in better insights into underlying dysfunctions.

For most kinds of dementia, the etiology remains obscure. In syndromes such as Huntington's disease, genetics plays an important role (Brackenridge, 1971); but more diverse factors are relevant in other conditions. Multi-infarct dementia, for example, can be classified by the distribution of the infarcts (such as cortical, subcortical, basal ganglia, brain stem); by the underlying disease process (for example, atherosclerosis, Fabry disease, hypertension, and others); or by onto-genetic and developmental circumstances (for example, vascular malformation, cigarette smoking).

Several hypotheses, not mutually exclusive, have emerged concerning the etiology of Alzheimer's disease. Genetic factors have been implicated, although the mode of transmission remains controversial (Matsuyama, 1983). Brain reactive antibodies have been described (Nandy, 1983; Ihara et al, 1983). A transmissible agent may be involved, analogous to the Creutzfeldt-Jakob agent (Roos, 1981). The term "prion" has been suggested to denote this small *proteinaceous infectious* particle, resistant to inactivation by most procedures that modify nucleic acids (Prusiner, 1982; Merz et al, 1983); further investigations may have significance for our understanding of the cause of several degenerative diseases such as DAT (Prusiner, 1984). External factors, such as head trauma (Corsellis, 1978) and aluminum toxicity (Banks and Kastin, 1983; Crapper, 1980), are also being investigated, but require further epidemiologic and experimental studies (Mortimer and Schuman, 1981).

Deficiency of acetylcholine (Ach) synthesizing enzymes, especially choline acetyl transferase (CAT), has been a consistent finding in DAT, although Ach receptor density is essentially unchanged (Coyle et al, 1983). Furthermore, anticholinergic drugs, such as atropine, transiently provoke a memory disturbance similar to that in DAT. The discovery that most of the cholinergic innervation of the cerebral cortex arises from the nucleus basalis of Meynert (a small region of the basal forebrain) and that these neurons are largely lacking in patients with DAT, suggests a possible neuroanatomical basis for the disease. The cause of these changes, their relation to the clinical findings and to the standard pathological hallmarks of the disease (plaques and tangles) remain conjectural.

Other leads consist of the dearth of adrenergic cells in locus ceruleus described for patients with early-onset but not late-onset dementia (Bondareff et al, 1982); abnormalities in the immune system (Matsuyama et al, 1978; Walford, 1982); in HLA antigens (Walford, 1980; Weitkamp et al, 1983); in the philothermal response of polymorphonuclear leukocytes (Jarvik et al, 1982); in red blood cells (Sorbi and Blass, 1983); in lithium countertransport rates (Diamond et al, 1983); and in other neurotransmitter systems (Greenwald et al, 1983). Development of new imaging techniques, such as positron emission tomography (PET) (Reivich and Alavi, 1983) and nuclear magnetic resonance (James et al, 1982) offer promise of additional leads toward refining our understanding of etiology.

CONCLUSION

Psychiatrists have an important contribution to make if health care is to adapt to the challenge posed by patients with dementia. Behavioral and emotional symptoms of dementia, as well as the reactions of family members, are major concerns in treatment.

The greatest challenge we face as psychiatrists is to prevent the spectre of thousands of institutions housing millions of our citizens maimed in mind, chained to chair or cot, incontinent of urine and feces, incapable of communicating their desires, and dependent upon frustrated, hostile, overworked, undercompensated, and uncomprehending "attendants" for their most elementary wants—such as food and water—and their most intimate needs. Only research offers the hope to free us from such a scenario of horror; only research which will yield the means of effective treatment and successful prevention.

REFERENCES

Albert ML: Subcortical dementia, in Alzheimer Disease: Senile Dementia and Related Disorders. Edited by Katzman R, Terry RD, Bick KL. New York, Raven Press, 1978

Albert ML: Geriatric neuropsychology. J Consult Clin Psychol 49:835-850, 1981

Albert ML, Feldman TG, Willis AL: The "subcortical dementia" of progressive supranuclear palsy. J Neurol Neurosurg Psychiatry 37:121-130, 1974

American Psychiatric Association: Diagnostic and Statistical Manual of Mental Disorders, 2nd ed. (*DSM-II*). Washington, D.C., Committee on Nomenclature and Statistics, American Psychiatric Association, 1968

American Psychiatric Association: Diagnostic and Statistical Manual of Mental Disorders, 3rd ed. (*DSM-III*). Washington, D.C., Task Force on Nomenclature and Statistics, American Psychiatric Associaton, 1980

Appell J, Kertesz A, Fisman M: A study of language functioning in Alzheimer patients. Brain Lang 17:73-91, 1982

Arie T: Confusion in old age. Age Ageing 7 (Suppl):72-76, 1978

Banks WA, Kastin AJ: Aluminum increases permeability of the blood-brain barrier to labelled DSIP and beta-endorphin: possible implications for senile and dialysis dementia. Lancet II:1227-1229, 1983

Benson DF, Cummings JL, Tsai SY: Angular gyrus syndrome simulating Alzheimer disease. Arch Neurol 39:616-620, 1982

Blessed G, Tomlinson BE, Roth M: The association between quantitative measures of dementia and of senile change in the cerebral grey matter of elderly subjects. Br J Psychiatry 114:797-811, 1968

Bondareff W, Mountjoy CQ, Roth M: Loss of neurons of origin of the adrenergic projection to cerebral cortex (nucleus locus ceruleus) in senile dementia. Neurology 32:164-168, 1982

Bonhoeffer K: Exogenous psychoses (1909), in Themes and Variations in European Psychiatry. Edited by Hirsch SR, Shepherd M. Charlottesville, University Press of Virginia, 1974

Brackenridge CJ: The relation of type of initial symptom and line of transmission to ages of onset and death in Huntington's disease. Clin Genet 2:287-297, 1971

Caine ED: Pseudodementia: Current concepts and future directions. Arch Gen Psychiatry 38:1359-1364, 1981

Chedru F, Geschwind N: Writing disturbances in acute confusional states. Neuropsychologia 10:343-353, 1972

Cohen DG: Historical views and evolution of concepts, in Alzheimer's Disease: The Standard Reference. Edited by Reisberg B. New York, The Free Press, 1983

Corsellis J: Post-traumatic dementia, in Alzheimer's Disease: Senile Dementia and Related Disorders. Edited by Katzman R, Terry RD, Bick KL. New York, Raven Press, 1978

Coyle JT, Price DL, Delong MR: Alzheimer's disease: a disorder of cortical cholinergic innervation. Science 219:1184-1190, 1983

Crapper DR, Quittkat SS, et al: Intranuclear aluminum content in Alzheimer's disease, dialysis encephalopathy and experimental encephalopathy. Acta Neuropathol 50:19-24, 1980

Crook T, Gershon S (Eds): Strategies for the Development of an Effective Treatment for Senile Dementia. New Canaan, Connecticut, Mark Powley Associates, Inc., 1981

Cummings JL, Benson DF: Dementia: A Clinical Approach. Boston, Butterworth Publishers, 1983

Cummings JL, Benson DF, Hill MA, et al: Aphasia in Alzheimer disease. Neurology (in press) 1984a

Cummings JL, Tomiyasu U, Read S, et al: Amnesia with hippocampal lesions after cardiopulmonary arrest. Neurology 34:679-681, 1984b

De Vaul RA: Acute organic brain syndromes: clinical considerations. Tex Med 72:51-54, 1976

Diamond J, Matsuyama S, Meier K, et al: Elevation of erythrocyte countertransport rates in dementia of the Alzheimer type. N Engl J Med 309:1061-1062, 1983

Engel GL, Romano J: Delirium, a syndrome of cerebral insufficiency. J Chronic Dis 9:260-277, 1959

Ernst P, Beran B, Safford F, et al: Isolation and the symptoms of chronic brain syndrome. Gerontologist 18:468-474, 1978

Fisher CM: Lacunar strokes and infarcts: a review. Neurology 32:871-876, 1982

Folstein MF, Folstein SE, McHugh PR: "Mini-mental state," a practical method for grading the cognitive state of patients for the clinician. J Psychiatr Res 12:189-198, 1975

Folstein MF, McHugh PR: Dementia syndrome of depression, in Alzheimer's Disease: Senile Dementia and Related Disorders. Edited by Katzman R, Terry RD, Bick KL. New York, Raven Press, 1978

Goodwin JS, Goodwin JM, Garry PJ: Association between nutritional status and cognitive functioning in a healthy elderly population. JAMA 249:2917-2921, 1983

Greenwald BS, Davis KL: Experimental pharmacology of Alzheimer disease. Adv Neurol 38:87-102, 1983

Greenwald BS, Mohs RC, David KL: Neurotransmitter deficits in Alzheimer's disease: criteria for significance. J Am Geriatr Soc 31:310-316, 1983

Gurland BJ, Cross PS: Epidemiology of psychopathology in old age: some implications for clinical services. Psychiatr Clin N Am 5:11-26, 1982

Hachinski VC, Lassen, NA, Marshall J: Multi-infarct dementia. A cause of mental deterioration in the elderly. Lancet II:207-210, 1974

Hachinski VC, Iliff LD, Zilhka E, et al: Cerebral blood flow in dementia. Arch Neurol 32:632-637, 1975

Hooshmand H, Escobar MR, Kopf SW: Neurosyphilis: a study of 241 patients. JAMA 219:726-729, 1972

Ihara Y, Abraham C, Selkoe D: Antibodies to paired helical filaments in Alzheimer's disease do not recognize normal brain proteins. Nature, 304:727-730, 1983

James AE, Price RR, Rollo FD, et al: Nuclear magnetic resonance imaging: a promising technique. JAMA 247:1331-1334, 1982

Jarvik LF, Eisdorfer C, Blum JE: Intellectual Functioning in Adults. New York, Springer Publishing Co., 1973

Jarvik LF, Ruth V, Matsuyama SS: Organic brain syndrome and aging: a six-year follow-up of surviving twins. Arch Gen Psychiatry 37:280-286, 1980

Jarvik LF, Matsuyama SS, Kessler JO, et al: Philothermal response of polymorphonuclear leukocytes in dementia of the Alzheimer type. Neurobiol Aging 3:93-99, 1982

Kahn RL, Goldfarb AI, Pollack M, et al: Brief objective measures for determination of mental status in the aged. Am J Psychiatry 117:326-328, 1960

Kral VA: Benign senescent forgetfulness, in Alzheimer's Disease: Senile Dementia and Related Disorders. Edited by Katzman R, Terry RD, Bick KL. New York, Raven Press, 1978

La Rue A: Memory loss and aging: distinguishing dementia from benign senescent forgetfulness and depressive pseudodementia. Psychiatr Clin N Am 5:89-103, 1982

Libow LS: Pseudo-senility: Acute and reversible organic brain syndrome. J Am Geriatr Soc 21:112-120, 1973

Libow, LS: Senile dementia and pseudosenility: clinical diagnosis, in Cognitive and Emotional Disturbance in the Elderly. Edited by Eisdorfer C, Friedel RO. Chicago, Year Book Medical Publishers, 1977

Lipowski, ZJ: Transient cognitive disorders (delirium, acute confusional states) in the elderly. Am J Psychiatry 140:1426-1436, 1983

Liston EH: Delirium in the aged. Psychiatr Cl N Am 5:49-66, 1982

Liston EH, La Rue A: Clinical differentiation of primary degenerative and multi-infarct dementia: a critical review of the evidence. Part I: clinical studies. Biol Psychiatry 18:1451-1465, 1983a

Liston EH, La Rue A: Clinical differentiation of primary degenerative and multi-infarct dementia: a critical review of the evidence. Part II: pathological studies. Biol Psychiatry 18:1466-1484, 1983b

Lloyd GG, Lishman WA: Effect of depression on the speed of recall of pleasant and unpleasant experiences. Psychol Med 5:173-180, 1975

Loeb C, Gandolfo C: Diagnostic evaluation of degenerative and vascular dementia. Stroke 14:399-401, 1983

McAllister TW: Overview: pseudodementia. Am J Psychiatry 140:528-533, 1983

Matsuyama SS: Genetic factors in dementia of the Alzheimer type, in Alzheimer's Disease: The Standard Reference. Edited by Reisberg B. New York, Free Press, 1983

Matsuyama SS, Cohen D, Jarvik LF: Hypodiploidy and serum immunoglobulin concentrations in the elderly. Mech Ageing Dev 8:407-412, 1978

Merz P, Somerville RA, Wisniewski HM, et al: Scrapie-associated fibrils in Creutzfeldt-Jakob disease. Nature 306:474-476, 1983

Mortimer JA, Schuman LM: The Epidemiology of Dementia. New York, Oxford University Press, 1981

Nandy K: Immunologic factors, in Alzheimer's Disease: The Standard Reference. Edited by Reisberg B. New York, Free Press, 1983

Nott PN, Fleminger JJ: Presenile dementia: the difficulties of early diagnosis. Acta Psychiatr Scand 51:210-217, 1975

Plum F: Dementia: an approaching epidemic. Nature 279:372-374, 1979

Pro JD, Wells CE: The use of the electroencephalogram in the diagnosis of delirium. Diseases of the Nervous System 38:804-808, 1977

Prusiner SB: Novel proteinaceous infectious particles cause scrapie. Science 216:136-144, 1982

Prusiner SB: Some speculations about prions, amyloid and Alzheimer disease. N Engl J Med 310:661-663, 1984

Raskind M, Peskind E, Rivard M-F, et al: Dexamethasone suppression test and cortisol circadian rhythm in primary degenerative dementia. Am J Psychiatry 139:1468-1471, 1982

Read SL, Jarvik LF: Cerebrovascular disease in the differential diagnosis of dementia. Psychiatric Annals 14:100-108, 1984

Reivich M, Alavi A: Position emission tomographic studies of local cerebral glucose metabolism in humans in physiological and pathophysiologcal conditions. Adv Metab Disord 10:137-176, 1983

Robinson RG: Investigating mood disorders following brain injury: an integrative approach using clinical and laboratory studies. Integrative Psychiatry 1:35-39, 1983

Ron MA, Toone BK, Garralda ME, et al: Diagnostic accuracy in presenile dementia. Br J Psychiatry 134:161-168, 1979

Roos, RP: Alzheimer disease and the lessons of transmissible virus dementia, in The Epidemiology of Dementia. Edited by Mortimer JA, Schuman LM. New York, Oxford University Press, 1981

Rosen WG, Terry RD, Fuld PA, et al: Pathological verification of ischemic score in differentiation of dementias. Ann Neurol 7:486-488, 1980

Rosvold HE, Mirsky AF, Sarason I, et al: A continuous performance test of brain damage. J Consult Clin Psychology 20:343-350, 1956

Roth M: The natural history of mental disorder. Journal of Mental Sciences 101:281-301, 1955

Sachar EJ: Endocrine abnormalities in depression, in Handbook of Affective Disorders. Edited by Paykel ES. New York, The Guilford Press, 1982

Schifler RB, Caine ED, Bamford KA, et al: Depressive episodes in patients with multiple sclerosis. Am J Psychiatry 140:1498-1500, 1983

Shapiro MF, Lehman AF, Greenfield S: Biases in the laboratory diagnosis of depression in medical practice. Arch Intern Med 143:2085-2088, 1983

Small GW: Multi-infarct dementia: the ischemic score revised. Syllabus and Scientific Proceedings, American Psychiatric Association 137th Annual Meeting, 1984

Small GW, Jarvik LF: The dementia syndrome. Lancet II: 1443-1446, 1982

Small GW, Liston EH, Jarvik LF: Diagnosis and treatment of dementia in the aged. West J Med 135:469-481, 1981

Sorbi S, and Blass J. Fibrolast phosphofructokinase in Alzheimer disease and Down syndrome, in Biological Aspects of Alzheimer's Disease Banbury Report. Edited by Katzman R. 15:297-308, 1983

Spar JE, Gerner R: Does the dexamethasone suppression test distinguish dementia from depression? Am J Psychiatry 139:238-240, 1982

Sternberg DE, Jarvik ME: Memory functions in depression. Arch Gen Psychiatry 33:219-224, 1976

Steuer J, Jarvik LF: Cognitive functioning in the elderly: influence of physical health, in Aging: Biology and Behavior. Edited by McGaugh JL, Kiesler SB. New York, Academic Press, 1981

Strub RL, Black FW: The Mental Status Examination in Neurology. Philadelphia, F.A. Davis, 1977

Task Force sponsored by the National Institute on Aging: Senility reconsidered: treatment possibilities for mental impairment in the elderly. JAMA 244:259-263, 1980

Tomlinson BE, Blessed G, Roth M: Observations on the brains of demented old people. J Neurol Sci 11:205-242, 1970

Walford RL: Immunological studies of Down's syndrome and Alzheimer's disease. Ann NY Acad Sciences 396:95-106, 1982

Walford RL, Hodge SE: HLA distribution in Alzheimer's disease, in Histocompatability testing in 1980. Edited by Terasaki P.I. Los Angeles, UCLA Tissue Typing Laboratory, 1980

Wechsler D: Manual for the Wechsler Adult Intelligence Scale. New York, Psychological Corp., 1955

Weingartner H, Silberman E: Models of cognitive impairment: cognitive changes in depression. Psychopharmacol Bull 18:27-42, 1982

Weitkamp LR, Nee L, Keats B, et al: Alzheimer disease: evidence for susceptibility loci on chromosomes 6 and 14. Am J Hum Genet 35:443-453, 1983

Wells CE: Dementia. Philadelphia, F.A. Davis, 1977

Wells CE: Pseudodementia. Am J Psychiatry 136:895-900, 1979

Wilkie FL, Eisdorfer C: Systematic disease and behavioral correlates, in Intellectual Functioning in Adults. Edited by Jarvik LF, Eisdorfer C, Blum JE. New York, Springer Publishing Co., 1973

Wilson RS, Fox JH, Huckman MS, et al: Computed tomography in dementia. Neurology 32:1054-1057, 1982

Winograd CH, Jarvik LF: The demented patient and the primary care physician: management challenges. Ann Intern Med (in press)

Zis AP, Goodwin FK: The amine hypothesis, in Handbook of Affective Disorders. Edited by Paykel ES. New York, The Guilford Press, 1982

Chapter 12

Substance Induced Organic Mental Disorders

by Mark S. Gold, M.D., Todd Wilk Estroff, M.D. and A.L.C. Pottash, M.D.

In this chapter we review some of the causes of substance induced organic mental disorders, or the so-called "secondary psychiatric disorders" caused by prescribed medications, illicit medications and exogenous poisons. Naturally occurring medical, neurological, endocrinological and other diseases, which are the great mimickers of psychiatric diseases, have been previously reviewed by our group (Estroff and Gold, 1984b) and others (Hall, 1980; Jefferson and Marshall, 1981) and, for the most part, are beyond the scope of this paper.

Substance induced organic mental disorders are often misdiagnosed because many psychiatrists and other physicians are neither aware of these disorders, nor order appropriate follow-up laboratory testing to help make the diagnosis clear.

The exact incidence and prevalence of these disorders is often not known, because it is an area of medicine and psychiatry that has been virtually ignored. Few studies of any sort exist and, in many cases, the psychiatric symptoms reported in this chapter are the result of single case reports. Therefore, though the symptoms must be considered rare, it must be emphasized that not enough studies have been done. Where studies have been done, percentages are included in the text. These disorders are more common in inpatients and in refractory chronic cases.

PRESCRIBED MEDICATIONS

Psychiatric symptoms occur in at least 2.7 percent of patients taking prescribed medication on a regular basis according to the Boston Collaborative Drug Surveillance Study of 9,000 patients (Boston Collaborative Drug-Related Program, 1971). The spectrum of adverse psychiatric reaction is well known, and extensive lists have been compiled and published (Anonymous, 1981; Hall et al, 1980). During a diagnostic psychiatric evaluation it is preferable to discontinue all medications for as long as possible and to evaluate the patient after a washout period.

Psychotropic Agents

Antidepressants (AD) can induce new psychiatric symptomatology in patients being treated for depression, and persons who abuse or accidentally take this medication. Toxic effects may include visual hallucinations and delirium. Anticholinergic toxicity may be caused by antidepressants, antihistamines, belladona alkaloids, antipsychotics, certain plants, benzotropine and trihexyphenidyl.

Suspected diagnosis can sometimes be confirmed by quantitative urine and blood testing. Patients who are schizophrenic may become more psychotic when an AD is added (Siris et al, 1978). AD withdrawal symptoms have been reported and have been described as being similar to influenza.

Antipsychotics (AP) produce behavioral side effects, from oversedation to total mutism and severe catatonia (Gelenberg, 1976). Akathisia and akinesia are common, but are often misinterpreted as anxiety and depression (Klein et al, 1980). APs can also cause neuroleptic malignant syndrome, a toxic syndrome that produces fever, muscular rigidity, akinesia, delirium and elevated creatinine phosphokinase (CPK) levels (Klein et al, 1980). Like ADs, anticholinergic delirium is well documented, especially when APs are used in combination with other drugs with anticholinergic properties. This may be misinterpreted as a worsening of the psychosis (Hall, 1980). Withdrawal symptoms can occur when these medications are discontinued, and can include restlessness, insomnia, increased appetite and giddiness (Gardos et al, 1978).

Lithium induced organic mental disorders include decreased concentration, decreased mood and a toxic delirium, especially if blood lithium levels are not monitored carefully (Rifkin et al, 1973; Hall, 1980). Hypothyroidism, nephrotoxic and permanent neurotoxic damage have been reported, especially in association with elevated serum lithium levels (Sellers et al, 1982; Donaldson and Cunningham, 1983).

Monoamine oxidase inhibitors have a spectrum of behavioral side effects similar to those of the previously mentioned antidepressants; but since many of them are more structurally related to epinephrine and amphetamine, they are more likely to induce anxiety, nervousness, agitation, insomnia and euphoria. In vulnerable individuals, they may induce symptoms indistinguishable from *DSM-III*'s description of cocaine or amphetamine intoxication, or mania or schizophrenia (Sheehy and Maxman, 1978).

Benzodiazepines and other sedative hypnotic compounds' chief behavioral symptoms (which occur while the drug is being administered) include oversedation and disinhibition. Severe depression with suicidal ideation, depersonalization and frank psychosis have been reported but are rare (Hall, 1980). Delirium may occur, especially in the elderly. The most common psychiatric misdiagnosis occurs not while the drugs are being administered, but when they are withdrawn in dependent individuals.

Disulfiram can produce a classic *DSM-III* delirium without associated psychiatric symptoms, or a delirium with associated psychiatric features, including severe depression, paranoid ideation and delusions. Psychiatric symptoms also occur in the absence of delirium and include anxiety, severe depression with successful suicide, psychoses that are indistinguishable from those described in *DSM-III*, bipolar mania and schizophrenia (Rainey, 1977; Hall 1980). Antipsychotic medication is contraindicated and may worsen the symptoms (Hall, 1980).

Antihypertensive Agents

Reserpine's (RP) organic mental disorder—depression—made it the father of the catecholamine hypothesis. Many other antihypertensives share the ability to precipitate depression in five to 20 percent of all patients (Pottash et al, 1981).

The patients most vulnerable to developing depression have a prior history of depression and have been on medication from two to eight months (Goodwin et al, 1972; Goodwin and Bunney, 1971). Alpha–methyldopa commonly causes psychiatric side effects, including sleep disorders (0.8 percent); dreams and nightmares (1.9 percent); and depression (3.6 percent). With clonidine, the most frequently reported psychiatric side effects are sedation and fatigue (47.6 percent), followed by sleep disturbances (4.7 percent) and depression (1.5 percent) (Paykel et al, 1982). Clonidine abuse and overdose can present with psychomotoric retardation. Propranolol's side effects include drowsiness and fatigue (3.1 percent); sleep disorders (0.4 percent); dreams and nightmares (1 percent); hallucinations—mostly hypnagogic and hypnopompic (0.5 percent)—and depression (0.7 percent) (Paykel et al, 1982).

Antiarrhythmic Drugs

Lidocaine and procainamide are reported to cause psychosis (Turner, 1982; McCrum and Guidry, 1978). Disopyramide causes acute transient toxic psychosis, including delusions of persecution and auditory and visual hallucinations (Padfield et al, 1977; Ahmad et al, 1979). Mental symptoms can occur as the first sign of digitalis toxicity, or in association with other well-documented toxic symptoms—such as arrhythmia, nausea and vomiting and yellow tinted vision—as was first reported by Duroziez in 1874. Sometimes this digitalis toxicity may be overlooked and misdiagnosed as a Coronary Care Unit delirium and end in death (Marriott, 1968). Patients have demonstrated visual hallucinations (Volpe and Soave, 1979), auditory hallucinations, paranoid ideation (Church and Marriott, 1959; Gorelick et al, 1978), thought disorder, mutism and labile mood swings (Shear and Sacks, 1978); these symptoms frequently occur in conjunction with some degree of disorientation and agitation, but can occur with clear consciousness.

Anticonvulsant Medications

There are many psychiatric side effects that are caused by anticonvulsant medications (Tollefson, 1980; Stores, 1975; Franks and Richter, 1979). They include sedation, confusional states, mood changes, changes in psychiatric motor energy levels, schizophrenia, psychosis, mania, depression, excitement, irritability, tearfulness, aggression and hyperactivity. Psychotic features range from somatic and paranoid delusions to auditory, visual and tactile hallucinations; these may be indistinguishable from schizophrenia or may be part of a delirious, acute, confusional state. In many instances the psychiatric symptoms are difficult to attribute to an individual medication. Epileptic patients have a higher incidence of associated psychiatric disturbance and are often on two or more anticonvulsants at a time. Psychiatric side effects of phenytoin include sedation, acute delirium with hallucinations, encephalopathy, tactile and visual hallucinations (Glaser, 1972; Stores, 1975), somatic delusions and schizophrenic-like psychoses (Stores, 1975; Tollefson, 1980).

In adults, drowsiness, sedation, depression and acute confusional states are reported with barbiturates; in children, excitement, irritability, tearfulness, aggression and a hyperkinetic syndrome are reported (Stores, 1975; Tollefson, 1980). Tolerance and withdrawal states produce the most common misdiagnosis.

Confusional states, major mood swings, paranoid psychoses, personality changes and confusional psychoses have all been reported with Primidone (Booker, 1972; Stores, 1975; Tollefson, 1980). Ethosuximide can induce anxiety, depression, delusions, hallucinations, psychosis (Roger et al, 1968; Buchanan, 1972), lethargy, euphoria (Stores, 1975), night terrors, aggression and paranoia (Tollefson, 1980). The infrequent reports of adverse psychiatric side effects of carbamazepine are drowsiness, anxiety, restlessness and rare reports of increasing psychosis (Stores, 1975; Tollefson, 1980; Dalby, 1971).

Other Prescribed Medications

Jones and Lance (1976) report prominent psychiatric side effects in patients being treated with baclofen (Lioresal), including hallucinations, illusions, paranoia, euphoria, aphrodisiac effects, depression, anxiety and suicidal ideation. Paranoia, auditory and visual hallucinations and *DMS-III* mania have also been reported (Arnold et al, 1980; Lees et al, 1977).

Goodwin (1971) found a 20 percent rate of psychiatric symptoms in parkinsonian patients who were treated with L–dopa. They included confusion or delirium (4.4 percent); depression (4.2 percent); agitation or activation (3.6 percent); psychosis, delusions or paranoia (3.6 percent); hypomania (1.5 percent); hypersexuality (0.9 percent) and other symptoms (1.5 percent). These results were confirmed and expanded to include vivid dreams, hallucinations and a model psychosis (12.5 percent) (Presthus and Holmsen, 1974; Moskovitz et al, 1978).

The side effects of bromocriptine are similar to L–dopa, and include confusion, vivid dreams, paranoid delusions and auditory, visual and olfactory hallucinations. A dose related psychosis (Parkes, 1980; Calne et al, 1978), as well as mania (Vlissides et al, 1978), have been reported. Atropine can produce a toxic psychosis that can mimic any psychiatric syndrome. In most cases it is actually an acute delirium limited to the time course of the drugs, clears rapidly and is physostigmine reversible.

Indomethacin and sulindac (which are structurally similar) have been reported to cause psychiatric symptoms after as little as one dose. Indomethacin has caused anxiety, agitation, hostility, paranoia, depersonalization, depression, hallucinations and psychosis (Thompson and Percy, 1966; Rothermich, 1966). Sulindac (Clinoril) has been reported to cause bizarre behavior, obsessive delusions, paranoia and combative/homicidal behavior after one 50 mg dose (Kruis and Barger, 1980).

Corticosteriods, especially prednisone, are well known to produce the entire range of research diagnostic criteria (RDC) indistinguishable disorders, ranging from depression to mania and schizophreniform psychoses (Estroff and Gold, 1984b). Decarbazine has been noted to cause confusion and/or depression in five percent of patients (Peterson and Popkin, 1980). Hexamethylamine has been noted to cause confusion, depression, hallucinations and suicide attempts in 20 percent of patients (Peterson and Popkin, 1980). Methotrexate has been noted to cause a dementing multifocal leukoencephalopathy accompanied by confusion, tremor, ataxia, irritability and somnolence. Those patients treated with folic acid showed stabilization and some improvement of the disease process. A reversible syndrome of decreased concentration and mood lability is induced by 5 Fluorouracil 5 FU (Peterson and Popkin, 1980). Vincristine is well known as a neurotoxin, causing late occurring irritability, depression and hallucinations (Peterson and Popkin, 1980). Vinblastine has been reported to cause anxiety and depression in up to 80 percent of patients within two to three days of the treatment. Mithramycin causes anxiety, irritability and increasing agitation during treatment. L–asparaginase has been reported to cause confusional states, delirium, stupor, personality changes and severe depression (Holland et al, 1974). Procarbazine, a monoamine oxidase (MAO) inhibitor can cause symptoms ranging from drowsiness to stupor. A manic episode has also been reported (Mann and Hutchison, 1967). Mitotane has been reported to cause confusional states.

Certain preanesthetics, especially opiates, have been found to cause acute psychiatric and behavioral symptoms. Nalorphine has been found to cause feelings of suffocation, panic, fear of impending death, delusion, and both auditory and visual hallucinations. Levallorphan causes "queer behavior" and fear, while pentazocine produces overactive, rambling or "crazy" thoughts or fear of dying (Hamilton et al, 1967). Cyclopropane and ether produce the greatest amounts of postanesthetic excitement when used for general anesthesia (Eckenhoff et al, 1961). Halothane and isoflurane cause transient increases in fatigue, depression, confusion, anger and tension, and corresponding decreases in friendliness and vigor, peaking two days after general anesthesia and resolving by the 30th day (Davison et al, 1975).

From the first reports of iproniazid's use it became clear that this medication could elevate a patient's mood. It can cause delirium alone (Hall, 1980) as well as toxic psychoses (with or without confusional features), and can be accompanied by irritability, paranoid ideation, thought disorder, and auditory and visual hallucinations (Hall, 1980; Wallach and Gershon, 1972). In one of the few studies using cycloserine alone, cycloserine caused psychiatric symptomatology of increasing severity as serum levels increased, mimicking naturally occurring depression, mania, schizophrenia and other psychoses (Wallach and Gershon, 1972; Hall, 1980a).

Intramuscular Penicillin G Procaine causes brief, severe psychiatric symptoms in a small number of patients. The symptoms can be so severe that the patient appears psychotic. The patient can become disoriented and extremely agitated; almost all of these patients have the idea that they are going to die immediately. The clearing of symptoms corresponds to the rapid fall of serum procaine to nontoxic levels (Green et al, 1974). Amphotericin B, chloroquine and quinacrine produce reversible psychoses (Winnetal, 1979; Engel, 1966).

There have been numerous reports associated with treatment using cimetidine, of either acute mental confusion (Kimelblatt et al, 1980), or a more severe syndrome consisting of confusion, agitation and auditory and visual hallucinations, which clears within one to two days of stopping of this substance. Bizarre speech and fluctuating levels of consciousness with or without extreme paranoia can accompany these symptoms (Barnhart and Bowden, 1979; Adler et al, 1980). Over-the-counter diet or asthma medications containing aminophylline, ephedrine, or phenylpropanolamine (an amphetamine analogue) have been reported to induce a variety of psychiatric symptoms, including psychosis.

TOXIC POISONINGS

The subject of heavy metals deserves special emphasis because it is an area of little knowledge, and the toxic potential of many metallic substances remains unknown. Heavy metals are defined as those of a high specific gravity (5.0 or more). Some are absolutely essential to health, forming vital parts of life processes and leading to significant disease when deficient from body systems. These include iron, copper, zinc, manganese, chromium, nickel, magnesium, molybdenum, cobalt, strontium, vanadium, and selenium.

Lead poisoning has been well known for over 2,000 years. In the past, blood levels above 60 μg/dl in adults have been universally acknowledged to be toxic (Hall, 1980; Needleman, 1982). This has been recently lowered to 40 μg/dl (Baker et al, 1983; Cullen et al, 1983), when behavioral and psychiatric symptoms are accounted the endpoint. This lowering of acceptable blood levels of lead points to the need for psychiatrists to work with researchers to adjust the "normal" ranges to include to cognitive, mood and behavioral symptoms. In children, lower IQs are reported for lead levels above 13 μg/dl (Yule et al, 1981). Adults have demonstrated that the brief exposure of three months to lead sources will cause progressive but reversible increases in tension, fatigue, confusion, anger and depression as blood levels rise between 40 and 60 μg/dl (Baker et al, 1983). Cullen also reported 13 percent of adult lead-poisoned patients had a presenting complaint of depression, and 22.6 percent were depressed and met *DSM-III* criteria for a major depressive disorder.

Psychiatric symptoms have been known for centuries among workers exposed to mercury. The psychiatric symptoms appear to be blood level related (Maghazaji, 1974). Most frequently reported are mood changes, severe irritability, anxiety, prominent depression and a unique form of xenophobia—a disorder in which the patient develops extreme self-consciousness to the point of avoiding strangers and becoming unable to function in front of his superiors.

Chronic arsenic intoxications usually present with a peripheral neuropathy, but in ten percent of cases the central nervous system (CNS) is predominately involved (Jenkins, 1966).

The manganese induced organic mental disorder has been called manganic madness (Hall 1980), locura manganica (describing a hypomanic syndrome of Chilean miners) (Mena et al, 1967) and manganese mania. These victims have been labeled schizophrenic and manic (Chandra, 1983).

Bismuth is contained in many skin lightening creams and can be absorbed transdermally, producing toxic levels. Psychiatric symptoms are the first prominent signs: They include depression, anxiety, apathy, slowed mentation and delusions (Supino-Viterbo et al, 1977), followed by the abrupt onset of a myoclonic encephalopathy, including a delirium tremens-like syndrome.

Psychiatric symptoms are the rule in thallium ingestion and include poor concentration, irritability, somnolence, fatigue, anorexia, psychosis (with vivid auditory and visual hallucinations) and organic brain syndrome.

Dialysis dementia is a disorder linked to aluminum levels (O'Hare et al, 1983) occurring among patients on hemodialysis. In its more subtle form it may present initially in up to 25 percent of patients as "behavioral changes" or "mental changes," including major depression and even hallucinations (O'Hare et al,

1983). Some of these psychiatric symptoms have been diagnosed as major depression and have been treated unsuccessfully with tricyclic antidepressants (O'Hare, 1983).

Ross et al (1981) reported bouts of severe depression lasting several hours to several days, alternating with attacks of temper and rage, touched off by minor incidents such as accidentally spilling salt, among workers exposed to organic tins.

There are a few reports of psychiatric symptoms resulting from hypermagnesiumia. Reversible lassitude, depression and psychotic and nonpsychotic organic brain syndromes are reported to occur in patients with elevated magnesium levels (Hall, 1980).

Almost every Wilson's Disease patient develops a psychiatric disorder during the course of the disease. The symptoms may range from mild anxiety through depression to bipolar disorder and schizophrenia. Diagnosis is made by simultaneous demonstrations of decreased serum copper and decreased ceruloplasmin.

The psychiatric effects of bromide preparations are well known, and can include extreme agitation and manic excitement requiring sedation and restraint; psychosis, including a thought disorder; delusions; and auditory and visual hallucinations (Hanes and Yates, 1938; Jefferson and Marshall, 1981).

Agents that produce anticholinesterase activity include organophosphate insecticides, nerve gases used in chemical warfare and drugs used to treat myasthenia gravis. They all act by inhibiting the enzyme acetylcholinesterase. This can be either reversible or permanent. The acute effects of these agents in normals include irritability, tension, anxiety, jitteriness, restlessness, giddiness, emotional withdrawal, depression, drowsiness, decreased concentration, confusion and unusual dreams (Bowers et al, 1964). Chronic exposure to organophosphate insecticides causes increased anxiety (Levin et al, 1976; Dille and Smith, 1964), increased irritability (Dille and Smith, 1964), depression (Dille and Smith, 1964) and decreased memory and attention.

Carbon monoxide poisoning can be unintentional, resulting from combustion of wood, charcoal, coal, tobacco, propane, or vinyl plastic, producing hypoxia through the body. The symptoms fluctuate frequently and have been mistaken for hysterical psychosis, borderline personality, schizophrenia, psychotic depression, catatonia and hysteria.

DRUGS OF ABUSE

Illicit drug use should be in the differential diagnosis of almost every patient presenting to the psychiatrist. Although most physicians agree with this concept, few take a complete history from the patient and family and follow this with a comprehensive laboratory testing for drugs of abuse, using a methodology sensitive to the low dosage and abuse of illicit drugs.

Frequently reported adverse psychiatric reactions to marijuana and THC include panic attacks and anxiety reactions usually lasting less than 24 hours (Smith, 1968; Jefferson and Marshall, 1981; Knight, 1976), depression severe enough to require psychiatric hospitalization (Knight, 1976), and acute toxic psychoses with or without clouding of consciousness, which clear within a few weeks (Knight,

1976; Tennant and Groesbeck, 1972; Rottanburg et al, 1982). Many of these reactions have a marked manic or schizoaffective manic quality (Rottanburg et al, 1982; Knight, 1976). The "marijuanaholic" diagnosis is made by observing behavioral change and 9–THC levels in blood and/or urine (Bloodworth, 1983).

Chronic opiate administration is associated with high rates of major and minor depressions (Weissman et al, 1977; Croughan et al, 1982; Rounsaville et al, 1982; Dackis and Gold, 1983). Three weeks after opiate detoxification (Dackis and Gold, 1983) there is 32 percent prevalence of RDC major depression and 10 percent minor depression. During opiate withdrawal we have noted transient depressed moods, manic behavior and, in very rare cases, emergence of a schizophreniform psychosis that cleared when opiates were again administered. Behavioral outbursts, when they occur, are carefully examined as possible signs of undetected withdrawal from another drug of abuse or from alcohol (Gold and Estroff, 1984).

The acute effects of amphetamines are dose dependent and can range from increased alertness, decreased fatigue and need for sleep; to severe anxiety and panic; to euphoria and hypomanic behavior; to acute psychoses that are limited to the presence of amphetamine in the body, and which can be indistinguishable from *DSM-III* bipolar disorder—manic phase. A misdiagnosis of schizophrenia and mistreatment are common (Beamish and Kiloh, 1960; Snyder, 1973; Jefferson and Marshall, 1981). There is also a characteristic "crash" or "discontinuation syndrome" characterized by hypersomic, psychomotoric retarded major depression.

As cocaine's abuse has skyrocketed, especially in middle and upper middle class populations (Gold, 1984), more attention has been paid to the acute toxic psychiatric effects that often present as psychosis, mania, or extreme paranoia, indistinguishable from classic *DSM-III* psychiatric disorders (Estroff and Gold, 1984a; Post and Kopanda, 1976; Gawin and Kleber, 1983).

Phencyclidine (PCP) can cause an acute psychosis of several days duration that clears rapidly. Yago et al (1981) have found a high prevalence of misdiagnosed PCP-induced manias, schizophrenias, and other "psychiatric disorders."

When psychiatric symptoms occur in association with LSD use, they may include a severe panic and anxiety reaction. A chronic psychosis of medium and sometimes prolonged duration, which can be indistinguishable from schizophrenia, has also been reported (Jefferson and Marshall, 1981). LSD abuse has been associated with bipolar manic disorders, schizoaffective disorders, major depressions (Bowers, 1977; Varday and Kay, 1983) and successful suicide (Bowers, 1977; Hensala et al, 1967). Flashbacks may occur weeks to months after the last injection of LSD; the symptoms of an LSD trip may recur at unpredictable times (Blumenfield, 1971; Schick and Smith, 1970).

The best studied group of those who inhale volatile fumes are persons exposed to these substances occupationally, such as painters, refinery workers and persons who directly fuel airplanes. Less well studied are children and adolescents who intentionally abuse glue, toluene, gasoline, cleaning fluid (trichloroethane) and nitrous oxide in order to experience euphorigenic effects. Immediate effects include euphoria, hallucinations in 50 percent of cases and conduct disordered behavior (Wyse, 1973). Personality changes, irritability, anxiety, panic, disorder symptoms, somatic complaints, fatigue, depression and organic brain syndromes have also resulted from the inhalation of volatile fumes (Struwe et al, 1983; Struwe and Wennberg, 1983).

Alcohol

Alcohol is rapidly absorbed from the GI tract, metabolized by the liver, and excreted unchanged in breath, urine and sweat in small amounts. It can be given as intravenous solution, as well (Schuckit, 1979; Jefferson and Marshall, 1981). Blood levels of alcohol are useful at the time of an evaluation, since they correlate with degree of acute intoxication (Schuckit, 1979).

Alcohol idiosyncratic intoxication is a syndrome of extreme reactions to small amounts of alcohol, which include aggressive assaultive and destructive behavior. Partial complex seizures concomitant with barbiturates, sedative hypnotic or stimulant abuse must be ruled out. Unfortunately, rather than alcoholism being identified early in its course, it is usually identified just prior to dissolution of the family, loss of career, or contraction of severe alcohol related physical disorders or substance induced organic mental disorder. Alcohol withdrawal states occur after days to weeks of heavy alcohol ingestion. They may range from mild symptoms, such as nausea and diarrhea, to irritability, headaches and mental sluggishness. Delirium tremens is a life-threatening medical condition, occurring two to four days after the end of alcohol ingestion. It is characterized by delirium, hallucinations, agitations, tremens, tachycardia and elevated blood pressure. Alcohol hallucinosis (auditory hallucinations in the presence of clear consciousness) often occurs during a period of decreased or no alcohol consumption. These states can be confused with anxiety disorders, mania, schizophrenia and other forms of psychosis. Other substance(s), medical diseases, and vitamin and nutritional deficiencies must be identified and treated.

Poly Drug Abuse

Drug abusing individuals generally abuse more than one substance. Differential diagnosis of poly drug intoxication/withdrawal is difficult, since the patient's symptoms can range from those of alcohol intoxication, to hallucinogens and to naturally occurring psychiatric diseases. Diagnosis is only possible with sensitive antibody or computer assisted gas chromatography/mass spectrometry (GC/MS) comprehensive drug testing.

The great danger of poly drug abuse is that there can be a synergistic effect among drugs that can produce a severe toxic, even lethal, result; any one drug taken alone would not have this effect (Schuckit, 1979).

Irritability and attacks of anger (Ayd, 1962; Griffiths et al, 1983), depressed mood and decreased social interaction may be seen in patients taking benzodiazepines or drinking. More severe and prolonged psychiatric reactions occur during the withdrawal phase of alcohol or sedative hypnotic use. A syndrome indistinguishable from the delirium tremens (DTs) or schizophrenia can develop with auditory and visual hallucinations, confusion and even seizures during withdrawal from any sedative hypnotic, including the barbiturates (Anonymous, 1981; Preskorn and Denner, 1977). Glutethimide (Doriden) and Ethchlorvynol (Placidyl) are particularly notorious for the development of similar reactions (Flemenbaum and Gunby, 1971; Hesten and Hastings, 1980; Gold and Estroff,

1984). To uncover a psychiatric disorder caused or precipitated by a prescribed medication, illicit medication or poison, the psychiatrist must (on the basis of the physical, neurological and endocrinological examination and review of the history given by the patient and others) generate a formal differential diagnosis and exclude all viable competing diagnoses through testing or other active processes of investigation.

A complete discussion of medical diseases that commonly present to a psychiatrist and imitate naturally occurring psychiatric syndromes are beyond the scope of this paper, but are fully reviewed in a recent publication (Estroff and Gold, 1984b).

CONCLUSION

In summary, recognition of these disorders is important because patients may exhibit psychiatric symptoms early, and many of the conditions are treatable and reversible. Psychiatrists have a special role in identifying patients with toxic or medical causes for their psychiatric symptoms. It is incorrect to assume that the consulting internist will be able to thoroughly address this complicated differential diagnosis. As the use of clinical laboratory tests in psychiatry becomes more common, and as the tests become more sophisticated, psychiatrists will increasingly identify patients with toxic and medical syndromes who previously would have been misdiagnosed (Pottash et al, 1982; Gold et al, 1984). The unique role of the psychiatrist will be to attempt to rule out these organic disorders prior to psychiatric treatment, thereby improving the response rate. Increasingly, psychiatrists in clinical practice are willing to accept this responsibility.

REFERENCES

Adler LE, Sadja L, Wilets G: Cimetidine toxicity manifested as paranoia and hallucinations. Am J Psychiatry 137:1112-1113, 1980

Ahmad S, Sheikh AI, Meeran MK: Disopyramide-induced acute psychosis. Chest 76:712, 1979

Anonymous: Drugs that cause psychiatric symptoms. The Medical Letter 23:9-12, 1981

Arnold ES, Rudd SM, Kirshner H: Manic psychosis following rapid withdrawal from baclofen. Am J Psychiatry 137:1466-1467, 1980

Ayd F: A critical appraisal of chlordiazepoxide. Journal of Neuropsychiatry 3:177-180, 1962

Baker EL, Feldman RG, White RF, et al: The role of occupational lead exposure in the genesis of psychiatric and behavioral disturbances. Acta Psychiatr Scand 67:38-48, 1983

Barnhart CC, Bowden CL: Toxic psychosis with cimetidine. Am J Psychiatry 136:725-726, 1979

Beamish P, Kiloh LG: Psychoses due to amphetamine consumption. Journal of Mental Sciences 106:337-343, 1960

Bloodworth RC: Medical Aspects of Marijuana Abuse. Psychiatry Letter, 1983

Blumenfield M: Flashback phenomena in basic trainees who enter the US Air Force. Military Medicine 39-41, 1971

Booker HE: Primidone toxicity, in Antiepileptic Drugs. Edited by Woodbury DM, Penry JK, Schmidt RP. New York, Raven Press, 1972

Boston Collaborative Drug-Related Programs: Psychiatric Side Effects of Non-psychiatric drugs. Seminars in Psychiatry 3:406-420, 1971

Bowers MB: Psychoses precipitated by psychotomimetic drugs: a follow-up study. Arch Gen Psychiatry 34:832-835, 1977

Bowers MB, Goodman E, Sim VM: Some behavioral changes in man following anticholinesterase administration. J Nerv Ment Dis 138:383-389, 1964

Buchanan RA: Ethosuximide toxicity, in Antiepileptic Drugs. Edited by Woodbury DM, Penry JK, Schmidt RP. New York, Raven Press, 1972

Calne DB, Plotkin C, Williams AC, et al: Long-term treatment of parkinsonism with bromocriptine. Lancet 1:735-738, 1978

Chandra SV: Psychiatric illness due to manganese poisoning. Acta Psychiatr Scand 67:49-54, 1983

Church G, Marriott HJL: Digitalis delirium: a report on three cases. Circulation 20:549-553, 1959

Croughan JL, Miller JP, Wagelin D, et al: Psychiatric illness in male and female narcotic addicts. J Clin Psychiatry 43:225-228, 1982

Cullen MR, Robins JM, Eskenazi B: Adult inorganic lead intoxication: presentation of 31 new cases and a review of recent advances in the literature. Medicine (Baltimore) 62:221-247, 1983

Dackis CA, Gold MS: Opiate addiction and depression—cause or effects. Drug and Alcohol Dependence, 11:105-109, 1983

Dalby MA: Antiepileptic and psychotropic effects of carbamazepine (Tegretol) in the treatment of psychomotor epilepsy. Epilepsia 12:325-334, 1971

Davison LA, Steinhelber JC, Eger EI, et al: Psychological effects of halothane and isoflurane anesthesia. Anesthesiology 43:313-324, 1975

Dille JR, Smith TW: Central nervous system effects of chronic exposure to organophosphate insecticides. Aerospace Medicine 35:475-478, 1964

Donaldson IMG, Cuningham J: Persisting neurologic sequelae of lithium carbonate therapy. Arch Neurol 40:747-751, 1983

Duroziez P: De delire et du coma digitaliques. Gazette Hebdomadaire de Medecine et de Chirurgie 11:780-783, 1874

Eckenhoff JE, Kneale DH, Dripps RD: The incidence and etiology of postanesthetic excitment. Anesthesiology 22:667-673, 1961

Engel GL: Quinacrine effects on the central nervous system. JAMA 197:235, 1966

Estroff TW, Gold MS: Medical and Psychiatric Complications of Cocaine Abuse and Possible Points of Pharmacologic Intervention. Advances in Alcohol and Substance Abuse, 1984a

Estroff TW, Gold MS: Psychiatric misdiagnosis, in Advances in Psychopharmacology: Predicting and Improving Treatment Response. Edited by Gold MS, Lydiard RB, Carman JS. Boca Raton, CRC Press, 1984b

Flemenbaum A, Gunby B: Ethchlorvynol (Placidyl) abuse and withdrawal (review of clinical picture and report of 2 cases). Diseases of the Nervous System 32:188-192, 1971

Franks RD, Richter AJ: Schizophrenia-like psychosis associated with anticonvulsant toxicity. Am J Psychiatry 136:873-974, 1979

Gardos G, Cole JO, Tarsy D: Withdrawal syndromes associated with antipsychotic drugs. Am J Psychiatry 135:1321-1324, 1978

Gawin FH, Kleber HD: Cocaine abuse treatment. Yale Psychiatric Quarterly 6:4-15, 1983

Gelenberg AJ: The catatonic syndrome. Lancet 1:1339-1341, 1976

Glaser GH: Diphenylhydantoin toxicity, in Antiepileptic Drugs. Edited by Woodbury DM, Penry JK, Schmidt RP. New York, Raven Press, 1972

Gold MS: 800-Cocaine. Edited by Gold MS. New York, Bantam Books, 1984

Gold MS, Estroff TW: The Comprehensive Evaluation of Cocaine and Opiate Abusers, in Handbook of Psychiatric Diagnostic Procedures, vol. 2. Edited by Hall RC, Beresford TP. New York, Spectrum Publications Inc., 1984

Gold MS, Pottash AC, Extein, I: The Psychiatric Laboratory, in Clinical Psychopharmacology. Edited by Bernstein JG. John Wright PSG Inc., 1984

Goodwin FK: Behavioral effects of L-dopa in man. Seminars in Psychiatry 3:477-492, 1971

Goodwin FK, Bunney WE: Depressions following reserpine: a reevaluation. Seminars in Psychiatry 3:435-448, 1971

Goodwin FK, Ebert MH, Bunney WE: Mental effects of reserpine in man: a review, in Psychiatric Complications of Medical Drugs. Edited by Shader RI. New York, Raven Press, 1972

Gorelick DA, Kussin SZ, Kahn I: Single case study paranoid delusions and auditory hallucinations associated with digoxin intoxication. J Nerv Ment Dis 166:817-818, 1978

Green RL, Lewis JE, Kraus SJ, et al: Elevated plasma procaine concentrations after administration of procaine penicillin G. N Engl J Med 291:223-226, 1974

Griffiths RR, Bigelow GE, Liebson I: Differential effects of diazepam and pentobarbital on mood and behavior. Arch Gen Psychiatry 40:865-873, 1983

Hall RCW, Stickney SK, Gardner ER: Behavioral toxicity of nonpsychiatric drugs, in Psychiatric Presentations of Medical Illness: Somotopsychic Disorders. Edited by Hall RCW. New York, Spectrum Publications, 1980

Hamilton RC, Dundee JW, Clarke RSJ, et al: Studies of drugs given before anesthesia XIII: Pentazocine and other opiate antagonists. Br J Anaesth 39:647-656, 1967

Hanes FM, Yates A: An analysis of four hundred instances of chronic bromide intoxication. South Med J 31:667-671, 1938

Hensala JD, Epstein LJ, Blacker KH: LSD and psychiatric inpatients. Arch Gen Psychiatry 16:554-558, 1967

Heston LL, Hastings D: Psychosis with withdrawal from ethchlorvynol. Am J Psychiatry 137:249-250, 1980

Holland J, Fasanello S, Ohnuma T: Psychiatric symptoms associated with L-asparaginase administration. J Psychiat Res 10:105-113, 1974

Jefferson JW, Marshall JR: Neuropsychiatric Features of Medical Disorders. New York, Plenum Publishing Corp., 1981

Jenkins RB: Inorganic arsenic and the nervous system. Brain 89:479-498, 1966

Jones RF, Lance JW: Baclofen (Lioresal) in the long-term management of spasticity. Med J Aust 1:654-657, 1976

Kimelblatt BJ, Cerra FB, Callero G, et al: Dose and serum concentration relationships in cimetidine associated mental confusion. Gastroenterology 78:791-795, 1980

Klein DF, Gittelman R, Quitkin F, et al: Diagnosis and Drug Treatment of Psychiatric Disorders: Adults and Children. Baltimore, Williams and Wilkins, 1980

Knight F: Role of cannabis in psychiatric disturbance. Ann NY Acad Sci 282:64-71, 1976

Kruis R, Barger R: Paranoid psychosis with sulindac. JAMA 243:1420, 1980

Lees AJ, Clarke CRA, Harrison MJ: Hallucinations after withdrawal of baclofen. Lancet 1:858, 1977

Levin HS, Rodnitzky RL, Mick DL: Anxiety associated with exposure to organophosphate compounds. Arch Gen Psychiatry 33:225-228, 1976

Maghazaji HI: Psychiatric aspects of methyl mercury poisoning. J Neurol Neurosurg Psychiatry 37:954-958, 1974

Mann AM, Hutchinson JR: Manic reaction associated wih procarbazine hydrochloride therapy of Hodgkin's disease. Can Med Assoc J 97:1350-1353, 1967

Marriott HJL: Delirium from digitalis toxicity. JAMA 203:178, 1968

McCrum ID, Guidry JR: Procainamide-induced psychosis. JAMA 240:1265-1266, 1978

Mena I, Marin O, Fuenzalida S, et al: Chronic manganese poisoning clinical picture and manganese turnover. Neurology 17:128-136, 1967

Moskovitz C, Moses H, Klawans HL: Levodopa-induced psychosis: A kindling phenomenon. Am J Psychiatry 135:669-675, 1978

Needleman HL: The neuropsychiatric implications of low level exposure to lead. Psychol Med 12:461-463, 1982

O'Hare JA, Callaghan NM, Murnaghan DJ: Dialysis encephalopathy: clinical, electroencephalographic and interventional aspects. Medicine 62:129-141, 1983

Padfield PL, Smith DA, Fitzsimos EJ, et al: Disopyramide and acute psychosis. Lancet 1:1152, 1977

Parkes D: Mechanisms of bromocriptine-induced hallucinations. N Engl J Med 302:1479, 1980

Paykel ES, Fleminger R, Watson JP: Psychiatric side effects of antihypertensive drugs other than reserpine. J Clin Pharmacol 2:14-39, 1982

Peterson LG, Popkin MK: Neuropsychiatric effects of chemotherapeutic agents for cancer. Psychosomatics 21:141-153, 1980

Post RM, Kopanda RT: Cocaine kindling and psychosis. Am J Psychiatry 133:627-634, 1976

Pottash ALC, Black HR, Gold MS: Psychiatric complications of anti-hypertensive medication. J Nerv Ment Dis 169:430-438, 1981

Pottash ALC, Gold MS, Extein I: The use of the clinical laboratory, in Inpatient Psychiatry Diagnosis and Treatment. Edited by Sederer LI. Baltimore, Williams and Wilkins, 1982

Preskorn SH, Denner LJ: Benzodiazepines and withdrawal psychosis. JAMA 237:36-38, 1977

Presthus J, Holmsen R: Appraisal of long-term levodopa treatment of parkinsonism with special reference to therapy limiting factors. Acta Neurol Scand 50:774-790, 1974

Rainey JM: Disulfiram toxicity and carbon disulfide poisoning. Am J Psychiatry 134:371-378, 1977

Rifkin A, Quitkin F, Klein DF: Organic brain syndrome during lithium carbonate treatment. Comprehensive Psychiatry 14:251-254, 1973

Roger J, Grangeon H, Guey J, Lob H: Psychological and psychiatric symptoms in treatment of epileptics with ethosuximide. Encephale 57:407-438, 1968

Ross WD, Emmett EA, Steiner J, et al: Neurotoxic effects of occupational exposure to organotins. Am J Psychiatry 138:1092-1095, 1981

Rothermich NO: An extended study of indomethacin. I. Clinical Pharmacology. JAMA 195:123-128, 1966

Rottanburg D, Robins AH, Ben-Arie O, et al: Cannabis associated psychosis with hypomanic features. Lancet 2:1364-1366, 1982

Rounsaville BJ, Weissman MM, Crits-Christoph K, et al: Diagnosis and symptoms of depression in opiate addicts: Course and relationship to treatment outcome. Arch Gen Psychiatry 39:151-156, 1982

Schick JFE, Smith DE: Analysis of the Flashback. Journal of Psychedelic Drugs 3:13-19, 1970

Schuckit MA: Drug and Alcohol Abuse: A Clinical Guide to Diagnosis and Treatment. New York, Plenum Medical Book Co., 1979

Sellers J, Tyre RP, Whiteley A, et al: Neurotoxic effects of lithium with delayed rise in serum lithium levels. Br J Psychiatry 140:623-625, 1982

Shear MK, Sacks MH: Digitalis delirium: Report of two cases. Am J Psychiatry 135:109-110, 1978

Sheehy LM, Maxmen JS: Phenelzine-induced psychosis. Am J Psychiatry 135:1422-1423, 1978

Siris SG, Van Kammen DP, Docherty JP: The use of antidepressant drugs in schizophrenia. Arch Gen Psychiatry 35:1368-1377, 1978

Smith DE: Acute and chronic toxicity of marijuana. J Psychedelic Drugs 2:37-47, 1968

Snyder SH: Amphetamine psychosis: a "model" schizophrenia mediated by catecholamines. Am J Psychiatry 130:61-67, 1973

Stores G: Behavioral Effects of Anti-epileptic Drugs. Dev Med Child Neurol 17:647-658, 1975

Struwe G, Wennberg A: Psychiatric and neurological symptoms in workers occupationally exposed to organic solvents—results of a differential epidemiological study. Acta Psychiatr Scand 67:68-80, 1983

Struwe G, Knave B, Mindus P: Neuropsychiatric symptoms in workers exposed to jet fuel—a combined epidemiological and casuistic study. Acta Psychiatr Scand 67:55-67, 1983

Supino-Viterbo V, Sicard C, Riszegliato M, et al: Toxic encephalopathy due to ingestion of bismuth salts: clinical and EEG studies of 45 patients. J Neurol Neurosurg Psychiatry 40:748-752, 1977

Tennant FS, Groesbeck CJ: Psychiatric effects of hashish. Arch Gen Psychiatry 27:133-136, 1972

Thompson M, Percy JS: Further experience with indomethacin in the treatment of rheumatic disorders. Br Med J 1:80-83, 1966

Tollefson G: Psychiatric implications of anticonvulsant drugs. J Clin Psychiatry 41:295-302, 1980

Turner WM: Lidocaine and Psychotic reactions. Ann Intern Med 97:149-150, 1982

Vardy MM, Kay SR: LSD psychosis or LSD-induced schizophrenia? A multimethod inquiry. Arch Gen Psychiatry 40:877-883, 1983

Vlissides DN, Gill D, Castelow J: Bromocriptine—induced mania? Br Med J 1:510, 1978

Volpe BT, Soave R: Formed visual hallucinations as digitalis toxicity. Ann Intern Med 91:865-866, 1979

Wallach MB, Gershon S: Psychiatric sequelae to tuberculosis chemotherapy, in Psychiatric Complications of Medical Drugs. Edited by Shader RI. New York, Raven Press, 1972

Weissman MM, Pottenger M, Kleber H, et al: Symptom patterns in primary and secondary depression: a comparison of primary depressives with depressed opiate addicts, alcoholics, and schizophrenics. Arch Gen Psychiatry 34:854-862, 1977

Winn RE, Bower MJ, Richards MJ: Acute toxic delirium neurotoxicity of intrathecal administration of amphotericin B. Arch Intern Med 139:706-707, 1979

Wyse DG: Deliberate inhalation of volatile hypocarbons: a review. CMA Journal 108:71-74, 1973

Yago KB, Pitts FN, Burgoyne RW, et al: The urban epidemic of phencyclidine (PCP) use: clinical laboratory evidence from a public psychiatric hospital emergency service. J Clin Psychiatry 42:193-196, 1981

Yule W, Lansdown R, Millar IB, et al: The relationship between blood lead concentrations, intelligence and attainment in a school population: a pilot study. Dev Med Child Neurol 23:567-576, 1981

Chapter 13

Future Interfaces Between Psychiatry and Neurology

by Robert M. Post, M.D.

The historical roots for the interface between psychiatry and neurology are deep and intertwined. The early psychiatrists emerged from a neurological tradition. Freud himself, in 1895, predicted a neurology of psychiatry in which: "The intention is to furnish a psychology that shall be a natural science: that is, to represent psychical processes as quantitatively determinant states of specifiable material particles. . . ." (Freud, 1954). Psychiatry may impinge on neurology, which is defined as the science dealing with the nervous system; specifically, with diseases of the nervous system. Because there is increasing evidence that the psychosis in major mental disorders may relate to nervous system dysfunction, one can begin to imagine an increasing emergence of "psychiatric neurology."

One of the first major treatment modalities for acute manic-depressive illness—electroconvulsive therapy (ECT)—was borrowed from neurology and based on clinical observations of apparently reciprocal relationships between seizures and psychosis in epileptic patients (Trimble, 1984; Robertson and Trimble, 1983). Paradoxically, drugs useful in the treatment of seizure disorders are now gaining prominence in the treatment of psychiatric disorders, particularly in manic-depressive illness. Carbamazepine (Tegretol) is emerging as an alternative treatment to lithium carbonate for acute (Post et al, 1983a) and prophylactic (Post et al, 1983b) management of manic-depressive illness (Ballenger and Post, 1980; Okuma, 1983; Kishimoto et al, 1983; Post et al, 1984a; Post and Uhde, 1984). Other anticonvulsants, including valproic acid and clonazepam, have been reported in double-blind clinical trials to have acute antimanic effects (Emrich et al, 1980; Chouinard et al, 1983). The early suggestions that phenytoin might also be useful for treatment of some neuropsychiatric disorders (Kalinowsky and Putnam, 1943; Freyhan, 1945; Kubanek and Rowell, 1946) remain to be confirmed in carefully controlled, double-blind studies.

This chapter reviews the implications of the convergence of common therapeutic tools for both psychiatry and neurology. This convergence also marks the beginning of major interactions between psychiatry and neurology in the areas of technical development, diagnosis and treatment. Psychiatry and neurology should mutually benefit from the current explosion in neuroscience technology, and from our increasing knowledge of brain biochemistry and function. The technical advances of the computerized axial tomography (CAT), positron emission tomography (PET) and nuclear magnetic resonance (NMR) offer great potential, not only in differential diagnoses, but in separating psychiatric from neurological disorders. This chapter highlights one new area of biochemistry that may provide a new generation of therapeutic biochemical treatments for neurology and psychiatry: the recently discovered and localized neuropeptide systems. Future technological advances—including the use of recombinant DNA techniques and basic neuroscience advances that should pave the way for major interactions between psychiatry and neurology—will also be considered.

THE ANTICONVULSANT CONNECTION

As already noted, carbamazepine is rapidly becoming recognized as a clinically effective treatment for manic-depressive (Post et al, 1984a) and secondary affective illness (Dalby, 1971; 1975). Mechanisms of action of the anticonvulsants in the treatment of either seizure disorders or the affective disorders are not yet known (Post et al, 1983c; 1984a); but elucidation of their mechanisms of action promises to be clinically and theoretically rewarding for both disciplines.

Different classes of anticonvulsants are useful in the treatment of different types of seizure disorders: major motor, complex partial, and petit mal or absence (Porter and Penry, 1978). Preliminary data suggest that the drugs that are effective in the treatment of major and complex partial seizures are also effective in manic-depressive illness (Post et al, 1984a). Thus, this differential responsivity should provide conceptual hints as to the important regional, biochemical and physiological effects of these agents, which may relate to important mechanisms in the affective disorders. Moreover, there is some early, indirect evidence that ability to inhibit limbic discharges (Albright and Burnham, 1980) might be associated with psychotropic effects in affective illness (Post et al, 1984a); but this hypothesis remains to be directly tested. The impact of anticonvulsants and related "membrane stabilizers" on other psychiatric syndromes, such as schizophrenic psychosis and aggression, also requires further study (Roy-Byrne and Post, 1984; Williams et al, 1982; Yudofsky et al, 1984).

In another study it was observed that electroconvulsive seizures (ECS) in the rat were also potent inhibitors of amygdala seizures (Post et al, 1984b). That is, the major motor seizures of ECS are, paradoxically, anticonvulsant. ECS (compared to sham ECS), administered prior to once-daily amygdala stimulation, completely blocked the development of kindling. Moreover, a series of seven ECS suppressed fully developed kindled seizures for up to five days. These data suggest that biochemical properties associated with the anticonvulsant effects of ECT in man might, in common with anticonvulsants such as carbamazepine, mediate its positive effects in affective illness. The psychiatric aspects of epileptic disorders have been reviewed by David Bear and colleagues in Chapter 10 of this volume. Understanding the complex interactions between the psychiatric disturbances accompanying seizure disorders, as well as a better understanding of the fundamental mechanisms underlying seizure disorders themselves, should prove rewarding for psychiatry. Neurology is generally considered to deal with structural alterations in the brain; however, in the epilepsies, structural pathology has not yet been defined (although there are often clear-cut physiological and electroencephalographic markers of the disease process). Pathological activation of neurotransmitter pathways observed during the epilepsies (Engel et al, 1982) may provide the most delineated map possible of critical neural circuits involved in emotional and behavioral disorders.

As in the epilepsies, consistent electrophysiological changes have been observed in some psychiatric illnesses. Alterations in the sleep structure, as seen in all night electroencephalographic recordings, have been documented in multiple studies of patients with primary affective illness (Kupfer et al, 1976; Gillin et al, 1984). Neurovegetative alterations accompanying the depressive process are equally well documented, with alterations in motor and appetite functions particularly noteworthy (see Post and Ballenger, 1984). In addition there are now, for the first time in psychiatry, well-documented biochemical abnormalities that occur in a substantial subgroup of patients with major affective illness. For example, cortisol hypersecretion is evident from 24-hour urinary excretion of free cortisol, altered patterns and amplitude of plasma cortisol secretion, as well as the well-documented data of an increased escape from dexamethasone suppression (Carroll et al, 1981; Rubinow et al, 1984).

ENDOCRINOLOGY AND THE BRAIN

While controversy continues regarding the specificity of escape from dexamethasone suppression in primary affective illness and its pathophysiological and diagnostic implications, there is little argument that the abnormality has been documented in multiple studies, in many countries, in hundreds of patients. Blunted thyroid stimulating hormone (TSH) response to thyrotropin releasing hormone (TRH) has also been well documented in a subgroup of depressed patients (Extein et al, 1984). These endocrinological abnormalities should provide important areas for further study. Clarification of the biochemical mechanisms involved in these alterations, and their relationship to clinical subgroups and treatment response, will be of considerable clinical and theoretical import. Studies by Gold and associates (1984), using the recently discovered peptide corticotropin releasing factor (CRF), may help to define the nature of the cortisol abnormality in depression. Preliminary evidence suggests that there may be "CRF overdrive" with an abnormality in feedback at the hypothalamic level (Gold et al, 1984). Depressed patients show blunted adrenocorticotropic hormone (ACTH) response to CRF, presumably because of desensitized CRF receptors.

Studies of CRF in depression and other psychiatric disorders forecast a science of neurological endocrinology related to behavior. In these areas, psychiatry is again competing with neurology as a science of neuropathology, since CRF has been localized in specific neurons of the brain. Not only is it localized in cell bodies of hypothalamic neurons related to the control of the hypothalamic–pituitary–adrenal axis (with terminals reaching the pituitary to control secretion of ACTH and cortisol), but cell bodies and terminals have also been localized in many other areas of the brain (Jacobowitz, 1983). Hokfelt and associates (1980) documented a most interesting property of the newly discovered cerebral peptides: They are often colocalized in neurons with classic neurotransmitters, such as dopamine, serotonin, norepinephrine, acetylcholine, or GABA. Alterations in many of these neurotransmitter systems have been postulated, both in major psychiatric disorders (Post et al, 1980) and in such neurological disorders as the epilepsies. Thus, as advances in neuroscience begin to define the physiological interactions between classic neurotransmitter and peptide systems occurring within the same and different neuronal elements, important information relevant to both disciplines should emerge. Most peptides and classic neurotransmitters are currently measurable in cerebrospinal fluid (CSF) (Post et al, 1982); but more precise techniques for their evaluation in the brain are anticipated.

Not only has there been evidence of colocalization of classic and peptide neurotransmitters within the same neurons, but recent data suggest that several peptides may also be localized within the same neurons. For example, CRF has been colocalized with substance P and vasopressin (Olschowka et al, 1983. Roth et al, 1982) within the neural elements. Swanson (1984) reported seven peptides in these neurons of the paraventricular nucleus: CRF, vasopressin, angiotensin, enkephalin, substance P, NPY and neurotensin. Increased fluorescence of CRF, vasopressin and angiotensin was observed following adrenalectomy, suggesting that peptide hormone progression and production may be altered by the endocrine milieu. Most recently, the coexistence of cholecystokinin (CCK) and CRF has been documented (Mezey et al, 1984).

SOMATOSTATIN AND NEUROPSYCHIATRIC ILLNESS

The explosion in knowledge of peptide function in the brain in the last decade is so impressive that it warrants another example of its potential clinical relevance. Much research in psychiatry has focused on measurement and delineation of the role of the noradrenergic system in psychiatric disorders, such as depression and anxiety. It is worth noting that noradrenergic neurons in the brain account for an extraordinarily small proportion (approximately 10,000 cells) of the estimated 10,000,000,000 cells in the brain. It is now apparent that neuropeptides have substantially added to our catalogue of putative neurotransmitter candidates defined in the brain. Somatostatin is a peptide originally described in the gastrointestinal tract that has now been specifically localized to a variety of neural elements in the brain (Reichlin, 1983). It is of particular interest to this discussion, since alterations in somatostatin have now been documented in a variety of neuropsychiatric conditions.

Brain somatostatin has consistently been reported to be decreased in autopsy specimens of the brains of patients with Alzheimer's dementia (Davies et al, 1980; Rossor et al, 1980). This is noteworthy, since somatostatin and acetylcholine have been shown to coexist in neurons (Delfs, 1984), and depletion of acetylcholine in the basal forebrain (substantia innominata) is widely recognized as a major defect in Alzheimer's disease. At the same time, somatostatin has been reported increased in the basal ganglia of patients with Huntington's Chorea (Aronin et al, 1983; Nemeroff et al, 1983). The decreases in somatostatin in the brain are paralleled by decreases in CSF of patients with Alzheimer's dementia (Serby et al, 1983; Wood et al, 1982; Oram et al, 1981).

Three studies have documented decreased somatostatin in the CSF of patients with depression (Gerner and Yamada, 1982; Rubinow et al, 1983; Agren and Lundgvist, 1984; Black et al, 1984). These studies provide further evidence that this decrease during depression is state related, and normalizes either with improvement or with the switch into hypomania or mania (Rubinow et al, 1983, 1984). In the study by Rubinow and associates (1984), higher levels of CSF somatostatin were associated with increased sleep disturbance, paralleling similar findings reported in animal studies.

The transient changes in somatostatin in CSF of depressed patients contrasts with the presumed permanent alterations in brain somatostatin observed during Alzheimer's disease and Huntington's Chorea. In this regard it is noteworthy that in acute exacerbations of multiple sclerosis (MS), decreases in somatostatin, which normalize during well intervals, have been noted (Sorensen et al, 1980). These findings suggest the possibility that neuropsychiatric syndromes involving either direct neuropathology (MS) or presumed functional alterations in neurotransmission (primary depression) are associated with fluctuations in somatostatin that can be detected in CSF.

MANIPULATION OF BRAIN PEPTIDES

The permanent changes as well as the state related changes in the neuropsychiatric syndromes raise the possibility that manipulations of somatostatin function may ultimately be of therapeutic value in several of these illnesses. Neurotransmitter and peptide replacement, and neural implants and nerve transplant techniques, have already been utilized in experimental animals (Freed, 1983); and two neural implants have been performed in man for the potential treatment of the dopaminergic defects of Parkinson's disease (Olson et al, 1983). In this way, a direct manipulation of somatostatin or acetylcholine function, through similarly derived transplant techniques, may be one form of treatment to be considered for patients with Alzheimer's dementia in the foreseeable future.

In depresson, where the changes are presumably transient and state related, other technologies might be employed in treatment. These could include direct manipulation of somatostatinergic functions through alteration in its biosynthesis, or inhibition of enzymes involved in its degradation. Techniques such as these have already been employed in treatment strategies in the classical neurotransmitter pathways. For example, our use of monoamine oxidase (MAO) inhibitors involves the strategy of inhibiting enzymes in the degradation of monoamine function, resulting in the potentiation of both catecholamine and indoleamine systems. The peptide hormones appear to be rather uniformly formed by cleavage of long prepromolecules, similarly raising the possibility that altering their synthesis or later degradation by appropriate peptide enzyme manipulations may be successful in changing central nervous system (CNS) peptide function (Snyder, 1983). Captopril—an inhibitor of angiotensin converting enzyme—and enkephalinease—already a well-accepted antihypertensive agent—have recently been reported in a preliminary communication to have mood elevating effects in three depressed patients (Zubenko and Nixon, 1984).

Another possible route for manipulating CNS peptide systems involves use of the CSF. Recently, this fluid pathway has been used to treat patients with severe pain syndromes through the intrathecal administration of beta-endorphin and its analogs (Hosobuchi and Li, 1978; Foley et al, 1979; Oyama et al, 1980; Pickar et al, 1984). These preliminary clinical trials provide the initial verification that altering the peptide composition of this fluid system (which has wide access to CNS structures and potentially different neurotransmitter receptors) may ultimately be of clinical use in a variety of neuropsychiatric syndromes (Post et al, 1982).

NEUROBEHAVIORAL DEVELOPMENT

Hubel and Weisel (1979) and others have documented that environmental alterations in visual input have lasting impact on the development and function of this system. Depending upon the time of onset and duration of deprivation of the visual input, marked physiological and anatomical changes occur within visual pathways that may be irreversible. Now that there is increasing definition of the neural systems (both classical and peptide) involved in emotional regulation and, specifically, in stress responsivity, one can look forward to the possibility that the impact of environmental alterations and stresses on biochemistry and physiology can also be defined. Perhaps there would be long-term and, at times, irreversible changes in functional as well as structural elements in these neural pathways (similar to those demonstrated by Hubel and Weisel) if the degree of early deprivation or enhancement is severe enough. In this fashion, one can conceive of an increasingly sophisticated neurobiology of behavior and emotional function that might become accurate enough to deal with psychoanalytic concepts that have long emphasized the importance of early childhood development on subsequent emotional and personality development. It is conceivable that fixation and regression may ultimately have definable biochemical, physiological, and perhaps even anatomical neural substrates.

Kandel (1983) has begun to study the molecular biology of anxiety in his model using *aplysia*, in which each neural element of the snail's simplified CNS is known. Direct changes in synaptic efficacy (probably mediated by serotonin, adenylate cyclase, protein phosphorylation, and calcium channels) and in synaptic structure have been observed in two forms of learned fear—sensitization and aversive classical conditioning.

MANIPULATION OF PEPTIDES WITH RECOMBINANT DNA TECHNIQUES

Another possible approach might involve the use of recombinant DNA techniques. The gene for somatostatin has already been isolated (Montminy et al, 1984) and transferred from one mammalian species to another (Lowe et al, 1984). It is disappointing that, in contrast to the transfer of the gene for growth hormone (Palmiter et al, 1983), the size of the animal was not altered. However, the technology of molecular biology now exists for such genetic manipulations, raising the possibility that critical genetic alterations could be identified and modified. It is also of interest that these techniques have been used to localize the gene involved in the production of Huntington's Chorea. Similarly, Sutcliffe et al (1980) have reported the identification of a brain specific peptide using recombinant DNA techniques. This, too, raises the possibility that important alterations in brain functions relevant to neurological and behavioral dysfunction might be achieved by direct recombinant DNA techniques, rather than by the more cumbersome techniques of the recent neurobiological era (which involve identification and isolation of the brain chemicals themselves). The investigative group of Guillemin and associates (1983) required six tons of brain tissue to isolate 1 mg of the tripeptide thyrotropin releasing factor (TRF). Recombinant DNA techniques have greatly simplified the process of identifying and sequencing behaviorally relevant brain proteins and peptides (Bloom, 1984).

BRAIN IMAGING

In the past decade there has been a parallel advance in the ability of neuro-scientists to image the brain. A short time ago, skull films provided a highly inadequate index of the nature of the underlying brain tissue. Skull deformities, fractures and erosions of the sella turcica might be observed with routine skull films, but little else could be observed. This has dramatically changed with the advent of the computerized axial tomography (CAT) scan images. Now, brain structures can be directly visualized, as well as the size of the cerebral ventricles and adjacent caudate bulge into the ventricles. In this fashion, the atrophy of Huntington's Chorea can be directly assessed and alterations in cerebral ventric-ular volume can be measured. Based on this new capability, a large number of studies have now documented increased ventrical:brain ratio (VBR) in a subgroup of acutely psychotic patients (Weinberger and Wyatt, 1982). A substantial proportion of schizophrenics were initially noted to have enlarged VBRs. More recently, patients with other psychotic diagnoses, including manic-depressive illness, have also emerged with large ventricles (Pearlson and Veroff, 1981, 1984; Pearlson et al, 1984; Targum et al, 1983; Nasrallah et al, 1982).

An additional caveat is in order in relation to many other biological findings in schizophrenia. It is possible that this structural alteration in the brains of schizophrenics may not only be not specific for schizophrenia, but also may be reversible. Kellner and colleagues (1983) have noted that affectively ill patients with the largest excretion of urinary free cortisol had the largest VBRs. These data are consistent with many studies in the neurological literature, indicating that treatment with glucocorticoids or ACTH markedly alters the appearance of the brain, producing a picture of apparent atrophy and increased VBR. Thus, it is possible that biochemical alterations associated with acute or chronic psychotic illness may be sufficient to alter the appearance of the brain and ventricular system on the CAT scan. It is also possible that these alterations themselves lead to dysregulated biochemical processes such as cortisol hypersecretion. Nonetheless, while increased CAT scan VBR has been associated with altered and deficient performance on a variety of neuropsychological tasks, the precise pathophysiology of increased VBR and its clinical correlates remain to be delin-eated. Recently, Reus and colleagues (1984) have confirmed the relationship between cortisol hypersecretion (measured by escape from dexamethasone suppression) and increased VBR, as well as cognitive impairment in depression.

NMR promises to yeild an even more detailed picture of brain structure in awake man. With this technique, white and gray matter can be differentiated, and the fine structure of the brain can be delineated, almost approximating the appearance of brain-slice techniques at autopsy. With this and related technol-ogies, many of the old distinctions between neurology and psychiatry will either be substantiated or fall by the wayside, as subtle alterations in cerebral pathology are documented in psychiatric illnesses. Whichever will be the case, this tech-nique holds great promise for the differential diagnosis of functional versus structural alterations in the brain; either type of alteration may emerge within the realm of neurology or psychiatry.

Regional alterations in brain function can be examined indirectly by using regional measures of blood flow (Risberg et al, 1981; Ingvar et al, 1984). A relative deficit in activation of the frontal lobes has been suggested in schizophrenia, and Ingvar reported increased frontal blood in mania.

Great excitement has been generated by the technique of positron emission tomography (PET), which has elucidated changes in brain function (that is, glucose utilization) in awake man with a regional neuroanatomy (and resolution approximating 0.7 cm), that was not even imagined a decade ago. With this technique, changes in brain functions during sleep and wakefulness have been documented. Different areas of brain glucose utilization can be clearly seen during resting, thinking, listening, viewing, remembering and performing motor tasks (Phelps, 1984)! Subtle alterations in the processing of information—such as the type of processing of music by trained professionals or naive subjects— can be differentiated in localized areas of the brain (Mazziotto et al, 1983). Marked increases in regional glucose utilization have been documented during seizures, while decreases in these same areas are seen during interictal periods (Engel et al, 1982). Specific regional alterations have not yet been consistently documented in either schizophrenia or manic-depressive illness. However, an interesting yet apparently nonspecific pattern of hyperfrontality has been noted in many studies of schizophrenic and affectively ill patients (Buchsbaum et al, in press). Phelps (1984) reported globally decreased cortical glucose utilization in depression, with increase following the switch into euthymic or manic states. DeLisi, Buchsbaum, Post and associates (unpublished data, 1984) have observed temporal lobe hypofunction relative to other brain areas in the same slice, in depressed patients compared to controls.

Since PET scan methodology is highly sensitive to the type of information processing occuring at the time of deoxyglucose injection (Mazziotto et al, 1982; Phelps, 1984), more discrete areas of pathology may be revealed once neuro-psychological tasks specifically designed for psychiatric patients are used in conjunction with the PET scan methodology. Buchsbaum (1983) has demon-strated that there are convergences between topographic mapping of the brain structure on an electrophysiological basis, and regional changes in glucose utili-zation based on PET scan methodology. However, in other illnesses (such as complex partial seizures), there can be discrepancies in localization of the epilep-tic focus based on electrophysical compared to PET scan methods. It is inter-esting that the localization using PET scan appears to be more accurate, in this instance, than that based on EEG findings—even those using depth electrode localization (Engel et al, 1982). Caution is urged in the application of these techniques, since changes in glucose utilization can be associated with mismatches with cerebral blood flow (as documented during seizure states); and increased glucose utilization in a given area, particularly if it is in an inhibitory pathway, may not relate to increased excitation.

Nonetheless, these techniques hold great promise for the future; we will be able, for the first time, to localize structural and functional pathology deep within the brain of awake, living man. With the increasing sophistication of psycho-logical paradigms used during PET scan, as well as the application of new tracers that label specific biochemical pathways—such as cholinergic (Eckelman et al, 1984), dopaminergic (Wagner et al, 1983; Garnett et al, 1983), or opiate (Snyder, 1984)—progress is expected that will elucidate regional selective neurotrans-mitter alterations in neuropsychiatric syndromes.

The brain—shielded by its unyielding structure of the skull, and in a cushion of cerebrospinal fluid—just a few short years ago did not appear to be accessible to any but the most invasive neurosurgical and electrophysiological techniques for assessing function of deep structures. This has changed dramatically within the past decade; wider application of the present methodologies should be of great clinical value for both neurology and psychiatry. Advances in technology in the decades to follow may be expected to bring even greater elucidation of the fine structure and function of the brain.

ELECTROPHYSIOLOGICAL AND ELECTROMAGNETIC ALTERATION OF BRAIN FUNCTION

Before 1970, one might understandably have believed that the elucidation of deep intracerebral pathology might not, in the end, be worthwhile or financially justifiable because of the inability to directly alter this pathology without gross destruction of brain tissue. However, several techniques already mentioned are almost ready for clinical application in man, and many other techniques are on the horizon. In addition to CSF, chemitrode and implant techniques, it is conceivable that with the appropriate manipulation of electromagnetic fields, local changes in brain activity may be achieved in a nonintrusive fashion. Barth et al (1982, 1984) have recently mapped electromagnetic potentials of the brain in both normal and epileptic patients.

Sophisticated means of electrical pacing of cardiac tissue have been employed in the past several decades, to the point where cardiac pacemakers are a relatively routine treatment of cardiac dysrhythmias; they provide a supplemental and safeguard backup for existing pharmacological treatments for cardiac arrhythmias. One can imagine similar technologies being used for the cerebral dysrhythmias. These might have particular application, not only in the epilepsies (in which inhibitory circuits might be stimulated), but in psychiatric syndromes (in which functional neural traffic, in pathways shown to be dysregulated, might be altered). Heath (1980) has used electrical stimulation on the midline cerebellar nuclei to attempt to alter psychiatric dysfunction. Electrophysiological stimulation or biochemical alterations, achieved either intraventricularly or intracerebrally through the use of chemitrodes, might be efficacious. These later techniques may be most useful in treating psychiatric syndromes in which neural alterations appear to involve "functional", rather than structural alterations usually associated with the major neurological diseases (and for which other techniques, including brain implants and transplants, may be required).

Brain transplant techniques, only a short time ago subjects for horror movies, now appear on the verge of clinical (if only experimental) application. We should be reminded of similar yet rapid strides in transplant technology that have taken kidney transplants from the highly experimental to the almost routine surgical procedure in a matter of a very few years. Several years ago, interface of the ultimate human computer—the brain—with biologically based electronic computers was a subject only for science fiction. Yet, at this time, Wyatt and associates at St. Elizabeths Hospital in Washington, D.C., are experimenting with computer interfaces with living tissue (Wyatt, 1983); and one can envision, in a short period of time, the possibility that computer prostheses may supplement and interact with natural brain function. Following several years of heart transplants, the world was startled by the introduction of the first mechanical heart. One might similarly predict that, after a period of experimental neurosurgical approaches to brain implants for discrete areas of neuropathology in man, a variety of experimental neural implants (including interfaces with computer-based systems) may be employed in attempts to supplement and ameliorate deficiencies in brain function.

REFERENCES

Agren H, Lundqvist G: Low levels of somatostatin in human CSF mark depressive episodes. Psychoneuroendocrinology 9:233-248, 1984

Albright PS, Burnham WM: Development of a new pharmacological seizure model: effects of anticonvulsants on cortical- and amygdala-kindled seizures in the rat. Epilepsia 21:681-689, 1980

Aronin N, Cooper PE, Lorenz LJ, et al: Somatostatin is increased in the basal ganglia in Huntington's disease. Ann Neurol 12:519-526, 1983

Ballenger JC, Post RM: Carbamazepine (Tegretol) in manic-depressive illness: a new treatment. Am J Psychiatry 137:782-790, 1980

Barth DS, Sutherling W, Engel J Jr, et al: Neuromagnetic localization of epileptiform spike activity in the human brain. Science 218:891-894, 1982

Barth DS, Sutherling W, Engel J Jr., et al: Neuromagnetic evidence of spatially distributed sources underlying epileptiform spikes in the human brain. Science 223:293-296, 1984

Bear D, Levin K, Blumer D, et al: Interictal behavior in hospitalized temporal lobe epileptics: relationship to idiopathic psychiatric syndromes. J Neurol Neurosurg Psychiatry 45:481-488, 1982

Black PM, Ballantine HT, Carr DB, et al: Beta-endorphin and somatostatin concentrations in the cerebro-spinal fluid of patients with depressive disorder. Proceedings of the Society of Biology and Psychiatry, Los Angeles, May 2-6, 1984

Bloom F: Molecular approaches to the characterization of neuronal function. Marjorie Guthrie Lecture in Genetics, NIH (Bethesda, MD, April 19, 1984)

Buchsbaum MS: Brain imaging in psychiatry. Abstracts of American College of Neuropsychopharmacology (Puerto Rico, Dec 12-16, 1983)

Buchsbaum MS, LeLisi LE, Holcomb HH, et al: Anteroposterior gradients in cerebral glucose use in schizophrenia and affective disorders. Arch Gen Psychiatry, in press

Carroll BJ, Feinberg M, Greden JF, et al: A specific laboratory test for the diagnosis of melancholia. Arch Gen Psychiatry 38:15-22, 1981

Chouinard G, Young SN, Annable L: Antimanic effect of clonazepam. Biol Psychiatry 18:451-466, 1983

Dalby MA: Antiepileptic and psychotropic effect of carbamazepine (Tegretol) in the treatment of psychomotor epilepsy. Epilepsia 12:325-334, 1971

Dalby MA: Behavioral effects of carbamazepine, in Complex Partial Seizures and Their Treatment: Advances in Neurology, vol 11. Edited by Penry JK, Daly DD. New York, Raven Press, 1975

Davies P, Katzman R, Terry RD: Reduced somatostatin-like immuno-reactivity in cerebral cortex from cases of Alzheimer disease and Alzheimer senile dementia. Nature 288:279-280, 1980

Delfs JR, Zhu C-H, Dichter MA: Coexistence of acetylcholinesterase and somatostatin-immunoreactivity in neurons cultured from rat cerebrum. Science 223:61-63, 1984

Eckelman WC, Reba RC, Rzeszotarski WJ, et al: External imaging of cerebral muscarinic acetylcholine receptors. Science 223:291-292, 1984

Emrich HM, von Zerssen D, Kissling W, et al: Effect of sodium valproate in mania. The GABA-hypothesis of affective disorders. Arch Psychiatr Nervenkr 229:1-16, 1980

Engel J Jr, Kuhl DE, Phelps ME: Patterns of human local cerebral glucose metabolism during epileptic seizures. Science 218:64-66, 1982

Extein I, Pottash ALC, Gold MS, et al: Changes in TSH response to TRH in affective illness, in Neurobiology of Mood Disorders. Edited by Post RM, Ballenger JC. Baltimore, Williams & Wilkins Co, 1984

Foley KM, Kourides IA, Inturrisi CE, et al: Beta-endorphin: analgesic and hormonal effects in humans. Proc Natl Acad Sci USA 76:5377-5381, 1979

Freed WJ: Functional brain tissue transplantation: reversal of lesion-induced rotation by intraventricular substantia nigra and adrenal medulla grafts, with a note on intracranial retinal grafts. Biol Psychiatry 18:1205-1267, 1983

Freud S: Project for a scientific psychology, in The Origins of Psychoanalysis: Letters to Wilhelm Fliess, Drafts and Notes: 1887-1902. New York, Basic Books, 1954

Freyhan FA: Effectiveness of diphenylhydantoin in management of nonepileptic psychomotor excitement states. Arch Neurol Psychiatry 53:370-374, 1945

Garnett ES, Firnau G, Nahmias C: Dopamine visualized in the basal ganglia of living man. Nature 305:137-138, 1983

Gerner, Yamada T: Altered neuropeptide concentrations in CSF of psychiatric patients. Brain Res 238:298-302, 1982

Gillin JC, Sitaram N, Wehr T, et al: Sleep and affective illness, in Neurobiology of Mood Disorders. Edited by Post RM, Ballenger JC. Baltimore, Williams & Wilkins Co, 1984

Gold PW, Chrousos GP, Kellner CK, et al: Psychiatric implications of basic and clinical studies with corticotropin-releasing factor. Am J Psychiatry 141:619-627, 1984

Guillemin R: A plethora of peptides in the brain. Abstract of the Annual Meeting, American College of Neuropsychopharmacology (Puerto Rico, Dec 12-16, 1983)

Heath RG, Llewellyn RC, Rouchell AM: The cerebellar pacemaker for intractable behavioral disorders and epilepsy: follow-up report. Biol Psychiatry 15:243-256, 1980

Hokfelt T, Johansson O, Ljungdahl A, et al: Peptidergic neurons. Nature 264:515-521, 1980

Hosobuchi Y, Li CH: The analgesic activity of human beta-endorphin in man. Commun Psychopharmacol 2:33-37, 1978

Hubel DH, Wiesel TN: Brain mechanisms of vision. Sci Am 241:150-162, 1979

Ingvar DH: Epilepsy related to cerebral blood flow and metabolism. Acta Psychiatr Scand 69:21-26, 1984

Jacobowitz DM: Localization of CRF and GRF in the brain: coexistence of other peptides in CRF neurons. Abstracts of the American College of Neuropsychopharmacology (Puerto Rico, Dec 12-16, 1983)

Kalinowsky LB, Putnam TJ: Attempts at treatment of schizophrenia and other non-epileptic psychoses with dilantin. Arch Neurol Psychiatry 49:414-420, 1943

Kandel ER: From metapsychology to molecular biology: explorations into the nature of anxiety. Am J Psychiatry 140:1277-1292, 1983

Kellner CH, Rubinow DR, Gold PW, et al: Relationship of cortisol hypersecretion to brain CT scan alterations in depressed patients. Psychiatry Res 8:191-197, 1983

Kishimoto A, Ogura C, Hazama H, et al: Long-term prophylactic effects of carbamazepine in affective disorder. Br J Psychiatry 143:327-331, 1983

Kubanek JL, Rowell RC: The use of dilantin in the treatment of psychotic patients unresponsive to other treatment. Dis Nerv Syst 7:47-50, 1946

Kupfer DJ: REM latency: a psychobiological marker for primary depressive disease. Biol Psychiatry 11:159-174, 1976

Lowe M, Goodman RH, Brinster R, et al: Expression of a metallothinine somatostatin fusion gene in transgenic mice (Abs). American Association of Clinical Research, May 1984

Mazziotto JC, Phelps ME, Carson RE, et al: Tomographic mapping of human cerebral metabolism: auditory stimulation. Neurology 32:921-937, 1982

Mezey E, Reisine TD, Skirboll L, et al: Cholecystokinin in the medial parvocellular subdivision of the paraventricular nucleus: coexistence with cortocotropin releasing hormone. Ann NY Acad Sci, 1984, in press

Montminy M, Goodman RH, Horovitz S, et al: Primary structure of the gene encoding rat preprosomatostatin. Proc Natl Acad Sci USA, 81:3337-3340, 1984

Nasrallah HA, McCalley-Whitters M, Jacoby CG: Cerebral ventricular enlargement in young manic males. J Affective Disord 4:15-19, 1982

Nemeroff CB, Youngblood WW, Manberg PJ, et al: Regional brain concentrations of neuropeptides in Huntington's chorea and schizophrenia. Science 221:972-975, 1983

Okuma T: Therapeutic and prophylactic efficacies of carbamazepine in affective disorders. Proc VIIth World Congress of Psychiatry (Vienna, July 11-16, 1983)

Olschowka JA, Diz DI, Jacobowitz DM: Coexistence of substance P, corticotropin releasing factor and acetylcholinesterase in neurons of the nucleus tegmenti dorsalis lateralis. Society for Neuroscience Abstracts, vol 9 (13th Annual Meeting, Boston, Nov 6-11, 1983)

Olson L, Backlung E-O, Sedvall G, et al: Intrastriatal chromaffin grafts in experimental and clinical parkinsonism: first impressions. Abstracts of the 5th International Catecholamine Symposium (Goteborg, Sweden, June 12-16, 1983)

Oram JJ, Edwardson J, Millard PH: Investigation of cerebrospinal fluid neuropeptides in idiopathic senile dementia. Gerontology 27:216-223, 1981

Oyama T, Jin T, Yamaya R, et al: Profound analgesic effects of beta-endorphin in man. Lancet 1:122-124, 1980

Palmiter RD, Norstedt G, Gelinas RE, et al: Metallothionin- human GH fusion genes stimulate growth of mice. Science 222:809-814, 1983

Pearlson GD, Veroff AE: Computerized tomographic scan changes in manic-depressive illness. Lancet 2:470, 1981

Pearlson GD, Garbacz DJ, Thompkins RH, et al: Clinical correlates of lateral ventricular enlargement in bipolar affective disorder. Am J Psychiatry 141:253-257, 1984

Phelps ME: The biochemical basis of cerebral function and its investigation in humans with positron CT. Proceedings of the American Psychiatric Association 137th Annual Meeting (Los Angeles, May 5-11, 1984)

Pickar D, Dubois M, Cohen MR: Behavioral change in a cancer patient following intrathecal beta-endorphin administration. Am J Psychiatry 141:103-104, 1984

Porter RJ, Penry JK: Efficacy and choice of antiepileptic drugs, in Advances in Epileptology, 1977: Psychology, Pharmacotherapy, and New Diagnostic Approaches. Edited by Meinardi H, Rowan AJ. Amsterdam, Swetz & Zeitlinger, 1978

Post RM, Ballenger JC: Neurobiology of Mood Disorders. Baltimore, Williams & Wilkins Co., 1984

Post RM, Uhde TW: Carbamazepine as a treatment for depressive illness: lithium nonresponsive rapid cyclers, in Special Treatments for Resistant Depression. Edited by Zohar J, Belmaker RH. New York, Spectrum Press, 1984

Post RM, Ballenger JC, Goodwin FK: Cerebrospinal fluid studies of neurotransmitter function in manic and depressive illness, in Neurobiology of Cerebrospinal Fluid, vol 1. Edited by Wood JH. New York, Plenum Press, 1980

Post RM, Gold PW, Rubinow DR, et al: Peptides in the cerebrospinal fluid of neuropsychiatric patients: an approach to central nervous system peptide function. Life Sci 31:1-15, 1982

Post RM, Uhde TW, Ballenger JC, et al: CSF carbamazepine and its −10, 11-epoxide metabolite in manic-depressive patients: relationship to clinical response. Arch Gen Psychiatry 40:673-676, 1983a

Post RM, Uhde TW, Ballenger JC, et al: Prophylactic efficacy of carbamazepine in manic-depressive illness. Am J Psychiatry 140:1602-1604, 1983b

Post RM, Uhde TW, Rubinow DR, et al: Biochemical effects of carbamazepine: relationship to its mechanisms of action in affective illness. Prog Neuropsychopharmacol Biol Psychiatry 7:263-271, 1983c

Post RM, Ballenger JC, Uhde TW, et al: Efficacy of carbamazepine in manic-depressive illness: implications for underlying mechanisms, in Neurobiology of Mood Disorders. Edited by Post RM, Ballenger JC. Baltimore, Williams & Wilkins Co., 1984a.

Post RM, Putnam F, Contel NR, et al: Electroconvulsive seizures inhibit amygdala kindling: implications for mechanisms of action in affective illness. Epilepsia 25:234-239, 1984b

Reichlin S: Somatostatin (first of two parts). N Engl J Med 309:1495-1501, 1983

Reus VI, Deicken R, Miner C, et al: Correlates of marked non-suppression. New Research Abstracts of the American Psychiatric Association 137th Annual Meeting (Los Angeles, May 5-11, 1984)

Risberg J, Gustafson L, Prohovnik I; rCBR measurements by ^{133}Xe inhalation: applications in neuropsychology and psychiatry. Prog Nucl Med 7:82-94, 1981

Robertson MM, Trimble MR: Depressive illness in patients with epilepsy: a review. Epilepsia 24:5109-5116, 1983

Rossor MN, Emson PC, Mountjoy CQ, et al: Reduced amounts of immunoreactive somatostatin in the temporal cortex in senile dementia of Alzheimer type. Neurosci Lett 20:373-377, 1980

Roth KA, Weber E, Barchas JD: Immunoreactive corticotropin releasing factor (CRF) and vasopressin are localized in a subpopulation of the immunoreactive vasopressin cells in the paraventricular nucleus of the hypothalamus. Life Sci 31:1857-1860, 1982

Roy-Byrne PP, Post RM: Carbamazepine in aggression, schizophrenia and other non-affective psychiatric syndromes. Submitted to *International Drug Therapies in Psychiatry*. Edited by Ayd F, 1984

Rubinow DR, Gold PW, Post RM, et al: Somatostatin in affective illness. Arch Gen Psychiatry 40:403-412, 1983

Rubinow DR, Post RM, Gold PW, et al: The relationship between cortisol and clinical phenomenology of affective illness, in Neurobiology of Mood Disorders. Edited by Post RM, Ballenger JC. Baltimore, Williams & Wilkins Co, 1984

Serby M, Richardson SB, Twente S, et al: CSF somatostatin in Alzheimer's Disease. Abstract of the Annual Meeting, American College of Neuropsychopharmacology (Puerto Rico, Dec 12-16, 1983)

Snyder SH: Neuroscience strategies for drug development. Abstracts of the Society for Neuroscience, 13th Annual Meeting, Presidential Symposium (Boston, Nov 6-11, 1983)

Snyder SH: Drug and neurotransmitter receptors: new perspectives. Presented at conference on "Mechanisms of Synaptic Regulation," NIMH (Bethesda, MD, May 31, 1984)

Sorensen KV, Christensen SE, Dupont E, et al: Low somatostatin content in cerebrospinal fluid in multiple sclerosis. Acta Neurol Scand 61:186-191, 1980

Sutcliffe JG, Shinnick TM, Green N, et al: Chemical synthesis of a polypeptide predicted from nucleotide sequence allows detection of a new retroviral gene product. Nature 287:801-805, 1980

Swanson LW: role of norepinephrine in the brain: from lab to man. Anatomy. Presented at American Psychiatric Association 137th Annual Meeting. (Los Angeles, May 5-11, 1984)

Targum SD, Rosen LN, De Lisi LE, et al: Cerebral ventricular size in major depressive disorder: association with delusional symptoms. Biol Psychiatry 18:329-336, 1983

Trimble MR: Interictal psychoses of epilepsy. Acta Psychiatr Scand 69:9-20, 1984

Wagner HN, Burns D, Dannals RF, et al: Imaging dopamine receptors in the human brain by positron tomography. Science 221:1264-1266, 1983

Weinberger DR, Wyatt RJ: Cerebral ventricular size: a biological marker for subtyping chronic schizophrenia, in Biological Markers in Psychiatry and Neurology. Edited by Usdin E, Hanin I. New York, Pergamon Press, 1982

Williams DT, Mehl R, Yudofsky S, et al: The effect of propranolol on uncontrolled rage outbursts in children and adolescents with organic brain dysfunction. J Am Acad Child Psychiatry 21:129-135, 1982

Wood PL, Etienne P, Lal S, et al: Reduced lumbar CSF somatostatin levels in Alzheimer's Disease. Life Sci 31:2073-2079, 1982

Wyatt RJ: Producing functional repair in the central and peripheral nervous system of mammals. Abstracts of the American College of Neuropharmacology (Puerto Rico, Dec 12-16, 1983)

Yudofsky SC, Stevens L, Silver J, et al: Propranolol in the treatment of rage and violent behavior associated with Korsakoff's psychosis. Am J Psychiatry 141:114-115, 1984

Zubenko GE, Nixon RA: Mood-elevating effect of Captopril in depressed patients. Am J Psychiatry 141:110-111, 1984

This chapter was written by the author in his private capacity. No official support or endorsement by NIMH is intended or should be inferred.

Afterword
The Paradox of Broca
by Stuart C. Yudofsky, M.D.

In medicine, much of what we know about the so-called normal derives from our study of the abnormal. This is particularly true in the specialties of psychiatry and neurology. For example, Broca's region of the brain is a relatively small locus in the posterior-inferior part of the frontal lobe, and it consists of the posterior portion of the foot of the third frontal convolution, the frontal operculum and the immediately adjacent cortical zone. As early as 1861, Paul Broca realized that this cortical region was involved in specific aspects of "articulated language" (Broca, 1861a and 1861b). He arrived at his conclusion by relating the language dysfunction of a patient to the particular location of his lesion. Despite almost unfathomable technological breakthroughs over the succeeding 120 years, today's scientists can neither chemically nor morphologically distinguish neurons in Broca's area from the contiguous cortical neurons that have distinct functions. Thus, the precise function of the neurons in Broca's area, to this day, can only be revealed through lesions. In a similar fashion, Freud related past experiences to psychopathology and thereby derived such theories as role conflict and the unconscious in symptom formation. Freud later applied these insights to gain understanding of normal development and normal function. How much would Freud have discovered about the workings of the mind if there were not childhood trauma and the resultant psychopathology?

It is my opinion that future discoveries about normal brain function—regardless of whether expressed through sensory or motor behavior, perception, mood, cognition, intellect, personality, social capacity, or otherwise—will directly relate to insights derived from neurologic and psychiatric illnesses. The silver lining of the scourge of psychiatric and neurologic illness is that these devastating diseases provide both the impetus and substrate whereby we can learn about ourselves. Through Alzheimer's disease we will eventually gain vital insights into the minute particles of matter and their complex spatial arrangements that regulate unimpaired memory and learning. Through our investigations of bipolar illness, we will gain vital insights into the chemistry and physics of healthy feelings, temperament and mood. One of life's bitter paradoxes is that, through the painful and disabling lesions treated by psychiatrists and neurologists, we are discovering ourselves. In this discovery we, ultimately, will not only free ourselves of illnesses but also free ourselves from limitations—ranging from anxiety to aging—that have been accepted for millennia as the human condition.

REFERENCES

Broca, P: Perte de la parole. Remollissement chronique et destruction partielle du lobe anterieur gauche du cerveau. Bull Soc Antrop (Paris) 2:219, 1861a

Broca, P: Remarques sur le siege de la faculte du langage articule suivie d'une observation d'aphemie. Bull Soc Anat (Paris) 6:330, 1861b

III

Sleep Disorders

Contents

Section III

Sleep Disorders
Introduction

by David J. Kupfer, M.D., Section Editor

Sleep and its mysteries have always held a certain fascination. The discovery by Aserinsky and Kleitman in the 1950s that rapid eye movement (REM) sleep was associated with the phenomenon of dreaming encouraged scientists who were rapidly discovering that the brain is as active during sleep as it is during waking hours (Aserinsky and Kleitman, 1953). There are several reasons that this update is particularly timely. First, while we have long had clinical information about sleep disorders, that experience is now augmented by objective information via psychophysiological measures. In the past, if an individual complained of disturbed sleep, the clinician could only take his word for it. However, through the new objective sleep laboratory techniques, we have since learned that a surprising number of clinically convincing insomnia complainers have normal amounts of sleep. This does not mean that these individuals have *no* disorder: they simply have a different disorder than subjective accounts indicate. Second, it is now easier to ascertain the true incidence of sleep disorders. For example, although many patients with affective illness may not complain of problems with their sleep, certain physiological changes in sleep architecture are associated with these conditions. Third, and of enormous practical importance, treatments now exist for many sleep disorders where none were previously available—especially in the major categories of the DIMS (disorders of initiating and maintaining sleep) and DOES (disorders of excessive sleep).

The relevance of sleep disorders to psychiatry and other medical specialties was recently highlighted by the National Institute of Health's (NIH) Office of Medical Applications of Research (OMAR), which held a consensus development conference on "Drugs and Insomnia: The Use of Medications to Promote Sleep." Conferences such as this one are designed to improve the lines of communication from the health research community to the practicing physician and the public by bringing together biomedical researchers, practicing physicians, consumers, and others in an effort to reach general consensus on whether a given medical technology is safe and effective. This national focus on sleep disorders further underscores the need to share current understanding of these illnesses and their treatment with practicing clinicians and has guided our selection of material for these seven chapters.

The current interest in sleep disorders represents the convergence of new developments in diagnosis, epidemiology, and treatment coupled with an intensive public—or at least medical—education effort. Quite simply, a psychiatrist practicing in the 1980s can and should know about these disorders.

Psychiatrists are no longer surprised when biomedical or physiological abnormalities are found to be associated with emotional and cognitive problems.

Indeed, scientists are actively searching for a physical cause or "markers" for many psychiatric diagnostic entities. Thus, the clinician should not be surprised to learn that the development of the sleep evaluation laboratory, largely in the past decade, has made possible the search for and, for some diagnoses, the identification of such markers in the area of sleep disorders. Polysomnography (PSG) allows a number of physiological systems to be monitored simultaneously during sleep without disturbing the sleeper. With these measures, investigators have not only plotted the architecture of normal sleep as it changes with advancing age but have also identified specific sleep parameters that vary in predictable directions in association with given psychiatric disorders. This new knowledge has facilitated a refined and more descriptive nosological system for diagnosing sleep disorders, allowing the physician more accurately to target a treatment intervention with some hope of success (ASDC, 1979).

A recent national survey found that one-third of the U.S. population reported some degree of insomnia; one-half of this group considered the insomnia serious. Half of the group with "serious insomnia" reported a high level of emotional distress. Yet insomnia is just one symptom of a symptom complex, the cause of which may be an underlying medical or psychiatric disorder. Evaluation of a patient's medical and sleep history and, when appropriate, application of sleep laboratory procedures to evaluate day and night sleep and their physiological patterns, may lead to the diagnosis of a sleep disorder and appropriate intervention. In the case of many insomnias, for example, use of benzodiazepines has been shown to be an effective treatment. Patients whose insomnia or hypersomnia is traced to an affective illness can be started on the appropriate antidepressant therapy. Patients who are not judged to be appropriate candidates for pharmacological intervention might show improvement with a nonpharmacological therapy such as relaxation training, biofeedback, systematic desensitization, or something as simple as discussion of good sleep hygiene habits.

The emphasis in this section—and what is important for the practicing clinician—is that treatments *are* available. The following seven chapters do not provide a comprehensive review of sleep. Rather, they provide an update on the sleep disorders that are of greatest relevance to the clinical psychiatrist, offering practical information in the areas of: sleep physiology as we know it from the latest PSG techniques; the nosology of sleep disorders recently put forth by the Association of Sleep Disorders Centers (ASDC); sleep changes and disturbances in those psychiatric disorders for which we have some knowledge of sleep parameters; and the treatment of sleep disorders with both pharmacological and nonpharmacological interventions.

While we have selected topics related to sleep disorders that should be of interest to psychiatrists, these disorders have a broad and overlapping boundary with many other medical specialties. Although psychiatrists are frequently consulted to evaluate insomnia and sleep problems, sleep disorders are not the exclusive domain of any one specialty of medicine. Organic insomnias often mimic psychologically generated sleep disturbances. The patient may tell the physician that the probable cause of his or her difficulty in sleeping is excessive worry or anxiety; but it is only in the sleep lab that the patient's myoclonus, sleep apnea, or bruxism may be revealed. The area of sleep disorders should be approached from the perspective of using this class of problem for collaboration and continued research among medicine, neurology, psychiatry, and other relevant specialties.

We have taken a developmental approach to the organization of this section, guiding the reader from an understanding of the parameters of sleep in normal individuals to the treatment of specific problems in a clinical population.

In Chapter 14, Drs. Karacan and Moore cover the history of sleep studies, sleep physiology as observed in various bodily systems and the sleep-wake cycle, in order to give the reader enough background to appreciate the significance of the work described in subsequent chapters. They review the deafferentiation paradigm, whereby sleep was assumed to be the temporary shutting down of mental and biological activity, and the way that the development of electroencephalography led to the discovery that during sleep, the brain is engaged in *different* activity than it is during the waking state, but not *less* activity. Drs. Karacan and Moore also review the stages and cycles of sleep and physiological events occurring in various bodily systems during sleep. Finally, they review the effects of neurotransmitters—such as serotonin, norepinephrine and others that are just now being studied—on the sleep-wake cycle.

In Chapter 15, Drs. Roffwarg and Erman review the new ASDC nosology and offer guidelines to physicians for referring a patient for evaluation in a sleep lab, and what both the patient and the physician should expect from such an evaluation. Very important for the practicing physician are the factors that make up good sleep hygiene habits, changes which may be all that is required for minor sleep complaints. However, when a more thorough work-up is required, the diagnosis is likely to fall into one of the four ASDC categories: disorders of initiating and maintaining sleep (the insomnias); disorders of excessive somnolence (hypersomnia); disorders of the sleep-wake schedule; and dysfunctions associated with sleep (the parasomnias). The reliability and validity of the ASDC diagnostic system, based on the work done in two multicenter case series studies, are reviewed, and the practitioner is given guidelines on how to manage patients with insomnia.

Dr. Gillin reviews the normal development of sleep and dreaming, and discusses some sleep disorders occurring in childhood, in Chapter 16. He describes the developmental course of the 24-hour rest and activity cycle, noting that the duration and structure of sleep change dramatically over the life span. At birth, the infant has virtually no circadian organization; in the normal elderly, the circadian cycle may again partially break down. Changes also occur in the amount of sleep time and in the pattern of sleep between infancy and old age. The area of sleep disorders in children remains largely unexplored territory. Although almost all children complain at one time or another of being unable to sleep or having "bad dreams," these complaints are often minor and stop with nothing more than parental reassurance. However, studies have shown legitimate sleep disorders occurring in children; in fact, narcolepsy usually begins in adolescence. Clinicians should be prepared to evaluate, diagnose, and treat sleep disorders in children.

In Chapter 17, Drs. Reynolds and Shipley review sleep disturbances as manifest in patients with affective illness and discuss the clinical use of the sleep electroencephalogram (EEG) in diagnosing affective illness and predicting response to treatment. In this area, several REM sleep findings, such as the shortened

REM latency or increased REM activity in the first part of the night, are significantly different from the sleep of normals. Drs. Reynolds and Shipley conclude with a discussion of three models of the relationship of EEG sleep to the pathophysiology of depression: neurochemical, chronobiological, and developmental.

Drs. Gillin, Reynolds, and Shipley review, in Chapter 18, sleep studies in selected adult psychiatric disorders—obsessive-compulsive disorders, dementia, schizophrenia, anxiety disorders, and borderline personality disorders—and document the progress achieved in establishing well-described EEG sleep abnormalities in these disorders. While progress has been made in testing and sometimes in discovering EEG sleep abnormalities associated with some of these disorders, often these findings are more sensitive than diagnostically specific. Yet these leads do offer hope that work is progressing in the right direction, both to clinicians whose patients complain of sleep problems, and to researchers searching for evidence of biological abnormalities in psychiatric illness.

Patients with sleep disorders may require treatment. This treatment may be either nonpharmacological or pharmacological, or some combination of the two. In Chapter 19, Drs. Hauri and Sateia consider nonpharmacological factors and treatments in insomnia, paying particular attention to behavioral and cognitive modalities, as well as to good sleep hygiene. They point out that people suffering from any chronic illness react to the illness psychologically, habituate to it, and change their lifestyles to accommodate the disease. This process is particularly true of sleep disorders. However, the opposite is also true: In a number of patients, a change in patterns and habits, under clinical guidance, often significantly improves sleep problems.

Nevertheless, some patients are refractory to such approaches or respond only partially. For many of these individuals, drug treatment may be indicated. This area is reviewed by Dr. Mendelson in Chapter 20: He discusses the pharmacology of hypnotics and pays particular attention to the benzodiazepines, the drugs prescribed most often for insomnia. He also reviews the efficacy of various agents; and provides guidelines for prescribing a drug for a patient with a sleep problem, and guidelines for such an agent's withdrawal.

Finally, just as every door that is opened reveals a new series of doors to unlock, I will highlight the mysteries of sleep that still lie before us.

REFERENCES

Aserinsky E, Kleitman N: Regularly occurring periods of eye motility, and concomitant phenomena during sleep. Science 118:273-274, 1953

Association of Sleep Disorders Centers: Diagnostic classification of sleep and arousal disorders. Sleep 2:1-127, 1979

Chapter 14

Physiology and Neurochemistry of Sleep

by Ismet Karacan, M.D., D.Sc. (Med) and
Constance Moore, M.D.

More discoveries, more data collection and more momentum have appeared in the past 30 years of sleep study than in the previous 2,000. The excitement has come from new technology, from the development of a multidisciplinary approach to evaluating sleep complaints and, concurrently, from an enhanced understanding of the chemistry of the brain. These developments have advanced the clinical approach to diagnosis and treatment of sleep-related disorders and of certain non-sleep-related disorders as well. In 1975 the Association of Sleep Disorders Centers (ASDC) was created, and more than 50 such centers are currently in operation. The next decade may bring with it the establishment of sleep disorders centers in almost every major medical center. Sleep research offers valuable information to related fields as well. It promises to illuminate the relationships between the dream process and memory, and the relationships of both to certain biological events. The sleeping brain provides a promising opportunity for scientific study of the relationships among molecular biology, dreaming and behavior, the complex intervening variables which have long been secrets of nature.

This chapter will discuss important benchmarks in sleep study history and will describe the basic physiological processes of sleep, with special attention given to neurochemistry. It will provide the reader with sufficient background to permit appreciation of the other sleep-related chapters of this volume.

SLEEP STUDY HISTORY

The Deafferentiation Paradigm

From the writings of the Epicurean philosopher Lucretius to the mid-twentieth century, sleep was assumed to be the temporary and partial shutting down of mental and biological activity. According to this paradigm, waking functions were akin to the pumping action of a windmill: Just as the pumping continued as long as the wind blew, so the body functioned as long as stimuli such as daylight and visible objects were present. Sleep would come as a result of either sensory deprivation or the termination (via cerebral mechanisms) of afferent signals or, most probably, both.

Experiments of the nineteenth century provided what was taken to be proof of the deafferentiation theory. Flourens (1824) demonstrated the sleeping attitude of birds after ablation of the cerebral hemispheres. This research, along with the work of Rolando (1809) and Purkinje (1846), formed part of the search to pinpoint the exact sleep center of the brain. In this respect, Gayet in France (1875) and Mauthner in Austria (1890) were able to associate the "lethargic syndrome" with lesions in the mesencephalon. Von Economo (1926, 1928), studying brain degeneration during the world wide encephalitis epidemic, associated sleep disorders with lesions in the hypothalamus, the periventricular grey matter, and a mesodiencephalic area extending to the hypothalamus. Although it is now clear that no single "sleep center" exists as such, the results of these studies have all proved valuable in the study of cerebral function during sleep.

The Development of Electroencephalography

Electroencephalography (EEG)—the monitoring of electrical activities in the brain—was the technique that allowed objective study of sleep and, in so doing, helped to supplant the deafferentiation theory. Caton (1875) found currents in electrodes that had been placed on the heads of monkeys, and in 1892 Ladd obtained similar results with human beings. However, the first significant research involving the EEG phenomenon was that of Hans Berger (1929), which demonstrated that the brain's electrical currents originate in the neuron, that those currents respond to sensory stimulation, and that epileptic seizures produce abnormal brain activity.

The 1930s and 1940s were a period of much exploration into the relationship of EEG readings and consciousness. Major developments came from the Loomis Laboratory, where early studies established that EEG patterns during sleep are entirely different from waking patterns. Loomis and his colleagues (1935) further observed that EEG patterns change as sleep progresses, and they hypothesized from their observations that changes in EEG patterns reflect changes in levels of consciousness. Two years later Blake and Gerard (1937) confirmed the relationship between sleep levels and distinctive brain potentials and, on the basis of behavioral data, inferred that a parallel exists between sleep depth and brain potential pattern.

Loomis et al (1937) also made one of the most fundamental contributions to the taxonomy of sleep. Citing their results from all-night EEG monitoring sessions, they delineated five separate sleep stages distinguishable by amplitude and frequency of the electrical activity present.

Certainly the most famous support of the deafferentiation theory was the experiment of Moruzzi and Magoun (1949), who found that electrical stimulation of the mesencephalic reticular formation in a patient with a transection just below the medulla changed a sleeping EEG pattern to that of a waking EEG pattern. Moruzzi and Magoun inferred from their results that sleep was due to the reduction of the tonic barrage of ascending reticular impulses, and that the sleep syndrome after midbrain transection was due to the termination of the waking influence of the ascending reticular activating system.

Breakdown of the Deafferentiation Theory

Put simply, the active theory of sleep holds that sleep is not simply a reduction of neural activity but an alternate type of neural activity. Evidence contradicting the deafferentiation theory had appeared since 1927, although the active sleep theory itself did not become popular for some time. Hess (1927, 1933, 1944) induced sleep by low-rate electrical stimulation of selected diencephalic loci, thereby suggesting an active sleep mechanism. He posited the existence of a sleep-controlling center within the thalamus. Although criticized by contemporaries, Hess's work was eventually confirmed with the use of EEG recordings; and today Hess is considered a pioneer in the field of sleep research.

Further evidence contradicting the deafferentiation theory appeared in the late 1950s. Batini and colleagues (1958, 1959) found that brainstem transections immediately rostral to the trigeminal rootlets produced EEG and behavior patterns of the waking state. They hypothesized that the sleep syndrome was linked to the abolition of a wakefulness structure that lay just above the midpontine transection. The continued waking EEG suggested the presence of an active mechanism capable of synchronizing the EEG and inducing sleep; this mechanism evidently lay just below the level of the section. Other brain locations have since been identified as hypnogenic regions; these will be discussed later.

The paradigm of "active" sleep was bolstered by the discovery of bursts of rapid eye movements (REMs) during sleep (Aserinsky and Kleitman, 1953). REM sleep, it was demonstrated, is linked to increased level and variability of heart rate, increased variability of respiration, nocturnal penile tumescence (NPT), and dreaming. A definite neural activity was therefore present in sleep. Indeed, REM appears to be a period of heightened brain activity, an essential component in the sleep of all mammals, and a possible factor in the memory process (Hawkins, et al, 1962; Jouvet, 1962; Oswald, 1962). In sum, it appears that sleep, and particularly REM sleep, is far from being the state of physical and mental shutdown once imagined.

THE EEG AND ONTOGENY OF SLEEP

The Stages of Sleep

Loomis et al (1937), as already noted, introduced five sleep stage gradations; their system was modified by Dement and Kleitman (1957) and later by Rechtschaffen and Kales (1968). The latter authors' classification is the one in general use and is summarized as follows:

Stage 0. Wakefulness with eyes closed. Waking EEG recordings contain alpha waves (8–12 cycles per second) and/or low voltage, mixed frequency activity. Muscle tone is usually high and some eye movement may be seen.

Stage 1. Relatively low-voltage beta (14–35 cps) and theta activity (4–7.5 cps), mixed frequency EEG without REMs. Vertex sharp waves may be present, slow eye movements appear, and EMG activity is not suppressed.

Stage 2. Irregular theta waves form the background of stage 2 sleep. Two types of phasic activity periodically interrupt: first, sleep spindles (sinusoidal bursts of 12-14 cps) are prominent in the central region; second, K-complexes (high-amplitude negative waves followed by positive activity) appear both spontaneously and as the result of external stimuli. High amplitude delta waves (0.5–3.5 cps) may be found in stage 2, but they do not constitute more than 20 percent of an epoch (a measure of time variously fixed between 30 seconds and one minute).

Stage 3. Stage 3 is recognized primarily by its slow (0.5–3.5 cps) high amplitude waves. Delta or "slow" waves account for 20 to 50 percent of stage 3 sleep.

Stage 4. This stage contains predominantly (above 50 percent) slow-wave sleep. Sleepers at stage 4 have high thresholds of arousal and, after total sleep deprivation, will show a significant rebound effect in the absolute and relative amounts of stage 4. Growth hormone secretion is increased during this stage. Stages 3 and 4 are sometimes scored together as "slow-wave" or "¾" sleep.

Stages 1–4 are known collectively as non-REM (NREM) sleep in humans. In animals, the stages are not as well distinguished and are variously called NREM, slow wave sleep (SWS), or synchronized sleep.

REM. Also known as "desynchronized" sleep, "1REM" sleep and "paradoxical" sleep (PS) in animals, this stage is characterized by stage 1 EEG characteristics; extreme hypotonia as evidenced by EMG readings; short bursts of phasic activity such as rapid eye movements, blood pressure and heart rate variability, and muscle twitches; and episodes of nocturnal penile tumescence. Subjects awakened during REM sleep demonstrate high dream recall, and REM sleep shows significant rebound in terms of latency to onset, relative amount, and absolute amount after sleep deprivation (Dement, 1960).

The Cycles of Sleep

The cycle of sleep staging is fairly constant within the eight hour sleep period. On any given night the average adult aged 25 years has four to six cycles in the following sequence: 1–2–3–4–3–2–REM. In this age group, time from the beginning of one REM episode to the beginning of the next is approximately 90 minutes, while duration of initial REM episodes is approximately 15 minutes. Quantity of slow-wave sleep diminishes and duration of REM episodes lengthens in the third and fourth cycles of the night. Nighttime awakenings tend to occur after REM episodes.

Sleep Study Variables

In order to quantitatively analyze the nature of human sleep, sleep researchers and clinicians routinely examine such variables as the total amount of sleep in a single night, the number of shifts between sleep stages, the amount of time in bed actually spent in sleep, the latency to the different sleep stages, and the number of awakenings. An idea of the quality of sleep may also be obtained by presleep and postsleep questionnaires, morning coordination tests, daytime alertness checklists, and tests for mental alertness such as symbol copying tests and digit symbol substitution tests.

Ontogeny

All human sleep variables are dependent upon age and sex, and a discussion of "normal" sleep must therefore be qualified. This chapter presents a summary of the major changes that occur in sleep variables. For a thorough examination of sleep ontogeny the reader is referred to *EEG of Human Sleep: Clinical Applications* (Williams et al, 1974).

Because of the inherent difficulties of *in utero* EEG monitoring, and because there is no behavioral context to give meaning to the terms "sleeping" or "waking" in such a state, information concerning the EEG of human fetuses is difficult to interpret. However, Okamoto and Kirikae (1951) have shown 0.5 to 2 cps waves in three-month-old fetuses. Thus EEG patterns begin to develop long before birth. Sterman and Jeannerod (1967) found bursts of fetal motility during the mother's stage 1 and stage 2 sleep, but interpretation of this finding is, again, difficult.

Changes in the characteristics of sleep are found throughout one's lifetime. Although for the most part these characteristics change gradually, there is a period of more distinct change in sleep patterns after three years of age, after puberty, and after the fourth decade of life (particularly in men). To illustrate the ontogeny of sleep, let us examine three age groups: group A (men, ages 20-29), group B (men, ages 40-49), and group C (men, ages 70-79).

First, total sleep time is reduced, even though the amount of time in bed may remain the same (one percent awake time for group A; six percent for group B; 16 percent for group C). Thus the elderly person lies in bed awake for longer periods. Over the same period, the number of nighttime awakenings also increases (3.5 awakenings for group A; 4.7 for group B; 7.1 for group C). These findings confirm the common observation of restless sleep in the elderly.

Second, the proportion of the five sleep stages varies over a lifetime. Figures 1 and 2 depict the changes in absolute amounts of waking time, REM sleep,

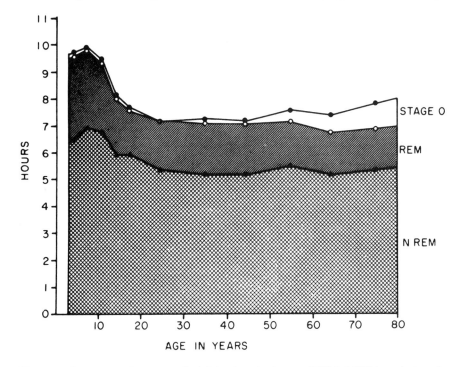

Figure 1. Average total amount of nightly sleep in terms of REM, NREM, and stage 0, for female age groups from 3 to 5 years through 70 to 79 years. (Reprinted from Robert L. Williams et al, *EEG of Human Sleep: Clinical Applications.* Copyright © 1974 by John Wiley & Sons, Inc. Reprinted by permission of John Wiley & Sons, Inc.)

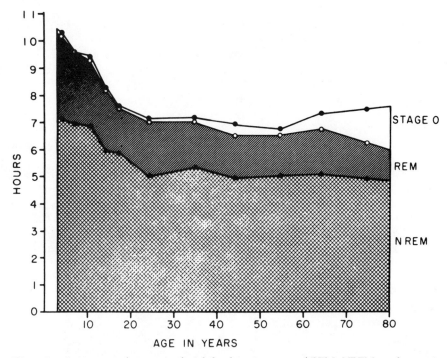

Figure 2. Average total amount of nightly sleep in terms of REM, NREM, and stage 0, for male age groups from 3 to 5 years through 70 to 79 years. (Reprinted from Robert L. Williams et al, *EEG of Human Sleep: Clinical Applications.* Copyright © 1974 by John Wiley & Sons, Inc. Reprinted by permission of John Wiley & Sons, Inc.)

and NREM sleep for men and women throughout an 80-year lifespan. Stage 4, which occupies 15 percent of sleep in group A, drops to three percent in group B and totally disappears in group C. REM sleep in group A (28 percent) is not as high as the 30 percent in boys ages three to five. However, group A does constitute the post-adolescent high range for REM sleep percentages. Succeeding groups show declines (23 percent for B; 18 percent for C). Although slight gain in the percentage of stage 1 and a fairly constant percentage of stage 2 are noted between groups A and B, there are *no* gains in absolute time for any of the five sleep stages, since the total sleep time declines (from 419 minutes for group A to 389 for group B to 373 for group C). This trend, in conjunction with the increase in nighttime awakenings, amounts to less time spent in actual sleep. The implications of these age-related changes are unknown. However, many researchers and clinicians believe they imply a "lighter" and less refreshing sleep.

ASPECTS OF PHYSIOLOGY IN SLEEP

Sleep is characterized by a change in the pattern of physiologic activity in organ systems. Historically, sleep was seen as a time of physiological slowdown, a time when the whole body "rested." We now know that sleep is characterized by a redistribution of the patterns of physiologic activity which may be not only sleep-related but sleep-stage-related. This section will summarize the changes seen in cardiovascular, pulmonary, cerebral and erectile physiology in sleep.

Cardiovascular Physiology in Sleep

Sleep-related cardiovascular function has been well studied, especially in cats and to a lesser extent in humans (Gassel et al, 1964; Guazzi and Zanchetti, 1965; Khatri and Freis, 1967; Reis et al, 1968; Richardson et al, 1968; Baccelli et al, 1969, 1974; Bristow et al, 1972; Coccagna et al, 1971; Mancia et al, 1971). These studies will be summarized.

Heart rate (HR) and arterial blood pressure (BP) progressively fall during NREM sleep and reach their lowest and least variable values in slow-wave sleep (SWS). In humans, the mean arterial BP in SWS decreases by about ten percent and the HR declines by about six percent in HR (Bristow et al, 1972). Cardiac output may (Khatri and Freis, 1967) or may not (Bristow et al, 1972) fall in humans in NREM sleep, and total peripheral resistance declines. Studies of regional blood flow in cats indicate that there is little vasodilation of mesenteric or renal vessels in synchronized sleep but marked vasodilation in paradoxical sleep (PS). There is also little change in skeletal muscle flow during synchronized sleep, but vasoconstriction with decreased flow to these muscles in PS (there is skeletal muscle hypotonia in PS).

Mean HR and BP remain at about the same levels in REM sleep as in SWS. However, there is greater variability in these parameters during REM sleep. Sharp, brief increases of up to 30-40 mm Hg occur in BP, probably due to phasic decreases in total peripheral conductance, and coincide with the onset of rapid eye movements and muscle twitches. HR declines tonically, but there may be brief tachycardias and bradycardias.

The cardiovascular changes just described may take on clinical relevance in patients with cardiovascular disease. Researchers have speculated that stroke, myocardial infarction, angina, and dysrhythmias may be precipitated in some patients by sleep-related cardiovascular changes, particularly the variable BP and HR of REM sleep.

There have been a number of case reports of patients suffering either increased arrhythmias or arrhythmias exclusively in sleep. However, the majority of studies have found that, overall, patients with known coronary artery disease or arrhythmias have a decrease in frequency of arrhythmias during sleep, with no significant difference between REM and NREM sleep (Smith et al, 1972; Lown et al, 1973; Karacan et al, 1977; Monti et al, 1975). However, there were some individuals from the study groups whose arrhythmias worsened with sleep. Studies of patients with fixed abnormal daytime S-T segment changes on EKG have yielded similar results. While a majority of the patients had improvement or no change in EKG findings, some (about 25 percent) had increased severity of the findings during sleep (Stern and Tzivoni, 1973). These may be helped by increased nighttime vasodilator and antiarrhythmic pharmacotherapy.

Lung and Upper Airway Physiology in Sleep

Sleep is accompanied by decreased respiratory function in normal subjects. In SWS, respiratory rate and minute ventilation decrease, as does the respiratory drive response to mild hypercapnia (Sullivan et al, 1979b). Breathing is generally more rapid, shallow, and erratic in REM sleep in association with the phasic components of that stage of sleep. Coughing and mucociliary clearance are reduced in SWS and REM sleep, leading to retention of lung secretions (Bateman et al, 1978). The partial collapse of the upper airway due to reduced smooth muscle tone (Sullivan et al, 1979a) further reduces respiratory function in REM sleep and, to a lesser degree, in NREM. The tone of the intercostal and geniog-lossal muscles also decreases in REM sleep. All of these functional changes are of little clinical significance in normal subjects but can be detrimental to patients with already impaired respiratory function, such as those with asthma or chronic obstructive lung disease, or in those with sleep apnea (see Chapter 15 of this volume).

Cerebral Circulation in Sleep

Brain circulation and metabolism are of particular interest to sleep researchers because the sleep-wake cycle is centrally regulated. The cerebral blood vessels are subject to autoregulation; that is, they are capable of dilating and constricting in response to brain tissue needs. In the resting waking state, cerebral blood flow (CBF) remains essentially constant over a wide range of systemic arterial blood pressures (mean BP between 60 and 150 mm Hg) via vasodilation and constriction. The vasculature is sensitive to changes in carbon dioxide tension (CO_2 is the main metabolic product of brain energy metabolism). Hypercapnea results in vasodilation and hypocapnia in vasoconstriction. The vasculature is much less sensitive to changes in arterial oxygen content.

CBF is related to cerebral metabolism. When systemic BP is maintained in a physiologic range and arterial pCO_2 and pO_2 are relatively stable, then the CBF should be an index of metabolically produced CO_2 from the brain. Increases in CO_2 lead to vasodilation and increased CBF. Thus, changes in CBF in sleep should imply corresponding changes in brain activity. It should be noted that the latter statement presumes that cerebrovascular autoregulation is not impaired in normal sleep—a presumption that has not been directly tested, although there is no evidence to suggest that it is impaired.

Reivich et al (1968) used an autoradiographic method to study regional blood flow during sleep in sleep-deprived cats. They used the highly diffusable inert tracer [^{14}C] antipyrine, which rapidly equilibrates between the arterial blood and cerebral tissue. Significant increases during synchronized sleep over waking were seen in a number of brainstem areas and in the association cortex. Increases of 50 percent or more over waking were found in all 25 cortical and subcortical areas measured during PS (the human REM equivalent). Townsend and colleagues (1973) used the [^{133}Xe] inhalation technique to study regional CBF in 11 healthy men. Only cerebral blood flow (not brainstem blood flow) was measured. They found reductions in all areas in SWS and increases in all areas in REM sleep, with the greatest increases in the temporal lobe regions. It should be noted that the latter method is less sensitive to changes in CBF than Reivich's autoradi-ographic method.

Using [^{133}Xe] inhalation, Sakai et al (1979) studied eight normal subjects in sleep stages 1 and 2 and narcoleptic patients in various sleep stages. Mean hemispheric CBF in normal subjects in stages 1 and 2 sleep was about ten percent less than while awake. Reductions of 25 percent occurred in the brainstem-cerebellar regions, with 23 percent, 20 percent, and 12 percent reductions in the right inferior temporal, right frontal, and right posterior temporal regions respectively. There was no significant difference in the flow reduction between the right and left hemispheres. Two narcoleptic patients entered REM sleep and showed increases of 35 percent in the brainstem-cerebellar regions. The six narcoleptic patients who entered stages 1 and 2 sleep showed an average of a 20 percent *increase* in mean hemispheric CBF and a 38 percent *increase* in brainstem-cerebellar blood flow, the opposite of the changes seen in normals.

A more direct measure of brain activity is determination of glucose utilization using the [^{14}C] deoxyglucose (2-DG) autoradiographic technique. Like glucose, 2-DG is transported across the blood-brain barrier and phosphorylated in cerebral tissues. However, unlike glucose, it is not metabolized for the production of energy—instead it remains trapped in the tissues. The 2-DG can be detected radiographically, and its presence in a given brain area is directly related to metabolic activity (Sokoloff, 1980).

A recent study in monkeys using the 2-DG autoradiographic technique revealed a reduction in metabolic rate in NREM sleep in the brain regions examined—a finding that does not support the hypothesis of active hypnogenic centers for NREM sleep (Nakamura et al, 1983). In this study (as in others measuring CBF or cerebral metabolism), the data could be biased if the subjects were extremely anxious in the waking state—because anxiety can increase cerebral metabolic demands. Another study in freely moving cats showed no significant differences in local 2-DG accumulation in NREM as compared to waking (Petitjean et al, 1982).

In summary, the data on cerebral activity and blood flow during NREM sleep suggest a global decrease in activity. Specific sites of increase have not been ruled out. In REM sleep, a global increase apparently occurs.

Sleep-Induced Erections

Episodes of nocturnal penile tumescence (NPT) are also present in sleep; these episodes occur during REM sleep in healthy men of all ages and are not significantly affected by degree of orgasmic satiation before sleep, by obvious neurosis, or by negative dream content (Fisher et al, 1965; Karacan, 1965, 1966, 1970; Karacan et al, 1966). For this reason, NPT serves as a biological marker for organically-related impotence: NPT episodes that are abnormal in terms of frequency, duration, or rigidity in the context of adequate REM sleep imply organic contributions such as vascular disease, neuropathy, endocrinopathy, or drug/alcohol abuse regardless of whatever psychological contributions may be present. Since NPT episodes can be measured quantitatively (Karacan, 1969), NPT evaluation serves as a cornerstone in the differential diagnosis of impotence. It also proves useful in documenting the effects of various drugs, such as antihypertensive medications and hypnotics, on erectile capacity.

Like all sleep-related variables, NPT changes gradually throughout the course of a lifetime. On a given night, a healthy 25-year-old man could be expected to have his first NPT episode after 90 minutes of NREM sleep; after that, episodes recur within approximately 90 minutes from the beginning of one episode to the beginning of the next. Duration of each episode for this age group is typically

30 minutes, with longer and more intense episodes toward the second half of the eight-hour sleep period. Men ages 20 to 29 will have an average of four episodes per night, while frequency declines to 2.6 per night in men ages 70 to 79 years (Karacan et al, 1976).

CIRCADIAN RHYTHMS AND THE SLEEP-WAKE CYCLE

Research in chronobiology has a long history, beginning with the recognition that the physiological functions of plants and animals have biological rhythms. These rhythms range in periodicity from a second or less to years, but the circadian rhythm is the one of most interest in terms of the sleep-wake cycle. In humans, the sleep-wake cycle, one of the circadian rhythms, is established some time after birth (Davis, 1981; Webb and Dube, 1981). It is genetically determined, not learned (Richter, 1971; Possidente and Hegmann, 1980; Davis, 1981). The periodicity is due to two separate factors: (1) zeitgebers and (2) endogenous pacemakers or central rhythm generating mechanisms. A zeitgeber is a signal from the environment which entrains or synchronizes the pacemaker to a periodic cycle, thereby helping establish the proper phasing of internal to external cycles. The most powerful zeitgeber in animals is the light-dark cycle. In humans, the knowledge of time of day and other social cues is also important. But even when zeitgebers are experimentally removed, circadian rhythms continue in a free-running pattern that is usually not very different from a 24-hour cycle (Richter, 1967, 1971; Aschoff, 1979; Weitzman et al, 1979). For example, in humans the sleep-wake cycle will generally develop about a 25-hour periodicity in the absence of zeitgebers.

In temporal isolation studies in humans (when the biological rhythms are free-running), the ratio of time asleep to total time remains fairly constant at about 30 percent, irrespective of period length. The REM sleep phase advances relative to sleep onset; that is, there is a shortened latency to the onset of the first REM period while the timing of stages 3 and 4 remains linked to sleep onset time (Weitzman et al, 1980). No differences are found in the 80–100 minute REM-NREM cycle length. Although the core temperature and sleep-wake cycle rhythms separate from each other during temporal isolation, the length of a sleep episode is correlated with the phase of the temperature rhythm. Long sleep episodes occur when subjects choose to sleep at the peak of the temperature cycle, and shorter episodes at the nadir (Czeisler et al, 1980).

There has been much interest in locating the circadian pacemaker(s). Research indicates that the suprachiasmatic nuclei (SCN) are a pacemaker. Lesions of the SCN bilaterally in rodents result in the loss of many circadian rhythms, including those of food intake, locomotor activity, pineal serotonin N-acetyltransferase, adrenal corticosterone, and estrous cycling (Raisman and Brown-Grant, 1977). Circadian sleep-wake cycles are abolished in SCN lesions in the rat while the amount of time spent in waking, SWS, and PS remains the same (Coindet et al, 1975; Ibuka and Kawamura, 1975). Lesions of the various afferent inputs do not produce arrhythmicity, but destruction of efferent fibers does. Furthermore, the SCN in rats show a circadian rhythm in electrical activity which persists with little period change in continuous light or dark (Inouye and Kawamura, 1979).

Are the SCN unique? Are they the sole circadian oscillators? Evidence suggests that circadian pacemakers are composed of multiple oscillators (Aschoff and Wever, 1976; Moore-Ede et al, 1976). For example, in the absence of zeitgebers, different physiological rhythms may separate from each other and develop somewhat different periods. In humans entrained to a 24-hour circadian cycle, the sleep-wake, temperature, cortisol, growth hormone (GH), and prolactin (PRL) cycles are linked. Temperature falls with sleep onset and rises sharply at the end of the sleep period, GH is mainly secreted during sleep stages 3 and 4, a large pulse of PRL secretion occurs shortly after sleep onset, and cortisol levels are at a nadir in early sleep and peak at the end of sleep. However, in the free-running state, the temperature and cortisol levels separate from the sleep-wake cycle, while the GH and PRL linkage is altered very little (Sassin et al, 1973; Aschoff and Wever, 1976; Weitzman et al, 1979). Also, rhythms of rectal temperature and cortisol levels persist after SCN lesions in primates (Fuller et al, 1981; Reppert et al, 1981). These findings imply that there is more than one circadian oscillator.

The pineal gland may also be involved in circadian cycling. Mammalian pineal glands synthesize and release melatonin at various rates, which are entrained by the 24-hour light-dark cycle (Quay, 1974). In rats, the enzyme that regulates melatonin synthesis, N-acetyltransferase, shows a 50-fold increase in activity at night. This activity appears to be regulated by beta-adrenergic receptors (Axelrod and Zatz, 1977). Chronic doses of melatonin given to birds have dose dependent effects on the locomotor activity cycles (Turek et al, 1976). Pinealectomy in birds abolishes free-running locomotor activity rhythmicity in darkness, but entrainment to light-dark cycles persists (Gaston and Menaker, 1968; Binkley et al, 1971).

It is of clinical interest that depression may be considered in terms of circadian time-keeping. During major depression, rhythms of temperature, REM sleep, and cortisol may be abnormally phase-shifted; that is, advanced with respect to the sleep-wake or light-dark cycle. Lithium, imipramine, and clorgyline, which are used in the treatment of affective illness, all have been shown to lengthen free-running rhythms in animals (Englemann, 1973; Johnsson et al, 1979; Wirz-Justice et al, 1980, 1982).

THE EFFECTS OF NEUROTRANSMITTERS AND OTHER ENDOGENOUS FACTORS ON SLEEP

Although the sleep-wake cycle is influenced by circadian factors, these appear to have a smaller role in regulating human sleep than do some specific neural systems. Despite the many studies in animals and humans which have attempted to pinpoint these neural systems and the neurochemicals involved, the intrinsic control mechanisms of sleep have not been identified with certainty. The following sections will focus on the neurotransmitters and peptides implicated in regulation of the sleep-wake cycle.

Neurotransmitters released from presynaptic neurons act to excite (depolarize) or inhibit (hyperpolarize) postsynaptic neurons by interacting with receptor sites on the postsynaptic neuron. The released neurotransmitter may also "feed back" onto receptors in the presynaptic neuron membrane, thereby influencing further release (or synthesis) of the neurotransmitter. Induction of sleep is believed to require both the inhibition of the arousal systems and activity in the sleep-inducing systems.

The sleep-wakefulness cycle depends on factors other than the neurotransmitter actions just described. Other substances such as hormones and drugs may act to influence neuronal activity by increasing or decreasing neurotransmitter synthesis, release, re-uptake, or degradation; by influencing receptor numbers or sensitivity to neurotransmitter; or by some other means.

Knowledge of the neurochemistry of the sleep-waking cycle is rapidly growing, but it is still in its infancy. Research is hampered by the multitude of technical problems encountered when any neurotransmitter research is conducted (for example, blood-brain barrier blocking passage of peripherally administered transmitter, anesthesia in experimental animals affecting neurotransmitter levels, deterioration of neurotransmitters after animal sacrifice, and so forth). Sleep-wake cycle research is further complicated by the lack of an animal species whose electroencephalographic sleep is equivalent to that of humans.

Since sleep is a spontaneous physiological phenomenon, it is sometimes difficult to prove that an experimental factor actually induces sleep (rather than sleep-onset being facilitated or occurring spontaneously). Also complicating the evaluation of putative sleep-inducing factors is the fact that certain chemicals such as general anesthetics, sedatives, and neurotoxins may produce EEG changes reminiscent of SWS and suppressed PS—in the extreme case, a coma—but these actions do not qualify as induction of physiologic sleep.

A distinction should be made between sleep-inducing and sleep-facilitating factors. Jouvet (1983) characterizes the sleep-facilitating and sleep-inducing factors as follows: A sleep-facilitating factor may be endogenous or exogenous and is not necessary, sufficient, or exclusive in producing sleep onset; but its presence may cause drowsiness and facilitate sleep onset and/or increased sleep duration in the presence of sleep-inducing factors. Examples are comfortable sleep environment, the post-prandial state, and sedative drugs. Removal of sleep-facilitating factors may temporarily delay sleep onset, but a secondary rebound of sleep should occur. Sleep-inducing factors are endogenous and are defined as acting directly on the executive mechanisms of sleep. Their administration at the receptor level should cause sleep onset and increase SWS, PS, or both. Inactivation of these factors should lead to suppression of SWS, PS, or both, which is not followed by secondary rebound and which is not reversed by sleep-facilitating factors. The distinction between sleep-facilitating and sleep-inducing factors becomes important when evaluating the basic research on the executive mechanisms of sleep.

The Monoamine Neurotransmitters

The monoamines—serotonin, norepinephrine, and dopamine—have been studied in terms of their influence on the sleep-wake cycle. Data are derived mainly from animal experiments, which have focused on (1) enhancement of amine activity by electrical stimulation of neurons, central or peripheral injection of the transmitter itself, or peripheral administration of a precursor of the transmitter to enhance neurotransmitter synthesis; or (2) reduction of the neurotransmitter activity via electrolytic or pharmacologic lesions, synthesis inhibitors, or receptor blockers. There are also some more "physiologic" experiments, which quantify the amount of neurotransmitter released during waking, paradoxical sleep, and synchronized sleep, or the amount of neuronal unit activity.

SEROTONIN. The research on serotonin as a sleep-inducing factor is more extensive than is research on other transmitters. The main area of the brain containing serotonergic neurons is the median raphe, which extends from the medulla to the midbrain. Serotonergic neurons are also found in the medullary and mesencephalic reticular formation (RF). The raphe neurons innervate the locus coeruleus (LC) and may, in addition, have a modulating effect on norepinephrine (NE) synthesis (Kostowski et al, 1974; Pickel et al, 1977). Electrical stimulation of the raphe in rats leads to sleep, reduces serotonin levels, and increases the serotonin metabolite 5-hydroxyindoleacetic acid (Kostowski et al, 1969). Electrolytic lesions lead to a reduction of SWS and PS about equally, in extensive lesions to the point of total insomnia without rebound (Jouvet, 1969, 1972; Morgane and Stern, 1974).

Injection of the sertonin precursor 5-hydroxytryptophan (5-HTP), which can cross the blood-brain barrier, suppresses PS and increases SWS in cats (Koella et al, 1968; Jouvet, 1969, 1972), and injection into the nucleus tractus solitarius is followed by SWS (Ledebur and Tissot, 1966). L-tryptophan, another serotonin precursor, has been used as a hypnotic drug in humans. It decreases the latency to sleep onset and increases the percentage of SWS (Wyatt et al, 1970b; Hartmann, 1974). In humans, L-tryptophan may also decrease REM latency and increase the amount of REM sleep when given in high doses (Oswald, 1969; Williams, 1971). In rabbits, L-tryptophan suppresses PS (Tabushi and Himwich, 1970).

Applying serotonin directly to areas of the brain by various methods also induces EEG sleep. Intra-arterial infusion of the area postrema (near the caudal end of the fourth ventricle) leads to EEG synchrony (as seen in SWS) in the rat, while saline, norepinephrine, acetylcholine, and lactic acid do not (Roth et al, 1970). Similar results with different techniques occur in cats (Koella and Czicman, 1966; Koella, 1974).

Central serotonin levels can be reduced by synthesis inhibition (parachlorophenylalanine [PCPA]), receptor blockade (methysergide), or destruction of serotonergic neurons (5, 6 or 5, 7–dehydroxytryptamine [DHT]). PCPA in cats causes dose dependent drops in both SWS and PS, which gradually return to control levels without rebound. The serotonin precursor 5–HTP restores the SWS (Delorme et al, 1966; Koella et al, 1968). Similar results occur in other animals.

Acute administration of methysergide to rabbits causes a dose dependent decrease in total sleep, with PS being more profoundly affected. Both PS and SWS return to normal levels with chronic use of methysergide; rebound occurs on drug withdrawal (Tabushi and Himwich, 1971).

DHT injection into the ventricular systems of rats (Ross et al, 1976) and cats (Froment et al, 1974) causes a large reduction in brain serotonin levels. The latter researchers found reductions in both SWS and PS which continued after ten days. Kiianmaa and Fuxe (1977) found a reduction in SWS in DHT-injected rats, while PS was not decreased significantly from that of control animals. Ross and colleagues (1976) found an acute drop in SWS and PS in both the DHT-injected rats and vehicle-injected controls.

The serotonin research cited thus far provides the basis for the theory that serotonin and the serotonergic raphe nuclei have a major role in the induction of sleep—that serotonin is a hypnogenic neurotransmitter for NREM sleep. Jouvet (1972) also proposed that REM sleep is "primed" by serotonergic neurons and then relayed through cholinergic neurons and the "REM-executive" NE neurons in the LC. However, some evidence contradicts this theory. Several studies using differing techniques (Sheu et al, 1974; McGinty and Harper, 1976; Puizillout et al, 1979; Trulson and Jacobs, 1979; Cespuglio et al, 1981) have found a decrease in the activity of serotonergic neurons of the raphe complex during SWS as compared to waking, and a further decrease during PS. These findings raise doubts about the hypothesis that serotonergic raphe neurons are crucial to the control of SWS and that they are necessary for the "priming" of REM sleep.

Koella (1981) resolves this apparent contradiction by suggesting that serotonergic systems act to dampen vigilance in waking (via inhibition of the ascending arousal system by means of a reticulo-solitario-reticular feedback loop) and trigger SWS by a short surge of activity, followed by a decrease in activity. Jouvet (1983) has discussed the paradoxical evidence from the perspective that serotonin may act as both a neurotransmitter and a neurohormone, and gives the following evidence. Some of the evidence for serotonin being a *neurotransmitter* affecting the sleep-wake cycle comes from its effect on ponto-geniculo-occipital (PGO) activity. PGO activity normally appears immediately before and during PS and is inhibited during waking. During PCPA-induced insomnia PGO activity is sustained. There is strong evidence that in cats serotonergic neurons exert a tonic inhibitory influence at the brainstem level, regulating or gating REM-type PGO waves (Koe and Weissman, 1966; Delorme et al, 1966; Brooks et al, 1972). Injection of the serotonin precursor 5-HTP is followed by almost immediate disappearance of PGO activity. The rapidity of the response is consistent with a neurotransmitter effect. There is a delay of 20 to 30 minutes prior to SWS and an hour or more prior to PS. In this delayed effect serotonin may behave as a *neurohormone*, leading to the synthesis and/or release of other hypnogenic factors. It must be noted that PCPA did not affect the frequency of PGO waves in waking in one study of rats (Kaufman and Morrison, 1983).

Injection of CSF from sleep-deprived cats into PCPA-treated insomniac cats leads to the reappearance of PS episodes after about half an hour (Sallanon et al, 1981), despite the fact that the level of indoleamine (serotonin plus 5-HTP) in the CSF was 1,000 times smaller than that required to elicit PS when injected intracisternally into PCPA-treated cats. This experiment and another in PS-deprived PCPA-treated cats (Sakai, 1981) suggest that there is a non-serotonergic PS factor and that serotonergic mechanisms may affect its synthesis and/or release. The possibility of a corresponding serotonin-responsive SWS factor will be discussed later.

NOREPINEPHRINE (NE) AND AROUSAL. Noradrenergic neurons are located in the medulla and pons, with the major source being the locus coeruleus (LC). The LC has widespread projections to the cortex and to all levels of the spinal cord. It may contain dopaminergic neuron cell bodies and has cholinergic input.

The ascending activating system (AAS), also called the reticular activating system, also contains noradrenergic neurons (along with cholinergic, serotonergic, and dopaminergic neurons).

NE neurons are probably involved in tonic cortical arousal. Electrical stimulation of the LC or AAS in cats produces EEG arousal and behavioral signs of vigilance (Moruzzi and Magoun, 1949; Koella, 1977, 1978). The induced arousal is accompanied by NE release (Tanaka et al, 1976) and is blocked by beta-adrenergic blockers, substantiating the adrenergic basis of the effect.

Blocking presynaptic alpha$_2$-adrenergic receptors increases NE activity by preventing release-inhibiting "feedback" onto the presynaptic neurons. Such blockade increases waking time in rats (Fuxe et al, 1974; Leppavuori and Putkonen, 1980). Other methods of increasing central NE (and dopamine), such as peripheral administration of amphetamine or L-dopa, also enhance waking time and EEG arousal.

Intraventricular infusion of NE in low doses in rats leads to enhanced behavioral activity (Segal and Mandell, 1970; Geyer et al, 1972). Higher doses in cats produce somnolence but not physiologic sleep (Feldberg and Sherwood, 1954). Also, recordings of neuronal activity in the LC and AAS show reduced activity with the onset of sleep.

Thus, NE neurons may mediate cortical arousal. However, there is evidence to the contrary. Lesions that destroy most of the LC and spare the pontine tegmentum have minor effects on cortical arousal; EEG arousal quickly returns to normal levels despite continued depletion of NE. Also, permanent depletion of cortical NE in rats achieved by injecting the neurotoxin 6-hydroxydopamine neonatally does not affect the EEG pattern of low voltage fast activity (Robinson et al, 1977).

NOREPINEPHRINE AND PS.   Paradoxical sleep in cats is facilitated by small increases of central NE caused by alpha$_2$-adrenergic blockade (Leppavuori and Putkonen, 1980). Moderate blockade of alpha$_1$-adrenergic receptors by prazosin (implying a moderate level of alpha$_1$ activation) favors the occurrence of PS (Hilakivi et al, 1983), while intense alpha$_1$ activation favors aroused waking and reduced PS. Complete blockade of alpha$_2$-adrenergic function with prazosin plus clonidine (an alpha-adrenergic agonist) dramatically reduces sleep (SWS and PS) and leads to a drowsy, waking state in the cat (Hilakivi et al, 1983).

The effects of experimental reduction of central NE activity ($\pm$ reduced dopaminergic activity) on PS are conflicting. Alpha$_2$-adrenergic agonism, which reduces NE release, decreases PS (Kleinlogel et al, 1975; Depoortere et al, 1977). Reserpine-induced reduction of PS in cats (reserpine depletes central monoamines) is reversed by L-dopa. The NE and DA synthesis inhibitor alphamethylparatyrosine has been found to decrease or increase PS in rats and cats (Torda, 1968; Hartmann et al, 1971; Stern and Morgane, 1973). However, mesencephalic injection of 6-hydroxydopamine leading to severe depletion of rostral NE and serotonin leads to increased PS and SWS (Panksepp et al, 1973). Norepinephrine denervation in the rat has less effect on PS than in the cat. Since 6-hydroxydopamine has more specific effects on NE neurons in the rat than in the cat (in which other monoaminergic systems are affected), Ramm (1979) suggests that the REM-disrupting effects of the drug result from nonspecific damage of neuronal systems rather than from primarily noradrenergic neuron damage.

INTERPRETATION OF NE EFFECTS ON AROUSAL AND ON REM SLEEP.
Cortical arousal, low voltage fast activity on the EEG, occurs in both waking and REM sleep; and it has been suggested that NE neurons participate in both. Evidence has been presented that NE neurons influence cortical arousal. Jouvet (1972) implies that NE neurons of the pontine tegmentum increase arousal by inhibition of certain serotonergic raphe neurons. There is other evidence, however, that NE neurons do not mediate cortical arousal. The data concerning possible noradrenergic influence on PS are also conflicting and the debate is not resolved. Interpreting the available data, some researchers believe that PS occurrence probably requires NE neurotransmission (Monnier and Gaillard, 1980; Koella, 1981). Ramm (1979) reasons that catacholaminergic neurons may play a modulatory but not essential or primary role in PS occurrence.

DOPAMINE (DA).   Central DA-producing neurons are found mainly in three areas: (1) the hypothalamo-hypophyseal portal systems, (2) the substantia nigra-ventral tegmental area, and (3) the periaqueductal grey area (also containing NE and serotonin cells). Research to elucidate possible dopaminergic influences on the sleep-wake cycle is not extensive. Often the technique used to reduce or enhance central DA levels pharmacologically also affects NE levels, making it difficult to differentiate the relative roles of the DA and NE systems. Nevertheless, there is some support for the hypothesis that DA neurons may be involved in maintaining arousal. Apomorphine is a dopamine agonist that may act either pre- or post-synaptically, depending on the dose. It induces sleep at lower doses and delays sleep onset and PS onset and duration in high doses (Kafi and Gaillard, 1976; Mereu et al, 1979; Cianchetti et al, 1980). Neuroleptics block these effects. Somewhat specific dopamine agonists such as bromocriptine and piribedil given acutely have also been shown to delay PS onset and reduce its duration (Wyatt et al, 1970a; Post et al, 1978; Radulovacki et al, 1979). Chronically, they may increase REM sleep duration in patients with Parkinson's disease (Passouant, 1981). However, most evidence suggests that the level of DA activity is directly related to the level of motor activity and less to the sleep-wake cycle per se (Jones et al, 1973; Adams, 1977; Roberts et al, 1975).

Gamma-Aminobutyric Acid (GABA)

GABA is an inhibitory neurotransmitter found widely in cortical, subcortical, and spinal areas of the CNS. Intracisternally injected GABA in rats leads to reduced locomotor activity (Freed and Michaelis, 1976) and antagonizes DA-induced hyperactivity (Pycock and Horton, 1979). Convulsants in high doses inhibit GABA synthesis and cause enhanced motor activity in lower doses (Wood and Peesker, 1972; Arnt and Scheel-Kruger, 1980). Mucimol, a GABA receptor agonist (Scheel-Kruger et al, 1978), and benzodiazepines, which facilitate GABAergic transmission, lead to sedation or decreased vigilance.

Acetylcholine (ACh)

Cholinergic transmission is probably involved in the production and maintenance of arousal. Systemic injection of ACh and of cholinomimetics produces EEG arousal in cats (Bremer and Chatonnet, 1949; Domino and Yamamoto, 1965), and ACh release is increased during waking over SWS (Gadea-Ciria et al, 1973).

Atropine, an antimuscarinic agent, produces EEG synchrony in dogs, cats, and monkeys, while the animals appear alert. The apparent dissociation between EEG and behavior is only partial, however, because there is an impairment in conditioned behavior (Wikler, 1952; Rougeul et al, 1969). Paradoxically, high doses of ACh applied directly to the brains of cats (Hernandez-Peon, 1965) and of ACh, nicotine, and pilocarpine injected intravertebrally in dogs induce an SWS-like state, as do cholinergic blockers (Haranath et al, 1977). The latter authors postulate that cholinergic *agonists* can inhibit transmission by overloading the receptor system.

A number of animal studies suggest that enhanced cholinergic transmission induces and prolongs PS or induces components of REM sleep such as EEG activation, EMG suppression, or PGO spikes (George et al, 1964; Hernandez-Peon et al, 1967; Karczmar et al, 1970; Hobson et al, 1976). Atropine has been found to block these effects (Domino et al, 1968; Magherini et al, 1971). Also, ACh output is increased during PS as compared to waking in the cat striatum (Gadea-Cirea et al, 1973) and in the cortex of cats treated with an anticholinesterase agent (Jasper and Tessier, 1971).

In humans 0.5 and 1.0 mg of arecholine (a muscarinic agonist) and 0.25, 0.5, and 1.0 mg physostigmine shortened the time to the next REM period when injected during the first or, in general, the second NREM period (Sitaram et al, 1977, 1978). However, the effects were actually more complex. A 0.5 mg dose of physostigmine induced REM sleep when given in the first NREM period but induced arousal when given in the second. Furthermore, the REM latency was shorter when physostigmine was given 35 minutes rather than five minutes after sleep onset.

Other Endogenous Sleep Factors

Although research is more limited than that concerning the previously mentioned neurotransmitters, and results are far from conclusive, there is evidence that some brain peptides are involved in the regulation of sleep.

DELTA SLEEP-INDUCING PEPTIDE (DSIP). Delta sleep-inducing peptide (DSIP) is a nonapeptide that has been isolated from cerebral venous blood of rabbits in which sleep was induced by electrical stimulation of the thalamus (Schoenenberger and Monnier, 1977). Intraventricular administration of DSIP enhances delta and spindle patterns in the EEG. In cats, intravenous DSIP augments SWS and, to a greater extent, PS (Scherschlicht, 1983). There seems to be a bell-shaped dose reponse curve to DSIP (and other brain peptides) so that doses that are too high or too low are ineffective (Kastin et al, 1980). DSIP has a short plasma half-life in rat brain, and elevated levels after systemic injection return to baseline in minutes (Kastin et al, 1979). Nonetheless, DSIP-induced EEG changes have a delayed and prolonged time course.

ARGININE VASOTOCIN (AVT). Arginine vasotocin (AVT) is a nonapeptide found in the pineal gland. AVT, unlike the closely related polypeptides vasopressin and oxytocin, induces SWS and suppresses PS when injected intraventricularly in cats (Pavel et al, 1977). AVT's effects in rats vary (Mendelson et al, 1980; Tobler and Borbely, 1980). In humans, AVT increases the amount of REM sleep and decreases REM sleep latency (Pavel, 1980; Pavel et al, 1980, 1981). Methergoline, a serotonin receptor blocker, prevents AVT induction of

REM sleep (Pavel et al, 1981). Despite these findings, the status of AVT as a sleep inducer awaits definite confirmation that AVT is found in the human pineal gland, 24-hour sleep-wake cycle monitoring with use of AVT, determination of whether AVT has effects beyond influence on serotonergic neurons, and explanation of its contradictory effects in rats.

FACTOR S. Pappenheimer et al (1967) first described the accumulation of a sleep-promoting factor in the CSF of sleep-deprived goats. This substance (factor S), a muramylpeptide of molecular weight less than 500, was later purified from the CSF and urine of sleep-deprived animals (Pappenheimer et al, 1975; Krueger et al, 1982). Intraventricularly administered factor S increases SWS and the amplitude of delta waves in rabbits (Krueger et al, 1982) and increases SWS in rats and cats (Pappenheimer et al, 1967; Krueger et al, 1980; Garcia-Arraras, 1981). The next step in the evaluation of factor S as a sleep inducer should be studies thoroughly evaluating its effect on the 24-hour sleep-wake cycle.

SLEEP-PROMOTING SUBSTANCE (SPS). Sleep-promoting substance (SPS) has been obtained from the brainstems of sleep-deprived rats (Uchizono et al, 1982). It has not yet been purified or characterized but contains at least two active fractions, SPS-A and SPS-B. The data about SPS are too preliminary to merit extensive discussion, but SPS in rats may promote SWS and suppress or promote PS, depending on the point in the circadian rhythm (Inoue et al, 1983).

VASOACTIVE INTESTINAL POLYPEPTIDE (VIP). Vasoactive intestinal polypeptide (VIP) is another polypeptide that has recently been studied in terms of its possible hypnogenic effects. The data are very preliminary, and must be verified. In brief, Riou et al (1983) have injected VIP intravenously into PCPA pretreated rats. VIP greatly enhanced both SWS and PS in PCPA insomniac cats. VIP also increased SWS and PS when injected at night (active time for rats) in non-PCPA-treated animals.

Protein Synthesis and Sleep

There is evidence that protein synthesis may be involved in the mechanisms that trigger sleep. Chloramphenicol, a protein synthesis inhibitor, given to REM-sleep-deprived cats prevents the typical REM sleep rebound (Drucker-Colin, 1981). Chloramphenicol applied to the medial pontine or midbrain reticular formation (RF) decreases the RF neuron unit activity and at the same time leads to abortive transitions to REM sleep (Drucker-Colin, 1981). Moreover, protein concentrations in perfusates from the midbrain RF peak during the times of REM sleep (Drucker-Colin et al, 1975). The cyclic release of proteins disappeared when insomnia was induced by lesions of the preoptic area (Drucker-Colin and Gutierrez, 1976).

Interpretation

NREM SLEEP. Onset of NREM sleep requires both the reduction of generalized arousal and the increase of certain hypnogenic factors. A critical level of serotonergic activity is probably necessary for onset of NREM sleep, and this level of activity may act directly or via facilitation of other sleep factors. A number of possible sleep factors have been identified, such as DSIP, AVT, factor S, SPS, and VIP. The "dewaking" or reduction of generalized arousal probably involves reductions in noradrenergic and cholinergic activity and perhaps changes in serotonergic activity. GABA probably facilitates dewaking, and GABA and DA are involved in the reduction of behavioral arousal and motor activity.

REM SLEEP. REM sleep is influenced by a complex interaction of structural and neurotransmitter systems, whose relationships are unclear. One can tentatively conclude that protein synthesis is necessary for the triggering of REM sleep. A certain level of noradrenergic activity is probably either necessary, or at least permissive, for the occurrence of REM sleep. The same can be said for cholinergic activity. Jouvet (1983) believes that serotonergic mechanisms may be involved, perhaps by enhancing the elaboration of a nonserotonergic REM factor. Hobson and McCarley (Hobson, 1974) propose a simple model of (1) an aminergic "REM-off" system composed of serotonergic and noradrenergic neurons that have their lowest discharge rates in early REM sleep and (2) a cholinergic "REM-on" system in the RF whose activity is highest in REM sleep. They believe these two systems interact to produce the NREM-REM cycle. However, the "REM-on" cells also fire whenever the animal moves (Seigel, 1979), and total destruction of the gigantocellular tegmental field (part of the proposed "REM-on" system) does not disrupt REM sleep (Sastre et al, 1979). Thus, the controversy continues and much research still needs to be done to determine the bases of the sleep-wake and NREM-REM cycles.

CONCLUSION

In summary, several neurotransmitters are relevant to sleep and sleep cycles, and their interactive relationship has been established. The definite sleep mechanisms and all related additional transmitters or intervening variables remain to be determined. However, research activities are underway in the proper areas, and technological advances are still appearing. Although sleep study is still in an early stage, an abundance of pragmatic information relating to sleep disorders is appearing in response to public demand.

Sleep disorders centers now offer proper differential diagnosis and treatment and are able to check for certain biological markers during sleep to assist in the identification of disorders not directly relating to sleep, such as depression and impotence. Thus, although sleep study has a definite benefit in and of itself, it is also of use to other medical disciplines. We can only believe that the sensitivity and specificity of our methods will improve over time, and we expect that sleep research will enable us to locate ever more specific drugs to help the practicing psychiatrist to induce or dilute certain types of behavior.

REFERENCES

Adams K: Cellular energy charge, synthesis and degradation, in Sleep and Memory—Sleep 1976. Edited by Koella WP, Levin P. Basel, Karger, 1977

Arnt J, Scheel-Kruger J: Intranigral GABA antagonists produce dopamine-independent biting rates. Eur J Pharmacol 62:51–61, 1980

Aschoff J: Circadian rhythms: influences of internal and external factors on the period measured in constant conditions. Z Tierpsychol 49:225–249, 1979

Aschoff J, Wever R: Human circadian rhythms: a multioscillator system Fed Proc 35:2326–2332, 1976

Aserinsky E, Kleitman N: Regularly occurring periods of eye motility, and concomitant phenomena during sleep. Science 118:273–274, 1953

Axelrod J, Zatz M: The beta-adrenergic receptor and regulation of circadian rhythms in the pineal gland, in Biochemical Actions of Hormones, Vol IV. Edited by Litwack G. New York, Academic Press, 1977

Baccelli G, Albertini R, Mancia G, et al: Neural and non-neural mechanisms influencing circulation during sleep. Nature (London) 223:184–185, 1969

Baccelli G, Albertini R, Mancia G, et al: Central and reflex regulation of sympathetic vasoconstrictor activity of limb muscle during desynchronized sleep in the cat. Circ Res 35:625–635, 1974

Bateman JRM, Clarke Sw, Pavia D, et al: Reduction of clearance of secretions from the human lung during sleep. J Physiol 284:55, 1978

Batini C, Moruzzi G, Palestini M, et al: Persistent patterns of wakefulness in the pretrigeminal mid-pontine preparation. Science 128:30–32, 1958

Batini C, Moruzzi G, Palestini M, et al: Effects of complete pontine transection on the sleep-wakefulness rhythm: the mid-pontine pretrigeminal preparation. Arch Ital Bio 97:1–12, 1959

Berger H: Uber das elektrenkephalogramm des menschen. Arch Psychiatr Nervenkr 87:527–570, 1929

Binkley S, Kluth E, Menaker M: Pineal function in sparrows: circadian rhythms and body temperature. Science 174:311–315, 1971

Blake H, Gerard RW: Brain potentials during sleep. Am J Physiol 119:692–703, 1937

Bremer F, Chatonnet J: Acetylcholine et cortex cerebral. Arch Intern Physiol Biochim 57:106–109, 1949

Bristow JD, Honour As, Pickering TG, et al: Cardiovascular and respiratory changes during sleep in normal and hypertensive subjects. Cardiovasc Res 3:476–485, 1972

Brooks DA, Gershon MD, Simon RP: Brain stem serotonin depletion and ponto-geniculo-occipital wave activity in the cat treated with reserpine. Neuropharmacol 11:511–520, 1972

Caton R: The electric currents of the brain. Br Med J 2:278 (Abstract), 1875

Cespuglio R, Faradji H, Gomez ME, et al: Single unit recordings in the nuclei raphe dorsalis and magnus during the sleep waking cycle of semi-chronic prepared cats. Neurosci Lett 24:133–138, 1981

Cianchetti C, Masala C, Mangoni A, et al: Suppression of REM and delta sleep by apomorphine in man: a dopamine mimetic effect. Psychopharmacol 67:61–65, 1980

Coccagna E, Mantovani M, Brignoni E, et al: Arterial pressure changes during spontaneous sleep in man. Electroencephalogr Clin Neurophysiol 31:277–281, 1971

Coindet J, Chouvet G, Mouret J: Effects of lesions of the suprachiasmatic nuclei on paradoxical sleep and slow wave sleep circadian rhythms in the rat. Neurosci Lett 1:243–247, 1975

Czeisler CA, Weitzman ED, Moore-Ede MC, et al: Human sleep: its duration and organization depend on its circadian phase. Science 210:1264–1267, 1980

Davis FC: Ontogeny of circadian rhythms, in Handbook of Behavioral Neurobiology, vol 4. Edited by Aschoff J. New York, Plenum Press, 1981

Delorme F, Froment JL, Jouvet M: Suppression des sommeil par la p-chloromethamphetamine et la p-chorophenylalanine. C R Soc Biol (Paris) 160:2347–2351, 1966

Dement WC: The effect of dream deprivation. Science 131:1705–1707, 1960

Dement WC, Kleitman N: The relation of eye movements during sleep to dream activity: an objective method for the study of dreaming. J Exp Psychol 53:339–346, 1957

Depoortere H, Honore H, Jalfre M: EEG effects of various imidazoline derivatives in experimental animals, in 3rd European Congress on Sleep Research. Edited by Koella WP, Levin P. Basel, Karger, 1977

Domino EF, Yamamoto K: Nicotine: effect on the sleep cycle of the cat. Science 150:637–638, 1965

Domino EF, Yamamoto K, Dren AT: Role of cholinergic mechanisms in states of wakefulness and sleep, in Progress in Brain Research, vol 28: Anticholinergic Drugs and Brain Function in Animals and Man. Edited by Bradly PB, Fink M. Amsterdam, Elsevier, 1968

Drucker-Colin R: Endogenous sleep peptides, in Psychopharmacology of Sleep. Edited by Wheatley D. New York, Raven Press, 1981

Drucker-Colin RR, Spanis CW, Cotman CW, et al: Changes in protein in perfusates of freely moving cats: relation to behavioral state. Science 187:963–965, 1975

Drucker-Colin RR, Gutierrez MC: Effects of forebrain lesions on release of proteins from the midbrain reticular formation during the sleep-wake cycle. Exp Neurol 52:339–344, 1976

Economo C von: Die pathologie des schlafes, in Bethes Handbuch der normalen und pathologischen Physiologie 17:591–621, 1926

Economo C von: Theorie du sommeil. J Neurol Psychiatr 28:437–464, 1928

Englemann W: A slowing down of circadian rhythms by lithium ions. Z Naturforsch 28:733–736, 1973

Feldberg W, Sherwood SL: Injections of drugs into the lateral ventricle of the cat. J Physiol (Lond) 123:148–165, 1954

Fisher C, Gross J, Zuch J: Cycle of penile erection synchronous with dreaming (REM) sleep. Arch Gen Psychiatry 12:29–45, 1965

Flourens P: Determination du role qui jouent les diverses parties du systeme nerveux dans les mouvements dits volontaries, ou de locomotion et de prehension. Memoires lus a l'Academie Royale des Sciences de l'Institut le 31 Mars et 27 Avril 1822, publies dans Recherches experimentales sur les proprietes et les fonctions du systeme nerveux dans les animaux vertebres. Paris, Crevot, 1824

Freed WJ, Michaelis EK: Effects of intracisternal GABA and glutamic acid upon behavioral activity in the rat. Pharmacol Biochem Behav 5:11–14, 1976

Froment JL, Petijean F, Bertrand N, et al: Effets de l'injection intracerebrale de 5.6–hydroxytryptamine sur les monoamines cerebrales et les etats de sommeil du chat. Brain Res 67:405–417, 1974

Fuller CA, Lydic R, Sulzman FM, et al: Circadian rhythm of body temperature persists after suprachiasmatic lesions in the squirrel monkey. Am J Physiol 241:R385–391, 1981

Fuxe K, Lindbrink P, Hokfelt T, et al: Effects of piperoxane on sleep and waking in the rat: evidence of increased waking by blocking inhibitory adrenaline receptors on the locus coeruleus. Acta Physiol Scand 91:566–567, 1974

Gadea-Ciria M, Stadler H, Lloyd KG, et al: Acetylcholine release within the cat striatum during the sleep-wakefulness cycle. Nature 243:518–519, 1973

Garcia-Arraras JE: Effects of sleep-promoting factor from human urine on sleep cycle of cats. Am J Physiol 241:E296–E274, 1981

Gassel MM, Ghelarducci B, Marchiafava PL, et al: Phasic changes in blood pressure and heart rate during the rapid eye movement episodes of desynchronized sleep in unrestrained cats. Arch Ital Biol 102:530–544, 1964

Gaston S, Menaker M: Pineal function: the biological clock in the sparrow? Science 160:1125–1127, 1968

Gayet M: Affection encephalique (encephalite diffuse probable) localise aux etages superieurs des pedoncules cerebraux et aux coches optiques ainsi qu'au plancher du quatrieme ventricule et aux parois laterales du troisieme. Arch Physiol Normal Pathol Series 2:341–351, 1875

George R, Haslett WL, Jenden DJ: A cholinergic mechanism in the brain stem reticular formation: induction of paradoxical sleep. Int J Neuropharmacol 3:541–552, 1964

Geyer MA, Segal DS, Mandell AJ: Effects of intraventricular infusion of dopamine and norepinephrine on motor activity. Physiol Behav 8:653–658, 1972

Guazzi M, Zanchetti A: Blood pressure and heart rate during natural sleep of the cat and their regulation by carotid sinus and aortic reflexes. Arch Ital Biol 103:789–817, 1965

Haranath PSRK, Indira G, Krishnamurthy A: Effects of cholinomimetic drugs and their antagonists injected into vertebral artery of unanaesthetized dogs. Pharmacol Biochem Behav 6:259–263, 1977

Hartmann E: Hypnotic effects of L-tryptophan. Arch Gen Psychiatry 31:394–397, 1974

Hartmann E, Bridwell TJ, Schildkraut JJ: Alpha-Methyl-paratyrosine and sleep in the rat. Psychopharmacologia 21:157–164, 1971

Hawkins DR, Puryeer HB, Wallace CD, et al: Basal skin resistance during sleep and "dreaming." Science 136:321–322, 1962

Hernandez-Peon R: Central neuro-humoral transmission in sleep and wakefulness. Prog Brain Res 18:96–117, 1965

Hernandez-Peon R, O'Flaherty JJ, Mazzuchelli-O'Flaherty AC: Sleep and other behavioral effects induced by acetylcholinergic stimulation of basal temporal cortex and striate structures. Brain Res 4:243–267, 1967

Hess WR: Stammganglien-Reizversuche. Berichte Über die Gesamte Biologie. Abt. B: Berichte Über die Gesamte Physiologie und experimentelle Pharmakologie. 42:554–555, 1927

Hess WR: Der Schlaf. Klin Wochenschr 12:129–134, 1933

Hess WR: Hypothalamische Adyamie. Helvetica Physiologica et Pharmacologica Acta 2:137–147, 1944

Hilakivi I, Leppavouri A, Pulkonin P: Alpha$_1$-adrenergic modulation of vigilance states in the cat, in Sleep 1982: 6th European Congress of Sleep Research, 1982. Edited by Koella WP. Basel, Karger, 1983

Hobson JA: The cellular basis of sleep cycle control, in Advances in Sleep Research, Vol 1. Edited by Weitzman ED. New York, Spectrum, 1974

Hobson JA, McCarley RW, McKenna TM: Cellular evidence bearing on the pontine brainstem hypothesis of desynchronized sleep control, in Progress in Neurobiology, vol 6: Neuronal Activity During the Sleep-Wake Cycle. Edited by Steriade M, Hobson JA. Oxford: Pergamon Press Ltd., 1976

Ibuka N, Kawamura H: Loss of circadian rhythm in sleep-wakefulness cycle in the rat by suprachiasmatic nucleus lesions. Brain Res 96:76–81, 1975

Inoue S, Honda K, Komoda Y: A possible mechanism by which the sleep-promoting substance induces slow wave sleep but suppresses paradoxical sleep in the rat, in Sleep 1982: 6th European Congress of Sleep Research, 1982. Edited by Koella WP. Basel, Karger, 1983

Inouye ST, Kawamura H: Persistence of circadian rhythmicity in a mammalian hypothalamic 'island' containing the suprachiasmatic nucleus. Proc Natl Acad Sci USA 26:5962–5966, 1979

Jasper HH, Tessier J: Acetylcholine liberation from cerebral cortex during paradoxical (REM) sleep. Science 172:601–602, 1971

Johnsson A, Pflug B, Englemann W, et al: Effect of lithium carbonate on circadian periodicity in humans. Pharmacopsychiatria 12:423–425, 1979

Jones BE, Bobillier P, Pin C, et al: The effect of lesions of catecholamine-containing neurons upon monoamine content of the brain and EEG and behavioral waking in the cat. Brain Res 58:157–177, 1973

Jouvet M: Recherches sur les structures nerveuses et les mecanismes responsables des differentes phases du sommeil physiologique. Arch Ital Biol 100:125–206, 1962

Jouvet M: Biogenic amines and the states of sleep. Science 163:32–41, 1969

Jouvet M: The role of monoamines and the acetylcholine-containing neurons in the regulation of the sleep-waking cycle. Ergebnisse der Physiologie, biologischen Chemie und experimentellen Pharmakologie. 64:166–307, 1972

Jouvet M: Hypnogenic indoleamine-dependent factors and paradoxical sleep rebound, in Sleep 1982: 6th European Congress Sleep Research, Zurich, 1982. Edited by Koella WP. Basel, Karger, 1983

Kafi S, Gaillard JM: Brain dopamine receptors and sleep in the rat: effects of stimulation and blockade. Eur J Pharmacol 38:357–363, 1976

Karacan I: The effect of exciting presleep events on dream reporting and penile erections during sleep. New York, State University of New York, Downstate Medical Center, Department of Psychiatry, 1965 (doctoral dissertation)

Karacan I: The developmental aspect and the effect of certain clinical conditions upon penile erection during sleep. Excerpta Medica International Congress Series, No 150, Proceedings of the IV World Congress of Psychiatry, Madrid, 1966

Karacan I: A simple and inexpensive transducer for quantitative measurements of penile erection during sleep. Behavior Research Methods and Instrumentation 1:251–252, 1969

Karacan I: Clinical value of nocturnal erection in the prognosis and diagnosis of impotence. Medical Aspects of Human Sexuality 4:27–34, 1970

Karacan I, Goodenough DR, Shapiro A, et al: Erection cycle during sleep in relation to dream anxiety. Arch Gen Psychiatry 15:183–189, 1966

Karacan I, Salis PJ, Thornby JI, et al: The ontogeny of nocturnal penile tumescence. Waking and Sleeping 1:27–44, 1976

Karacan I, Guinn G, Mathur V, et al: The incidence of premature ventricular contractions during sleep in patients with coronary artery disease. Sleep Res 6:189, 1977

Karczmar A, Longo VG, Scotti de Carolis A: A pharmacological model of paradoxical sleep: the role of cholinergic and monoamine systems. Physiol Behav 5:175–182, 1970

Kastin AJ, Nissin C, Schally AV, Coy DJ: Additional evidence that small amounts of a peptide can cross the blood-brain barrier. Pharmacol Biochem Behav 11:717–719, 1979

Kastin AJ, Olson GA, Schally AV, et al: DSIP—more than a sleep peptide? Trends in Neuroscience 3:163–165, 1980

Kaufman LS, Morrison AR: PGO spikes in rats: the effects of PCPA and a comparison with the acoustic startle response, in Sleep 1982: 6th European Congress of Sleep Research, 1982. Edited by Koella WP. Basel, Karger, 1983

Khatri IM, Freis ED: Hemodynamic changes during sleep. J Appl Physiol 22:867–873, 1967

Kiianmaa K, Fuxe K: The effects of 5.7–dihydroxytryptamine-induced lesions of the ascending 5–hydroxytryptamine pathways on the sleep-wakefulness cycle. Brain Res 131:287–301, 1977

Kleinlogel H, Scholtysik G, Sayers AC: Effects of clonidine and BS 100-141 on the EEG sleep pattern in rats. Eur J Pharmacol 33:159–163, 1975

Koe BK, Weissman A: p–Chlorophenylalanine: a specific depletor of brain serotonin. J Pharmacol Exp Ther 154:499–516, 1966

Koella WP: Serotonin—a hypnogenic transmitter and an antiwaking agent. Adv Biochem Psychopharmacol 11:181–186, 1974

Koella WP: Beta-blockers and sleep, in Beta-Blockers and the Central Nervous System. Edited by Kielholz P. Berlin, Hans Huber, 1977

Koella WP: Central effects of beta-adrenergic blocking agents: mode and mechanism of action, in A Therapeutic Approach to the Psyche via the Beta-Adrenergic System. Edited by Kielholz P. Berlin, Hans Huber, 1978

Koella WP: Neurotransmitters in sleep, in Psychopharmacology of Sleep. Edited by Wheatley D. New York, Raven Press, 1981

Koella WP, Czicman J: Mechanism of the EEG-synchronizing action of serotonin. Am J Physiol 211:926–934, 1966

Koella WP, Feldstein A, Czicman J: The effect of parachlorophenylalanine on the sleep of cats. Electroencephalogr Clin Neurophysiol 25:481–490, 1968

Kostowski W, Giacalone E, Garattini S, et al: Electrical stimulation of midbrain raphe: biochemical, behavioral and bioelectrical effects. Eur J Pharmacol 7:170–175, 1969

Kostowski W, Samanin R, Bareggi SR, et al: Biochemical aspects of the interaction between midbrain raphe and locus coeruleus in the rat. Brain Res 82:178–182, 1974

Krueger JM, Bacsik J, Garcia-Arraras J: Sleep-promoting material from human urine and its relation to factor S from brain. Am J Physiol 238:E116–E123, 1980

Krueger JM, Pappenheimer JR, Karnovsky ML: The composition of sleep-promoting factor isolated from human urine. J Biol Chem 257:1664–1669, 1982

Ledebur IX, Tissot R: Modification de l'activite electrique cerebrale du lapin sous l'effet de micro-injections de precurseurs des monoamines dans les structures somnogens bulbaires et pontiques. Electroencephalogr Clin Neurophysiol 20:370–381, 1966

Leppavouri A, Putkonen PTS: Alpha-adrenoceptive influences on the control of the sleep-waking cycle in the cat. Brain Res 193:95–115, 1980

Loomis AL, Harvey EN, Hobart GA: Potential rhythms of the cerebral cortex during sleep. Science 81:597–598, 1935

Loomis AL, Harvey EN, Hobart GA: Cerebral states during sleep as studied by human brain potentials. J Exp Psychol 21:127–144, 1937

Lown B, Tykocinski M, Garfein A: Sleep and ventricular beats. Circulation 4:691–701, 1973

Magherini PC, Pompeiano O. Thodeu U: The neurochemical basis of REM sleep: a cholinergic mechanism responsible for rhythmic activation of the vestibulo-oculomotor system. Brain Res 35:565–573, 1971

Mancia G, Baccelli G, Adams DB, et al: Vasomotor regulation during sleep in the cat. Am J Physiol 220:1086–1093, 1971

Mauthner L: Zur Pathologie und Physiologie des Schlafes, nebst Bemerkungen uber die Nona. Wien Med Wochenschr 40:961–964, 1001–1004, 1049–1052, 1093–1094, 1144–1146, 1185–1188, 1890

McGinty DJ, Harper RM: Dorsal raphe neurons: depression of firing during sleep in cats. Brain Res 101:569–575, 1976

Mendelson WB, Gillin J, Pisner G, Wyatt RJ: Arginine vasotocin and sleep in the rat. Brain Res 182:246–249, 1980

Mereu GP, Scarrati E, Puglietti E, et al: Sleep induced by low doses of apomorphine in rats. Electroencephalogr Clin Neurophysiol 46:214–219, 1979

Monnier M, Gaillard JM: Biochemical regulation of sleep. Experientia 36:21–24, 1980

Monti JM, Folle LE, Peluffo C, et al: The incidence of premature contractions in coronary patients during the sleep-wake cycle. Cardiology 60:257–264, 1975

Moore-Ede MC, Schmelzer WS, Kass DA, et al: Internal organization of the circadian timing systems in multicellular animals. Fed Proc 35:2333–2338, 1976

Morgane PJ, Stern WC: Chemical anatomy of brain circuits in relation to sleep and wakefulness, in Advances in Sleep Research, Vol 1. Edited by Weitzman ED. New York, Spectrum, 1974

Moruzzi G, Magoun HW: Brainstem reticular formation and activation of the EEG. Electroencephalogr Clin Neurophysiol 1:455–473, 1949

Nakamura RK, Kennedy C, Gillin JC, et al: Hypogenic center theory of sleep: no support from metabolic mapping in monkeys. Brain Res 268:372–376, 1983

Okamoto Y, Kirikae T: Electroencephalographic studies on brain of foetus of children of pre-birth and new-born, together with a note on reactions of foetus brain upon drugs. Folia Psychiatr Neurol Jap 5:135–146, 1951

Oswald I: Sleeping and Waking: Physiology and Psychology. New York, Elsevier, 1962

Oswald I: Sleep, dreams and drugs, in Modern Trends in Psychological Medicine. Edited by Price HG, London, Butterworth, 1969

Panksepp J, Jalowiec JC, Morgane PJ, et al: Noradrenergic pathways and sleep-waking status in cats. Exp Neurol 41:233–245, 1973

Pappenheimer JR, Miller TB, Goodrich CA: Sleep promoting effects of cerebrospinal fluid from sleep-deprived goats. Proc Natl Acad Sci USA 58:513–517, 1967

Pappenheimer JR, Koski G, Fencl V, et al: Extraction of sleep promoting factor S from cerebrospinal fluid and from brains of sleep deprived animals. J Neurophysiol 38:1299–1311, 1975

Passouant P: Effect on sleep on dopaminergic agonists, in Apomorphine and Other Dopaminomimetics, vol 2, Clinical Pharmacology. Edited by Corsini GU, Gessa GL. New York, Raven Press, 1981

Pavel S: Pineal arginine vasotocin: an extremely potent sleep inducing nonapeptide hormone. Evidence for the involvement of 5–hydroxytryptamine containing neurons in its mechanism of action, in Sleep 1978. Edited by Popoviciu L, Asgian B, Badiu G. Basel, Karger, 1980

Pavel S, Psatta D, Goldstein R: Slow-wave sleep induced in cats by extremely small amounts of synthetic and pineal vasotocin injected into the third ventricle of the brain. Brain Res Bull 2:251–254, 1977

Pavel S, Goldstein R, Petrescu M: Vasotocin, melatonin and narcolepsy: possible involvement of the pineal gland in its pathophysiological mechanism. Peptides 1:281–284, 1980

Pavel S, Goldstein R, Petrescu M, et al: REM sleep induction in prepubertal boys by vasotocin: evidence for the involvement of serotin containing neurons. Peptides 2:245–250, 1981

Petitjean F, Seguin S, Des Rosiers MH, et al: Local cerebral glucose utilization during waking and slow wave sleep in the cat. A [^{14}C] deoxyglucose study. Neurosci Lett 32:91–97, 1982

Pickel VM, Joh TH, Reis DJ: A serotonergic innervation of noraderenergic neurons in the locus coeruleus: demonstration by immunocytochemical localization of the transmitter specific enzymes tyrosine and tryptophan hydroxylase. Brain Res 131:197–214, 1977

Possidente B, Hegmann JP: Circadian complexes: circadian rhythms under common gene control. J Comp Physiol 139:121–126, 1980

Post RM, Gerner RH, Carnan JS, et al: Effects of a dopamine agonist piribedil in depressed patients. Relationship of pretreatment homovanillic acid to antidepressant response. Arch Gen Psychiatry 35:609–615, 1978

Puizillout JJ, Gaudinchazal G, Daszuta A, et al: Release of endogenous serotonin from encephale isole cats. 2. Correlations with raphe neuronal activity and sleep and wakefulness. J Physiol (Paris) 75:531, 1979

Purkinje JE: Wachen, Schlaf, Traum und verwandte Zustande. In Handworterbuch der Physiologie mit Ruksicht auf physiologische Pathologie, Vol III. Edited by Wagner R von, Braunschweig, Vieweg und Sohn, 1846

Pycock CJ, Horton RW: Dopamine-dependent hyperactivity in the rat following manipulation of GABA mechanisms in the region of the nucleus accumbens. J Neural Transm 45:17–33, 1979

Quay WB: Pineal chemistry in cellular and physiologic mechanisms. Springfield, IL, Charles C Thomas, 1974

Radulovacki M, Wojcik WJ, Fornal C: Effects of bromocriptine and a-flupenthixol on sleep in REM sleep deprived rats. Life Sci 24:1705–1712, 1979

Raisman G, Brown-Grant K: The "supra-chiasmatic syndromes": endocrine and behavioral abnormalities following lesions of the supra-chiasmatic nuclei of the female rat. Proc R Soc Lond (Biol) 198:297–314, 1977

Ramm P: The locus coeruleus, catacholamines, and REM sleep: a critical review. Behav Neural Biol 25:415–448, 1979

Rechtschaffen A, Kales A: The manual of standardized terminology, techniques and scoring system for sleep stages of human subjects, NIH Publication No 204. Washington, DC. National Institutes of Health, 1968

Reis DJ, Moorhead D, Wooten GF: Redistribution of visceral and cerebral blood flow in the REM phase of sleep. Neurology 18:282, 1968

Reivich M, Isaacs G, Evarts E, et al: The effect of slow wave sleep and REM sleep on regional cerebral blood flow in cats. J Neurochem 15:301–306, 1968

Reppert SM, Perlow MJ, Ungerleider LG, et al: Effects of damage to the suprachiasmatic area of the anterior hypothalamus on the daily melatonin and cortisol rhythms in the rhesus monkey. J Neurosci 1:1414–1425, 1981

Richardson DW, Honour AJ, Goodman AC: Changes in arterial pressure during sleep in man, in Hypertension, Vol XVI, Neural Control of Arterial Pressure. Edited by Wood JE. New York, American Heart Association, 1968

Richter CP: Sleep and activity: their relation to the 24-hour clock. Sleep and altered states of consciousness. Proceedings of the Association for Research in Nervous and Mental Disease 45:8–27, 1967

Richter CP: Inborn nature of the rat's 24 hour clock. J Comp Physiol Psychol 75:1–4, 1971

Riou F, Cespuglio R, Jouvet M: Sleep-facilitating effect of vasoactive intestinal polypeptide in the rat, in Sleep 1982: 6th European Congress of Sleep Research, 1982. Edited by Koella WP. Basel, Karger, 1983

Roberts DCS, Zis AP, Fibiger HC: Ascending catecholamine pathways and amphetamine-induced locomotor activity: importance of dopamine and apparent non-involvement of norepinephrine. Brain Res 93:441–454, 1975

Robinson TE, Vanderwolf CH, Pappas BA: Are the dorsal noradrenergic bundle projections from the locus coeruleus important for neocortical or hippocampal activation? Brain Res 138:75–98, 1977

Rolando P: Saggio sopra la vera struttura del cervello dell'uomo e degli animali e sopra la funzioni del sistema nervoso. Sassari Stamperie i S.S.R.M., 1809

Ross CA, Trulson ME, Jacobs BL: Depletion of brain serotonin following intraventricular 5.7–dihydroxytryptamine fails to disrupt sleep in the rat. Brain Res 114:517–523, 1976

Roth GI, Walton PL, Yamamoto WS: Area postrema: abrupt EEG synchronization following close intraarterial perfusion with serotonin. Brain Res 23:223–233, 1970

Rougeul A, Verdeaux J, Letalle A: Effets electrographiques et comportementaux de divers hallucinogenes chez le chat libre. Rev Neurol (Paris) 120:391–394, 1969

Sakai K: Some anatomical and physiological properties of pontomesencephalic tegmental neurons with special reference to the PGO waves and postural atonia during paradoxical sleep in the cat, in The Reticular Formation Revisited. An IBRO Symposium. Edited by Brazier MAB. New York, Raven Press, 1981

Sakai F, Meyer JS, Karacan I, et al: Narcolepsy: regional cerebral blood flow during sleep and wakefulness. Neurology 29:61–67, 1979

Sallanon M, Buda C, Janin M, et al: L'insomnie provoquee para lo p-chlorophenylalanine chez le chat. Sa reversibilite par l'injection intraventriculaire de liquide cephalorachidien preleve chez des chats prives de sommeil paradoxal. C R Seances Acad Sci (Paris) 292:113–117, 1981

Sassin JF, Frantz AG, Kapen S, et al: The nocturnal rise of human prolactin is dependent on sleep. J Clin Endocrinol Metab 37:436–440, 1973

Sastre JP, Sakai K, Jouvet M: Persistence du sommeil paradoxal chez le chat apres destruction de l'aire gigante cellulaire de tegmentum pontique par l'acide kainique. C R Seances Acad Sci (Paris) 289:959–964, 1979

Scheel-Kruger J, Arnt J, Braestrup C, et al: GABA-dopamine interaction in substantia nigra and nuceus accubens—relevance to behavioral stimulation and stereotyped behavior. Adv Biochem Psychopharmacol 19:343–346, 1978

Scherschlicht R: Pharmacological profile of delta sleep-inducing peptide (DSIP) and a phosphorylated analogue, (Ser-PO₄) DSIP, in Sleep 1982: 6th European Congress of Sleep Research, 1982. Edited by Koella WP. Basel, Karger, 1983

Schoenenberger GA, Monnier M: Characterization of a delta-electroencephalogram (sleep) inducing peptide. Proc Natl Acad Sci USA 74:1282–1286, 1977

Segal DS, Mandell AJ: Behavioral activation of rats during intraventricular infusion of norepineprine. Proc Natl Acad Sci USA 66:289–293, 1970

Seigel JM: Reticular formation activity and REM sleep, in The Functions of Sleep. Edited by Drucker-Colin R, Sckurovich M, Sterman BM: New York, Academic Press, 1979

Sheu YS, Nelson JP, Bloom FE: Discharge patterns of the cat raphe neurons during sleep and waking. Brain Res 73:263–276, 1974

Sitaram N, Mendelson WB, Wyatt RJ, et al: Time dependent induction of REM sleep and arousal by physastigmine infusion during human sleep. Brain Res 122:562–567, 1977

Sitaram N, Moore AM, Gillin JC: Induction and resetting of REM sleep rhythm in normal man by arecholine: blockade by scopolamine. Sleep 1:83–90, 1978

Smith R, Johnson L, Rothfeld D, et al: Sleep and cardia arrhythmias. Arch Intern Med 130:342–349, 1972

Sokoloff L: The ^{14}C deoxyglucose method for the quantitative determination of local cerebral glucose metabolism: theoretical and practical considerations, in Cerebral Metabolism and Neural Function. Edited by Passonneau JV, Hawkins RA, Lust WD, et al. Baltimore, Williams & Wilkins, 1980

Sterman MB, Jeannerod M: Relationship of fetal activity to maternal EEG sleep stage. Electroenceph Clin Neurophysiol 23:81 (abstract), 1967

Stern S, Tzivoni D: Dynamic changes in the ST–T segment during sleep in ischemic heart disease. Am J Cardiol 32:17–20, 1973

Stern WC, Morgane PJ: Effects of alpha-methyltyrosine on REM sleep and brain amine levels in the cat. Biol Psychiatry 6:301–306, 1973

Sullivan CE, Zamel N, Kozar LF, et al: Regulation of airway smooth muscle tone in sleeping dogs. Am Rev Respir Dis 119:87–99, 1979a

Sullivan CE, Murphy E, Kozar LF, et al: Ventilatory responses to CO_2 and lung inflation in tonic versus phasic REM sleep. J Appl Physiol 47:1304–1310, 1979b

Tabushi K, Himwich HE: 5–hydroxytryptophan and the sleep-wakefulness cycle in rabbits. Biol Psychiatry 2:183–188, 1970

Tabushi K, Himwich HE: Electroencephalographic study of the effects of methysergide on sleep in the rabbit. Electroencephalogr Clin Neurophysiol 31:491–497, 1971

Tanaka C, Inagaki C, Fujiwara H: Labeled noradrenaline release from rat cerebral cortex following electrical stimulation of locus coeruleus. Brain Res 106:384–389, 1976

Tobler I, Borbely A: Effect of delta sleep inducing peptide (DSIP) and arginine vasotocin (AVT) on sleep and motor activity in the rat. Waking Sleeping 4:139–153, 1980

Torda C: Effect of changes of brain norepinephrine content on sleep cycle in rat. Brain Res 10:200–207, 1968

Townsend RE, Prinz PN, Obrist WD: Human cerebral blood flow during sleep and waking. J Appl Physiol 35:620–625, 1973

Trulson ME, Jacobs BL: Raphe unit activity in freely moving cats: correlation with levels of behavioral arousal. Brain Res 163:135–150, 1979

Turek FW, McMillan JP, Menaker M: Melatonin: effects on the circadian locomotor rhythm of sparrows. Science 194:1441–1443, 1976

Uchizono K, Ishikawa M, Iriki M, et al: Purification of sleep-promoting substances (SPS). Adv Pharmacol Chemother 2:217–225, 1982

Webb WB, Dube MG: Temporal characteristics of sleep, in Handbook of Behavioral Neurobiology, vol 4. Edited by Aschoff J. New York, Plenum Press, 1981

Weitzman ED, Czeisler CA, Moore-Ede MC: Sleep-wake, neuroendocrine and body temperature circadian rhythms under entrained and nonentrained (free-running) conditions in man, in Biological Rhythms and Their Central Control Mechanism. Edited by Suda M, Hayaishi O, Nakagawa H. New York, Elsevier, 1979

Weitzman ED, Czeisler CA, Zimmerman JC, et al: Tuning of REM and stages 3 and 4 during temporal isolation in man. Sleep 2:391–407, 1980

Wikler A: Pharmacologic dissociation of behavior and EEG "sleep patterns" in dogs; morphine, N-allylmorphine and atropine. Proc Soc Exp Biol Med 79:261–265, 1952

Williams HL: The new biology of sleep. J Psychiatr Res 8:445–478, 1971

Williams RL, Karacan I, Hursch CJ: EEG of Human Sleep: Clinical Applications. New York, John Wiley & Sons, 1974

Wirz-Justice A, Wehr T, Goodwin SK, et al: Antidepressant drugs slow circadian rhythms in behavior in brain neurotransmitter receptor. Psychopharmacol Bull 16:45–47, 1980

Wirz-Justice A, Kafka MJ, Naber D, et al: Clorgyline delays the phase-position of circadian neurotransmitter receptor rhythms. Brain Res 241:115–122, 1982

Wood JD, Peesker SJ: A correlation between changes in GABA metabolism and isonicotenic acid hydrazide-induced seizures. Brain Res 45:489–498, 1972

Wyatt RJ, Chase TN, Scott J, et al: Effect of L-Dopa on the sleep of man. Nature 228:999–1001, 1970a

Wyatt RJ, Engelman K, Kupfer DJ, et al: Effects of l-tryptophan (a natural sedative) on human sleep. Lancet 7678:842–846, 1970b

Chapter 15

Evaluation and Diagnosis of the Sleep Disorders: Implications for Psychiatry and Other Clinical Specialties

by Howard Roffwarg, M.D. and Milton Erman, M.D.

Psychiatrists are frequently and traditionally consulted to evaluate insomnia and sleep problems because both patients and referring doctors are aware of the broad interface between emotions and sleep. This chapter, therefore, has two objectives: to explain the requirement for a systematic approach by psychiatrists to the multiple etiologies of the sleep disorders, and to contribute a working orientation toward sleep complaints, their diagnostic evaluation, and therapeutics.

The study of sleep pathology is evolving into an area of diagnostic and therapeutic concentration which has attracted clinician-investigators from several medical specialties, notably, psychiatry, neurology and, more recently, pulmonary medicine. Encouraged and supported since the early 1960s by departments of psychiatry throughout the country and assisted by the new tool of sleep electrophysiology (polysomnographic recording, or PSG), many psychiatrists with clinical/research interests in sleep have made significant findings relating to the neurobiology of sleep, dreaming, and sleep disorders. As interest in sleep pathology as a clinical subspecialty increases, sleep disorders centers continue to be developed in psychiatry departments. These diagnostic units encourage comprehensive psychologic and physiologic assessment of patients with sleep difficulties (Dement and Guilleminault, 1973; Reynolds et al, 1979). This orientation is consistent with psychiatry's role as a medical discipline.

Though research has uncovered a pivotal role for organic and heritable phenomena in some psychiatric conditions, untoward experience alone is, at times, sufficient to provoke psychopathologic and psychophysiologic reactions. In regard to insomnia, for example, both acute anxiety and depression interfere massively with previously normal sleep; subtler shifts in psychophysiological equilibrium may also mobilize more concealed pressures that disturb normal sleep. Conceding its sensitivity to psychophysiologic disruption, sleep is inevitably a physiologic process.

Until recently, most physicians took little notice of intermittent snoring or unusual body movements in sleep and doubted their medical significance. Though medical technology was enthusiastically applied to the measurement of almost every known body function, it long remained medically acceptable to let physiological aberrances during sleep pass unnoticed. That era is fortunately coming to a close. With the advent of nocturnal sleep recording, the reasons for these and other sleep complaints, and the disorders of which they are symptoms (for example, sleep apnea, narcolepsy, nocturnal myoclonus) are being clarified (Zarcone, 1973; Ferriss, 1984). The tendency to trivialize patient and bed partner stories of unusual somatic activity in sleep has, in turn, diminished.

As chronic insomnia has been brought under combined psychiatric, medical, and polysomnographic scrutiny in the last decade (Schmidt, 1983), it has become clear to all observers that, more than any other single factor, psychologic disruption, wholly or in part, is most frequently responsible for insomnia (Kales et al, 1974; Coleman, 1983).

Advances in knowledge notwithstanding, sleep remains a neglected arena of scientific understanding. Wide gaps persist in our understanding of metabolic and physiological derangements in sleep: More people die at night than by day; more drugs are used in connection with sleep than for any other therapeutic purpose (Institute of Medicine, 1979); our life support systems are at their most unpredictable and unreliable as they daily swing through the supposed rest cycle; and we are just now discovering some of the true physiological causes of poor sleep in old age (Coleman, 1983). Far from taking refuge in blanket psychological explanations of disordered sleep (Kales et al, 1981), we must draw on psychiatry's growing psychobiological awareness and acknowledge how much there is to learn about the dysfunctions of sleep. Psychiatry should insist on an affirmative and searching psychologic and biologic exploration into the mechanisms of insomnia.

Psychiatrists have come to accept that organically provoked disruptions of sleep are the usual cause of excessive daytime sleepiness. On the other hand, emphasizing the belief that symptomatic sleep disturbance is almost invariably a product of "psychiatric" difficulties, some psychiatrists (Kales JD et al, 1982; Tan et al, 1984) are disinclined to credit the same or similar somatic phenomena (breathing interruptions, leg jerks) with giving rise to insomnia complaints, though such events irrefutably disrupt polygraphically recorded sleep.

This refusal is puzzling. For, if certain somatically induced disruptions of sleep finally eventuate in the symptom of daytime somnolence, may not some of the provoked awakenings earlier be recallable by the patient? Recent data, in fact, indicate that, as sleep loss accrues in nocturnal myoclonus, the awareness of sleep disturbance by the patient becomes blurred and the presenting symptom ultimately shifts over to daytime sleepiness (Rosenthal et al, 1984). It is a clinical reality that patients with indisputable central apnea awakenings usually present with disturbed sleep, whereas obstructive apnea patients, who show more arousals, sleep loss and hypoxemia, complain of daytime sleepiness. Beyond this fact, other physical phenomena, like pain or limitation of motion, are well known to instigate insomnia (Williams et al, 1974).

The Hershey investigators dispute that central apnea and nocturnal myoclonus may symptomatically disturb sleep and point to their single finding that noncomplaining sleepers (called normals) show no more of these activities in sleep than professed insomniacs (Bixler et al, 1982a, b; Kales A et al, 1982). But pathology is often asymptomatic and symptoms may be misperceived, minimized or denied. As much as anything, we should be alerted by these data to the perils of deciding solely on the basis of patient allegation whether or not insomnia exists. When *asymptomatic* and *normal* are confounded, we are put in danger of coming to the medically unsound conclusion that pathology (in this case, organically provoked sleep disruption) exists only if it is apparent to the individual. Be that as it may, the Hershey data, in fact, showed signs of poorer sleep in the so-called normals with myoclonus than in those without. There was much worse sleep in the insomnia complainers but also in the noncomplainers with organic perturbations than would be expected in normals (Williams and Karacan, 1974; Kales et al, 1984). These investigations were conducted in younger people than those who show the highest incidences of these pathologies (Coleman, 1983) and, further, they lacked other sleep scoring analyses that can reveal subtly disturbed sleep in the PSG (Carskadon et al, 1980). In work that holds promise for greater future understanding of the effects of numerous but brief disturbances of sleep, several recent studies have found that it may be possible to predict the form and severity of symptoms connected with organic disturbances of sleep by careful analysis of the number and duration of PSG arousals (Carskadon et al, 1980, 1982; Moldofsky et al, 1984; Rosenthal et al, 1984; Stepanski et al, 1984).

Accordingly, it is now almost universally recognized that sleep in psychologically healthy individuals can be extensively and symptomatically disturbed by somatic phenomena of which the sleeper is unaware. The patient does not know *why* he awakens; but he is aware of at least some of the awakenings, probably the longer ones (Rosenthal et al, 1984). Several independent studies (Guilleminault et al, 1973, 1975; Hauri and Hawkins, 1973; Zorick et al, 1981; Coleman, 1983) and two large case series (Coleman et al, 1982; Coleman, 1983) document that shallow or stopped breathing in sleep (usually central apnea but also mild obstructive apnea), leg jerking (nocturnal myoclonus), persistence of alpha rhythm, gastroesophageal reflux, and other medical and neurologic conditions hold off or fragment the continuity of sleep. The somatic source of the arousals can remain unsuspected for decades but operate nightly.

A cardinal characteristic of chronic insomnias not associated with psychiatric symptoms is the stability of the sleep disturbance. The insomnia is seemingly unaffected by vicissitudes of mental state, a feature that is perplexing to patient and doctor alike. Discovery and treatment of an often covert organic factor is critical to elimination of the insomnia. To complicate matters, conditioned arousing tendencies may not only coexist independently with an organic cause of insomia, but their effects may also be grafted onto and aggravate organic sleep disturbances, owing to the patient's growing apprehension and negative expectation about ever experiencing restful sleep (persistent psychophysiological insomnia).

Complete elucidation of organic contributions to insomnia symptoms is not possible without laboratory recording, although excellent clues to their existence can be obtained from an observant bed partner. In one recent experience with individuals who were applying to participate in an insomnia study, sleep disorder specialists had conducted complete sleep and psychiatric interviews; however, they failed to identify that approximately 30 percent of the potential subjects had insomnia that proved to be definitively attributable to physiological abnormalities in subsequent sleep recordings (Roffwarg et al, 1982). On further examination, it became clear that the subjects lacked any subjective awareness that organic factors were operating. When asked what they thought had delayed sleep onset or caused midsleep awakenings, they invariably brought up their concerns and stresses.

Apart from some patients having no idea that their insomnia is caused by organic factors, other patients who also have clinically convincing insomnia complaints astonishingly do not show objectively insufficient sleep when recorded. No office diagnostic procedure is capable of identifying this condition, *subjective insomnia complaint without objective findings.*

At the recent Consensus Development Conference on Drugs and Insomnia sponsored by the National Institute of Mental Health (NIMH) (1984), broad acknowledgment was made of the complexity of sleep disorders diagnosis and of the necessary diagnostic procedures undertaken in sleep disorders evaluation centers. Similar judgments were made in the Institute of Medicine study on sleeping pills, insomnia and medical practice. (Solomon et al, 1979).

SLEEP LABORATORY EVALUATION, THE PATIENT AND THE DOCTOR

In psychiatry and to some degree in medicine, a bias lingers that recording the sleep of a patient at night in the laboratory is likely to be inefficacious and, in any event, unseemly. The psychiatrist may catch himself feeling that in sending a patient to a sleep laboratory he is violating a confidence, or causing the patient to be observed in overly intimate and unprotected circumstances.

The family physician is admonished that sleep disorder referral ". . . often detracts from treating the patient in a holistic manner" (Kales JD et al, 1980). Sleep laboratory evaluations are portrayed in this view as ". . . expensive and time consuming, and often contributing only minimally to the overall management of the insomniac patient. In fact, they (the evaluations) may even detract from the comprehensive psychiatric, neurological, pharmacological and general medical approach that is necessary for the effective management of insomnia" (Soldatos et al, 1979). Correspondingly, Tan et al (1984) calls attention to the high correlation between psychopathology and insomnia, which in their view strongly suggests a "causal relationship between psychiatric disorders and insomnia." They reassure the psychiatrist that, by making a *DSM-III* diagnosis in every patient, he can diagnose, with great confidence and without sleep recording, cases of sleep disturbances in office practice.

Undoubtedly, such a causal relationship frequently exists between psychiatric disorders and insomnia. However, one needs to keep in perspective whether covariance between the prevalence rates of *general psychopathology* and *insomnia* necessarily indicates that insomnia has a specific and single etiology (Kales A et al, 1983; 1984). Psychopathology can result *from* insomnia as well as *fomenting* it. For example, when MMPI patterns are differentially analyzed for separate subgroupings of organic and "psychiatric" insomnias, the data reveal clearly discriminable patterns of psychopathology pertaining to the two types of insomnia (Zorick et al, 1981). Finally, though we must give weight to the correlation, for example, of alcohol and drug abuse as well as poor sleep hygiene with psychologic disability, we must also acknowledge their *independent* sleep-disrupting effects. Coexistent psychologic problems often play less of a role in sleep disturbance than their associated *behaviors*, which require specific reversal if the sleeplessness is to ameliorate. Some insomnia complainers require study because they are sleeping much better than they realize.

A fundamental issue, then, is whether reliance by the practitioner, solely upon his diagnostic capabilities within the "office setting", is any longer acceptable either as a proper standard of diagnosis or as a suitable objective of modern medical practice.

Sleep laboratory recording or polysomnography (PSG) is a highly professional and practical means of obtaining diagnostically critical information. An extraordinary number of relevant physiological systems may be monitored easily in sleep without significant perturbation of the patient. The recording is unimpeded by the artifactual reactivity that often distorts laboratory monitoring in the conscious patient. In this sense, sleep physiology recordings are among the most versatile of laboratory biomedical assessments.

Any biological function that is measurable in the waking state can and should be recorded in sleep if the data are germane to the patient's health and functioning. Monitoring of EEG, EKG, leg muscle activity, body movement, fine motor behaviors (video), respiration, expired gases, blood oxygen saturation, cerebral blood flow, body temperature, gastric acid, and galvanic skin response may all be obtained in sleep, many concurrently registered.

Recording multiple physiological systems in the sleep-disturbed subject makes it much less likely to overlook a secondary source of insomnia (e.g., central apnea), which may require special treatment even if the primary diagnosis (e.g., insomnia due to depression) has been accurately surmised by the referring psychiatrist. Confirming the *primary* diagnosis is also, of course, not without value.

An additional consideration in support of sleep laboratory assessment relates to the medical wisdom that diagnostic laboratory monitoring is best carried out when the pathological events are manifest, not when they are latent. This is exemplified in two situations: In apnea, patients breathe well when awake and usually have normal blood gases; only in sleep can the blocked ventilation and plummeting blood oxygen levels that are characteristic of the condition be recorded. In nocturnal myoclonus, the patient cannot tell the doctor anything about his leg jerks; they appear just at the threshold of or during sleep, and are out of the patient's awareness.

How A Sleep Disorders Center Operates

Sleep disorders centers are, by and large, diagnostic units. The patient is seen "in consultation" for a requested, specialized investigation. A comprehensive sleep disorders center accepts medical responsibility for the patient while he or she is being studied but does not "take the patient over." Of course, the polysomnographer might recommend additional recording variables to the referring doctor, as any consultant might. The patient is returned to the referring physician for treatment with an account of the test results. Centers generally do not engage in long-term care of patients, except as part of research protocols.

Discussion usually takes place after the laboratory assessment and interpretation of the studies. If the patient's doctor requests it, a sleep disorders specialist will begin a recommended treatment to help the referring doctor evaluate preliminary results. If a psychiatrist's patient is found to have an "organic sleep disorder," the psychiatrist continues to treat the psychiatric problem. The psychiatrist may, if he wishes, assume follow-up of the sleep condition as well, or he may prefer to have another doctor do so.

In reference to diagnostic accuracy and treatment specificity, laboratory recording is recommended for the chronically symptomatic sleep disorders patient. While a careful interviewer can pick up highly informative clinical signs suggesting particular disorders, these possibilities can be confirmed only in the sleep lab.

Diagnosis represents only the first step in the care of the patient. Treatment of an organic condition requires additional information (psychiatric sleep disturbances may also benefit from such data), which includes: severity of pathology (number of apneas, leg jerks, arousals, etc.); possibility of additional or secondary conditions that are treatable; absence versus occurrence of arrhythmias and major oxygen desaturations (in apnea); changes in the pathological events during the course of the night; effects of sleeping position on the pathological events; relationship of the episodes to particular stages of sleep; objective analysis of total sleep, sleep latency, number of arousals, stage percentages, and stage shifts; REM sleep latency, which can be a useful biological identifier of primary or endogenous depression (Kupfer and Thase, 1983); relationship of the recorded sleep parameters to the patient's subjective sleep estimations on the same night (an extremely important datum); documentation and quantification of daytime tendency to sleep; and determination of actual REM onsets in narcolepsy.

With the exception of the last item, all of these variables are provided by sleep lab recording. While they are valuable in selection of optimal treatment, they are equally significant in establishing a baseline of pathology against which the results of treatment may be measured.

THE PSYCHIATRIST AND SLEEP LABORATORY ASSESSMENTS

When psychiatric factors cause insomnia, psychiatric treatments aimed at the primary pathology are also the treatment of choice for the associated insomnia. Poor sleep should dissipate with psychiatric improvement. Diagnostic specificity and therapeutic attention to the underlying disorder are axioms of both good psychiatry and good medicine. However, no sleep disorders specialist would advocate suspension or diversion of suitable psychiatric treatment if a psychiatric patient turned out to have a sleep disturbance explained in large part by a nonpsychiatric element. Psychiatric factors—whether they are wholly or only partially, primarily or secondarily, related to the insomnia—must be addressed vigorously, or the sleep problem will attract psychiatric overlay.

It is important for psychiatrists to understand that there are no controversies in the sleep field regarding psychiatric factors that are significant and frequent in insomnia, or the urgency of their being resolved therapeutically. In support, two national surveys, comprising thousands of sleep center patients, document that half of all primary insomnia diagnoses made in sleep disorders diagnostic centers fall into psychologic and psychiatric categories (Coleman, 1983). The perceived need in the sleep field is not to convince the psychiatrist that his area of professional concern is not important to insomnia, only that it does not suffice as an exclusive causality. The psychiatrist's appreciation of the etiology of insomnia must be widened so that he is concerned also with whether his patient is breathing at night, whether the patient has stereotyped, repetitive leg jerks, brain wave abnormalities, gastroesophageal reflux, nonemotion-laden sleep-schedule disturbances, sleep hygiene problems, or whether he *only thinks he is insomniac* (ASCD, 1979).

It is neither necessary nor desirable to send every insomnia complainer with psychiatric problems to a sleep laboratory. The examining psychiatrist, however, must be reasonably well-informed of the fundamentals of sleep symptom presentation in order to select the minority of patients in whom polygraphic sleep recording is required to provide necessary information.

Guidelines have been established to assist the practitioner in using sound clinical judgment, in combination with the patient's treatment responses, to confirm tentative diagnoses before considering referral to a sleep laboratory (Coleman et al, 1982). It need only be added that validation is required for a confirmed diagnosis. History from the patient and office examination are indispensable, but clinical diagnosis requires verification either in the laboratory or from the patient's long-term response to a course of treatment. This feedback suffices as confirmation in the clinical situation and, in fact, adds important new data.

Accordingly, the psychiatrist does not require protection or relief from consideration of sleep laboratory investigation for a patient when diagnostically advisable. There is no reason why psychiatrists should be less comfortable when obtaining technical information about patients in a sleep laboratory than when requesting a neurological examination, or an EEG, CAT scan, psychometrics, neuropsychological testing, thyroid indices, and plasma levels of lithium and psychotropic drugs, all of which have become customary "out of the office" referrals.

Physiologic monitoring, which is noninvasive, comfortable, and private (as well as the diagnostic sleep interview and psychological tests, if requested), appear to pose no problem either for concurrent psychiatric evaluation or for long-term psychotherapy. Because sleep centers use psychologically trained personnel the opportunity exists to denote *both* waking and sleeping behaviors of patients in relation to their anticipations about sleep recording, a situation that might mobilize unexpected emotions. This capability permits a sleep laboratory to provide psychodiagnostically data to the referring doctor and to "fill in" particular medical/psychiatric information that is sought by the referring specialist.

NEED FOR A SPECIFIC SLEEP DISORDERS CLASSIFICATION SYSTEM

Neither excessive daytime somnolence nor disturbed sleep are trifling problems for the great numbers of people who are afflicted. They are crippling and their effects are unremitting.

For reasons that are not yet understood, individuals differ sharply from one another in terms of their requirement for sleep. Not everyone is enlightened about these individual differences, and the idea that an absolute amount of sleep is necessary for all persons still has some advocates.

The stimulus to develop diagnostic specificity for disturbed sleep and sleepiness emerged from a growing recognition of nosological confusion and therapeutic frustration. The inefficacy of strictly psychiatric therapies, as applied to the mass of insomnia complainers, had become apparent. There simply seemed to be more to learn about the contexts in which insomnia occurs and about the possibilities of detecting specific diagnostic characteristics in certain insomnia presentations.

Similar to the thrust leading to *DSM-III*, construction of the diagnostic classification of the sleep disorders (ASDC, 1979) focused, first, on the formal naming and describing of some clinical polysomnographic condition, encountered in patients but never before comprehensively annotated; and, second, on the development of operation criteria to help delineate and standardize their diagnoses. Reliable diagnostic differentiation was viewed as unquestionably vital to establishing diagnostic validity and to elucidating pathological mechanisms, both indispensible prerequisites for advances in treatment. Inability to suspect or correctly diagnose a specific sleep pathology insures no treatment, or worse, mistreatment of the condition.

Whether the insomnia complainer is seen by a practitioner or in a sleep disorders center, the general problem should be dealt with in the same way: that is, to establish the patient's average nightly sleep need when he was not insomniac, using the criterion that the amount of sleep in question is the quantity required for full alertness and vigor the whole day. The quota of required sleep is calculated, adjusting for weekday/weekend variations, as if the same amount of sleep must be obtained every day. The average sleep need is then compared to the amount of sleep currently being obtained. Daytime symptoms of insomnia are also surveyed, keeping in mind that insomnia does not lead to morbid sleepiness during the day as much as might be expected.

Some individuals require only one to four hours of sleep each night to function pleasurably and capably all day, whereas others consistently require eight to 12 hours of sleep. Approximately 60 percent of the population obtain from six to eight hours of sleep nightly. Eight hours was formerly regarded as the "golden mean" of sleep need.

If a short-sleeping individual has no daytime symptoms of insomnia, such as fatigue, weakness, distractibility, poor concentration, and muscle aches, he should not be considered to have a functional insomnia irrespective of obtaining an unconventionally brief period of sleep at night. The insomnia complaint is valid, however, if a currently short-sleeping individual previously slept longer and felt good during the day, and now is feeling bad by day.

Sleep Hygiene Abuse

The doctor should be aware of the elements of "sleep-wake hygiene" and question the patient about his schedule and habits. Humans may wish to "sup and frolic with the gods"; but their mortal, circadian physiology soon brings them back to earth, or at least to poor sleep.

As discussed, individuals should have a reasonably accurate knowledge of daily sleep needs. The period of time spend in bed should not be substantially greater than the actual sleep requirement. Too much time spent in and around bed leads to the danger of random napping and the threat of an irregular or desultory sleep-wake cycle. With consequent deterioration of circadian sleep-wake bimodality, there is attendant flattening and disruption of the circadian hormone and temperature curves.

Regular arousal times and bedtimes are important because of the recruitment of other circadian rhythms to the sleep-wake cycle. Sleep becomes less efficient when moved to habitual waking hours, and, as every shift-worker knows, alertness and cognitive functioning are at risk whenever wakefulness must be voluntarily maintained during habitual sleep periods.

Sleep also suffers when there is excessive irregularity in the amount of daily exercise taken and wide variation in the quantity and types of foods eaten, particularly before bedtime. A steady amount of exercise, appropriate to the individual, should be maintained on a daily basis. Adequate nutrition promotes sleep by preventing hunger during the night and by providing some protein to the brain. Overly large intakes of food or difficult-to-digest items eaten late in the evening may cause poor sleep.

Alcohol must also be viewed as a problem. Although a "little nip" has been a favorite sleep-promoting agent since ancient times, alcohol loses its sleep-onset sedation powers if taken on a daily basis. However, even when alcohol is used regularly, it never loses its countervailing property of increasing the number of awakenings and reducing deep stages of sleep.

INSOMNIA COMPLAINT IS NOT INSOMNIA DISORDER

Insomnia is not a disorder; it is only a symptom, in that it marks the interruption of a normal function. In common with most symptoms, it is activated by a number of causes. The practitioner's failure to distinguish an insomnia *complaint* from an insomnia *disorder* is a major problem. Patients' accounts of insomnia have traditionally been accepted at face value by doctors as valid representations of disturbed or insufficient sleep. But the individual who is a "short sleeper" does not realize, as he complains of insomnia, that he is obtaining all the sleep he requires. To make matters worse, individuals who are "sleep hygiene abusers" or have delayed sleep phase syndrome also present with an insomnia complaint, but they definitely should not be given the general treatments for insomnia; these disorders require *specific* treatments. The usual insomnia therapies in these situations only delay proper treatment or create secondary problems.

Subjective Complaint Without Objective Findings

Insomnia patients as a group are reputed to overestimate the time it takes to fall asleep and also to underestimate the duration of sleep and its continuity. Doctors usually make general allowances for this tendency. More disturbing to clinicians, however, is the almost universal experience in sleep disorders centers (Dement et al, 1975; Carskadon et al, 1976; Zorick et al, 1981; Coleman, 1983) that seven to 20 percent of all insomnia complainers—patients with convincing accounts of chronic and severe inability to fall or remain asleep—make incredible misjudgments about their sleep. The patient's estimate stands in stark contrast to the absence of *any* sleep onset delay or sleep maintenance disturbance. This discrepancy between subjective and objective sleep is found repeatedly in both laboratory and home recordings.

In the opinion of all observers, subjective insomnia complainers are not malingerers; they genuinely believe they are not sleeping. The stories sound as authentic as the narratives of true insomnia patients. Because the patients show no apparent psychological or behavioral abnormalities, practitioners cannot divine from their office interviews that objective sleep monitoring will be in the normal range. Accordingly, this condition is given the non-insomnia disorder diagnosis, Subjective Insomnia Complaint Without Objective Findings (ASDC, 1979).

Carskadon et al (1976) studied 122 patients with the complaint of insomnia, most of whom had previously been screened for organic sources of insomnia. Of the 57 who stated that they generally slept five hours or less, only 17.5 percent conformed to that description in the laboratory. Fifty-four percent slept between six and seven hours when being recorded, and another 10.5 percent slept longer than seven hours. Almost half of the whole group fell asleep in less than 15 minutes, including 20 of the 46 who estimated their home sleep latencies at greater than 60 minutes. Many of the subjects had total sleep times and sleep latencies indistinguishable from noncomplaining individuals. Clearly, some, but not all, of this population of insomnia complainers fell into the "subjective only" category.

Research is underway in this "condition." It is widely believed that these patients have some sort of pathology, possibly excessive, brief arousals from sleep which generate a *sense* of wakefulness (Carskadon et al, 1976), a tendency to misperceive state of consciousness, or a need for displacement of psychopathology into a more acceptable guise, a sleep disturbance complaint. Showing the patients their sleep records and discussing with them some of the possible explanations for their idiosyncratic subjective estimates of sustained wakefulness often start movement toward their improved perception of sleep.

"Subjective complaint only" individuals must be identified, then further explored for the true sources of their complaints. They have sought help and require understanding and response. Nevertheless, their assertions of insomnia cannot be validated by reliable polysomnographic measures. These patients will not be well served if their problem is mislabeled as insomnia. Treatments will be given that, at best, are beside the point. In view of the finding that a considerable number of insomnia complainers do not have insomnia when recorded in the sleep laboratory, the suggestion (Kales JD et al, 1980; Soldatos et al, 1979) that insomnia complainers do not require sleep studies leaves the patients open to improper diagnosis and treatment.

Sleep History

In evaluating patients with sleep disorder complaints and attempting to gather diagnostic clues as to the nature of the problem, a sleep history is important. The Brief Sleep Disorders History (Table 1) samples most of the areas of concern that have been discussed in this section. Taking about 10-15 minutes to complete a brief sleep history has the advantage of being systematic. A more detailed history (Roffwarg and Altshuler, 1982) is necessary to characterize fully the features of a specific sleep disorder that may be presented by a patient. In connection with a comprehensive sleep disorders assessment, patients fill out

Table 1. Brief Sleep Disorders History

---

1. Times of retiring and arising. Variations between weekdays and weekends. Recent changes in this sleep-wake schedule.

2. Subjective quality (ie, soundness, restorativeness) of sleep.

3. Amount of daily sleep needed to feel ideally alert and energetic throughout awake functioning. Are drugs required?

4. How often is that amount of sleep obtained in relation to the nightly average? Disagreements with home observers about whether or not sleeping, or time spent asleep.

5. Sleep habits and requirements in childhood and other major periods of life. Subjective quality of sleep in those periods. Attitudes towards sleep.

6. Is sleep difficult to get into, disturbed during its course, or foreshortened? If so, effect on daily functioning. Daytime symptoms related to poor sleep.

7. Is sleepiness during waking hours a problem? Is the problem worsening? Is it impossible to resist falling asleep during the day? Episodes of muscle weakness with laughter. Snoring. Intermittent snoring and gagging. Leg jerking in sleep. Any other troublesome events in sleep.

8. Drugs and alcohol before 6 P.M.; after 6 P.M.

9. General emotional and physical problems. How treated?

10. Sleep-hygiene: eating, drinking, bed comfort, sleep environment, temperature, noise, light, etc.

---

a questionnaire which probes habits, phenomenology, and medication pertaining to their sleep history and current sleep. This history is reviewed in detail in the evaluation interview.

DIAGNOSTIC CLASSIFICATION OF SLEEP/AROUSAL DISORDERS

In view of the already known psychological factors in insomnia and the growing number of organic pathologies that were being uncovered as sources of sleep disturbance and daytime sleepiness symptoms, the Association of Sleep Disorders Centers (ASDC), in conjunction with the leading sleep research society, the Association for the Psychophysiological Study of Sleep (APSS), organized in 1976 the consensus development of a criterion-based diagnostic classification of sleep and arousal disorders (ASDC, 1979). The ASDC approach to categorization of the full spectrum of sleep disorders is recognized internationally and is the most frequently used diagnostic classification in Europe and Asia. It appears in outline form (Table 2) as Appendix E of *DSM-III*. The *DSM-III* sections on sleepwalking and sleep terror were prepared from the *ASDC Classification Manual*'s textual descriptions.

Table 2. Outline of Diagnostic Classification of Sleep and Arousal Disorders

A. DIMS: Disorders of Initiating and Maintaining Sleep (Insomnias)
  1. Psychophysiological
    a. Transient and Situational
    b. Persistent
  2. *associated with*
    Psychiatric Disorders
    a. Symptom and Personality Disorders
    b. Affective Disorders
    c. Other Functional Psychoses
  3. *associated with*
    Use of Drugs and Alcohol
    a. Tolerance to or Withdrawal from CNS Depressants
    b. Sustained Use of CNS Stimulants
    c. Sustained Use or Withdrawal from Other Drugs
    d. Chronic Alcoholism
  4. *associated with*
    Sleep-induced Respiratory Impairment
    a. Sleep Apnea DIMS Syndrome
    b. Alveolar Hypoventilation DIMS Syndrome
  5. *associated with*
    Sleep-related (Nocturnal) Myoclonus and "Restless Legs"
    a. Sleep-related (Nocturnal) Myoclonus DIMS Syndrome
    b. "Restless Legs" DIMS Syndrome
  6. *associated with*
    Other Medical, Toxic, and Environmental Conditions
  7. Childhood-Onset DIMS
  8. *associated with*
    Other DIMS Conditions
    a. Repeated REM Sleep Interruptions
    b. Atypical Polysomnographic Features
    c. Not Otherwise Specified
  9. No DIMS Abnormality
    a. Short Sleeper
    b. Subjective DIMS Complaint Without Objective Findings
    c. Not Otherwise Specified
B. DOES: Disorders of Excessive Somnolence
  1. Psychophysiological
    a. Transient and Situational
    b. Persistent
  2. *associated with*
    Psychiatric Disorders
    a. Affective Disorders
    b. Other Functional Disorders
  3. *associated with*
    Use of Drugs and Alcohol
    a. Tolerance to or Withdrawal from CNS Stimulants
    b. Sustained Use of CNS Depressants
  4. *associated with*
    Sleep-induced Respiratory Impairment
    a. Sleep Apnea DOES Syndrome

Table 2. Continued

---

      b. Alveolar Hypoventilation DOES Syndrome
    5. *associated with*
    Sleep-related (Nocturnal) Myoclonus and "Restless Legs"
      a. Sleep-related (Nocturnal) Myoclonus DOES Syndrome
      b. "Restless Legs" DOES Syndrome
    6. Narcolepsy
    7. Idiopathic CNS Hypersomnolence
    8. *associated with*
    Other Medical, Toxic, and Environmental Conditions
    9. *associated with*
    Other DOES Conditions
      a. Intermittent DOES (Periodic) Syndromes
        i. Kleine-Levin Syndrome
        ii. Menstrual-associated Syndrome
      b. Insufficient Sleep
      c. Sleep Drunkenness
      d. Not Otherwise Specified
   10. No DOES Abnormality
      a. Long Sleeper
      b. Subjective DOES Complaint Without Objective Findings
      c. Not Otherwise Specified
C. Disorders of the Sleep-Wake Schedule
    1. Transient
      a. Rapid Time Zone Change ("Jet Lag") Syndrome
      b. "Work Shift" Change in Conventional Sleep-Wake Schedule
    2. Persistent
      a. Frequently Changing Sleep-Wake Schedule
      b. Delayed Sleep Phase Syndrome
      c. Advanced Sleep Phase Syndrome
      d. Non-24-Hour Sleep-Wake Syndrome
      e. Irregular Sleep-Wake Pattern
      f. Not Otherwise Specified
D. Dysfunctions Associated with Sleep, Sleep Stages, or Partial Arousals
   (Parasomnias)
    1. Sleepwalking (Somnambulism)
    2. Sleep Terror (Pavor Nocturnus, Incubus)
    3. Sleep-related Enuresis
    4. Other Dysfunctions
      a. Dream Anxiety Attacks (Nightmares)
      b. Sleep-related Epileptic Seizures
      c. Sleep-related Bruxism
      d. Sleep-related Headbanging (Jactatio Capitis Nocturnus)
      e. Familial Sleep Paralysis
      f. Impaired Sleep-related Penile Tumescence
      g. Sleep-related Painful Erections
      h. Sleep-related Cluster Headaches and Chronic Paroxysmal
        Hemicrania
      i. Sleep-related Abnormal Swallowing Syndrome
      j. Sleep-related Asthma
      k. Sleep-related Cardiovascular Symptoms
      l. Sleep-related Gastroesophageal Reflux

Table 2. Continued

m. Sleep-related Hemolysis (Paroxysmal Nocturnal Hemoglobinuria)
n. Asymptomatic Polysomnographic Finding
o. Not Otherwise Specified

From Association of Sleep Disorders Centers Classification Committee: Diagnostic Classification of Sleep and Arousal Disorders, first edition. Copyright © 1979 by Raven Press. Reprinted by permission of the ASDC and Raven Press.

The ASDC sleep nosology was also applied to the *International Classification of Diseases 9th Revision, Clinical Modifications (ICD-9-CM)*, the North American version of *ICD-9*. Because it was completed late in the formulation of *ICD-9-CM*, the ASDC nosology could only be partially fit into *ICD-9-CM*.

A diagnostic framework was required which would encompass the entire spectrum of normal and abnormal sleep, one formulated from the shared experience of working experts and incorporating their consensus agreements concerning diagnostic criteria, terminology and the most fruitful categorization of disorders. The ASDC classification does not impose theoretical presuppositions on clinical knowledge, but rather reflects clinical observations about sleep disorders.

The new nosology is rooted at the most fundamental clinical level—patient complaint—because most etiological factors and mechanisms of sleep disorders still await full recognition. Vital to the classification system is the discriminability that it provides for the four major groupings of disorders in terms of symptom pattern. The patient's *type of presenting chief complaint* (for example, insomnia [DIMS], daytime sleepiness [DOES], intrusions of pathological events into sleep [Parasomnias], and disorders of sleep-wake schedule) dictates the organization of the four categorical rubrics of the nosology. Though clinically useful currently, this emphasis on *type* of symptom may ultimately be dispensable in later classifications.

This initiative in diagnostic standardization of sleep pathology represented an important step in providing an objective basis for dependable diagnosis, shared data collection, and research. In the spirit of *DSM-III*, the sleep nosology is highly specified with respect to identification and differentiation of conditions so that data can be gathered in relation to the validity of the diagnostic entities. This system is not fixed but serves as a standard for new concepts and findings.

The Four Types of Disorders

The ASDC Classification System categorizes four major types of disorders:

A. DIMS, OR DISORDERS OF INITIATING AND MAINTAINING SLEEP (INSOMNIAS). The DIMS are a heterogeneous group of conditions that are associated with situational, psychiatric, and organic conditions. They are brought together in one rubric because each is responsible for inducing disturbed or diminished sleep. Use of the term, Disorders of Initiating and Maintaining Sleep, though cumbersome, serves to remind us that insomnia is not one entity but rather a multiplicity of conditions, which vary considerably in their manifestations of sleep disturbance. Insomnia deserves to be considered as an *entity* only insofar as it may be a final common symptom pathway, which is triggered by a wide variety of arousing influences. Each condition in the DIMS grouping is marked by one or more distinctive features, allowing the use of a "logic tree" scheme of differentiation to locate a particular disorder among the group.

In considering the differential diagnosis of a DIMS, it is particularly useful to pay close attention to the distribution of wakefulness during the night: Is the difficulty in crossing the threshold into sleep, in repeated disruptions of sleep throughout its course, or in foreshortening of morning sleep? Whereas anxiety syndromes and situational disturbances frequently inhibit the capacity to fall asleep, endogenous depression generally exerts itself in awakenings that are increasingly more insistent after half to two-thirds of the normal nocturnal sleep period has transpired.

Organic insomnias often mimic the psychologically related sleep disturbances, particularly the sleep maintenance (middle) type of DIMS. They rarely cause *only* premature A.M. awakenings. However, some myoclonus and central apnea presentations, especially in young adults with mild, almost subdiagnostic, manifestations, are indistinguishable from classical "inability to fall asleep" (sleep onset) situational DIMS.

B. DOES, OR DISORDERS OF EXCESSIVE SOMNOLENCE. The disorders of excessive somnolence are a varied group of functional and organic conditions in which the chief symptoms may include one or all of the following: inappropriate and undesirable sleepiness during waking hours, decreased cognitive and motor performance, increase in actual tendency to sleep, unavoidable napping, increase in total 24-hour sleep, and difficulty in achieving full arousal on awakening. This category is heavily dominated by narcolepsy and obstructive upper airway syndrome (apnea). The fact that most of the pathological events occurring in sleep which cause excessive daytime sleepiness are *not* in the patient's awareness cannot be emphasized too greatly.

C. DISORDERS OF THE SLEEP-WAKE SCHEDULE. This category of disorders is composed of a collection of clinical syndromes, some exogeneously instigated and others, such as delayed sleep phase, apparently having an endogeneous contribution. These conditions warrant grouping as a separate cluster because of a shared, cardinal feature—every disorder represents one form or another of *misalignment* between the 24-hour, clock-time organization of an individual's behavioral sleep and wake periods and his internal circadian rhythm. Normally, most of our fundamental physiologic activities (e.g., hormone production, body temperature, brain metabolism) systematically conform in their circadian patterns to our regular, 24-hour, behavioral sleep-wake periodicity to which the physiologic oscillations have been recruited. When the behavioral periodicity alters, the internal rhythms attempt to readapt to the new pattern.

In two conditions, delayed sleep phase and advanced sleep phase, the misalignment is not between the sleep-wake behaviors of the individual and his own established internal periodicities (they remain aligned), but rather between the individual's behavioral/physiologic, circadian phase relationship, now slipped by three to six hours, and the conventional environmental pattern. For example, a premedical student with delayed sleep phase sleeps routinely from four A.M. to 12 noon and misses most morning classes. The student's problem is not in his physiologic mechanisms of sleep and waking *per se* so much as in the mismatch between his circadian placement of sleep (four A.M. to noon) and the pattern that is usual and necessary in his environment. To put it plainly, his sleep schedule disturbance is inhospitable to his required chemistry class, which begins at 8 A.M.

Unfortunately, sleep schedule disturbances are not proclaimed to the doctor as such. The patient usually complains of being either unable to sleep when he wants or to be awake and functioning when he wants. These complaints are less than routinely recognized for what they are and are usually interpreted and treated as an insomnia problem.

D. DYSFUNCTION ASSOCIATED WITH SLEEP, SLEEP STAGES, AND PARTIAL AROUSALS (PARASOMNIAS). The parasomnias are a group of clinical conditions that, like sleep schedule disorders, are not pathologies of the actual processes that support the sleep and wake states. Rather, they are physical phenomena that are undesirable with respect to sleep. They either appear exclusively in sleep (e.g., somnambulism) or are exacerbated by sleep (e.g., asthma, gastroesophageal reflux). These phenomena are, in the main, manifestations of atypical CNS activation during sleep discharged either into the skeletal musculature or into channels of autonomic activity. Table 2 outlines some of these conditions.

Sleep Classification and Psychiatric Diagnosis

The ASDC nosology is a categorization only of types of sleep pathology. It was not advanced as a substitute nosology for the many discrete psychologic and psychiatric states that are delineated in classifications of psychiatric disorders; in fact, it deals only with the psychopathologies known to be associated with sleep derangements.

The sleep syndromes in the ASDC classification which are linked to psychophysiologic/psychiatric conditions constitute a relatively small group of sleep abnormalities. Disturbances of sleep take fewer forms than the manifold types of emotional states that cause sleep disturbance. Each and every psychopathology does not cause a unique DIMS; in fact, one PSG type is common to several psychopathologic, drug, and organic conditions.

On the other hand, though it does not credit the existence of a sleep disturbance as *prima facie* evidence of an emotional disorder, the sleep classification system indisputably affirms, with the first two subcategories of DIMS and DOES, the psychiatric sources of sleeplessness and excessive sleepiness. The nosology encourages exploration of all the psychologic and organic mechanisms under consideration of insomnia as well as estimation of their relative weights in each case of insomnia. Multiple diagnoses for sleep disorders are used in the ASDC classification because more than one of either or both organic and mental factors may be part of the symptom story. This approach is parallel to the use of the multiaxial diagnostic system in *DSM-III*.

The ASDC manual prescribes the rendering of a *DSM-III* diagnosis whenever psychopathology is present, which would not be detailed adequately by the appropriate sleep disorder category. To illustrate, the subcategory DIMS associated with Affective Disorder is the only diagnosis slot available for an insomnia disorder related primarily to depressive (or manic) psychopathology. The psychopathology requires much greater delineation, which must be accomplished by co-classifying the depression with the suitable *DSM-III* or *ICD-9* category. Having secondary and tertiary ASDC diagnoses helps. Accordingly, a patient with DIMS due to Alcoholism may also be recognized and coded secondarily to take note of a longstanding obsessional syndrome.

In summary, the ASDC Classification of Sleep and Arousal Disorders prompts the physician to consider psychologic factors in the diagnosis of insomnia. A *DSM-III* diagnosis, which will help to specify the psychopathology, should be made conjointly with the appropriate designation of sleep pathology. Alone, however, the *DSM-III* diagnosis may be relevant to psychiatric status but not in all cases to the cause of the sleep disorder.

Multi-Center Case Series Studies

Specialists and practitioners have been able to learn and apply ASDC criteria for discrimination among disorders. This workability of the ASDC nosology is documented in two multi-center case series studies (Coleman et al, 1982; Coleman, 1983), which yielded virtually identical overall incidences of the conditions evaluated and recorded in sleep disorders centers.

In general, the disorders of excessive somnolence (DOES) comprised 50 percent of all patients seeking help (Figure 1). This percentage, however, does not reflect the relative prevalence of insomnia in the population, probably because of the more pressing nature of the excessive sleepiness disability and its cardiovascular sequelae, and the lesser tendency for physicians to refer patients with insomnia to sleep centers. Figure 2 shows that the combined proportion of psychophysiological and psychiatrically related insomnias averaged about half of all the DIMS patients studied. Only a small proportion of sleep laboratory studies done

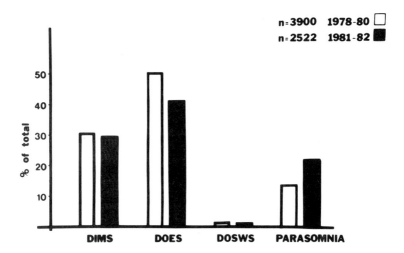

Figure 1. Summary of overall diagnostic categories for sleep-wake disorder patients (not including nocturnal penile tumescence cases). See text for explanation of the categories. From "Diagnosis, Treatment and Follow-up of About 8,000 Sleep/Wake Disorder Patients," by R.M. Coleman, in Sleep/Wake Disorders: Natural History, Epidemiology, and Long-Term Evolution. Edited by C. Guilleminault and E. Lugaresi. Copyright © 1983 by Raven Press. Reprinted by permission of Raven Press.

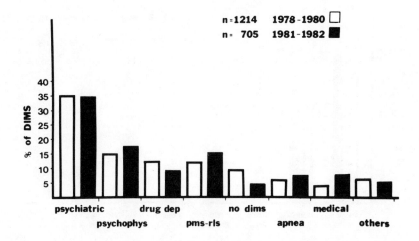

Figure 2. Differential diagnosis of DIMS (Insomnia). *Psychophys*—persistent psychophysiological DIMS, Ala; *Drug Dep*—use of drugs and alcohol, A3; *PMS—RLS*—periodic movements in sleep (nocturnal myoclonus) and "restless legs" syndrome, A5; *No DIMS*—comprises subjective insomnia complaint without objective findings and short sleeper, A9; *Apnea*—comprises mostly central apnea and hypopnea, and some mild obstructive conditions, A4; *Medical*—comprises other medical, toxic, and environmental conditions, A6; *Others*—comprises childhood onset DIMS, A7, repeated REM sleep interruptions, A8a, and atypical PSG features, A8b. From "Diagnosis, Treatment and Follow-up of About 8,000 Sleep/Wake Disorder Patients," by R.M. Coleman, in Sleep/Wake Disorders: Natural History, Epidemiology, and Long-Term Evolution. Edited by C. Guilleminault and E. Lugaresi. Copyright © 1983 by Raven Press. Reprinted by permission of Raven Press.

on patients presenting with excessive daytime sleepiness explored complaints considered to be due to psychological or psychiatric problems (see Figure 3). Narcolepsy and obstructive sleep apnea clearly predominate (about 75 percent of total) among the DOES syndromes.

Reliability and Validity of the Diagnostic System

There have been no methodologically flawless reliability and validity studies of the new sleep nosology. However, general agreement prevails, except in one quarter (see Kales JD et al, 1982), that the Diagnostic Classification of Sleep and Arousal Disorders is a successful system; physicians who face the task of diagnosing patients with sleep disorders claim that, with few exceptions, they are able to find a specific descriptive designation for every condition.

With respect to diagnostic reliability, the results of the first two multi-center case series studies of the ASDC, comprising 3,900 and 2,522 patients, respectively (Coleman et al, 1982; Coleman, 1983), show good stability of the diagnoses nationally in the two populations from more than 20 different centers. It is important to keep in mind that the first survey was carried out when the nosological system was first being used in many centers; the classification was only two years old at the start of the second case series. The chief reason, however, for some apparent discrepancies between centers in terms of the frequency of certain diagnoses is the specialization of certain centers for DIMS or DOES conditions in general (Coleman et al, 1982).

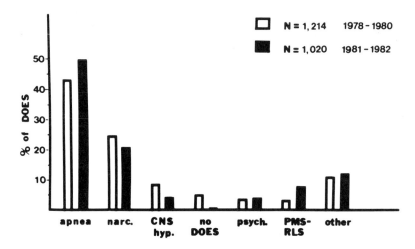

Figure 3. Differential diagnosis in DOES (hypersomnia). *Apnea*—mainly obstructive apnea and hypopnea, B4; *Narc*—narcolepsy, B6; *CNS hyp*—idiopathic central nervous system hypersomnia, B7, includes the non-narcoleptic hypersomnia variants; *No DOES*—comprises long sleeper and subjective DOES complaint without objective findings, A10; *Psych*— comprises both psychophysiological, B1, and psychiatric-associated DOES, B2; *PMS-RLS*— see Figure 2; *Other*—comprises use of drugs and alcohol, B3; and other DOES conditions, B9, including the periodic hypersomnia, insufficient sleep syndrome, sleep drunkenness. From "Diagnosis, Treatment and Follow-up of About 8,000 Sleep/Wake Disorder Patients," by R.M. Coleman, in Sleep/Wake Disorders: Natural History, Epidemiology, and Long-Term Evolution. Edited by C. Guilleminault and E. Lugaresi. Copyright © 1983 by Raven Press. Reprinted by permission of Raven Press.

In summary, the ASDC sleep disorders classification works because it is criterion-based and is open to reliability and validity assessments grounded in data (see Reynolds et al, 1981; Hauri, 1983; Zorick et al, 1981, 1982; Coleman et al, 1982; Coleman, 1983). However, like *DSM-III*, the sleep nosology is a working, descriptive system that has invited and predicted changes in its own composition in response to data.

WHAT STANCE FOR THE PRACTITIONER REGARDING INSOMNIA MANAGEMENT?

As we have seen, the office physician is vulnerable to overestimations of sleeplessness in one to two out of every ten nonorganic patients. He also cannot be expected to pick up any clues to concealed, organic insomnia conditions in another three out of every ten patients with insomnia complaints (Roffwarg et al, 1982).

Physicians are always tempted to carry out major tests on every patient and every symptom, yet most become aware of the impracticality of this course. Though distressed at times over diagnostic uncertainties, the experienced doctor learns the value of using good clinical judgment. The technique of therapeutic ·trial, with frequent follow-up, represents a time-honored medical strategy aimed at obtaining useful etiological information while attempting to provide therapeutic relief of symptoms.

The clinician has much more latitude in dealing with insomnia in which the periods of disturbed sleep are transient or of short duration (a few days to three weeks). These are likely to be either actual but self-remitting bouts of psychologically related insomnia or the consequence of temporary physical illnesses. With longer-term insomnia pictures, however, the complaints that do *not* either reflect true insomnia disorders or constitute organic problems tend to be unresponsive to general insomnia treatments (allowing for brief improvements as each new course is begun). Ultimately, after repeated treatment failures, additional diagnostic work-up is warranted.

Organic pathologies are more frequent in older people, so therapists should not wait too long to obtain a sleep work-up if the insomnia is unresponsive. But, as in younger patients, the practitioner may choose first to try general therapies.

In the initial stage of evaluating a long-term insomnia, the physician should base therapeutic interventions on the statistical likelihood that the insomnia is due to one of the following: poor sleep hygiene (including use of drugs or alcohol), chronic stress, psychiatric problems, or self-fulfilling problems (negative conditioning to sleep).

Briefly, a first step is to withdraw drugs and alcohol slowly; supervise sleep hygiene; schedule regular bedtimes and waking times with the advice and cooperation of the patient; and, a bit later, if indicated, recommend a course of biofeedback/relaxation or some other behavioral or retraining therapy. There is relatively little harm, alternatively, in trying a *temporary* course of a short-acting, benzodiazepine hypnotic so long as the physician receives adequate feedback from the patient within two weeks. These measures may sometimes be astonishingly successful, and their effects are also heuristically valuable.

In cases in which situational or psychological issues are prominent, psychiatric evaluation is indispensible. Depending on the nature of the problem, treatments such as stress reduction, psychotropic drugs for target psychiatric symptoms, and/or short-term psychotherapy for conflict resolution or support should be used.

If the patient-appropriate modalities of treatment just mentioned have been used with no effect on the patient's sleep disturbance, or if the sleep-related symptoms persist despite successful psychiatric therapy, referral to a sleep center is advisable for further evaluation of a possibly unrecognized cause of insomnia.

SLEEP DISORDERS OF CONCERN TO PSYCHIATRISTS

In the next several pages, the sleep disorders of leading interest to psychiatrists will be selectively reviewed.

It is worth clarifying that, although not all insomnia complaints prove to be insomnia disorders, it is equally true that not all insomnia-presenting sleep disorders appear in the ASDC Classification under DIMS: Disorders of Initiating and Maintaining Sleep. This is because the DIMS category is reserved for conditions that are primarily responsible for inducing disturbed or insufficient sleep. The disorders that will be mentioned now cause other pathology primarily along with insomnia, or only apparently cause insomnia as part of a sleep-wake schedule disturbance. Putting aside transient and short periods of disturbed sleep, the non-insomnia disorders that seem to the patient and are presented to the physician as insomnia are (from ASDC nosology, sections B, C, and D): delayed and advanced sleep-phase syndromes and all other persistent disorders of the sleep-wake schedule, sleep-related epilepsy, gastroesophageal reflux, and other parasomnias, such as bruxism, which may secondarily disturb sleep.

The non-insomnia disorders that may present as insomnia as well as the organic insomnia disorders that are frequently offered by patients as a "stress or psychological problem" may be assembled into a list of conditions that can "masquerade" as functional insomnia (see Table 3). The practitioner will not be able to identify the first four "conditions" without laboratory assistance. Whether the sleep problem is apparent or real, the risk of a patient's developing a secondary psychiatric problem is much greater than in the normally sleeping population.

The chronic sleepiness of narcolepsy convinces many individuals with that disorder (and many psychiatrists until recently) that psychological reasons explain their "withdrawals." If the patients do not feel that way, many of their family members and co-workers do. Accordingly, when a sleepiness syndrome or a DIMS is unremitting, a sleep laboratory work-up, in helping to clarify what is truly wrong, helps the patient to "identify" the problem.

Table 3. Conditions That by History Alone Are Frequently Mistaken for Psychologically Related Disorders of Initiating and Maintaining Sleep (DIMS)

- Subjective DIMS Complaint With No Objective Findings
- Sleep Apnea DIMS Syndrome (Central Apnea)
- Sleep-related (Nocturnal) Myoclonus
- Atypical Polysomnographic Features (Alpha Sleep)

The following conditions may also be mistaken but can usually be correctly identified through careful history of patient's sleep pattern, drug intake, and medical status:

- Short Sleeper
- Advanced Sleep Phase
- Delayed Sleep Phase
- Irregular Sleep-Wake Pattern
- Non-24-Hour Sleep-Wake Syndrome
- Secondary Depression
- Sustained Use of Stimulant Drugs, Alcohol, or Sleeping Pills
- Sustained Use of Medical Drugs
  (e.g., thyroid, chemotherapeutic agents, antimetabolites, oral contraceptives, propranolol, nasal sprays, decongestants, theophylline)
- Other Medical Conditions
  (e.g., gastroesophageal reflux, sleep epilepsy, sleep-related cardiovascular symptoms, incipient dementia, endocrine and metabolic diseases, hypoglycemia, nutritional disorders, food allergies)

DIMS: Disorders of Initiating and Maintaining Sleep (Insomnias)

TRANSIENT, SHORT-TERM AND SITUATIONAL PSYCHOPHYSIOLOGI-CAL DIMS. This is the category of insomnia that is seen most frequently in the general population and by the practicing psychiatrist. The *transient* type refers to sleep disturbances of one to several days, whereas *short-term* corresponds to insomnia lasting less than three weeks. The former is provoked, for example, by jet lag or brief hospitalizations; the transient and short-term may both arise from emotional arousal or conflict caused by loss or perceived threat.

This insomnia is typically seen during periods of interpersonal or intrapsychic conflict, preceding major life changes (marriage, divorce, birth of a child), in the course of intense job or career demands, or following sudden disappointments and frightening events. The disturbances may present with any combination of sleep disruptions such as difficulty falling asleep, intermittent awakenings, and premature early morning arousal (notably when a depressive component is present). The patients have a history of preceding normal sleep. The insomnia may recur when the susceptible individual again experiences a threshold level of stress.

This usually unambiguous, real sleep disturbance may be viewed as an "insomnia of everyday life," expectable and predictable considering the many possibilities for emotional upsurge from which few people can shield themselves completely in the course of a lifetime. However, individuals who are insecure and vulnerable to emotional arousal are most frequently and severely affected. In them, the frequency and severity of sleep disruption can reach the level of a serious clinical problem requiring intervention.

PERSISTENT PSYCHOPHYSIOLOGICAL DIMS. This condition is usually at least two months in duration, more typically many months or years. This source of sleep disturbance has gained considerable notice among medical sleep disorders specialists. Though psychologists have long recognized the influence of conditioning on sleep (Bootzin and Nicassio, 1978), psychiatrists have been relatively unaware of it in the formal sense, preferring to think of insomnia as caused by conflict and emotional excess. However, the shared awareness that insomnia has a tendency to "feed itself" fits well in a conditioning model.

This diagnosis requires understanding as a condition. Its increasing use relates to our sudden recognition that the conditioning component of this insomnia is an independent element that may become "attached" to almost any other insomnia, including the psychiatric group. This process constitutes the mechanism of long-term entrenchment of insomnia (Hauri, 1982).

The linkage of emotional excess, either covert or overt, and sleep disturbance is so well established that it is no longer open to question. The sequence of emotional upset leading to insomnia is likely to be the purest representation available of the influence of mental events on neurophysiology. However, after annotating the psychiatrically classifiable conditions associated with insomnia, there remains a sizable group of patients without organic DIMS conditions who are also not subject to severe or well-defined psychopathological categorization. They also do not sleep well. The persistent psychophysiological DIMS diagnosis encompasses this population and describes a specific kind of behavioral-pathophysiological combination of elements.

Before diagnosing persistent psychophysiological DIMS, however, clinicians should exclude a classifiable psychiatric disorder. Patients with a persistent psychophysiological DIMS are more the "high tension" type, lacking subjectively perceived anxiety and tending to somaticize their inner emotionality or perceived stress. Persistent psychophysiological DIMS should be reserved for people who do not demonstrate generalized anxiety syndromes, phobic disorder, obsessive-compulsive disorder, major or minor depression, or other clinically diagnosable psychiatric states. Yet they persist in a sleep disturbance without organic explanation. Why?

The hallmark of this DIMS syndrome is the focused absorption of the patient *on the sleep problem itself*. They tend to minimize other mental/emotional concerns. Consequently, this DIMS disorder is rather fixed. It does not vary with the waxing and waning of emotion as with other psychologically induced sleeplessness. The patients show good family and work relationships and functioning, not the general maladaptive behavior of the conventional psychiatric patient.

Due to the self-fulfilling disintegration in confidence that one *can* sleep and corresponding development of apprehension about sleeping may reinforce an earlier tendency of these patients to sleep poorly. The insomnia may become persistent under these circumstances and takes on "a life of its own." The patient develops a virtual "neurosis" about the *process* of sleeping. These patients continually make great efforts to sleep when lying in bed, unaware of the arousing effect of the concentrated trying. They become overanticipatory about sleeping, and, though last to realize it because they consciously so wish to sleep, the patients develop a negative expectation (an internal conditioning factor) that they will sleep in their bedrooms. The bedroom (an external conditioning factor), in fact, often becomes associated with the difficulty in sleeping, and the patient paradoxically sleeps better in other rooms of the house and away from his home, whereas normal sleepers routinely report sleeping worse away from their customary sleep environments.

Persistent psychophysiological DIMS patients sleep better than any other individuals in the sleep laboratory, an experience that always embarrasses them, for they believe the staff will see them as "subjective only" patients who do not really have a problem. But, unlike the latter, they are well aware of times when they sleep poorly *or* well and are quite accurate in their estimates. They tend to sleep better in any situation in which they are not expecting to sleep and/or are relieved of trying.

Anxious, obsessional, or depressed patients, if they consult their feelings, know *why* they do not sleep; the psychophysiological DIMS patient typically claims to have *no idea* why he does not sleep. This is because conditioning factors responsible for poor sleep are not experienced subjectively. The tendency not to sleep, however, emerges every time the patient is in a situation associated with earlier sleep difficulties. These patients do tend to experience tension, if not frank anxiety, and are prone to somatization.

Persistent psychophysiological DIMS is the only diagnosis in the ASDC Classification of Sleep and Arousal Disorders that explicitly takes conditioning phenomena into account. It gives these subtle but tenacious shapers of our behavior and feelings a deserved place of importance in explaining the development of a unique type of chronic insomnia. The diagnosis of persistent psychophysiological DIMS should be used when insomnia-reinforcing mechanisms, such as apprehensive overconcern in relation to trying to sleep or to insufficient sleep, are strongly represented in the patient's history.

The diagnosis of persistent psychophysiological DIMS does not preclude additional psychological characterization of the patient when indicated; rather, it can be part of a multiple diagnostic assessment of an insomnia disorder. For example, patients who worry about not being able to sleep ("Doctor, believe me, I kneel down and pray every night that I'll sleep.") also may be, for example, mildly depressed, or use small amounts of drugs and alcohol. However, persistent psychophysiological DIMS is basically an insomnia arising primarily from overattention to the process of sleeping and excessive, worried attempts to sleep.

How does the clinician decide whether an insomnia is more fundamentally associated with a chronic depression that is largely "masked" or better explained by persistent psychophysiological DIMS? The discrimination may not be simple, but it usually can be made by considering somatic symptoms of depression (in the absence of sadness): recent life events that predictably lead to depression; a pattern of sleeplessness featuring early morning arousability; the finding that depression, though covert, was a *first event* rather than a reaction to the frustrations of poor sleep and resultant fatigue; and biological correlates of depression such as short REM latency and dexamethasone nonsuppression.

DIMS ASSOCIATED WITH PSYCHIATRIC DISORDERS. A number of psychiatric illnesses are patently correlated with sleep complaints. Of great interest to the psychiatrist and sleep researcher alike are the depressive disorders. Without question, depression accounts for the greatest incidence of chronic insomnia so that sleep centers are on the alert to apprehend it in all its forms and gradations.

From the clinical perspective, depressed patients may present with several specific sleep complaints—hypersomnia in the depressed bipolar patient, difficulty falling asleep (relatively less likely), fragmented and unrefreshing sleep, and early morning awakening (more likely in the unipolar patient). The relationship of depressive and nondepressive psychiatric disorders to sleep variables is discussed in more detail in succeeding chapters of this section.

Insomnia complaints are also frequently seen in patients with generalized anxiety disorders, panic and phobic disorders, hypochondriasis, obsessive-compulsive disorders, and several types of personality disorders in which suppressed or repressed anger or anxiety probably play leading roles.

DIMS ASSOCIATED WITH USE OF DRUGS AND ALCOHOL. The psychiatrist has considerable contact with these problems. Drugs and alcohol have negative influences on sleep in several ways. Insomnia associated with the chronic use of barbiturates and similar types of hypnotic drugs (Kales et al, 1979) and of alcohol (Adamson and Burdick, 1973; Gross and Hastey, 1975) has been recognized for some time, as having minor and major withdrawal syndromes associated with physiologic habituation to these agents. Interrupted sleep may also be seen in association with sustained use or withdrawal from other drugs that influence the sleep cycle, including cancer chemotherapeutic agents, thyroid preparations, anticonvulsants, opiates, and hallucinogens.

The sustained use of stimulant agents understandably may disrupt sleep. Patients using these types of drugs may not inform physicians of their drug use, or may not recognize the negative influence that the drug has on sleep maintenance. Whereas a thorough medical history and physical examination may suggest the presence of such a problem, it may, on occasion, be necessary to use toxicologic screens of blood or urine to confirm occult drug use with absolute certainty. The sleep EEG also sensitively detects drug use by displaying 16-18 Hz and 20-22 Hz bands prominently.

SLEEP-INDUCED RESPIRATORY IMPAIRMENT. The propensity of respiratory disturbances to interrupt sleep has already been reviewed. Sleep apnea syndromes are most frequently associated with complaints of excessive sleepiness, especially in patients with predominant obstructive and mixed apnea disturbances. However, apnea (cessation of breathing) and hypopnea (hypoventilation) of the central type (disturbances of ventilatory drive and frequency) may be occult causes of disturbed nocturnal sleep. The impairment in ventilatory drive need not be complete, and hypopneas also can lead to sufficient falls in oxygen saturation to evoke arousals on a frequent and recurrent basis throughout the night. As mentioned, the central apnea/hypopnea patient is often unaware of his respiratory problems because he breathes without difficulty when awake. The interrupted snoring so characteristic of the obstructive apneic patient may be less severe but rarely entirely absent. Central apnea usually is worst in REM sleep because the hypercapnic respiratory (elevated CO_2) drive is suspended during that stage. As a result, interruptions in breathing are longer in REM sleep and falls in oxygen are lower than in NREM stages. The severity of central apnea is increased by alcohol use. In patients with cardiac problems, the falls in oxygen may provoke nocturnal arrhythmias and elevation in blood pressure, but these effects are less frequently seen than in obstructive apnea.

Some patients with obstructive sleep apnea may also present with predominant complaints of disturbed nocturnal sleep. In the early stages of the disorder, before sleepiness becomes overwhelming, some of the nocturnal awakenings can be remembered. In some cases, individuals who are aware of their obstructive apnea and frightened of the possible health consequences of this disorder have a secondary insomnia due to forcing themselves to remain awake at night, despite their sleepiness.

NOCTURNAL MYOCLONUS AND "RESTLESS LEGS" SYNDROME. These disorders both fragment nocturnal sleep but are often not fully recognized or appreciated by the patient. Restless legs syndrome derives from a disagreeable sensory phenomenon in the legs which patients experience as they sit still for any period of time or lie down at night. They report an almost irresistible urge to move their legs about in order to relieve the sensation. When symptoms occur at bedtime, they interfere with sleep onset.

Nocturnal myoclonus is a syndrome of repetitive, stereotyped leg muscle jerks of variable duration and frequency during the night, not associated with disagreeable leg sensations and most often not remembered. Usually, the episodes occur with a frequency of 20 to 40 seconds for several minutes to an hour or more at a time (see Figure 4). These periods occur repetitively during the night. The degree of arousability associated with each myoclonic episode is variable; however, in most patients, sleep is continually disrupted. Even if frank awak-

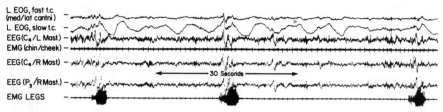

L EOG, fast t.c.
(med/lat cantni)
L EOG, slow t.c.
EEG(C₄/L Mast.)
EMG (chin/cheek)

EEG(C₄/R Mast)

EEG (P₃/R Mast.)
EMG LEGS

30 Seconds

Figure 4. Sleep-related (nocturnal) myoclonus. Approximately 90 seconds of a continuous polysomnographic record, showing characteristic myoclonic leg jerks in an insomnia complainer, occurring semirhythmically every 20 to 40 seconds.

enings do not occur in association with every myoclonic episode, consolidation and depth of sleep suffer; and sleep is perceived as light, broken, and restless.

Information obtained from a spouse or other bed partner is often helpful concerning the presence of myoclonic twitching in an insomnia complainer. The partner's sleep may be disturbed as much as the sleep of the patient. These disorders account diagnostically for ten to 15 percent of all the investigated complaints (Coleman, 1983).

Antidepressant and anticonvulsive medications and sleep medications in withdrawal excite exacerbations of nocturnal myoclonus.

MEDICAL, TOXIC AND ENVIRONMENTAL DIMS. A host of medical, toxic, and environmental conditions are associated with objective disturbances of sleep. Common problems in this group include acute or chronic pain, hyperthyroidism, shortness of breath, and persistent nocturnal cough. Rarer conditions (such as hypothyroidism, neoplasms), particularly those that influence or impair central nervous functioning, may also lead to the complaint of insomnia. An extensive survey of sources of impaired sleep is provided in the Diagnostic Classification of Sleep and Arousal Disorders (ASDC, 1979).

CHILDHOOD-ONSET DIMS. This entry was established in the ASDC nosology to characterize those individuals with a distinctive history of otherwise unexplained sleeplessness prior to puberty and persistence into adulthood. In the adult, the clinical appearance is similar to that of persistent psychophysiological DIMS, with the exception of relative absence of the conditioning factors that are closely allied with persistent psychophysiological DIMS. It is speculated that this condition may develop out of early emotional turmoil or psychological disturbance, but it is difficult to make a determination in many of the cases as to whether the insomnia was secondary to longstanding psychological difficulties or a "primary" (i.e., constitutional) insomnia. In these patients, sleep difficulties tend to remain relatively constant, as in persistent psychophysiological DIMS and in the organically caused insomnias, during periods of both poor and good emotional adaptation. Childhood DIMS patients are often resistant to treatment, suggesting that their longstanding symptoms may reflect a CNS dysfunction of sleep-arousal mechanisms.

REPEATED REM SLEEP INTERRUPTIONS. Much less frequent than originally anticipated, this condition is one of recurrent selective arousals from REM sleep. These awakenings often occur about 90 minutes after sleep onset, during the first REM sleep period, and recur in rhythmic fashion in each later REM period of the night. Patients do not usually report the type of dysphoric or frightening dream content seen in dream anxiety attacks (nightmares) and may not be aware that these awakenings are occurring from dreaming sleep. At other times, these patients have experienced the conventional periods of disturbing dreams or nightmares. The REM sleep interruptions that develop may represent a learned avoidance of nightmares, with progression to a fixed sleep continuity insomnia. In this obvious conditioning, the parallels to persistent psychophysiological DIMS are obvious.

ATYPICAL POLYSOMNOGRAPHIC FEATURES (ALPHA SLEEP). In Atypical polysomnographic features, sleep is experienced as interrupted and nonrestorative by the patient, who may or may not have psychopathology. Key to the disorder are the associated, unusual, or abnormal polysomnographic findings. The most common of these conditions is alpha sleep, characterized by the presence of alpha (high voltage) waves that are superimposed on the NREM sleep EEG and persist all through sleep. REM sleep is usually spared. Some segments of sleep unaccountably show relative sparing of this alpha "riddling."

These patients typically report being fatigued and insufficiently rested during the day. They describe their sleep as unrefreshing, and, although sleep duration in alpha sleep tends to be within normal limits, the patients may seriously underestimate the amount of sleep actually obtained. This may be because the alpha activity gives the sleeper the "sense" of continuous vigilance. This diagnosis is used only if alpha sleep persists after a prolonged period of abstinence from drug or alcohol use, which may cause alpha sleep in withdrawal periods.

Another type of atypical polysomnographic feature is low sleep spindle activity, observed in an appreciable number of otherwise situational DIMS.

NO DIMS ABNORMALITY. Two types of patients may be given this diagnosis. Subjective DIMS Complaint Without Objective Findings is used to describe the individuals who attest to severe insomnia but in whom the narrative is not supported in sleep studies. Polysomnography reveals relatively normal sleep length, architecture, and physiology. Nevertheless, the patient's subjective perception of sleep is that it is as disturbed in the laboratory as at home. This condition is a significant cause of overdiagnosis of insomnia and has already been discussed.

Short sleepers require less sleep in a 24-hour period than is conventional or assumed for individuals their age. Their sleep, though short, is unbroken and normal. No true complaints regarding sleep quality or daytime functioning exist. Rather, these people can be unhappy about being up alone, and may express concern about the amount of sleep they are obtaining based on myths or commonly held expectations about "normal" sleep needs. The short sleeper category of no DIMS abnormality is reserved for individuals whose regular pattern of nighttime sleep totals less than 75 percent of the amount typically seen for their age group.

DOES: Disorders of Excessive Somnolence

PSYCHOPHYSIOLOGICAL DOES. Unlike its counterpart in the DIMS group, psychophysiological DOES is not frequently diagnosed. It is associated with some degree of psychopathology but generally not to such an extent that a *DSM-III* psychiatric diagnosis is appropriate. The transient episodes, which may be compared to periods of conservation-withdrawal, are characterized by professed drowsiness and a tendency to remain in bed or return to bed frequently during the day. The pattern begins suddenly and is a response to an identifiable life change, conflict, or loss. Although total sleep time may increase somewhat at the onset of such a reaction, actual extension of sleep over a long period has not been documented and is not expected to be a feature of this reaction. Psychophysiological DOES lasts for less than three weeks. It is not clear whether this "condition" has sufficient independent validity to be differentiated adequately from minor depressive reaction.

Such reactions may develop into a *persistent* complaint characterized by reports of chronic weariness, excessive sleeping, and daytime napping while under stress. They are not associated with *objective* findings of increased sleep. Some patients with depleted, "neurasthenic" personality features may be appropriately placed in this diagnostic category, although they may present with predominant complaints of disturbed nocturnal sleep and daytime fatigue.

DOES ASSOCIATED WITH PSYCHIATRIC DISORDERS. These syndromes of daytime sleepiness are reviewed in Chapters 16, 17 and 18. One important point should be made here, however. Patients with bipolar depression who are hypersomnic rarely, if ever, show the degree of "major league" sleepiness and daytime sleep behavior characteristic of the leading DOES syndromes: narcolepsy, obstructive apnea, and drug ingestion.

DOES ASSOCIATED WITH USE OF DRUGS AND ALCOHOL. Hypersomnia complaints may also be related to drugs and alcohol. Stimulant medications, taken over a protracted period of time, may lead to a degree of physiological dependence or habituation. When this occurs, tolerance to or withdrawal from these drugs may lead to such complaints as daytime sleepiness, sleep "attacks," impaired arousal from sleep, and extended nocturnal sleep periods. While such tolerance is most likely to occur in drug abusers who have used medications over long periods of time, it may also be seen in individuals who take stimulant or appetite-suppressant agents only under medical supervision. Hypersomnia complaints, which are less severe and shorter in duration, may be seen in association with mini-withdrawals—"crashing"—when lower doses of stimulant medication are taken on an infrequent or intermittent basis.

Sustained use of medications with CNS suppressant effects may also be associated with hypersomnia complaints. Whereas the drug-abusing population is at high risk for this symptom—the "nodding off" heroin addict perhaps being the prime example—patients may also develop DOES symptoms when using drugs for therapeutic purposes, even while under medical supervision. Medications commonly prescribed by psychiatrists which frequently lead to such complaints include sleeping medications, anti-anxiety drugs, tricyclic and reserpine antidepressants, and antihistamine compounds. Ethanol is the most widely used substance leading to hypersomnia complaints (Renner, 1978).

SLEEP-INDUCED RESPIRATORY IMPAIRMENT (OBSTRUCTIVE APNEA). Disturbances in nocturnal respiration are an important cause of daytime hypersomnia. Obstructive sleep apnea has only in recent years been appreciated as a significant medical disturbance as well as frequent cause of excessive sleepiness. Virtually all patients with significant degrees of obstructive apnea will report a longstanding history of loud, continuous snoring. Though they may not be aware of the significance of the apneic pauses (interruptions in breathing during which snoring is absent), spouses or family members are quick to report "gasping, choking, snorting" breakthroughs for air concurrent with brief arousals.

Most such patients are moderately obese and have hypertrophied oro- and hypopharangeal structures, but relatively few have a classic Pickwickian habitus or retain CO_2 during waking hours. The vast majority of apnea patients are men, and most are over the age of 50. Some patients are at or below a normal weight for their height. When significant apnea is seen in a thin individual—young adult, child, or woman—some degree of pathology of the upper airway is likely. This can include hypertrophic tonsils and adenoids, a low-set palatal rim or webbing (almost back to the posterior pharangeal wall), large uvula, large tongue (macroglossia), small and retro-set mandible, and a number of other anatomic abnormalities.

It is uncommon that a patient with substantial obstructive upper airway syndrome will not report *extreme and inappropriate daytime sleepiness*, though he or she may deny the severity of the problem. An overweight, snoring, hypertensive patient is at risk for obstructive apnea. Serious medical complications of the apnea develop if the syndrome persists for too long. These include pulmonary and systemic hypertension; congestive heart failure (corpulmonale); cardiac arrhythmias of various types (including runs of premature ventricular contractions and ventricular tachycardia); sinus arrests; impairments in memory, attention, and cognition; impotence; and changes in emotional regulation, such as irritability, emotional lability, and depression.

The dramatic health consequences and degree of functional impairment that obstructive apnea patients endure may explain why they make up the single largest group of patients presenting at sleep disorders centers (Coleman, 1983). The pathogenesis of this disorder probably relates both to significant disruption of nocturnal sleep associated with repetitive, continuous apneas throughout the night (and recurring from as low a frequency as ten episodes per hour to as many as 1,000 episodes in a single night) as well as to the resulting brain anoxia. Despite the severe nature of this disturbance, marked improvement and even complete cure may be accomplished through medical and/or surgical therapies.
NOCTURNAL MYOCLONUS. This disorder, discussed in the DIMS section, may also lead predominantly to hypersomnia complaints, with varying degrees of objective sleepiness. As is the case with the DIMS complainers, patients may be unaware of the presence or severity of their nocturnal myoclonic disturbance.
NARCOLEPSY. Narcolepsy is the flagship DOES syndrome about which physicians are most knowledgeable. It makes up the second largest group of patients presenting to sleep disorders centers for evaluation of hypersomnia complaints. The classic tetrad of excessive sleepiness, cataplexy, sleep paralysis, and hypnagogic imagery is often, but not always, seen. Cataplexy is a unique and characteristic feature of narcolepsy. When the patient describes cataplectic attacks of muscular weakness, typically triggered by expressions of emotion such as laughter or anger, the probability is very good that the diagnosis is narcolepsy.

Narcolepsy is now understood as a physiological disturbance, seen in mammalian species other than humans, and with at least a partial hereditary component. Abnormal manifestations of REM sleep account for much of the pathology of this disorder. Sleep onset REM periods may be subjectively appreciated as hypnagogic hallucinations, which may be accompanied by sleep paralysis. Dissociated REM sleep inhibition of the voluntary musculature leads to complaints of cataplexy and sleep paralysis.

This is not a rare disease; it is more frequent than chronic glomerulonephritis and is diagnosed all too slowly by the general physician. Psychiatrists may mistake the classical sleepiness in its mild, "workable" form as withdrawal, poor motivation, negativism, and hostility. The hypnagogic imagery and sleep paralysis symptoms, alone and in combination, may make for some bizarre, psychopathological-like histories. As is the case with many medical disorders, narcolepsy presents a wide range of severity, from mild cases to those that are so severe that employment is functionally impossible. Partial remissions and exacerbations occur. Sleep paralysis and hypnagogic imagery may be seen without cataplexy; cataplexy may present in isolation without other REM-associated phenomena. The presence of REM sleep onset at night or during daytime naps, an important sleep laboratory parameter, remains the most valid and reliable method available for diagnosing narcolepsy.

MEDICAL, TOXIC AND ENVIRONMENTAL CONDITIONS. Any of the above may induce hypersomnia. Although occurring relatively infrequently, conditions such as endocrine and metabolic disturbances, nutritional deficiency states, uremia, hypercapnia, liver failure, and CNS disorders (including space occupying lesions, intracranial hemorrhage, and CNS trauma or infections) should be ruled out whenever hypersomnolence, the patient's history, and physical signs arouse suspicion.

INTERMITTENT DOES (PERIODIC) SYNDROMES. Kleine-Levin syndrome and menstrual associated syndrome are rare causes of hypersomnia complaints. The bizarre nature of these disturbances may bemuse physicians into diagnosing these patients inappropriately as suffering from psychiatric disorders, despite the presence of classical symptomatology (Waller, 1984).

NO DOES ABNORMALITY. Long Sleeper, not truly a sleep disorder, is the DOES equivalent of the No DIMS, Short Sleeper. It is reserved for individuals who consistently sleep substantially more in 24 hours than is conventional for their age group. Sleep, though long, is normal in architecture and physiology. These individuals have no complaints about their sleep. In a fashion similar to the presentation of the short sleeper, they may seek evaluation because of the fear that they must be psychologically or medically abnormal. Others may believe they have a sleep disorder. As young adults, these patients regularly sleep more than nine hours per 24-hour period and may need as much as 14 hours' sleep nightly to feel alert during daytime functioning. If occupational or social demands lead to total sleep times below the individual's required amount, symptoms of insufficient sleep syndrome may occur.

SUBJECTIVE DOES COMPLAINT WITHOUT OBJECTIVE FINDINGS. This type of patient has been discussed earlier. Briefly, these patients' complaints of excessive sleepiness cannot be verified by close observation and polysomnographic studies (multiple daytime nap sleep latencies). Though most patients in this category appear sincere in their reports of hypersomnia and have no particular investment in any diagnosis or treatment regimen, some malingerers, hoping for a continuous supply of stimulant medications, report specific sleep complaints. They may even attempt to mimic REM eye movements during polysomnographic evaluation for a chance at a narcolepsy diagnosis and then medication.

Disorders of the Sleep-Wake Schedule

DELAYED SLEEP PHASE SYNDROME. Individuals with this disorder report bedtimes and rise times that are substantially later than desired, with difficulty falling asleep until even later in the night. If the patient tries to arise at "conventional" hours, he is unable fully to become alert. He feels well if able to get his "full night's" sleep, even at delayed hours (that is, 3-4 A.M.–11-12 A.M.).

This disorder is generally seen in younger patients and may be set off, in part, by work or social activities that intrude into the patient's normal sleep period. In part it may be constitutional. Susceptibility to this disorder varies, with some individuals able to tolerate regular delays in the sleep phase for several consecutive days without developing a permanently shifted sleep and wakefulness pattern. It may remain a persistent problem despite the patient's sincere efforts and desire to go to sleep at the desired sleep hour on a regular basis. This syndrome mimics sleep onset insomnia and is often treated unsuitably with drugs. A specific treatment, based on sleep-wake phase angle physiology called *chronotherapy*, is specific for the condition (Czeisler et al, 1981).

ADVANCED SLEEP PHASE SYNDROME. A disorder characterized by early sleep onset and a normal sleep length, this condition does not interfere with the work or school day, but leads to an inability to stay awake in the evening or to sleep in the morning until an hour that would be considered desired or "conventional" by most adults. This condition is rare, but can be confused with the premature morning awakening pattern of depression.

POOR SLEEP HYGIENE. Many patients with DIMS and DOES complaints do, in fact, have poor sleep hygiene, with quite irregular patterns of sleep and wakefulness which disrupt regular sleep-wake cycles and lead to diminished influence of circadian rhythmicity on sleep-wake schedules. In general, patients with these habits report frequent daytime naps at irregular times and excessive bedrest, but sleep per 24-hour period is normal for their age. Endocrine, temperature, and other circadian functions may lose much of their normally predictable nature. Clear sleep-wake rhythms are lost, and sleep is frequently broken into short blocks occurring several times per 24-hour period.

NON-24-HOUR SLEEP-WAKE SYNDROME. Rarely, individuals may have a sleep-wake schedule whose periodicity is greater than 24 hours. These patients report a pattern of *incremental* delays in sleep *and* wake times to steadily later times over successive days (the shift in Delayed Sleep Phase, once made, usually remains fixed). When the individual's internal biological rhythm is out of phase with his desired daily schedule, the chief complaint is difficulty falling asleep coupled with inability to remain awake during the day. When the cycles are in phase, there may be no complaint.

This disturbance represents the periodicity of circadian rhythms and has been studied in environments free of time cues. In these studies, which deprive subjects of awareness of time of day or of sunrise or sunset, individuals develop a "free running" pattern, with a typical periodicity of approximately 25 hours. Outside of these isolated environments, this type of pattern may be detected in blind individuals, as well as in individuals with schizoid personality who are so isolated from normal societal activity that they are no longer influenced by the types of time-associated cues that typically govern our lives.

IRREGULAR SLEEP-WAKE PATTERN. This syndrome is one of disorganized and variable sleep and waking behavior. Patients indulge in excessive bedrest and report frequent daytime naps at irregular times. Sleep at night is not of adequate length, and this condition may present with an insomnia complaint, although 24-hour sleep is normal for the patient's age. Endocrine, temperature, and other circadian function curves may also be disrupted. Various somatic complaints usually follow. The patient generally has no understanding that the sleep complaints are not the cause of the problem, but rather a result of the disordered, near-random 24-hour schedule.

The Parasomnias

Sleepwalking, sleep terrors, and enuresis are all examples of phenomena observed in specific stages of sleep. They are described in detail in *DSM-III*.

DREAM ANXIETY ATTACKS. These "nightmares" are awakenings from REM sleep with unmistakable, detailed recall (unlike Sleep Terror) of extended and disturbing dreams accompanied by anxiety and some autonomic arousal.

Nightmares typically occur in the latter portion of nocturnal sleep but may be seen in naps that are more than an hour long. They may be experienced at all ages by virtually everyone and tend to be more prevalent at times of emotional turmoil and after painful life events. Nightmares do not cause the post-arousal panic observed in sleep terrors nor is the autonomic arousal as great. Individuals awakening from nightmares are usually oriented to their environment and have a clear sensorium within a short period of time. Fear of nightmares sometimes causes an insomnia syndrome in anxious or psychotic patients.

EPILEPTIC SEIZURES. Epileptic seizures may at times be confused with episodes of sleep terror. Sleep-related seizures may take the form of generalized convulsions, or may be partial seizures with complex symptomatology. In some patients (25 percent), seizures occur exclusively during sleep. The attacks are most commonly seen during the first two hours after sleep onset or during a second peak period from around 4:00 to 6:00 A.M.

Sleep-related epileptic seizures may occur at any age, but are most frequent in children. The patient may offer a chief complaint of disturbed sleep or morning drowsiness (a post-ictal state). The course of sleep-related epileptic seizures is varied; usually no daytime deficits ensue, though impairment may be seen referable to underlying pathology.

SLEEP-RELATED BRUXISM. Bruxism is a parasomnia of nocturnal teeth grinding. It occurs predominantly during stage 2 sleep and is often accompanied by a loud grating or clicking sound. The patient has no awareness of the grinding and is rarely awakened by it. Episodes of bruxism may be associated with partial arousals, and overall sleep may be lightened in these patients. Bruxers often complain of aching jaws and other symptoms suggestive of temporo-mandibular joint (TMJ) syndrome. In general, emotional factors do not seem to be a major contributory factor in the development of bruxism, as was once thought. Dentists desperately try to prevent tooth erosion with various types of mouth guards because no way has been found to stop bruxing.

IMPAIRED SLEEP-RELATED PENILE TUMESCENCE. Impaired sleep-related penile tumescence describes a finding derived from sleep studies and refers to primary organic factors affecting neural or vascular investment of the penis. Though the force of tumescence gently declines with age, the presence of erections during REM sleep may be an expected finding through the elderly years. In psychogenic impotency, REM sleep-related tumescence is normal, or near normal, whereas it is impaired in certain waking sexual situations. The impairment is twofold with the organic impotencies (Williams and Karacan, 1975).

CLUSTER HEADACHES AND CHRONIC PAROXYSMAL HEMICRANIA. Both of these headaches are relatively rare types of vascular headaches. They appear to be triggered by the onset of REM sleep. Sleep-related gastroesophageal reflux, the less frequent sleep-related abnormal swallowing syndrome, and sleep-related asthma are all disturbances that may cause medical as well as insomnia complaints. Gastroesophageal reflux is a prominent cause of sleep disturbance in older patients.

SUMMARY

Sleep problems may be subtle but, nevertheless, life-crippling. Psychiatrists may evaluate sleep problems skillfully because of their psychophysiological training. Workable guidelines for dealing with insomnia should be followed first: incorporating the practitioner's sound clinical diagnoses and affirmation with therapeutic trials, using stress, drug, and alcohol reduction; relaxation; and temporary use of safe sedative medications. If such measures do not improve the sleep problem, specialized consultation and laboratory assessment are indicated.

As in many conditions that psychiatrists treat, consultative evaluation of patients is routinely requested to aid diagnosis and therapy. Patients find sleep studies pleasant; the yield of information is great; psychiatric treatment is not compromised, and the practitioner feels more confident in his management of the patient. The increasing biomedical sophistication of psychiatry permits fuller diagnostic exploration than is possible in routine office interviews.

The not infrequent situations when fragmentation of sleep may occur without awareness have been described, as well as subjective complaints of insomnia without evidence of sleep disruption. Further, organically induced sleep disruption frequently mimics psychologically related insomnias because patients, not usually cognizant of what awakens them under these conditions, attribute the cause to psychological factors. Of course, permutations of psychological and organic phenomena frequently lie behind an insomnia complaint. The clinician cannot always dissect the controlling factors. Simply making a psychiatric diagnosis may be relevant to current psychopathology but not always to the cause of the sleep disorder. *DSM-III* diagnoses, in combination with sleep disorder specifications made possible by a comprehensive sleep diagnostic system, make identification of individual sleep disorders highly reliable.

REFERENCES

Association of Sleep Disorders Centers Classification Committee: Diagnostic Classification of Sleep and Arousal Disorders, first edition. Sleep 2:1-137, 1979

Adamson J, Burdick JA: Sleep of dry alcoholics. Arch Gen Psychiatry 28:146-149, 1973

Bixler EO, Kales A, Soldatos CR, et al: Sleep apneic activity in a normal population. Res Commun Chem Pathol Pharmacol 36:141-152, 1982a

Bixler EO, Kales A, Vela-Bueno A, et al: Nocturnal myoclonus and nocturnal myoclonic activity in a normal population. Res Commun Chem Pathol Pharmacol 36:129-140, 1982b

Bootzin RR, Nicassio, PN: Behavioral treatments for insomnia, in Progress in Behavior Modification. Edited by Hersen M, Eisler R, Miller P. New York, Academy Press, 1978

Carskadon MA, Dement WC: Respiration during sleep in the aged human. J. Gerontol 36:420-423, 1981

Carskadon MA, Dement WC, Mitler MM, et al: Self-reports versus sleep laboratory findings in 122 drug-free subjects with complaints of chronic insomnia. Am J Psychiatry 133:1382-1388, 1976

Carskadon MA, Van den Hoed J, Dement WC: Sleep and daytime sleepiness in the elderly. J Geriatr Psychiatry 13:135-151, 1980

Carskadon MA, Brown, ED, Dement, WC: Sleep fragmentation in the elderly: relationship to daytime sleep tendency. Neurobiol Aging, 3:321-327, 1982

Coleman, RM: Diagnosis, treatment, and follow-up of about 8,000 sleep/wake disorder patients, in Sleep/Wake Disorders: Natural History, Epidemiology, and Long-Term Evolution. Edited by Guilleminault C, Lugaresi E. New York, Raven Press, 1983

Coleman RM, Roffwarg HP, Kennedy SJ, et al: Sleep-wake disorders based on a polysomnographic diagnosis: a national cooperative study. JAMA 247:997-1103, 1982

Coleman RM, Bliwise DL, Sajben N, et al: Epidemiology of periodic movements during sleep, in Sleep/Wake Disorders: Natural History of Epidemiology, and Long-Term Evolution. Edited by Guilleminault C and Lugaresi E. New York, Raven Press, 1983

Czeisler CA, Richardson GS, Coleman RM, et al: Chronotherapy: resetting the circadian clocks of patients with delayed sleep phase insomnia. Sleep 4:1-21, 1981

Dement WC, Guilleminault C: Sleep disorders: the state of the art. Hospital Practice 8:57-71, 1973

Dement W, Guilleminault C, Zarcone V: The pathologies of sleep: a case series approach, in The Nervous System, vol 2, The Clinical Neurosciences. Edited by Tower D. New York, Raven Press, 1975

Ferriss G: Sleep disorders. Neurologic Clinics 2:51-69, 1984

Gross MM, Hastey JM: A note on REM rebound during experimental alcohol withdrawal in alcoholics, in Advances in Experimental Medicine and Biology, vol 59. Edited by Gross MM. New York, Plenum, 1975

Guilleminault C, Eldridge FL, Dement WC: Insomnia with sleep apnea: a new syndrome. Science 181:856-858, 1973

Guilleminault C, Raynal D, Weitzman ED, et al.: Sleep-related periodic myoclonus in patients complaining of insomnia. Trans Am Neurol Assoc 100:19-21, 1975

Hauri P: The sleep disorders, in Current Concepts. Kalamazoo, MI, Upjohn Company, 1982

Hauri PJ: A cluster analysis of insomnia. Sleep 6:326-338, 1983

Hauri P, Hawkins DR: Alpha-delta sleep. Electroencephalogr Clin Neurophysiol 34:2333-2337, 1973

Institute of Medicine: Report of a study: sleeping pills, insomnia, and medical practice. Washington, DC, National Academy of Sciences, 1979

Kales A, Bixler EO, Tan T-L, et al: Chronic hypnotic-drug use: ineffectiveness, drug-withdrawal insomnia, and dependence. JAMA 227:513-517, 1974

Kales A, Scharf MB, Soldatos CR, et al: Clinical evaluation of hypnotic drugs: contributions from sleep laboratory studies. J Clin Pharmacol 19:329-336, 1979

Kales A, Soldatos CR, Kales JD: Sleep disorders: evaluation and management in the office setting, in American Handbook of Psychiatry, vol 7. Edited by Arieti S, Brodie HKH. New York, Basic Books Inc, 1981

Kales A, Bixler EO, Soldatos CR, et al: Biopsychobehavioral correlates of insomnia, part 1: role of sleep apnea and nocturnal myoclonus. Psychosomatics 23:589-600, 1982

Kales A, Bixler EO, Vela-Bueno A, et al: Biopsychobehavioral correlates of insomnia, III: polygraphic findings of sleep difficulty and their relationship to psychopathology. Int J Neurosci 23:43-56, 1984

Kales JD, Kales A, Bixler EO, et al: Sleep disorders: What the primary care physician needs to know. Postgrad Med 67:213-220, 1980

Kales JD, Soldatos CR, Kales A: Diagnosis and treatment of sleep disorders, in Treatment of Mental Disorders. Edited by Griest JH, Jefferson JW, Spitzer RL. New York, Oxford University Press, 1982

Kupfer DJ, Thase ME: The use of the sleep laboratory in the diagnosis of the affective disorders. Psychiatr Clin 6:3-25, 1983

Moldofsky H, Tullis C, Lue FA, et al: Sleep-related myoclonus in rheumatic pain modulation disorder (Fibrositis syndrome) and in excessive daytime somnolence. Psychosom Med 46:145-151, 1984

National Institute of Mental Health, Consensus Development Conference: Drugs and Insomnia: The Use of Medications to Promote Sleep. JAMA 251:2410-2414, 1984

Renner J: Drug addiction, in Massachusetts General Hospital Handbook of General Psychiatry. St. Louis, Mosby, 1978

Reynolds CF III, Coble P, Holzer B, et al: Sleep and its disorders. Primary Care 6:417-438, 1979

Reynolds CF, Shubin RS, Coble PA, et al: Diagnostic classification of sleep disorders: implications for psychiatric practice. J Clin Psychiatry 41:296-299, 1981

Roffwarg HP, Altshuler KZ: The diagnosis of sleep disorders, in Eating, Sleeping and Sexuality. Edited by Zales MR. New York, Brunner/Mazel Publishers, 1982

Roffwarg HP, Herman JH, Lettieri L: Recent experience in attempting to isolate a group of patients with pure functional insomnia. Presented to European Sleep Society, March, 1982

Rosenthal L, Roehrs T, Sicklesteel J, et al: Periodic leg movements, sleep fragmentation and sleep-wake complaints. Sleep Research 12:279, 1984

Schmidt HS: Disorders of sleep and arousal, in Psychiatry: Essentials of Clinical Practice. Edited by Gregory I, Smeltzer DJ. Boston/Toronto, Little, Brown and Company, 1983

Solomon F, White CC, Parron DL, et al: Sleeping pills, insomnia and medical practice. N Engl J Med 300:803-808, 1979

Stepanski E, Lamphere J, Badia P, et al: Sleep fragmentation and daytime sleepiness. Sleep 7:18-26, 1984

Tan T-L, Kales JD, Kales A, et al: Biopsychobehavioral correlates of insomnia, IV: diagnosis based on DSM-III. Am J Psychiatry 141:357-362, 1984

Waller D, et al: Recognizing and managing the adolescent with Kleine-Levin syndrome. Journal of Adolescent Health Care 5:139-141, 1984

Williams RL, Karacan I: Sleep disorders and disordered sleep, in American Handbook of Psychiatry Vol 4, Organic Disorders and Psychosomatic Medicine. Second edition. Edited by Reiser MF. New York, Basic Books, 1975

Williams RL, Karacan I, Hursch CJ (eds): EEG of Human Sleep. New York, John Wiley & Sons, 1974

Zarcone V: Narcolepsy. N Engl J Med 288:1156-1166, 1973

Zorick FJ, Roth T, Hartse KM, et al: Evaluation and diagnosis of persistent insomnia. Am J Psychiatry 138:769-773, 1981

Zorick F, Roehrs T, et al: Patterns of sleepiness in various disorders of excessive daytime somnolence. Sleep 5:S165-S174, 1982

Chapter 16

The Ontogeny of Sleep Disorders and Sleep Disorders in Childhood

by J. Christian Gillin, M.D.

The opening chapter of this section described the physiology and neurochemistry of sleep. The chapter on evaluation and diagnosis of sleep disorders laid out four major categories of sleep problems the physician is likely to see, and offered guidelines as to when to refer a patient to a sleep evaluation center and what to expect from such a work-up. With this foundation, the reader is ready for an introduction to the ontogeny of sleep and dreaming and to some of the sleep disorders found in childhood.

SLEEP AND DREAMING: NORMAL DEVELOPMENT

Ontogeny of Sleep

All pathological disorders must be viewed against the backdrop of normal human development; sleep disorders are no exception. The 24-hour organization of rest and activity, and the duration and structure of sleep, change dramatically over the life span (Roffwarg et al, 1966; Feinberg, 1974; Williams et al, 1974). At birth, the infant shows virtually no circadian organization of the rest-activity cycle; and, often to the consternation of his parents, he has a disposition to be awake at night as much as he is asleep during the day. About 12 to 14 weeks of extrauterine life are necessary before babies show fairly well organized sleep periods at night and prolonged wakefulness during the daylight hours. Napping persists, however, until about age three to five years in our country, although siestas are the norm throughout life in many cultures.

At the other extreme of life, the circadian cycle of sleep and wakefulness may partially break down in normal elderly individuals. Wakefulness at night and sleepiness and napping during the day may increase. Compared with young adults and middle-aged subjects, the elderly tend to show a pattern of "early-to-bed, early-to-rise." Many normal elderly also show subclinical sleep apnea (episodes when breathing ceases for periods of ten seconds or more many times throughout the sleep period) and leg-jerks (nocturnal myoclonus) in sleep; the reasons for and clinical significance of these observations are unknown at this time (Kripke et al, 1983). Clinicians should be aware of this possibility, however, when treating elderly patients who may show daytime sleepiness as a result of respiratory impairment during sleep. It is thought that the frequent awakenings or hypoxemia-hypercapnea associated with apnea may cause excessive sleepiness the next day. Nor should clinicians neglect the possibility that drugs—sedative hypnotics, tranquilizers, antidepressants, or others—could either induce or exacerbate sleep apnea (Mendelson et al, 1981). Thus, daytime drowsiness following the use of hypnotics may reflect either the continued presence of pharmacologically active compounds or the induction of respiratory impairment.

Other major changes in the amount and type of sleep also occur between infancy and old age. The newborn may sleep a total of 16 hours out of each 24, of which about 50 percent of sleep time is spent in rapid eye movement (REM) sleep. Moreover, sleep may begin with REM sleep, and the infant's non-REM (NREM) sleep may lack the EEG characteristics, such as K–complexes, sleep spindles, and delta waves, which define sleep stages 1 through 4. During the next months, NREM sleep matures in complexity of EEG patterns, duration, and timing, so that it occurs increasingly at the beginning of the nocturnal sleep period. Simultaneously, the infant shows longer and longer periods of wakefulness during the daylight hours, and this is taken at the expense of daytime REM sleep. Nocturnal REM latency, or time between falling asleep and the onset of the first REM period, gradually increases; and REM sleep tends to become relatively more prominent toward the end than the beginning of the night (Fagioli and Salzarulo, 1982; Navelet et al, 1982; Coons and Guilleminault, 1982; Schulz et al, 1983).

Even at an early age, there are considerable individual differences in sleep duration and other traits, which tend to be stable, at least for short to intermediate periods of time (Dittrichova et al, 1976), but may tend to weaken over many years (Klackenberg, 1982). Genetic factors may be important partial determinants for some sleep characteristics in adults (Webb and Campbell, 1983; Nurnberger et al, 1983). Individual differences in sleep duration and other characteristics have been related to temperament in infants and children (Carey, 1972; Weissbluth, 1981). Interestingly, "REM storms"—intense rapid eye movements during REM sleep—at age six months were found to be significantly, negatively correlated with Bayley Scales of Mental Development at age 12 months (Becker and Thoman, 1981).

During the early and middle years of childhood, sleep-related behaviors may be both charming and exasperating: the bedtime rituals, teddy bear, and "just one more drink of water" at age two; the stormy and grumpy wakening from the nap at two-and-a-half; the "wonderful sleeper" at ages six through seven; and the resistance to bedtime at age eight (Ames, 1964).

These behavioral characteristics are also accompanied by significant changes in EEG sleep patterns during the latency and pubertal years. Total stage 4 sleep and REM latency tend to fall from age six through the middle or end of adolescence (Carskadon 1982; Carskadon et al, 1980, 1983). In some ways, the preadolescent years represent the period of life in which the differences between sleep and wakefulness are maximal. During the daytime children tend to be alert, active, and almost unable to sleep; at night, they sleep deeply and soundly. Indeed, high intensity auditory stimuli of 123 dB, about 90 dB above waking threshold values, fail to arouse children aged eight to 12 during the first sleep cycle, and this is true for hyperactive children as well as normal controls (Busby and Pivik, 1983).

A number of important developments take place during the adolescent years. Sleep duration, at least on school nights, tends to decrease during the prepubertal years (Anders et al, 1978, 1980). The extent to which this pattern results from cultural influences (that is, academic pressures) as compared with physiological development is not entirely clear. It appears that children aged eight to 17 are averaging about 1.5 hours less sleep now than their great-grandparents 75 years ago (Webb and Agnew, 1975). While this reduction may reflect increased academic pressure, the widespread use of the electric light bulb, or other environmental factors, it could also be related to the earlier age of adolescence. In addition, midway through the adolescent period children develop daytime sleepiness, that is, the ability to sleep when offered the opportunity to nap (Carskadon, 1980, 1982), and this change may be importantly related to certain disorders of excessive daytime sleepiness. Narcolepsy, for example, typically but not invariably starts during the teenage years (Carskadon et al, 1981). Surveys reveal that prepubertal children rarely nap or experience irresistible urges to sleep during the day, but that both tendencies increase during adolescence (Carskadon, 1980, 1982; Simonds and Parraga, 1982).

The early phase of sexual maturation in adolescence is also accompanied by, and perhaps initiated by, an augmented release of luteinizing hormone (LH) and, in boys, of testosterone, during sleep (Boyar et al, 1972, 1974; Judd et al, 1977). Interestingly, women with anorexia nervosa show flat patterns of LH secretion, typical of normal preadolescence, when they are amenorrheic, but normal adult patterns when they have recovered.

As subjects pass from early adulthood to late middle age, REM latency tends to fall modestly, and stage 4 sleep eventually disappears almost completely, probably somewhat sooner in men than women (Williams et al, 1974; Gillin et al, 1981). It is well known that there is an inverse relationship between amplitude and frequency of EEG waves. Feinberg et al (personal communication) have recently shown that the amplitude at the lower frequencies—that is, those that define delta sleep (0.5–3.0 Hz)—is reduced more in normal elderly subjects than young ones. Since Feinberg (1974) had previously speculated that NREM sleep, and especially stage 4 sleep, reflects the intensity of an unknown metabolic process that reverses the effects of wakefulness, the loss of EEG amplitude in the delta frequency during NREM sleep could indicate a diminution in the intensity of these restorative processes. Moreover, growth hormone, which is normally secreted in association with stage 4 sleep and which probably has general anabolic effects, is no longer released during sleep after middle age (Carlson et al, 1972).

The Ontogeny of Dreaming

Although "dreams" may be reported as early as age two to three, there has been a reluctance to accept these accounts as true dream reports. It is often difficult to distinguish them from "tall tales" of actual or imagined events until about age seven (Ames, 1964). With the advent of EEG sleep laboratory studies of REM and NREM sleep, it has been possible to study the phenomenology of mental activity during sleep in much greater detail, and Foulkes (1983) has recently found a fascinating evolution of dreaming and thinking in children. When children aged three to five were awakened from REM sleep, dream reports were rare, occurring only about 15 percent of the time. When dreams did occur, they were typically short and static, with little evidence of a plot, movement, feeling, or self-portrayal. While animals were frequently mentioned, human characters were not. At older ages, the frequency of dream reports increased to about 30 percent at ages five to seven, 43 percent at seven to nine, and about 80 percent (the usual adult level) at ages nine to 11. Moreover, dream content, when it occurred, also matured with age. The child of five to seven reported several events in series, physical activity, and social interaction. The child of seven to nine described his own participation in the dream and some affect. Foulkes also found that abstract or thought-like thinking was not common in NREM sleep until children reached adolescence. He related the development of dreaming and thinking in children to other aspects of cognitive development in the tradition of Piaget.

At the other extreme of life, old age, the frequency of dream recall following REM awakenings declines. Kahn et al (1969), for example, found a rate of dream recall of 43.5 percent in the elderly (age 70 to 87) compared with 87 percent in the young adult population.

Kramer et al (1975) reported that dream recall was inversely related to severity of chronic brain syndrome: 57 percent in mildly demented patients, 35 percent in severely organic patients, and only eight percent in an older group with very severe chronic brain syndrome. With increasing dementia, dream content tended to become simpler and emotionally blander, with more references to family than strangers. Thus, both age and organic brain disorders affect REM sleep mechanisms. An obvious potential common mechanism could be cholinergic processes that are involved in aging, REM sleep, and memory.

SOME SLEEP DISORDERS OCCURRING IN CHILDHOOD

Although children are usually reported by their parents to sleep soundly and to be in a good mood upon awakening, most also occasionally exhibit some unusual sleep behavior or disorder (Simonds and Parraga, 1982). About 28 percent of a sample of 369 children from kindergarten through twelfth grade were reported to be restless sleepers at least once a week and 20 percent on a daily basis. At a frequency of at least once a week, about eight percent snored, eight percent ground their teeth, ten percent were fearful of the dark, four percent wet the bed, five percent insisted on sleeping with others, five percent were drowsy during the daytime, two percent had irresistible sleepiness, and two percent had nightmares or the more serious night terrors (pavor nocturnus). These complaints are often minor and self-limited; but clinicians should be prepared to evaluate, diagnose, and manage these problems in an appropriate manner.

Excessive Daytime Sleepiness

Excessive daytime sleepiness is not usually discussed in childhood sleep disorders since it is more commonly diagnosed in adults. It is discussed here for emphasis, since it may be present in children. The failure to recognize it as a disorder, in either children or adults, is a missed opportunity to end distress and disability.

The most common cause of short-term daytime sleepiness is probably sleep loss or the use of sedating medications (such as antihistamines). Chronic daytime sleepiness, however, should be carefully evaluated, with two diagnoses particularly in mind: narcolepsy and sleep-related respiratory impairment, such as sleep apnea. Psychiatrists should be aware that the sleepy child is often viewed as lazy, retarded, obstinate and disobedient, hyperactive, or emotionally disturbed. His or her academic and social performance often suffer, and the child may develop secondary problems of poor morale and self-esteem.

Narcolepsy

Narcolepsy is characterized by two major symptoms—excessive daytime sleepiness and cataplexy—and several less specific ones, such as vivid dreaming upon falling asleep (hypnogogic hallucinations) and sleep paralysis (brief periods of paralysis at the transitions between wakefulness and sleep). Excessive sleepiness can be distinguished from fatigue by irresistible sleep episodes when the child wishes to remain awake. Cataplectic attacks are brief episodes (seconds to minutes) in which voluntary control of muscle tone and movement is lost. They are frequently precipitated by emotional arousal, such as fright, anger, laughter, or excitement. Narcolepsy is a disorder of REM sleep, representing the inappropriate and irresistible appearance of REM sleep or certain of its components (such as muscle atonia and dreaming) during wakefulness.

The disorder usually begins insidiously before the age of 15, with vague symptoms of excessive daytime sleepiness or hypersomnia or, occasionally, cataplexy. The full syndrome is usually not apparent before the end of adolescence or the early twenties, but it has occasionally been seen in preadolescent children (Wittig et al, 1983). The etiology of narcolepsy is unknown, but it tends to run in families, and the development of narcoleptic signs has been followed longitudinally in a few susceptible adolescents (Carskadon et al, 1981).

Since narcolepsy is a lifelong disorder, the diagnostic process should include an evaluation in a sleep laboratory, particularly since treatment often involves administration of amphetamines and other stimulants. These drugs are tightly regulated, making it difficult for narcoleptics to obtain needed medications. In addition, some drug addicts may simulate narcolepsy in order to obtain prescriptions. EEG recordings reveal two major findings in narcolepsy. First, sleep onset is fast, both at night and during daytime multiple sleep latency tests. Secondly, REM latency is short.

Narcolepsy patients and their families benefit from education and support. Sleep "hygiene" principles—adequate sleep at night, regular hours, daytime exercise, and scheduled naps during the day in some patients—are sometimes useful. Stimulant medications—such as amphetamine, methylphenidate (Ritalin), and cylert (Pemoline)—may control daytime sleepiness but must be used conservatively in order to avoid the development of tolerance, dependence, and toxicity. Tricyclic antidepressants, usually in low doses, are often useful in reducing cataplexy.

Sleep-Induced Respiratory Impairment

The obstructive sleep apnea syndrome has received considerable attention in recent years. It typically occurs in the middle-aged, overweight, sleepy man with loud snoring and is often associated with hypertension and cor pulmonale. Sleep apnea has also been reported in children (Guilleminault et al, 1976) sometimes, but rarely, in association with childhood Pickwickian Syndrome (Simpser et al, 1977). The pathophysiology usually involves a compromise of the nasopharyngeal airway, although central nervous system abnormalities are thought to be involved in some cases in which frequent central apneas also occur. Sleep apnea may be especially common in children with large tonsils and adenoids, which may occlude the air passages, particulary during sleep. With the additional symptom of obesity, these children have the so called "Chubby Puffer" syndrome (Stool et al, 1977). There is some speculation that Sudden Infant Death Syndrome results from sleep apnea.

More recently, it has been recognized that the child with heavy snoring may experience disordered breathing and an increased respiratory resistive load, even though he or she does not suffer from completely obstructed episodes of sleep apnea. Compaints of excessive daytime sleepiness probably occur less frequently in children than in adults with apnea, but behavioral problems may be more frequent (Stool et al, 1977; Guilleminault et al, 1982; Mauer et al, 1983; Frank et al, 1983). For example, in a group of 25 children aged two to 14 referred to Stanford University Hospital, eight had hypersomnolence, 12 hyperactivity, ten aggressive and rebellious behavior, ten pathological shyness and social withdrawal, ten learning problems, and 11 clumsiness. In addition, six had frequent morning headaches and 12 had frequent upper airway infections (Guilleminault et al, 1982). Many of these children also had nocturnal symptoms of profuse sweating, restless sleep and abnormal movements, enuresis, and sleeping in abnormal positions.

These disorders may respond to various surgical procedures, including tonsillectomy, adenoidectomy, nasal septal reconstruction, or, in severe cases, tracheostomy, which relieve the airway obstruction. Medications, including nasal decongestants, tricyclic antidepressants, and respiratory stimulants, have also been useful in some patients. Physicians should establish whether their pediatric or adult patients are chronic snorers by asking parents, bedpartners, or others who have observed the patient asleep or by making an auditory tape recording of respiratory sounds during sleep. Positive evidence of persistent, heavy snoring should be a reason for concern and for further investigation. Referral to a sleep-disorders center may be indicated for complete documentation of respiratory patterns, cardiovascular functioning, and blood gases during sleep.

Sleep in Attention Deficit Disorder with Hyperactivity (ADDH)

Insomnia and difficulties going to bed have commonly been reported in children with attention deficit disorder with hyperactivity (ADDH). *DSM-III* criteria for diagnosis of this disorder include sleeping problems, and parents commonly mention them.

It is somewhat surprising, therefore, to find that all-night EEG sleep studies have not established any solid differences between the sleep patterns of children with ADDH and those of controls (see Greenhill et al, 1983; Chatoor et al, 1983; Khan, 1982; and Busby et al, 1981, for recent findings and reviews of the literature). No major differences in sleep time, sleep latency, sleep architecture, or autonomic activity have emerged when the studies are examined in aggregate, although some studies have found specific abnormalities. For example, REM latency was reported to be long in some studies (Haig et al, 1974; Busby et al, 1981) but short, especially in a subgroup of patients, in a more recent study (Khan, 1982).

Increased motor activity, as measured by EEG arousal, has been found in some sleep laboratory studies (Busby et al, 1981; Small et al, 1971). A recent naturalistic assessment of motor activity has confirmed and extended these observations. Porrino et al (1983a) had hyperactive boys and normal controls wear a small, solid-state ambulatory activity monitor on a waist belt for a week. The hyperactive boys were generally more active than the controls at 11 specific times, including the sleep period, especially on nights before school rather than weekends.

The effects of stimulant medications on sleep in the sleep laboratory have been surprisingly modest in these children, considering the amount of concern in clinical practice that children may be kept awake iatrogenically with these drugs. These children have often been treated with amphetamine or methyl-phenidate (Ritalin), and more recently, pemoline (Cylert). EEG sleep laboratory differences before and during chronic treatment with these drugs are usually small (Small et al, 1971; Greenhill et al, 1983; Nahas and Krylnicki, 1977). Never-theless, many clinicians administer the doses early in the day to avoid keeping the child awake at night. Increased sleep latency is commonly reported by these children's parents, has often been documented in the sleep laboratory in some children, and has recently been shown in the home environment, using the previously described ambulatory activity monitor (Porrino et al, 1983b). Amphet-amine (15 mg/day) or placebo was administered at eight A.M. Although active drugs decreased most motor activity for about eight hours, a "rebound hyper-activity" was observed in the evening and throughout the night, particularly on school nights as compared with weekends. This observation suggests that setting and anticipation may have some influence on the effect of amphetamine on sleep and may help explain why sleep laboratory studies have generally found little drug effect.

A recent preliminary study suggested that evening and bedtime rebound hyperactivity may be decreased by administration of a long-acting form of dextroamphetamine before bedtime. Even though the drug increased sleep latency and reduced sleep efficiency (by 4.5 percent), as well as showing a number of other effects on sleep architecture, the clinical impression, based on parental reports, was that children settled down more easily at bedtime (Chatoor et al, 1983). Clinicians may wish to prescribe stimulants in the late afternoon or evening to calm the hyperactive child.

Enuresis

Some basic concepts of enuresis have recently been re-evaluated. First, although primary enuresis is often associated with childhood psychiatric disorders, not all enuretic children are psychiatrically disturbed (Mikkelsen et al, 1980). Clini-cians should not assume *a priori* that enuresis is a symptom of an emotional or medical disorder. Secondly, recent findings have not supported the earlier hypothesis that enuresis is a "disorder of arousal" occurring in delta (especially stage 4) sleep (Broughton, 1968). Both Kales et al (1977) and the NIMH group (Mikkelsen et al, 1980; Gillin et al, 1982) found that enuretic episodes were not preferentially concentrated in specific sleep stages.

In the latter study, 40 boys with severe primary enuresis were compared with 17 normal boys. The enuretic children were equally divided into psychiatrically "disturbed" (two depression, one mixed anxiety-depression, six generalized anxiety disorder, three attention deficit disorder, seven unsocialized conduct disorder) and "nondisturbed" subgroups. Episodes tended to occur about four hours after sleep onset or, on nights when there was more than one episode, about four hours after the first one (Gillin et al, 1982). Since there is evidence that the capacity of the bladder is small in enuretic children and that the number and intensity of spontaneous detrusor contractions is high, four hours may be more or less the capacity of the small active enuretic bladder. Furthermore, in comparison with age matched controls, enuretic boys had more shallow sleep—increased stage 1, more intermediate wakefulness, and less stage 4 and delta sleep—even on "dry" nights. This observation did not support the idea that enuresis is associated with unusually deep sleep, at least as defined by conventional sleep staging. In addition, disturbed and nondisturbed boys did not differ in distribution of enuretic episodes by sleep stage, although there was a strong trend for more episodes to occur in REM sleep in the nondisturbed boys than in the disturbed ones. All night sleep patterns were similar in the two groups.

There is good evidence that bell-and-pad conditioning is efficacious in enuretic children and that it may eventually cure the problem. Drugs, in contrast, only suppress the problem. Psychotherapy does not appear to be beneficial for the enuresis *per se* but may be helpful when the child is emotionally upset or in secondary enuresis when continence has been lost following a traumatic event or other emotional disturbance (Mikkelsen and Rapoport, 1980). When the child is very distressed about the enuresis, the use of a tricyclic antidepressant medication can be considered. Rapoport et al (1980) found desipramine and imipramine (75-125 mg at bedtime, each) to be equally efficacious, but most boys were partial rather than complete responders. Clinical response began soon after onset of treatment, but tolerance developed in a substantial proportion of boys within two to six weeks. Both clinical efficacy and side effects correlated significantly with plasma levels of the drugs, but high plasma levels did not guarantee efficacy. If a child has not responded, the dose may be increased until a clinical response has been achieved or significant side effects have developed.

The mechanism of action of tricyclic antidepressants in enuresis is not known. Since children did not respond to methscopolamine, peripheral anticholinergic effects were apparently not involved (Rapoport et al, 1980).

The use of tricyclics in enuresis is not a trivial matter and should be considered only in severe cases and with careful monitoring. Unexpected deaths have occurred in children who have been treated with tricyclic antidepressants for enuresis. If these drugs are used, they should be prescribed for as short a period of time as possible (a visit or holiday) and in as low a dose as possible. Recent experimental evidence has shown that vasopressin analogues may be effective in enuresis and that this effect is partially independent of the drug's antidiuretic properties (Aladjem et al, 1982). More research is needed to establish its efficacy, safety, and mechanism of action.

Sleep in Children with Obsessive-Compulsive Disorder

Childhood obsessive-compulsive disorder is a relatively rare psychiatric illness that is found in only about one percent of child psychiatric inpatients (Judd, 1965). Its symptoms are similar to those found in adult obsessive-compulsive disorder.

As part of a systematic, prospective study on childhood obsessive-compulsive disorder, Rapoport et al (1981) have presented preliminary data on all-night EEG sleep recordings from nine adolescent patients (aged 13-17, seven boys, two girls) and 15 age- and sex-matched controls. Six of the nine patients reported sleep disturbance. Of 24 sleep measures, nine were statistically different. The patients showed less total sleep time, sleep efficiency, NREM sleep, stage 2 sleep, REM latency, and REM sleep, and greater sleep latency, stage four percentage and delta sleep percent. These sleep patterns are similar to those seen in adults with obsessive-compulsive disorder (see below) and also in middle-aged adults with moderate to severe endogenous depression. In particular, REM latency appeared to be low and was not associated with obvious depression. Interestingly, stage 4 sleep, which is typically low in a variety of medical and psychiatric conditions, was actually elevated, at least as a percentage of total sleep time; absolute minutes of stage 4 sleep were not different.

It should be emphasized that this was a preliminary report and that new patients are currently under study. The present result, together with other neuropsychological and CAT scan abnormalities, do suggest the presence of objective biological differences between patients with obsessive-compulsive disorder and controls.

CONCLUSION

While we are beginning to gain some knowledge of the ontogeny of sleep and of the manifestations of disturbed sleep in particular periods of life, the areas of sleep disorders in children and sleep-related symptoms in general psychiatric disorders in young patients remain largely uncharted. Perhaps some of the answers will be revealed in the next generation of sleep research.

REFERENCES

Aladjem M, Wohl R, Boichis, et al: Desmopressin in nocturnal enuresis. Arch Dis Child 57:137-140, 1982

Ames LB: Sleep and dreams in childhood, in International Series of Monographs on Child Psychiatry. Edited by Harms E. New York, MacMillin Co, 1964

Anders TF, Carskadon MA, Dement WC: Sleep habits of children and the identification of pathologically sleepy children. Child Psychiatry Hum Dev 9:56-63, 1978

Anders TF, Carskadon MA, Dement WC: Sleep and sleepiness in children and adolescents. Pediatr Clin North Am 27:29-43, 1980

Association of Sleep Disorder Centers, Diagnostic Classification of Sleep and Arousal Disorders. Sleep 2:1-137, 1979

Becker PT, Thoman EB: Rapid eye movement storms in infants: rate of occurrence at 6 months predicts mental development at 1 year. Science 212:1415-1416, 1981

Boyar R, Finkelstein J, Roffwarg H: Synchronization of augmented luteinizing hormone secretion with sleep during puberty. N Engl J Med 287:582-586, 1972

Boyar RM, Rosenfeld RS, Kapen S, et al: Human puberty. Simultaneous augmented secretion of luteinizing hormone and testosterone during sleep. J Clin Invest 54:609-618, 1974

Broughton RJ: Sleep disorders: disorders of arousal? Enuresis, somnambulism, and night-mares occur in confusional states of arousal, not in "dreaming sleep." Science 159:1070-1078, 1968

Busby K, Firestone P, Pivik RT: Sleep patterns in hyperkinetic and normal children. Sleep 4:366-383, 1981

Busby K, Pivak RT: Failure of high intensity auditory stimuli to affect behavioral arousal in children during the first sleep cycle. Pediatr Res 17:802-805, 1983

Carey WB: Night awakening and temperament in infancy. J Pediatr 84:756-758, 1972

Carlson HE, Gillin JC, Gorden P, et al: Absence of sleep related growth hormone peaks in aged normal subjects and in acromegaly. J Clin Endocrinol Metab 34:1102-1105, 1972

Carskadon MA: The second decade in Sleeping and Waking Disorders: Indications and Technique. Edited by Guilleminault C. Addison and Wesley Publishing Co., 99-125, 1982

Carskadon MA, Harvey K, Duke P, et al: Pubertal changes in daytime sleepiness. Sleep 2:453-460, 1980

Carskadon MA, Harvey K, Dement WC: Multiple sleep latency tests during the development of narcolepsy. West J Med 135:414-418, 1981

Carskadon MA, Oraz JE, Dement WC: Evolution of sleep and daytime sleepiness in adolescence, in Sleep/Wake Disorders: Natural History, Epidemiology and Long Term Evolution. Edited by Guilleminault C, Lugaresi E. New York, Raven Press, 1983

Chatoor I, Wells KC, Conners CK, et al: The effects of nocturnally administered stimulant medication on EEG sleep and behavior in hyperactive children. J Am Acad Child Psychiatry 22:337-342, 1983

Coons S, Guilleminault C: Development of sleep-wake patterns and non-rapid eye movement sleep stages during the first six months of life in normal infants. Pediatrics 69:793-798, 1982

Dittrichova J, Paul K, Vondracek J: Individual differences in infants' sleep. Dev Med Child Neurol 18:182-188, 1976

Fagioli I, Salzarulo P: Sleep states development in the first year of life assessed through 24-h recordings. Early Hum Dev 6:215-218, 1982

Feinberg I: Changes in sleep cycle patterns with age. J Psychiatr Res 10:283-306, 1974

Foulkes D: Dream ontogeny and dream psychophysiology, in Sleep Disorders: Basic and Clinical Research. Edited by Chase MH, Weitzman, ED. New York, SP Medical and Scientific Books, 1983

Frank Y, Kravath RE, Pollack CP, et al: Obstructive sleep apnea and its therapy: clinical and polysomnographic manifestations. Pediatrics 71:737-742, 1983

Gillin JC, Duncan WC, Murphy DC, et al: Age related changes in sleep in depressed and normal subjects. Psychiatry Res 14:73-89, 1981

Gillin JC, Rapoport JL, Mikkelsen EJ, et al: EEG sleep patterns in enuresis: a further analysis and comparison with normal controls. Biol Psychiatry 17:947-953, 1982

Greenhill L, Puig-Antich J, Goetz R, et al: Sleep architecture and REM sleep measures in prepubertal children with attention deficit disorder with hyperactivity. Sleep 6:91-101, 1983

Guilleminault C, Eldridge FL, Simmons FB, et al: Sleep apnea in eight children. Pediatrics 58:23-30, 1976

Guilleminault C, Winkle R, Korobkin R, et al: Children and nocturnal snoring: evaluation of the effects of sleep related respiratory resistive load and daytime functioning. Eur J Pediatr 139:165-171, 1982

Haig JR, Schroeder CS, Schroeder SR: Effects of methylphenidate on hyperactive children's sleep. Psychopharmacol Bull 37:185-188, 1974

Judd HL, Parker DC, Yen, SS: Sleep-wake patterns of LH and testosterone release in prepubertal boys. J Clin Endocrinol Metab 44:865-859, 1977

Judd L: Obsessive-compulsive neurosis in children. Arch Gen Psychiatry 12:136-146, 1965

Kahn E, Fischer C, Lieberman L: Dream recall in the normal aged. J Amer Geriatric Soc 17:1121-1126, 1969

Kales A, Kales JD, Jacobson A, et al: Effects of imipramine on enuretic frequency and sleep stages. Pediatrics 60:431-436, 1977

Khan AU: Sleep REM latency in hyperkinetic boys. Am J Psychiatry 139:1358-1360, 1982

Klackenberg G: Sleep behavior studied longitudinally. Data from 4-16 years on duration, night-awakening, and bedsharing. Acta Paediatr Scand 71:501-506, 1982

Kramer M, Roth T, Trinder J: Dreams and dementia: a laboratory exploration of dream recall and dream content in chronic brain syndrome patients. Int J Aging Human Dev 6:169-178, 1975

Kripke DF, Ancoli-Israel S, and Okudaira N: Sleep apnea and nocturnal myoclonus in the elderly. Neurobiol Aging 3:329-336, 1983

Mauer KW, Staats, BA, Olsen KD: Upper airway obstruction and disordered nocturnal breathing in children. Mayo Clin Proc 58:349-353, 1983

Mendelson WB, Garnett D, Gillin JC: A single case study: flurazepam-induced sleep apnea syndrome in a patient with insomnia and mild sleep-related respiratory changes. J Nerv Ment Dis 169:261-264, 1981

Mikkelsen EJ, Rapoport JL, Nee L, et al: Childhood enuresis. I. Sleep patterns and psychopathology. Arch Gen Psychiatry 37:1139-1144, 1980a

Mikkelsen EJ, Rapoport JL: Enuresis: psychopathology, sleep stages, and drug response. Urol Clin North Am 7:361-377, 1980b

Nahas AD, Krynicki V: Effect of methylpenidate on sleep stages and ultradian rhythms in hyperactive children. J Nerv Ment Dis 164:66-69, 1977

Navelet Y, Benoit O, and Bouard G: Nocturnal sleep organization during the first months of life. Electroencephalogr Clin Neurophysiol 54:71-78, 1982

Nurnberger JI, Sitaram N, Gershon ES, et al: A twin study of cholinergic REM induction. Biol Psychiatry 18:1161-1173, 1983

Porrino LJ, Rapoport JL, Behar D, et al: A naturalistic assessment of the motor activity of hyperactive boys. I. Comparison with normal controls. Arch Gen Psychiatry 40:681-687, 1983a

Porrino LJ, Rapoport JL, Behar D, et al: A naturalistic assessment of the motor activity of hyperactive boys. II. Stimulant drug effects. Arch Gen Psychiatry 50:688-693, 1983b

Rapoport JL, Mikkelsen EJ, Zavadil A, et al: Childhood enuresis. II. Psychopathology, tricyclic concentration in plasma, and antienuretic effect. Arch Gen Psychiatry 37:1146-1152, 1980

Rapoport J, Elkins R, Langer D, et al: Childhood obsessive-compulsive disorder. Am J Psychiatry 138:1545-1554, 1981

Roffwarg HP, Muzio JN, Dement WC: Ontogenetic development of the human sleep-dream cycle. Science 152:604-619, 1966

Schulz H, Salzarulo P, Fagioli I, et al: REM latency: development in the first year of life. Electroencephalogr Clin Neurophysiol 56:316-322, 1983

Simonds JF, Parraga H: Prevalence of sleep disorders and sleep behaviors in children and adolescents. J Am Acad Child Psychiatry 21:383-388, 1982

Simpser MD, Strieder DJ, Wohl ME, et al: Sleep apnea in a child with the Pickwickian Syndrome. Pediatrics 60:290-293, 1977

Small MH, Hibi S, Feinberg I: Effects of amphetamine sulfate on EEG sleep patterns of hyperactive children. Arch Gen Psychiatry 25:369-380, 1971

Stool SE, Eavy RD, Stein NL, et al: The "Chubby Puffer" Syndrome. Clin Pediatr 16:43-50, 1977

Webb W, Agnew H: Are we chronically sleep deprived? Bulletin of the Psychopharmacology Society 6:47-48, 1975

Webb WB, Campbell SS: Relationships in sleep characteristics of identical and fraternal twins. Arch Gen Psychiatry 40:1093-1095, 1983

Weissbluth M: Sleep duration and infant temperament. J Pediatr 99:817-819, 1981

Williams RC, Karacan I, Hursch CJ: Electroencephalography (EEG) of human sleep: clinical applications. John Wiley & Sons, New York, 1974

Wittig R, Zorick F, Roehrs T, et al: Narcolepsy in a 7-year-old child. J Pediatr 102:725-727, 1983

Chapter 17

Sleep in Depressive Disorders

by Charles F. Reynolds III, M.D. and
James E. Shipley, M.D.

It is useful to place a clinical review of sleep changes in depressive illness within the broader context of sleep disorders in general. A basic tenet of this discipline is that the physician should attempt to establish the major (and possibly etiologic) correlates of the patient's complaint of disturbed sleep, with the goal of formulating a specific treatment plan. When the patient's complaint of diminished, excessive, or otherwise disturbed sleep is measured objectively in the sleep laboratory (ideally as part of a comprehensive medical, neurological, and psychiatric evaluation), it becomes apparent that not all sleep disturbance is alike. With respect to psychiatric disorders, for example, the altered or disturbed sleep seen in psychiatric states possesses varied features of sleep continuity, sleep architecture or composition, and rapid eye movement (REM) sleep.

Both clinical and electrophysiological heterogeneity is emphasized in the nosology of sleep and arousal disorders recently developed by the Association of Sleep Disorders Centers (ASDC, 1979). This nosology sets forth the many types of disorders of initiating and maintaining sleep (the insomnias) associated with a variety of psychiatric and neuropsychiatric states, including depression. At the same time, it emphasizes the fact that some psychiatric patients, particularly those with anergic depression, may present with a disorder of excessive sleepiness. The nosology has now been applied in a multi-center study of patients presenting with sleep complaints, and data on more than 8,000 sleep disorder patients have now been published (Coleman et al, 1982). When one examines the distribution of medical, psychiatric, and psychophysiological diagnoses of patients presenting to sleep disorders centers ("treatment" prevalence, as opposed to general prevalence), a psychiatric condition, particularly anxiety and affective disorders, is the final diagnosis in 30 to 35 percent of patients presenting with a complaint of insomnia. The remaining 65 to 70 percent of diagnoses of insomnia include nocturnal periodic leg movements, sleep apnea syndromes, persistent psychophysiological or conditioned insomnia, substance abuse disorders, subjective insomnia without objective findings, and a variety of primary medical disorders.

This chapter will focus primarily on those disorders of initiating and maintaining sleep which are specifically psychiatric; within this category, depression is of major importance.

AREAS OF CONSENSUS

At present, four major areas of consensus have emerged from clinical sleep research in depression during the 1970s and early 1980s (Kupfer and Reynolds, 1983). First, the majority of depressed patients demonstrate *hyposomnia*; that is, a sleep continuity disturbance usually associated with increased wakefulness or difficulty maintaining sleep. The frequent report of early morning awakening is a manifestation of this difficulty which is seen in depression. A minority of depressed patients, perhaps 15 to 20 percent, show *hypersomnia*, manifested by both more time in bed and greater total sleep time during the 24-hour day. This clinical feature is usually associated with psychomotor slowing and anergia. When objectively measured in the laboratory, however, these patients do not have as great a physiological sleep tendency during the day as do patients with narcolepsy or obstructive sleep apnea syndrome.

A second area of consensus is that depressed patients show a reduction in slow-wave or "delta" sleep, usually reported as a reduction or absence of stages 3 and 4 sleep. Since it is also true that considerably more stage 1 sleep is present in depressed patients, reflecting in part the greater number of arousals and stage shifts, one might conclude that the major change in the non-REM (NREM) sleep of depressives is the presence of lighter sleep such as stages 1 and 2, to the exclusion of stages 3 and 4. Again, however, when compared to patients with such primary sleep disorders as narcolepsy or sleep apnea, depressed patients tend not to show as much stage 1 sleep, though they do frequently show more than normals.

The third finding, and the one that has become most prominent because of its considerable replicability, has been a shortened time from sleep onset to the first REM period. While this finding is somewhat contingent upon the criteria used to determine sleep onset, in almost all depressed states REM sleep latency is shortened. The relationship of REM latency and the severity of the illness is also established, in that more severely depressed patients usually have a shorter REM latency than do less severely depressed patients.

Finally, the fourth and most recent finding receiving considerable attention has been altered temporal distribution of REM sleep during the night. Depressed patients typically show a greater percentage of early REM sleep than do age-matched normal controls or insomniacs. Another way of describing this finding is that depressed patients show a shift of REM sleep time into the first third of the night, manifested usually by a long and "active" (that is, with a profusion of rapid eye movements) first REM period. In contrast, normal subjects usually show progressively longer and more active REM sleep periods during the course of the night.

These EEG sleep findings in depression are greatly affected by the age of the patient. In other words, age-dependent decreases in slow-wave sleep and in REM latency, as well as an increase in wakefulness after sleep onset, have been shown in both depressives and normal individuals. The implications of this age-related increase in the sleep disturbances of depression for both clinical practice and theory will be presented later in this chapter.

AREAS OF UNCERTAINTY

Several issues concerning the EEG sleep features of depression are still unresolved (Kupfer and Reynolds, 1983; Kupfer and Thase, 1983). First, it is unclear whether hyposomnia or hypersomnia will be found in bipolar depressive syndromes. The hyposomnic picture is found in most mixed depressed states and depressed bipolar patients requiring hospitalization, but in bipolar and/or anergic outpatients, the complaint of hypersomnia seems to be a much more common feature (Detre et al, 1972). The available data suggest that the sleep pattern of hyposomnia may be reflected in the level of severity; for example, affective psychoses are usually associated with profound hyposomnia.

Second, while diminished stages 3 and 4 slow-wave sleep and increased amounts of stage 1 sleep are found in depression, this feature is not specific to depression. The same changes are often present in other chronic psychiatric and medical conditions, including such primary sleep disorders as sleep apnea syndrome or narcolepsy. The development of computer-assisted techniques for analyzing and describing the EEG signal, however, is already permitting a more refined analysis of NREM sleep changes in depression and other disorders. Thus, it may be premature to conclude that the reported reduction of stages 3 and 4 sleep in depression means that EEG slow-waves per se are virtually not present in depressed patients. For example, if the major change in slow-wave sleep were a reduction in amplitude, it is still possible that the number of slow-waves could in fact be similar in depressive states, during remission, and even in controls, but that the intra-night temporal distribution of slow-wave sleep density could be distinctive for depression.

Third, while REM latency is considered to be the most frequent and consistent sleep phenomenon found in depressed patients, issues dealing with its specificity to depression and certain depressive subtypes (for example, primary versus secondary) remain to be resolved. For example, shortened REM latency has been considered to be a feature of primary major and endogenous depressions rather than secondary and nonendogenous depressions; however, when depressive states associated with alcoholism and drug abuse have been included in the secondary depressive group, there has often been an inability to separate primary and secondary depression (associated with substance abuse) on the basis of REM latency. Also, short REM latencies (particularly, multiple sleep onset REM periods) are seen in the nocturnal sleep of narcoleptics and occasionally in sleep apnea patients, as well as in patients withdrawing from CNS depressant or stimulant drugs. Another area of uncertainty is whether the increased severity in endogenous depression accounts for the more frequent findings of a shortened REM latency in this disorder. Finally, there remains the question of whether REM latencies have a bimodal distribution in depressed patients. Patients with particularly shortened REM latencies, that is, under 20 minutes, seem to represent those depressed patients with a greater severity of illness (including delusional depressives) and a greater resistance to treatment response. However, many elderly depressed patients may also have a very short REM latency, reflecting the effect of age on this particular measure. Thus, when age and psychosis are taken into account, a bimodal distribution of REM latency in primary depressives may be replaced by a more continuous unimodal distribution ranging from 0-65 minutes.

In summary, many of the sleep continuity disturbances of depression are probably nonspecific, including the prolonged sleep latency, increased number of awakenings after sleep onset, and decreased sleep efficiency (ratio of time spent asleep to total recording period) and maintenance. Likewise, the diminished slow-wave sleep of depression seems relatively nonspecific, with the important caveat that this generalization may require revision when the NREM sleep of depressed patients is further analyzed with computer-assisted techniques.

In contrast, the constellation of REM sleep findings in depression seems relatively specific, including the shortened latency to the first REM period, the increase in early REM percent (that is, prolongation of the first REM period), and the increase in number of rapid eye movements (REM density) for the night as a whole and during the first REM period particularly. It should be noted that these findings characterize the baseline sleep of depressed patients, apart from the effects of any challenge, such as the administration of pharmacologic compounds or the use of various sleep deprivation techniques. Further characterization of features specific to depression will probably emerge from the use of such challenge techniques. For example, studies that have used the infusion of cholinergic compounds (physostigmine or arecoline) have shown that some depressed patients may have a more rapid induction of the second REM sleep period than do patients who do not have an affective disorder when the cholinergic compound is infused during the second NREM period (Sitaram et al, 1982). Other studies using REM sleep deprivation have shown that the sleep of depressed patients on recovery nights is characterized by a higher percentage of early REM sleep than that of nondepressed insomniac controls (Vogel et al, 1980).

CLINICAL USE OF THE SLEEP EEG IN PSYCHIATRY

Diagnostic Sensitivity and Specificity

Currently available evidence suggests that EEG sleep studies have utility both in the diagnostic confirmation and in the differential diagnosis of depression. Most published studies in this area have used a quantitative approach for estimating the accuracy of EEG sleep studies by considering their sensitivity, specificity, and diagnostic confidence. "Sensitivity" refers to a test's ability to identify diagnostically true cases; "specificity" refers to a test's ability to exclude false cases. Finally, "diagnostic confidence" is the percentage of true positive test results over the total number of index cases plus the number of false positives. Studies using EEG sleep variables have demonstrated acceptable sensitivity (range: 61.0 to 90.0 percent) and specificity (range 72 to 100 percent) for different EEG sleep measures, in diverse settings, and across various comparison groups (Thase and Kupfer, in press). Similarly, these studies, which will be summarized below, have suggested that the diagnostic confidence of an abnormal EEG sleep study is relatively high (range: 83 to 100 percent) in the confirmation and differential diagnosis of depression.

Rush and colleagues (1982) were able to distinguish endogenous versus nonendogenous depressed outpatients with a diagnostic confidence of 83 percent (sensitivity: 71 percent; specificity: 83 percent) by using a REM latency cutoff score of 60 minutes or less for the endogenous depressives. Akiskal and Tashjian (1983) were able to classify correctly by diagnosis outpatients with primary depression versus either outpatients with secondary depression, nondepressed psychiatric, or normal controls, with a diagnostic confidence of 90 percent (sensitivity: 62 percent; specificity: 88 percent) by using a REM latency cutoff score of

70 minutes or less on two consecutive nights (Akiskal and Tashjian, 1983). Reynolds and colleagues (1983a) were able to show successful separation of outpatients with primary depression from outpatients with generalized anxiety disorder with a 90 percent diagnostic confidence (sensitivity: 90 percent; specificity 80 percent), by using REM latency and REM percentage in a discriminant function analysis. These same investigators were also able to classify correctly elderly primary depressives and elderly patients with senile dementia of the Alzheimer's type with a diagnostic confidence of 85.7 percent (sensitivity: 67 percent; specificity: 89 percent), by using a REM latency cutoff score of 30 minutes or less for the depressives (Reynolds et al, 1983b).

The diagnostic accuracy of EEG sleep studies compares favorably with studies using the dexamethasone suppression test (DST) reviewed by Carroll (1982). In fact, EEG sleep studies have generally shown greater sensitivity for the diagnostic confirmation of depression than that reported for the DST, particularly with outpatient samples. Several groups have now directly compared the diagnostic accuracy of EEG sleep and DST approaches. For example, Rush et al (1982) found greater sensitivity for detection of endogenous depression using shortened REM latency than an abnormal DST (76 percent versus 38 percent), but somewhat lower specificity (72 percent versus 94 percent). Significantly, shortened REM latency was present in all of the DST nonsuppressors.

EEG Sleep Correlates of Depressive Subtypes

EEG sleep measures may be useful not only in the diagnostic confirmation and differential diagnosis of depression from nonaffective psychiatric states, but also for distinguishing diagnostic subtypes of depression. For example, as already noted, a number of investigators have compared EEG sleep in patients classified as endogenously or nonendogenously depressed. Feinberg et al (1982) were able to classify correctly 75 percent of endogenous and nonendogenous depressives by using a discriminant function analysis based on shortened REM latency and increased REM density in the endogenous depressives. Rush and colleagues (1982) have also found REM latency to be significantly lower in endogenously depressed outpatients than in nonendogenously depressed outpatients.

Delusional depression represents a special subtype of endogenous depression, with a significantly poorer response rate to tricyclic antidepressants and often greater psychomotor disturbance. The sleep of these patients is characterized by an even greater decrease of sleep efficiency, more intermittent wakefulness, and less slow-wave sleep than that of other primary depressives. Patients with an RDC diagnosis of schizoaffective depression tend to show EEG sleep measures very similar to those of delusionally depressed patients. Both groups, for example, are characterized by similar reductions in REM sleep latency and degree of sleep continuity disturbance (Kupfer and Thase, 1983). Such findings may be taken as support of the controversial position that schizoaffective disorder is probably a variant of affective disorder rather than schizophrenia.

Regarding the distinction of unipolar versus bipolar primary affective disorder, sleep efficiency tends to be reduced in unipolar depression compared to bipolar depression (Detre et al, 1972); however, phase of illness needs to be considered when discussing hypersomnia in bipolar depression. For example, patients in a mixed state of bipolar disorder often have significant hyposomnia and sleep continuity disturbance. Conversely, a number of bipolar (II) depressives share common clinical features (i.e., anergia, hypersomnia, low levels of overt anxiety, and response to lithium) and genetic history with bipolar patients. Sleep studies in anergic unipolar depressives are often similar to those of bipolar patients, both showing evidence of hypersomnia, such as elevated sleep efficiency. Shortened REM latency has been reported in all series studying bipolar depressives. The difference in sleep efficiency between unipolar and bipolar depressives may parallel differences between these groups in psychomotor activity levels because bipolar depressives tend to show lower levels of daytime and nocturnal activity than unipolar depressives.

Another application of EEG sleep studies with both theoretical and clinical interest is for the differential diagnosis of severe character disorder and primary depressive symptomatology. There is a growing body of research suggesting that a portion of this heterogeneous group may have affective disorders responsive to antidepressant chemotherapy. As part of a prospective, longitudinal study of a large group of characterologic depressives, Akiskal and colleagues (1980) compared pretreatment EEG sleep in five characterologic depressives who subsequently responded to tricyclic antidepressants, with the sleep of eight nondepressed controls, seven characterologic depressives who did not respond to tricyclics, and six patients with unipolar depression. The authors found that REM latency was reduced to a mean of 57.6 minutes in the drug-responder group and thus was indistinguishable from that of the unipolar depressive comparison group (50 minutes).

The EEG sleep of patients with *DSM-III* diagnosable borderline personality disorder also tends to be similar in many regards to the sleep of age-matched primary depressives who do not meet criteria for borderline character disorder. The similarity of sleep measures suggests that, in some patients, there may be a relationship between borderline personality and the affective spectrum of disorders. EEG sleep studies can also be applied in cases in which the diagnosis of depression is masked by psychosomatic symptomatology. In this regard, Blumer et al (1982) studied EEG sleep in a sample of 20 chronic pain patients with insomnia. The mean REM latency for the entire sample was only 60.8 minutes, with eight patients' values falling below 60 minutes. REM latency was also inversely correlated to a significant extent with the post-dexamethasone four p.m. cortisol level.

In summary, EEG sleep measures have already shown considerable promise in the differential diagnosis of depression from nonaffective disorders and in the distinction of depressive subtypes. However, it is apparent that different sets of EEG sleep criteria are necessary to differentiate endogenous from nonendogenous depression, anxiety disorder, dementia, and so forth. Hence, improving diagnostic accuracy based on EEG sleep measures remains a priority for clinical research. Further study is also necessary to determine the best way to control for such potentially confounding and interactive variables as age, severity, and phase of illness. In addition, larger series of age-matched normal and psychiatric controls are needed to provide adequate comparison groups. Technical advances in EEG sleep methodology should also improve diagnostic utility. For example, the use of computer-assisted or automated rapid eye movement and delta analysis may lead to new methods for distinguishing subtypes of depression. Moreover, study of sleep during daytime naps shows some promise for further understanding the sleep-wake disturbances of depression.

Clearly, patients with an unambigious diagnosis of depression do not need to undergo EEG sleep evaluation in order to confirm the clinical diagnosis. Referral for EEG sleep studies should be considered in diagnostically difficult (for example, too many or too few symptoms) or treatment refractory cases. EEG sleep studies should also be considered when the differential diagnosis includes a medical-depressive (that is, "organic-affective," in *DSM-III* terminology) syndrome or primary degenerative dementia with depression. In these latter instances, EEG sleep findings are often distinguished by a reduction in the amount of phasic rapid eye movement activity, compared with primary depression uncomplicated by concurrent medical or neurological disorder (Reynolds et al, 1983a). Results of EEG sleep studies in such cases may provide important information affecting the risk-benefit ratio of antidepressant treatment. The finding of sleep EEG stigmata of primary depression in a patient with mixed symptoms should increase the clinician's confidence in undertaking a full trial of pharmacotherapy. In certain cases with delusions and extremely shortened REM latency, ECT may be the treatment of choice at the outset. In the elderly patient with mixed symptoms of depression and dementia, EEG sleep may also provide useful prognostic information concerning the likelihood of subsequent long-term institutionalization for progressive dementia, versus the relatively more normal existence of the recovered depressive.

Prediction of Treatment Response

In addition to their utility for distinguishing depression from nonaffective disorders and for distinguishing between subtypes of major depression, EEG sleep measures may also be useful in monitoring the neurophysiological effects of tricyclic antidepressant and in the prediction of treatment response.

All-night EEG sleep recordings during drug treatment have shown that a number of tricyclic antidepressants produce rapid suppression of REM sleep, as evidenced by REM latency prolongation, REM activity reduction, and REM percent decrease. Moreover, by using automated or computer-assisted REM sleep analyses, it can be shown that a drug-induced REM suppression is also reflected by an immediate reduction in the number, frequency, and size of rapid eye movements, with a redistribution of REM frequency and intensity such that once started on medication, the second REM period becomes more intense than the first. Tonic aspects of REM sleep, such as REM latency, REM percent, and the number of REM periods, tend to remain suppressed for weeks or even longer during maintenance treatment. In contrast, a partial or complete tolerance to suppression of REM phasic activity and intensity by amitriptyline (the drug for which the most data exist) appears to develop over several weeks of treatment. Correlations between steady-state plasma levels of amitriptyline and several measures of REM suppression during the third and fourth weeks of drug treatment have also been shown, particularly for the tonic aspects of REM, but not for the phasic aspects.

Patients who respond to amitriptyline tend to show a greater REM sleep suppression during the first two nights of drug administration than do nonresponders. Thus, final clinical response tends to be correlated significantly with the extent of REM percent reduction and prolongation of REM latency during the first two nights of drug treatment. Drug responders are significantly more likely than nonresponders to have an initial reduction in REM sleep time to ten percent or less, and a prolongation of REM latency to 100 minutes or longer. In addition, reduction in sleep latency also discriminates drug responders from nonresponders. Thus, in addition to relative lack of REM sleep suppressant effects, drug nonresponders also experience little improvement in initiating sleep during the early nights of amitriptyline treatment. The best prediction equation correctly classifies between 55 and 69 percent of patients as good, partial, or poor drug responders, compared to the 33 percent expected by chance alone. Additional research is necessary to find out whether clinical response characteristics for other antidepressants can be determined.

Another application of sleep measures lies in the assessment of treatment course beyond the immediate response to the acute episode. There is considerable interest in ascertaining the residual sleep abnormalities in depressed patients during remission. The hypothesis is essentially that those individuals who are at high risk for a relapse or the onset of a new episode will demonstrate either sleep abnormalities no different from the acute episode, or abnormalities found somewhere between the acute episode and the normal state. Unfortunately, it is not yet possible to determine whether such residual abnormalities in the sleep of depressed patients apparently in remission actually represent trait vulnerability or, simply, long-lasting CNS effects of an episode of affective illness. Furthermore, it is impossible to know whether such patients ever had normal EEG sleep. Clearly, longitudinal studies of EEG sleep in first-degree relatives of depressed patients with no personal history of affective disorder would help address this problem. For example, if it were found that first-degree relatives of depressed probands had an increased frequency of polysomnographic abnormalities (such as decreased REM latency) even in the absence of any personal history of affective disorder, then such abnormalities could be seen as markers of the vulnerability to affective disorder, and more powerful inferences could be made regarding the role of such abnormalities in the etiopathogenesis of depression. These speculations lend themselves to the following brief theoretical overview of the EEG sleep findings in depressive disorders, using several perspectives: developmental, chronophysiological, and neurochemical.

EEG SLEEP AND THE PATHOPHYSIOLOGY OF DEPRESSION

Neurochemical Models

The foregoing considerations suggest that EEG sleep studies in depression might help in understanding the pathophysiology of depression. McCarley (1982) has recently summarized evidence concerning EEG sleep disturbance in depression with respect to a balance between cholinergic and monoaminergic activity. He has proposed a reciprocal interaction model of state control, involving REM-inhibiting activity originating from the locus coeruleus (norepinephrine) and midbrain raphe (serotonin) nuclei, and REM-excitatory activity from the pontine reticular formation (acetylcholine). This cholinergic basis for REM sleep parallels the apparent cholinergic hypersensitivity of some depressed patients, as reflected by the faster induction of the second REM period by the muscarinic cholinergic agonist, arecoline, as well as by the increased sensitivity of some affective disorder patients to the dysphoriogenic effects of cholinergic compounds (Sitaram et al, 1982).

Chronobiological Models

A growing, though as yet inconclusive, body of research has also linked the EEG sleep abnormalities of depression to disturbances of biological rhythms. Thus, onset of REM sleep, distribution of REM density, body temperature, and serum cortisol levels appear to be abnormally phase-advanced in depression (Wehr, 1982). In addition, phase advancement of the sleep-wake cycle may temporarily induce clinical remission in some depressed patients.

A second chronobiological perspective is provided by the two-process model of sleep regulation, developed by Borbely (1982). This model posits that the sleep changes of depression depend upon the interaction of two processes, which themselves affect the timing and organization of sleep. First, process "S" (which represents sleep propensity or need) could reflect a hypothesized sleep factor that accumulates during wakefulness and is dissipated by sleep. Second, process "C," a circadian factor, is seen to reflect REM sleep propensity and may be linked to circadian temperature rhythm. In depression, it may be factor S that is specifically deficient, as evidenced by the overall short sleeptime, sleep maintenance difficulties, reduced slow-wave sleep and EEG delta wave activity, the early appearance of REM sleep, and clinical benefits of sleep deprivation. One might speculate that the waning ability to sleep which characterizes both normal aging and, to a much greater extent, depression, reflects a greater vulnerability of process "S" to aging, while process "C" may be relatively more age-resistant or stable. Perhaps, also, the apparent cholinergic hypersensitivity of some depressed patients reflects more fundamentally a disinhibition of REM mechanisms mediated through a weakened process "S," as a result of either normal aging, depression, or their interaction.

Developmental Models

According to the preceding view, depression can be considered as a correlate of aging, which naturally raises a developmental perspective. It is now known that decreases in slow-wave sleep (and its amplitude) and in REM latency, and increases in wakefulness after sleep onset, are the major age-related changes in the nocturnal sleep of normal individuals. These are the same changes that occur most predictably in major depressive illness, although to a much greater extent. In other words, the age-dependent decrease in slow-wave sleep and in REM latency and the increase in intermittent wake time seem to occur in depressed persons to a much greater extent than in normals. This observation raises the question of whether persons in whom these changes in sleep continuity and slow-wave sleep occur earlier in life are not therefore more vulnerable to the development of depression. As previously suggested, the question could be addressed by studying the sleep of children of depressed patients who themselves have no personal history of affective disorder (but are at increased risk), and comparing their sleep findings with those of normal controls who have no familial history of depression.

At this time, it seems unlikely that the issues raised here concerning sleep and its regulation in depression and in aging can be answered without the use of challenge strategies, whether nonpharmacological (for example, REM deprivation or total sleep deprivation, challenges to thermoregulation, or exposure to bright light at crucial intervals), or pharmacological (for example, the use of specific cholinergic probes). In any case, EEG sleep methods will continue to provide a noninvasive neurophysiological window for studying the pathophysiology of depression and mechanisms of drug action. Further development and wider application of EEG sleep methodology should continue to yield advances in the diagnosis, treatment, and understanding of depression.

REFERENCES

Akiskal HS, Rosenthal TL, Haykal RF, et al: Characterological depressions: clinical and sleep EEG findings separating subaffective dysthymias' from 'character-spectrum disorders.' Arch Gen Psychiatry 37:777–783, 1980

Akiskal HS, Tashjian R: Affective disorders: II. Recent advances in laboratory and pathogenetic approaches. Hosp Community Psychiatry 34:822–830, 1983

Association of Sleep Disorders Centers: Diagnostic classification of sleep and arousal disorders. Sleep 2:1–127, 1979

Blumer D, Zorick T, Heilbronn M, et al: Biological markers for depression in chronic pain. J Nerv Ment Dis 170:425–428, 1982

Borbely AA: A two-process model of sleep regulation. Human Neurobiology 1:155–204, 1982

Carroll BJ: The dexamethasone suppression test for melancholia. Br. J Psychiatry 140:292–304, 1982

Coleman R, Roffwarg H, Kennedy S, et al: Sleep-wake disorders based on a polysomnographic diagnosis: a national cooperative study. JAMA 247:997–1003, 1982

Detre TP, Himmelhoch J, Swartzburg M, et al: Hypersomnia and manic-depressive disease. Am J Psychiatry 128:1303–1305, 1972

Feinberg M, Gillin JC, Carroll BJ, et al: EEG studies of sleep in the diagnosis of depression. Biol Psychiatry 17:305–316, 1982

Kupfer DJ, Reynolds CF: Neurophysiologic studies of depression: state of the art, in The Origins of Depression: Current Concepts and Approaches. Edited by Angst J. Berlin, Springer-Verlag, 1983

Kupfer DJ, Thase ME: The use of the sleep laboratory in the diagnosis of affective disorders. Psychiatr Clin North Am 6:3–25, 1983

McCarley RW: Sleep and depression: common neurobiological control mechanisms. Am J Psychiatry 139:565–570, 1982

Reynolds CF III, Shaw D, Newton T, et al: EEG sleep in outpatients with generalized anxiety disorder: a preliminary comparison with depressed outpatients. Psychiatry Res 8:81–89, 1983a

Reynolds CF III, Spiker DG, Hanin I, et al: EEG sleep, aging, and psychopathology: new data and state of the art. Biol Psychiatry 18:139–155, 1983b

Rush AJ, Giles DE, Roffwarg HP, et al: Sleep EEG and dexamethasone suppression test findings in outpatients with unipolar major depressive disorder. Biol Psychiatry 17:327–341, 1982

Sitaram N, Nurnberger JI, Gershon E, et al: Cholinergic regulation of mood and REM sleep: potential model and marker of vulnerability to affective disorder. Am J Psychiatry 139:571–576, 1982

Thase ME, Kupfer DJ: Current status of EEG sleep in the assessment and treatment of depression, in Advances in Human Psychopharmacology, vol 6. Edited by Burrows GD, Werry JS. Greenwich, Conn, JAI Press, Inc., 1983

Vogel GW, Vogel F, McAbee RS, et al: Improvement of depression by REM sleep deprivation. Arch Gen Psychiatry 37:247–253, 1980

Wehr TA: Circadian rhythm disturbances in depression, in Rhythmic Aspects of Behavior. Edited by Brown FC, Graeber RC. Hillsdale, NJ, Erlbaum Associates, 1982

Chapter 18

Sleep Studies in Selected Adult Neuropsychiatric Disorders

by J. Christian Gillin, M.D., Charles F.
Reynolds III, M.D. and James E. Shipley, M.D.

Complaints of sleep disturbance are common in patients suffering from a variety of psychiatric and other disorders, and all-night EEG sleep studies have provided valuable, nonintrusive biological measures in clinical research. One measure— REM latency—has received particular attention. The following discussion reviews some sleep studies of disorders other than depression, which was covered in the previous chapter.

ADULT OBSESSIVE-COMPULSIVE DISORDER

Although sleep complaints apparently have not been included in classical clinical descriptions of adult obsessive-compulsive disorder, a recent study found that nine out of 14 patients did report sleep disturbance (Insel et al, 1982). Seven patients described both difficulty getting to sleep and staying asleep, while two mentioned hypersomnia (12 hours per night in each case). Obsessive worries and checking rituals were frequently blamed for poor sleep.

All night EEG sleep recordings were obtained from 14 patients with moderate to severe obsessive-compulsive symptoms and compared with normal controls and patients with depression. This study was an ordeal for some patients who were fearful of "contamination" or concerned that the sleep study would interfere with cleaning rituals. Not all obsessive-compulsive subjects were able to participate fully in the study.

The results showed that the sleep records of patients with obsessive-compulsive disorder were very similar to those obtained from patients with depression. In comparison to normal controls, both patient groups showed short REM latency, decreased total sleep time with more awakenings, less stage 4 sleep, and decreased sleep efficiency (sleep time over time in bed) and REM sleep efficiency (time in REM sleep over time from the beginning to end of a REM period). The patients with obsessive-compulsive disorder differed from those with depression on only two measures: They had more stage 1 and stage 3 sleep. In addition, there was a strong tendency toward lower REM density ($p < .07$) in the patients with obsessive-compulsive disorder.

Both the Hamilton Depression Rating Scale and the Global Anxiety Scale were negatively correlated with sleep efficiency, and positively correlated with awake-movement time in the patients with obsessive-compulsive disorder. The obsessional subscale of the Comprehensive Psychiatric Rating Scale correlated negatively with stage 4 sleep and positively with REM density. REM latency did not correlate with any of these three rating scales.

The severity of depressive symptoms did not appear to account for short REM latency in the patients with obsessive-compulsive disorder. First, the rating scales for depression did not correlate. Second, when patients were divided into depressed and nondepressed subgroups, both groups had significantly shorter REM latency than normal controls but did not differ significantly from each other. Indeed, the two patient groups, taken as a whole, had mean REM latency values that differed by only one minute.

In an additional study, ten patients with obsessive-compulsive disorder were studied with the dexamethasone suppression test (DST). Four of them were nonsuppressors, approximating the incidence of abnormal response in affective disorders. The presence of these biologic markers as well as good clinical response to tricyclic antidepressants, in both obsessive-compulsive disorder and depression, suggest that the two disorders may share some common pathophysiological mechanisms. Nevertheless, the two can be distinguished on the basis of clinical symptoms, natural history, and genetic studies. Further research is needed to understand the underlying psychobiological basis for these disorders and their common biological markers.

DEMENTIA

Night wandering, "sun-downing," disturbed sleep, and nocturnal use of hypnotics and tranquilizers are common in demented patients. Families frequently institutionalize their demented relatives when it becomes too difficult to care for them at night.

Disturbed sleep patterns are specifically mentioned in *DSM-III* as a symptom of delirium, which is often a complication of dementia and a differential diagnostic consideration. Sleep studies of delirium apparently have not been conducted on a systematic basis.

In comparison to normal, age-matched controls, patients with senile dementia of the Alzheimer's type (SDAT) appear to show a flattening of the circadian cycle of rest and activity, with major intrusions of wakefulness during the sleep period at night and major interruptions of wakefulness by sleep during the day (Prinz et al, 1982). In some ways these patterns are similar to those observed in animals with lesions in the suprachiasmatic nucleus (SCN), which display an "arrhythmic" succession of short bursts of sleep and wakefulness throughout the 24-hour day with little circadian organization of sleep and activity. In this vein, it is interesting to speculate that three closely situated anatomical structures that could be involved are found in the basal forebrain-anterior hypothalamic area: the SCN, which acts as a biological clock; the nucleus basilis of Meynert, which is the source of cholinergic innervation of the cortex and which appears to be somewhat selectively destroyed in SDAT; and the basal forebrain, which has been implicated in basic sleep mechanisms, particularly NREM sleep. The Cholinergic REM Induction Test (Gillin et al, 1983) may be useful in clinical investigations of cholinergic functioning in dementia but would have to be conducted carefully for reasons of safety.

Various disturbances of sleep stages and sleep architecture have also been observed in dementia. Sleep stages 3 and 4 show a particular attrition, and more detailed observations of EEG patterns reveal loss of delta waves, K-complexes, and sleep spindles. Loss of REM sleep has also been reported in relatively old, severely demented patients (Prinz et al, 1983) but not in a more recent study of younger, less severely demented patients (Lowenstein et al, 1983). In the first study, REM sleep was significantly and negatively correlated with measures of cognitive performance and memory, but not in the second study, which, in addition, did not report low REM sleep levels. Rather, delta sleep was positively correlated with memory performance (Lowenstein et al, 1983). These observations suggest that sleep stage changes may parallel the natural course of SDAT, with loss of stage 4 sleep early in the onset of the disorder and loss of REM sleep later with more severity.

Values for REM latency have been variable in SDAT. In apparently the only comparison of demented patients and age-matched depressed patients, Reynolds et al (1983) found no significant difference in mean REM latency, although short REM latencies tended to cluster more in depression than dementia. REM density was significantly lower in demented than depressed patients; and sleep continuity, although disturbed in both groups, was less so in dementia than depression.

Neither the treatment nor the pathophysiology of disturbed sleep-wake patterns in dementia is well understood at this time. Elderly patients, especially demented ones, are particularly at risk for the toxic side effects of the benzodiazepine hypnotics and major tranquilizers. Both classes of drugs have been associated with ataxia, cognitive and attentional impairment, "pseudo-dementia," and daytime sleepiness. The elderly tend to eliminate these drugs slowly and to show greater sensitivity at comparable blood levels than younger patients. They are also at greater risk for hypotensive and cardiovascular side effects, extrapyramidal side effects, and tardive dyskinesia with the major antipsychotic drugs.

While the therapeutic potential of chronobiological approaches has not been systematically studied in dementia, they are worthy of consideration. Such approaches would involve going to bed and getting up at regular times; minimizing naps; maximizing daytime activity and stimulation; and being exposed to bright lights and sunshine during the day, especially near the wake-up time and bedtime. The actual hours would probably be best tailored to the patient (that is, natural owls and larks, long and short sleepers) and would not impose unrealistic expectations (that is, sleep from 8:00 P.M. until 8:00 A.M.).

Since the sleep problems of the demented patient are, to some extent, an exaggeration of trends seen in many normal elderly, further research in these areas will help clarify certain issues about normal aging. To what extent are the "normal" sleep trends normal or pathological? Do changes in sleep duration and timing reflect altered "need to sleep" or "ability to sleep"?

SCHIZOPHRENIA

Following the discovery of REM sleep, there was considerable interest in the possibility that psychosis and, in particular, hallucinations, reflected an abnormality of REM sleep (see Gillin and Wyatt, 1975 and Feinberg and Hiatt, 1978). In general, cross sectional studies have failed to reveal any consistent, significant abnormalities of REM sleep.

However, two other findings of uncertain significance have emerged. First, two studies have suggested that actively ill schizophrenics fail to show a normal rebound of REM sleep following experimental REM deprivation (Zarcone et al, 1975; Gillin and Wyatt, 1975). This finding is somewhat controversial (Vogel, 1975). In any case, REM rebound has not been absent in every actively ill schizophrenic patient studied or present in every control subject (Gillin and Wyatt, 1975). Second, low amounts of stage 4 sleep have been reported consistently in a significant proportion of schizophrenic patients, particularly during the first REM period.

Preliminary computer analysis of delta wave activity suggests that, for the first NREM period, average amplitude of, number of, and time occupied by delta waves (0.5–3 Hz) were lower in patients than normal controls and that the average frequency of waves was significantly higher. These latter data have not yet been published. While the diagnostic specificity of low stage 4 sleep in schizophrenia is poor—this finding is common in many other pathological conditions—it is a relatively robust finding, and its pathophysiological and prognostic significance is unknown.

It would be particularly interesting to compare schizophrenics, depressed, normal aged, demented, and other groups with low amounts of stage 4 sleep by means of computer analyzed delta waves to determine whether they share common or separate phenomenological mechanisms that result in lowered stage 4 sleep scored by eye (that is, is it possible that low stage 4 could result from either a specific loss of amplitude or from a reduction in number of delta waves?). No consensus exists on whether low stage 4 sleep is a state or a trait marker of schizophrenia or whether it would be of value in high-risk or genetic studies of schizophrenia. Feinberg (1982) has speculated that the decline of stage 4 sleep in normal adolescence reflects a reduction in cortical synaptic density and a fall in daytime cerebral metabolic rate, and that a defect in this maturational process may be related to schizophrenia emerging in adolescence.

In addition, short REM latency has been reported in a number of studies comparing schizophrenics and normal controls (Feinberg et al, 1964; Stern et al, 1969; Jus et al, 1973). Since short REM latency has also been reported in patients with schizoaffective schizophrenia (Reich et al, 1975), it has been argued that earlier studies included patients whose diagnosis is in question according to more recent diagnostic criteria. Nevertheless, there apparently have been no recent studies with newer methods of diagnosis to settle these matters.

While REM density (a measure of eye movement intensity in REM sleep) has usually been reported to be normal in schizophrenia, Benson and Zarcone (1982) have recently reported on another method of measuring the phasic events of REM sleep—namely, middle ear muscle activity (MEMA)—which is recorded by tympanic acoustic impedance. Patients with schizoaffective disorder had significantly lower rates than normals and patients with schizophrenia, and a strong trend to lower rates than patients with depression. While the mean value for schizophrenic patients was not statistically different from normal controls, the schizophrenic patients showed greater variance, and a sizeable subgroup displayed values above those of any subjects from the three other groups. Further work is needed to confirm this observation.

ANXIETY DISORDERS

The nosology of sleep and arousal disorders developed by the Association of Sleep Disorders Centers (ASDC) (1979) recognizes anxiety states as "associated" with disorders of initiating and maintaining sleep. In support of this classification, a study by Kales and colleagues (1976) is cited which describes MMPI profiles in insomniacs. Similarly, other investigations have begun with patients who claim to be insomniacs or "poor sleepers," have documented their sleep polygraphically, and then have generated personality profiles. Such studies describe the incidence of anxiety in insomniacs but leave open the questions of incidence and nature of sleep disorder in anxious patients. To address this deficiency in our knowledge, some investigators (Reynolds et al, 1983) have recently begun studying the EEG sleep characteristics of patients with various types of anxiety disorders.

One area being studied is whether generalized anxiety disorder has definitive EEG sleep characteristics and whether they differ from the sleep characteristics of primary depression. The question of such psychobiological differences, if any, is pertinent to clinicians because the differential diagnosis of anxiety versus depression sometimes cannot be made with confidence, particularly in younger patients in whom depressive states frequently present with prominent anxiety symptoms.

In a preliminary study, both patients with generalized anxiety disorder (n = 10) and patients with primary depression (n = 20) showed similar patterns of sleep continuity disturbance when compared with controls, with difficulty falling asleep (prolonged sleep latency), difficulty maintaining sleep (increased intermittent wakefulness), and diminished sleep efficiency generally (Reynolds et al, 1983). Similarly, with respect to sleep architecture measures, both depressed and anxious patients had reduced amounts of delta sleep (stages 3 and 4) compared to controls. Thus, impairment in sleep continuity and reduction of delta sleep appear to be nonspecific, in the sense that they are seen in both generalized anxiety disorder and primary depression. In contrast, a reduction of REM sleep percent occurred in the anxious patients but not necessarily a short REM latency, while both a short REM latency and an increased REM percent were seen in depressives. Ninety percent of depressives and 80 percent of anxious patients were correctly classified by research diagnosis when two sleep variables (REM latency and REM percent) entered into a discriminant function analysis. These data furnish external validation for the clinical (*DSM-III*) distinction between generalized anxiety disorders and primary depression, and provide additional evidence for the concept that the sleep of psychiatric patients who complain of insomnia is not distinguished by one type of abnormality.

EEG sleep studies of patients with anxiety disorders other than generalized anxiety (e.g., obsessive-compulsive and panic) are needed. In a symposium on anxiety sponsored by the American Psychopathological Association (1980), Sachar cogently put the issue as follows: "Anxiety states in animals and in man are not simply an amalgam, a nonspecific mishmash, a spectrum of arousal that is purely a matter of graded intensity; on the contrary, there are qualitatively different anxiety systems that are possible to dissect on a number of grounds." A recent report on psychobiologic measures (including EEG sleep) in childhood obsessive-compulsive disorder (Rapoport et al, 1981) indicated that the EEG sleep measures of nine adolescents with primary obsessive-compulsive disorder resembled those of young adults with primary depressive disorder. The authors report that "all subjects would have met *DSM-III* criteria for major depressive disorder at some time in their life." Insel and colleagues (1982) have also found similarities between the EEG sleep of adult obsessive-compulsive patients (n = 14) and patients with primary depression, pointing to a possible biological link between obsessive-compulsive disorder and affective illness.

BORDERLINE PERSONALITY DISORDER

Disorders of personality are also recognized by the ASDC nosology (1979) as associated with sleep disturbances, either insomnia or excessive sleepiness. In the case of personality disorders, the nature of the association with sleep disturbance is complex and multifaceted. Many such patients will develop a sleep disturbance in association with a chaotic life style, which entails an irregular sleep-wake schedule, poor nutrition and exercise habits, living environments that are physically and temporally adverse to good sleep, and use or abuse of central nervous system depressants or stimulants. Some of these patients may be caught up in the vicious cycle of "trying too hard" to sleep, a form of psychophysiological insomnia. Insomnia is rarely a straightforward problem since it usually involves some or all of these factors. In addition, patients with personality disorders may become clinically anxious or depressed and develop a sleep disturbance associated with this change of affective state.

Several EEG studies on patients with a borderline personality disorder have been completed (Akiskal, 1981; Bell et al, 1983; McNamara et al, 1984). *DSM-III* diagnostic criteria for this disorder include a longstanding pattern of impulsive behavior (particularly physically self-damaging acts such as suicidal gestures or self-mutilation), a pattern of unstable interpersonal relationships, intense anger or loss of control of anger, pervasive uncertainty about issues relating to identity (such as sexual preference or long-term goals), chronic feelings of emptiness or boredom, and affective instability and dysphoria. *DSM-III* views the affective instability and dysphoria of borderline personality patients as part of a characterologic disorder. A second viewpoint, represented by Akiskal (1981), is that borderline psychopathology is a manifestation of an atypical affective disorder. A third viewpoint in this nosologic argument, espoused by Carroll et al (1981), is that borderline psychopathology represents *both* an affective disorder and a personality disorder.

The development of EEG sleep studies and the application of short REM latency as a biological marker in primary affective disorder, together with the development of a reliable assessment method for the clinical research diagnosis of borderline personality disorder, make possible an investigation into the nature of depression in these patients. Akiskal (1981) has reported that REM latency is short in outpatients with borderline personality disorders, comparable to values seen in outpatients with primary depression. In a pilot investigation by Reynolds et al (1984) the EEG sleep of borderline patients and primary depressives was compared. In both groups, evidence of sleep continuity disturbance (difficulty in getting to sleep and maintaining sleep) and increased REM activity and density during the night as a whole, and particularly during the first REM period, were present when compared with age-matched controls (McNamara et al, 1984). First-night REM latencies were more variable in the borderline group than in the depressives, but by the second night in the laboratory both groups showed short REM latencies of around 50 minutes in comparison to control values of 75 minutes. These similarities in EEG sleep suggest a relationship for some borderline personality patients to the affective spectrum, and cast doubt on the definition of the borderline syndrome as a pure character type.

The relationship between borderline personality disorder and primary major depression has been further studied prospectively using EEG sleep studies, SADS-L interviews, and family history data (Reynolds et al, 1984). Ten consecutively admitted borderline patients (prospective sample), defined by Gunderson's Diagnostic Interview for Borderlines (DIB), underwent EEG sleep studies on two consecutive nights and were compared to previously reported samples of RDC-defined depressed patients, normal controls, and DIB-defined borderlines who had been referred "to rule out major depression" (retrospective sample) (McNamara et al, 1984). REM latency values were similar in depressed and both borderline groups but significantly different from controls. Eighty-five percent of REM latency values in RDC major depressives were less than 65 minutes, compared to similar rates of 75 percent in the prospective sample of borderlines and 65 percent in the retrospective sample, versus 35 percent for controls (X^2 = 10.7, p <.005). The REM latency in borderline patients did not vary with the severity of depression as measured by the Hamilton Rating Scale. In the prospective borderline sample, the major SADS-L diagnoses were chronic intermittent depression (n = 5), current major depression (n-4) (two unipolar, two bipolar II), and labile personality (n = 1). Family history data revealed high rates of clinical depression, alcohol abuse, and suicide attempts in both the retrospectively and prospectively studied borderline samples, with a combined rate of 53 percent of the families having definite depression, 41 percent having alcohol abuse, and 23.5 percent suicide attempts. This convergence of nosologic, family history, and biologic data supports the concept of a close relationship between criteria-defined borderline personality disorder and affective illness.

CONCLUSION

From these brief reviews, it is clear that considerable progress has been made in establishing relatively well described EEG sleep abnormalities (that is, short REM latency and low stage 4 sleep) in some psychiatric disorders and in testing leads in others. Like the dexamethasone suppression test and thyrotropin releasing hormone test, these findings are often more sensitive than diagnostically specific. Knowledge about age-related sleep changes in health and sickness has also grown, and the entire field of sleep disorders medicine has arisen more or less de novo in the past 15 years. These developments offer increasing hope to clinicians who face patients complaining of sleep disorders as well as to researchers seeking evidence of biological abnormalities in psychiatric illness.

Nevertheless, many issues remain to be resolved through future research. The state and trait sensitivity and specificity of specific abnormal measures or clusters of measures need to be clarified in relation to diagnosis and clinical characteristics. For example, does the flattened sleep-wake circadian cycle and loss of stage 4 sleep separate patients with senile dementia of the Alzheimer's type from all other diagnostic groups? What is the significance of short REM latency in so many diagnostic groups; and would the combination of short REM latency, high REM density, and prolonged duration of the first REM period provide better diagnostic discrimination between primary depressives, obsessive-compulsives, and schizoaffectives? What are the pathophysiological mechanisms involved in these various disturbances? Both basic and clinical research efforts over the coming years should provide some answers to these questions and enrich the scientific basis of psychiatry.

REFERENCES

Akiskal HS: Subaffective disorders: dysthymic, cyclothymic and bipolar II disorders in the 'borderline' realm. Psychiatr Clin North Am, 4:25-46, 1981

Association of Sleep Disorders Centers: Classification of sleep and arousal disorders. Sleep, 2:1-153, 1979

Bell J, Lycaki H, Jones D, et al: Effects of pre-existing borderline personality on clinical and EEG sleep correlates of depression. Psychiatry Res 9:115, 1983

Benson KL, Zarcone VP, Jr.: Middle ear muscle activity during REM sleep in schizophrenic, schizoaffective, and depressed patients. Am J Psychiatry 139:1474-1476, 1982

Carroll BJ, Greden JF, Feinberg M, et al: Neuroendocrine evaluation of depression in borderline patients. Psychiatr Clin North Am, 4:89-99, 1981

Feinberg I: Schizophrenia: caused by a fault in programmed synaptic elimination during adolescence? J Psychiatr Res 17:319-334, 1982

Feinberg I, Koresko RL, Gottlieb F: Sleep electroencephalographic and eye movement patterns in schizophrenic patients. Psychiatry 5:44, 1964

Feinberg I, Hiatt JF: Sleep patterns in schizophrenia: a selective review, in Sleep Disorders: Diagnosis and Treatment, Edited by Williams RC, Karacan I. New York, John Wiley & Sons, 1978

Gillin JC, Wyatt RJ: Schizophrenia: perchance a dream? Int Rev Neurobiol 17:297-342, 1975

Gillin JC, Sitaram N, Nurnberger JI, et al: The Cholinergic REM Induction Test (CRIT). Psychopharmacol Bull 19:668-670, 1983

Insel TR, Gillin JC, Moore A, et al: The sleep of patients with obsessive-compulsive disorder. Arch Gen Psychiatry 39:1372-1377, 1982

Jus K, Bouchard M, Jus AK: Sleep EEG studies in untreated long term schizophrenic patients. Arch Gen Psychiatry 29:386-390, 1973

Kales A, Caldwell AB, Preston TA, et al: Personality patterns in insomnia. Arch Gen Psychiatry, 33:1128-1134, 1976

Lowenstein RJ, Weingartner H, Gillin JC, et al: Disturbances of sleep and cognitive functioning of patients with dementia. Neurobiol Aging 3:371-177, 1983

McNamara E, Reynolds CF, Soloff PH, et al: Electroencephalographic Sleep Evaluation of Depression in Borderline Patients. Am J Psychiatry 141:182-186, 1984

Prinz PN, Vitaliano PP, Vitiello MV, et al: Sleep EEG and mental function changes in senile dementia of the Alzheimer's type. Neurobiol Aging, 3:361-370, 1983

Rapoport J, Elkins R, Langer DH, et al: Childhood obsessive-compulsive disorder. Am J Psychiatry 138:1545-1554, 1981

Reich L, Weiss BL, Coble P. Sleep disturbance in schizophrenia: a revisit. Arch Gen Psychiatry 32:51-55, 1975

Reynolds CF, Shaw DH, Newton TF, et al: EEG sleep in outpatients with generalized anxiety disorder: a preliminary comparison with primary depression. Psychiatry Res 8:81-89, 1983a

Reynolds CF, Spiker DG, Hanin I, et al: Electroencephalographic sleep, aging, and psychopathology: new data and state of the art. Biol Psychiatry 18:139-155, 1983b

Reynolds CF, Soloff PH, Taska LS, et al: EEG sleep evaluation of depression in borderline patients: a prospective replication. Sleep Research 13:125, 1984

Sachar EJ: Anxiety: New Research and Changing Concepts, Edited by Klein DG, Rabkin J. New York, Raven Press, 1980

Stern N, Fram D, Wyatt RJ, et al: All night sleep studies of acute schizophrenics. Arch Gen Psychiatry 20:470-477, 1969

Vogel GW: A review of REM sleep deprivation. Arch Gen Psychiatry 32:749-761, 1975

Zarcone V, Azumi K, Dement WC, et al: REM phase deprivation and schizophrenia II. Arch Gen Psychiatry 32:1431-1438, 1975

Chapter 19

Nonpharmacological Treatment of Sleep Disorders

by Peter J. Hauri, Ph.D. and Michael J. Sateia, M.D.

People who suffer from chronic diseases react to them psychologically. The longer the disease lasts, the more the patient habituates to it, changes his or her lifestyle, and develops new behavioral patterns that fit the disease. To improve the chronic condition, these adaptations, as well as the original causes of the disorder, need to be examined and treated. This is especially true in the sleep disorders because sleep, itself, is exquisitely sensitive to psychological disturbances. This chapter examines the nonpharmacological treatment approaches for chronic sleep disorders and outlines the range of skills and considerations that are necessary for their treatment.

PSYCHOLOGICAL FACTORS IN CHRONIC INSOMNIA

Life experience suggests that some relationship exists between sleep disturbance and one's psychological state. While the Association of Sleep Disorders Centers (ASDC) nosology clearly accounts for disorders of initiating and maintaining sleep which are secondary to specific psychiatric illness, it also leaves room for speculation regarding possible psychological determinants of other types of insomnia, most notably, the psychophysiological variety.

There is evidence that a significant number of insomniacs demonstrate a pattern of psychopathology characterized by neurotic depression, anxiety, a proclivity to ruminate, and a marked tendency to internalize emotion and to somaticize their psychological distress. This psychological profile, or components of it, is likely to play a causative role for some insomniacs. Adverse experiences in childhood serve to establish the psychological disturbance, while a period of major life stresses may precipitate the onset of the insomnia. Studies have suggested that different psychological profiles may exist for different subsets of insomnia, although current information is not conclusive.

Many authors have made efforts to expand our understanding in this area, most often by using psychometric testing to obtain psychological profiles of insomniacs. Although these studies suggest some areas of agreement, many are fraught with contradictions. One of the most frequent sources of confusion is the diversity of problems the term "insomnia" has been used to explain. Considerable variation also exists with respect to the use of polysomnography (PSG) to provide objective sleep parameters with which to correlate psychological variables. Finally, psychopathology, demonstrated by whatever method, is often assumed to cause the insomnia, despite the fact that few data have emerged which would allow one to distinguish primary factors from those that might occur as secondary effects of chronic insomnia. Most clinicians and researchers believe that personality and other related psychological factors play a prominent role in the etiology of insomnia. Even with its shortcomings, much research to date supports this viewpoint (Kales et al, 1983; Coursey et al, 1975; Monroe, 1967).

SLEEP HYGIENE

Some individuals can break any rule of sleep hygiene and still sleep soundly; others need to follow sleep hygiene rules more carefully. Excessive concern with sleep hygiene rules may not be beneficial, however. For example, although it is useful to establish regular sleeping and waking times, it is probably not harmful to sleep in on an occasional morning or to stay up late when the situation arises.

The following sleep hygiene guidelines have been established (Hauri, 1981): **SLEEP AS MUCH AS NEEDED TO FEEL REFRESHED AND HEALTHY DURING THE FOLLOWING DAY, BUT NOT MORE.** Insomniacs often seem to stay in bed too long, trying to squeeze the last drop of sleep out of each night (Monroe, 1967, Spielman et al, 1983). Curtailing the time spent in bed seems to solidify sleep. Excessively long times in bed seem related to sleep fragmentation and shallow sleep.

MAINTAIN REGULAR AROUSAL TIMES. Our internal, circadian cycle deviates from the 24-hour light-dark cycle established by the sun (Aschoff et al, 1975). It has to be synchronized almost daily, like a clock that loses about an hour per day. The best method of synchronizing our internal rhythm is to maintain a regular arousal time because this event can be controlled and because the process of waking up and getting out of bed in the morning is a strong biological stimulus (changing from sleeping to waking, from a horizontal to a vertical position, from inactivity to activity). Maintaining a regular bedtime is much less important because one cannot force sleep. Going to bed when one is not sleepy will usually lead to frustration and maladaptive learning; it will not synchronize the internal rhythm.

MAINTAIN A STEADY AMOUNT OF EXERCISE. A healthy body sleeps better and deeper than an unfit body (Griffin and Trinder, 1978). However, this association occurs over weeks and months; an occasional heavy workout will probably not deepen sleep on the following night (Hauri, 1969).

AVOID OCCASIONAL LOUD NOISES. Noise from aircraft flyovers or from trucks should be avoided. If one must sleep in an environment in which loud noises occur, they should be masked with a steady "white" noise such as an air conditioner or fan; the bedroom should be sound attenuated. Globus and colleagues (1974) have shown that people do not adjust to occasional loud noises, even if they no longer remember them in the morning.

KEEP THE ROOM TEMPERATURE COMFORTABLE. Either excessively warm rooms (above 75°F) or excessively cold rooms (below 40°F) disturb sleep (Schmidt-Kessen and Kendel, 1973; Ziegler, 1972).

HUNGER MAY DISTURB SLEEP. A light bedtime snack may help. Indeed, it has been shown that a high carbohydrate diet decreases waking and very light sleep (Porter and Horne, 1981). Others have shown that warm milk or Ovaltine at bedtime helps (Southwell et al, 1972). It is still debatable whether this effect involves tryptophan metabolism, gastric hormones (Fara et al, 1969), or other mechanisms.

CAFFEINE AND TOBACCO DISTURB SLEEP. This is true even for those who feel that this is not the case (Karacan et al, 1976; Soldatos et al, 1980). Caffeine is found not only in coffee, which contains up to 125 mg per cup, but also in freshly brewed tea (75 mg per cup), and cola drinks (up to 50 mg per eight ounces), according to Walker (1982). In addition, excessive use of stimulants complicates benzodiazepine intake because the substances contained in coffee, tea and tobacco stimulate the same hepatic enzymes that metabolize benzodiazepines (Downing and Rickels, 1981).

One frequently encounters insomniacs who claim they cannot sleep without a cup of coffee or some bedtime cigarettes. While atypical, paradoxical reactions cannot be ruled out; it seems more likely that these patients may be heavily addicted to coffee or tobacco. Not smoking or not drinking for a few hours starts a withdrawal process with its associated tension and agitation. Usually, such people sleep much better once they have overcome withdrawal.

AVOID ALCOHOL. Although alcohol allows tense people to relax and fall asleep, the ensuing sleep is fragmented and disturbed; as a result, less sleep is accumulated by morning than it would be without alcohol (Rundell et al, 1972).

DO NOT WORRY OR BROOD IN BED. Trying hard to sleep prevents sleep. It is usually better to keep one's mind occupied with nonthreatening stimuli such as reading, listening to records, or watching TV until one can no longer remain awake, than to lie in bed frustrated, seeking sleep. However, there are exceptions. For example, those who have established a conditioned association between the bed and arousal should not do their relaxing, reading, or T.V. watching in bed.

KEEP BUSY, EVEN AFTER A SLEEPLESS NIGHT. Good sleepers seem busier, more active, and more involved in their work and with other people than insomniacs, who focus more on themselves and various forms of passive relaxation (Marchini et al, 1983). The more one is sleep-deprived, the more one should seek large body activity (e.g., hiking, washing laundry) and avoid small muscle activity (e.g., needlepoint) or taxing mental work.

ADJUST NAPS. Some people benefit from a midday nap, functioning better in the afternoon and falling asleep more easily on a night after a nap. This may be because they do not try so desperately to sleep at night and therefore fall asleep more easily if they have had a nap. Such people should nap. Others feel groggy and nonfunctional after naps and sleep more poorly on that night. They should avoid naps. The reasons for these personal variations in napping behavior are not yet known.

Flexibility is needed in reviewing these rules with a given insomniac. One tries each rule for a few days or weeks. If it works, continue. If it seems to interfere with sleep, try something else.

BEHAVIORAL AND COGNITIVE TREATMENTS

The sheer number of behavioral techniques for insomnia is impressive. However, it appears that the type of approach one uses may be less important than the competence and thoroughness with which it is done. For example, while tension headaches can often be relieved by eight to ten EMG biofeedback sessions, insomniacs typically need two to four times that many sessions before improvement starts. The behavioral treatment of insomnia is not something that can be handled in a few short office visits; it takes patience, time, and skill. Insomniacs who need behavior therapy may benefit more from referral to the appropriate therapist than from management by a busy general physician.

There are currently four models of insomnia that have stimulated the development of behavioral techniques in this area (Borkovec, 1982):

INSOMNIACS ARE TOO TENSE. This is a common sense assumption. Most good sleepers find that they are tense and agitated when they occasionally experience sleep disturbance. By extrapolation, we assume that insomniacs are chronically in such a tense and agitated state. However, this theory has conceptual and empirical problems. "Tension" is often ill-defined; psychological agitation correlates poorly with an elevated muscle tonus, e.g., in the frontalis EMG. Also, numerous studies have found that time to sleep onset does not correlate well with frontalis EMG levels or assessments of psychological tension (Browman and Tepas, 1976; Good, 1975; Haynes et al, 1974).

INSOMNIACS ARE PHYSIOLOGICALLY HYPERAROUSED. While the original study by Monroe (1967) showed elevated physiological arousal in poor sleepers, subsequent studies have not always produced a consistent picture. Johns et al (1971) failed to replicate Monroe's rectal temperature differences. Frankel et al (1973) detected no difference in 17-hydroxycorticosteroids between insomniacs and controls. Although Freedman and Sattler (1982) did find a group of sleep-onset insomniacs who were physiologically hyperaroused when going to bed, these differences "washed out" quickly, before sleep started.

INSOMNIACS ARE COGNITIVELY HYPERAROUSED. Clinical experience, as well as many empirical studies, document a "racing mind," general worries and concerns about sleep, fears about insomnia, and other negative, worrisome thoughts (Geer and Katkin, 1966; Roth et al, 1976; Kales et al, 1976; Borkovec et al, 1979). However, it is often difficult to know what is cause and what is effect. Do thoughts occur because we cannot sleep, or do thoughts keep us from sleeping?

INSOMNIACS DO NOT STOP THINKING DURING THE LIGHTER PHASES OF SLEEP. Noted as early as 1969 by Rechtschaffen and Monroe, and later documented on numerous occasions (for example, Borkovec et al, 1981; Hauri and Olmstead, 1983), insomniacs often report having been awake and thinking when aroused from EEG-defined stage 2 sleep. Although the significance of this finding is still unclear, it seems conceivable that on a psychological level many insomniacs are still awake at a time when biologically their EEG indicates sleep.

Although most research papers on behavioral treatments of insomnia pay homage to one of these four models, in practice there is wide overlap. For example, frontalis EMG biofeedback was developed on the assumption that most insomniacs were muscularly tense. However, Borkovec (1982) as well as Hauri (1981) found that the amount of actual EMG relaxation in microvolts was poorly correlated with the insomniac's improvement in sleep. Rather, it seems that the cognitive focusing on a monotonous task may have been the crucial variable. Also, the four models of insomnia discussed above are not mutually exclusive. Kales et al (1983) have suggested that the repression and denial of emotional issues lead to cognitive activation in many insomniacs; this, in turn, causes both chronic, generalized, physiological arousal as well as increased muscle tension.

Relaxation Training

Numerous relaxation techniques have been shown more effective than credible placebo when treating sleep-onset insomnia. These techniques include progressive relaxation, a method of tensing and then relaxing various muscle groups throughout the body (Coursey et al, 1980; Nicassio et al, 1982); autogenic training, a complex technique of focusing one's attention on various parts of the body, coupled with auto-suggestions of heaviness, warmth, etc. (Coursey et al, 1980); and meditation (Woolfolk et al, 1976). However, it may not be the actual amount of muscle relaxation that is crucial. Based on a series of well-controlled studies, Borkovec (1982) concluded that "learning to focus one's attention on relatively pleasant, monotonous, internal sensations, especially those generated by attention-getting, discrete tension release of muscle groups, may be incompatible with worrisome thoughts and images that prevent sleep onset." This cognitive focusing may be the sleep-inducing mechanism rather than the actual tension release, according to Borkovec.

Hauri (1981) has shown that not all insomniacs are psychologically or physiologically tense. Those who are relaxed in both spheres but are still unable to sleep may actually become worse when pushed into relaxation training (Hauri et al, 1982). Thus, one needs a method of assessing tension. Clinically, this is usually done by observing the insomniac's behavior during an interview. More reliably, patients may be asked to recline on a bed in a darkened room while their frontalis EMG is recorded for ten to 20 minutes (using standard biofeedback equipment, but no actual feedback). Not only is the average level of muscle tonus of interest, but its change with time is, as well. Good sleepers decrease their frontalis tonus when asked to lie down for a few minutes, and they often fall asleep. Tense insomniacs, those who later profit from relaxation training, usually show a high and gradually increasing EMG over the 20 minutes of assessment.

Biofeedback

There are two modes in which biofeedback technology can be used for insomnia: the relaxation mode, and the training of specific biological parameters. In the relaxation mode, biofeedback is simply another method to teach relaxation. One measures a physiological parameter that is associated with relaxation; for example, muscle tension, EEG theta waves, or vasodilation (indexed by hand temperature). One then teaches the insomniac how to manipulate that variable in the hope that this will bring about a general state of relaxation. Insomniacs often benefit from such training (Borkovec and Weerts, 1976; Hauri, 1981), since many of them cannot accurately assess when they are tense and when they are relaxed. They are therefore unable to profit from admonitions to relax until biofeedback has identified and labelled their state of relaxation for them.

Sensory motor rhythm (SMR) training uses biofeedback technology in the second mode. Briefly, it has been shown that, compared with normals, chronic insomniacs are deficient in 14-16 cps power in the EEG, even when awake (Jordan et al, 1976). This may be important because the main characteristic of

NREM sleep is the sleep spindle in that 14–16 cps range. Sterman and MacDonald (1978) have shown that humans can be taught to strengthen their 14–16 cps rhythms with biofeedback; that is, to produce more EEG waves in that frequency range while awake. In the ten to 20 percent of psychophysiologic and childhood-onset insomniacs who are relaxed but still cannot fall asleep, SMR training has been shown effective for improving sleep (Hauri, 1981; Hauri et al, 1982). Moreover, in that group the amount of SMR learning was directly correlated with the amount of the patient's sleep improvement in both sleep onset and sleep maintenance insomniacs.

Stimulus Control Therapy

Stimulus control therapy is specifically designed for those insomniacs who show a conditioned arousal response to their own bedroom. One explains the thinking behind this therapy to the patient and then sets down the following rules (from Bootzin and Nicassio, 1978):

(a) Go to bed only when sleepy.
(b) Use the bed only for sleeping; do not read, watch television, or eat in bed.
(c) If unable to sleep, get up and move to another room. Stay up until really sleepy, then return to bed. If sleep still does not come easily, get out of bed again. The goal is to associate bed with falling asleep quickly.
(d) Repeat Step c as often as necessary throughout the night.
(e) Set the alarm and get up at the same time every morning regardless of how much sleep was obtained during the night. This helps the body acquire a constant sleep-wake rhythm.
(f) Do not nap during the day.

If these rules are followed, patients will usually sleep very little during the first few nights. This accumulated sleep deprivation is then used during later nights to help the patients fall asleep quickly, even in their own bedrooms. The treatment usually lasts a few weeks and is remarkably effective in those patients who suffer from conditioned arousals (Turner and Ascher, 1979; Lacks et al, 1983; Haynes et al, 1975). However, it does take willpower to get out of bed at night and go to another room, even though one feels extremely fatigued; therefore, almost daily follow-up is recommended with such insomniacs during the time they undergo this type of therapy.

Paradoxical Intention and Other Cognitive Therapies

As has already been said, the more one tries to sleep, the more one stays awake. Paradoxical intention tries to use the reverse of this process, with surprisingly good results. One tells the patient to stay awake for as long as possible, using a credible rationale. For example, one might tell insomniacs that their description of presleep mentation is lacking, that one needs to know *much* more about the thoughts that occur while they are lying in bed awake. The patients are then admonished to stay in bed awake as long as is humanly possible in an effort to notice all the details of their thinking. Ascher and Efran (1978) report success with this method in patients in whom more traditional relaxation training has failed. Others suggest that subjective sleep latencies in serious and chronic insomniacs can be reduced by 50 percent or more using this technique (Ascher and Turner, 1980; Relinger and Bornstein, 1979).

Other approaches try to deal with the ruminative, intrusive thinking that most insomniacs see as their main problem (Lichstein and Rosenthal, 1980; Nicassio and Gil, 1978). This may be done by "chunking"—connecting the randomly occurring thoughts into logical groups that are more easily managed (Lindsley, in press); by teaching structured fantasies to counteract these thoughts (Coates and Thoresen, 1979); or by problem-solving techniques to handle realistic worries during the day (Thoresen et al, 1981). Indeed, focusing one's attention on non-stressful matters may be effective. Haynes et al (1981) asked insomniacs and good sleepers to solve cognitive tasks while falling asleep (e.g., "count backwards from 347 by 18s as quickly as you can"). While these stressors, presented every 15 seconds, delayed sleep onset for good sleepers, they *shortened* sleep latency in insomniacs.

Monotonous Stimulation

Folklore has long held that monotonous stimulation (raindrops on the roof, a brook babbling, ocean waves) is conducive to sleep. Webb and Agnew (1979) found that intermittent tones (800 cps tones, two seconds on, two seconds off) induced sleep better than either total silence or a monotonous sound, and that this effect was enhanced further when subjects were asked to count to themselves at the beginning and at the end of each tone. Spinweber (1983) found that insomniacs fell asleep faster on the night when their auditory evoked potentials were measured by clicks delivered every 15 seconds. Thus, it appears that focusing on some repetitive, non-threatening stimulus (even counting sheep?) might be effective in inducing sleep.

Sleep Restriction

A new and potentially powerful treatment has recently been introduced by Spielman et al (1983). Observing that insomniacs lie in bed much longer than they are actually able to sleep, Spielman and colleagues first computed the average time per night that a person was actually sleeping, as reported in sleep logs filled out at home. Insomniacs were then allowed to stay in bed only for the length of this total sleep time. Initially, this curtailment of bedtime resulted in some sleep deprivation, which in itself caused the insomniacs to fall asleep faster and make more efficient use of the short time that they were allowed to spend in bed. As sleep efficiency (total time asleep per night divided by total time in bed) rose to .9 or greater for an average of five consecutive nights, each insomniac was then allowed 15 minutes' additional bedtime. After a few weeks, time in bed reached average levels, and most of it was now spent asleep.

Other Methods

Other behavioral methods have occasionally been reported as successful insomnia treatments, including hypnosis (Paterson, 1982); electrosleep (Ijima et al, 1983); and acupuncture (Dudukgian, 1974). Others have found such methods to be unsuccessful (for example, Coursey et al, 1980).

Overall, a surprising number of behavioral strategies are available. The challenge is to select the program that makes sense and is appropriate to a given patient, and then to be flexible enough to approach the problem from a different angle if the first method fails. Besides the benefits inherent in each method, working with a behavioral therapist on these strategies teaches the insomniac problem-solving skills and imparts the overall attitude that sleep difficulties are potentially solvable if one does not give up. This approach rekindles hope and, in itself, counteracts the passive, defeatist attitude so prevalent in insomniacs.

A THEORY OF PSYCHOPHYSIOLOGIC INSOMNIA

Behavioral treatment addresses the learned, maladaptive factors that are often involved in chronic insomnia. In some cases these factors may be central. In others (for example, insomnia secondary to nocturnal myoclonus, depression, or neurosis, or secondary to surgery and chronic pain), learning factors that maintain the insomnia may arise as secondary complications to other sleep disturbances. Because the psychological and behavioral issues can be examined most clearly in persistent psychophysiologic insomnia, a theory for that problem will be presented first.

Persistent psychophysiologic insomnia seems to arise in people who claim to have been weak but adequate sleepers throughout their lives and who then have undergone a serious crisis. In other words, patients with psychophysiologic insomnia typically report that they "always" had a few poor nights of sleep per month throughout their lives, but that they then developed a severe, relentless case of insomnia after some serious medical or psychological stress, possibly years or even decades before.

To understand persistent psychophysiological insomnia, one must first recall what happens to most of us during a serious, prolonged crisis: We sleep poorly. After a few nights of disturbed sleep, we cannot help but become concerned because the poor sleep affects our daytime functioning. It is natural, then, to try harder to sleep, and this sets up a vicious cycle: The more sleep we need, and the harder we try, the less we are able to sleep. Similarly, because we have laid in bed for a few nights, having become frustrated and upset about the crisis and about our inability to sleep, stimuli surrounding our bedroom environment gradually become associated with (conditioned to) frustration and arousal. Darkness, the pillows, a bed partner sleeping, or the act of brushing one's teeth can, by themselves, trigger frustration and arousal. People who suffer from trying too hard to sleep (internal arousal) will often report that they fall asleep whenever they do not want to; for example, while watching the news, driving a car, or in lectures. Patients who suffer mainly from conditioned insomnia (external arousal) will report that they sleep quite well away from their own bedroom; for example, on the living room couch, on vacation away from home, or in the sleep laboratory.

In most of us, the twin maladaptive habits of trying too hard to sleep and conditioned arousal will gradually disappear after the crisis has been resolved. Any learned habit extinguishes when not reinforced. However, if a predisposition toward an occasional poor night of sleep exists, these habits will not extinguish according to learning theory. Thus, a maladaptive sleep habit, learned decades before during a period of stress, will keep the insomnia alive in those who were weak sleepers to start with. In other words, one can never learn not to worry about sleep if this worry is justified by a few "naturally occurring" poor nights of sleep per month.

In addition to maladaptive learning, more complications arise with time, as the sleeper's self-concept changes to that of an insomniac. The person then thinks of himself or herself as being seriously flawed by an inability to sleep, and as a person who is weak in handling the stresses of life. Note that the learned, maladaptive habits that maintain such an insomnia do not need to be triggered by psychological stress alone. They can be equally well-released by a medical problem such as pain, a psychological problem such as depression, or an environmental problem such as excessive noise.

No universal treatment has been found to be effective in dealing with the learned behavioral aspects of insomnia. Rather, the challenge is to develop a specific treatment approach that is tailored to each individual insomniac. The literature is full of behavioral-psychological treatments that were effective "in a majority of cases," but no treatment claims efficacy with all insomniacs. Similarly, where one treatment fails, another is often successful. Ascher and Efran (1978), for example, have shown that the strategy of "paradoxical intention" was effective in patients who had not responded to relaxation therapy.

PSYCHOTHERAPY IN THE TREATMENT OF CHRONIC INSOMNIA

An attempt to define a single, suitable psychotherapeutic approach to the insomniac patient would be somewhat akin to suggesting a common, appropriate approach to the treatment of fever. The diversity of psychopathologies, personalities, lifestyles, and behavioral patterns exhibited by these patients is sufficient enough to defy any such attempt. Nevertheless, the available data on psychological disturbances, as well as clinical experience, do suggest some guidelines for psychotherapy with this population.

The importance of obtaining a detailed history as a basis for any psychotherapeutic intervention cannot be overemphasized. A thorough sleep history, which includes details of childhood sleep patterns and significant life events and stressors at the time of onset of the insomnia, is essential. An analysis of behavioral factors that may be relevant to the genesis and maintenance of the disorder requires careful attention (vide supra). The necessity of complete psychiatric and medical histories is obvious. Kales et al (1974) have pointed out that the failure to acquire an adequate psychological history is a common deficiency of many insomnia evaluations. Information regarding the individual's early development must be sought, and evidence of significant conflict arising from this period should be pursued. An analysis of the patient's predominant cognitive style and defenses is often indispensable to an understanding of the sleep disorder. Finally, the clinician must comprehend the significance of the insomnia in the life of the individual. What is the impact of the disturbance on social, occupational, and family function and how, in the patient's view, does the insomnia affect him or her psychologically?

From the outset, the clinician must recognize that psychotherapeutic intervention with these patients is, at best, a difficult task. A host of pitfalls will inevitably present themselves before the treatment process has even been initiated. Many of these complications are similar to those observed in the psychotherapy of patients with somatic illness. As Karasu (1978) has pointed out, such patients are generally not aware of the role that stress may play in the establishment and maintenance of the disorder, and will exhibit considerable denial of the psychological contributions to the somatic disturbance. The initial resistance the therapist confronts can be overwhelming. The patient with insomnia will frequently present an overt message of a desperate need for help, while simultaneously offering a covert message that he or she cannot (or will not) be helped. This strategy of resistance and nihilism is practically implemented by means of fixating on the symptom of insomnia to the exclusion of all else, especially discussion of psychological issues. In conjunction with this tactic, these patients may demand that the therapist focus an undue amount of attention on the issue of hypnotic medications. They will frequently express a fervent desire to be rid of or avoid such medication. However, any attempt by the therapist to comply with the overt request is often met with sabotage.

This apparent need for maintenance of the insomnia in some patients can be fueled by the secondary gain the individual derives from it. Cause and effect relationships become reversed in the patient's mind. The life stresses, conflict, and dysfunction they experience are not viewed as contributors to the insomnia but as results of sleep deprivation. This explanation provides a readily invoked excuse for current and past life difficulties, one that is largely, in their view, out of their control.

In designing a therapeutic approach for the insomnia patient, it is unwise to narrow the focus of treatment excessively, particularly during the early phase of treatment. Although psychological disturbance may play a major role in the disorder, the therapist who ignores proper behavioral and psychopharmacological management is not likely to succeed. Behavioral factors, in the form of conditioned arousal and poor sleep hygiene, will eventually complicate the overwhelming majority of insomnias. Many patients who present for evaluation and treatment of insomnia will benefit from short-term treatment with a benzodiazepine hypnotic. Such treatment may ease patient anxieties and provide a calmer atmosphere in which psychological issues can be explored more productively. Unfortunately, many chronic insomniacs will already have been treated, often overtreated, with a variety of hypnotics and will ultimately need to be withdrawn from these medications. As noted above, this issue has great potential for becoming a battleground. While the necessity for proper management and timely discontinuation of the hypnotic must be communicated by the physician, the prudent therapist will avoid a power struggle. Abrupt discontinuation may precipitate panic in patients for whom the hypnotic has become a way of life, and result in an equally abrupt termination from treatment by the patient. Gradual weaning, utilizing a steadily increasing interval between doses, may prove more tolerable.

Regardless of the particular psychotherapeutic approach chosen, education and reassurance are required. The patient must be provided with information regarding the multifactorial etiology of the sleep disorder and the necessity of a multifaceted approach to treatment. Soldatos et al (1979) have emphasized the need for reassurance to ameliorate the patient's fear of sleeplessness.

Selection of the proper psychotherapeutic approach must be based on careful consideration of the characteristics of the insomnia, as well as on thoughtful analysis of the patient's capacity to make meaningful gains within the framework of the prescribed therapy. Kales and colleagues (1982) strongly advocate insight-oriented psychodynamic psychotherapy in the treatment of insomnia. To the extent that psychopathology is a major determinant, this approach seems entirely appropriate, with the stipulation that the patient be screened properly. Clearly, patients who are not sufficiently motivated or who lack the necessary intelligence or psychological-mindedness will not derive significant benefit from this approach, and should not be treated in this manner.

The analytically oriented perspective on patients with psychophysiological disorders applies to many insomnia patients. This view, as summarized by Karasu (1978), holds that these individuals are prone to development of somatic disorders because of their inability to express emotional conflict directly. Neurotic feelings, especially aggression, lead to significant conflict; and physical symptoms are employed to ward off such conflict. Nemiah and Sifneos (1970) have suggested that the psychosomatic patient is characterized by an inability to describe feelings and a "preoccupation with the minutiae of their environment" (Nemiah et al, 1976). This behavior has been termed alexithymia (Sifneos, 1972).

In discussing the psychotherapeutic approach to the insomnia patient, Kales et al (1974) offer a similar profile. They suggest that sleep represents a loss of control, a state in which forbidden impulses may be destructively expressed. Their group advocates an active and direct exploration of the conflict with an ultimate goal of fostering the outward expression of emotion, particularly aggression. The goal of constructive therapy must be to shift the patient's attention away from the insomnia as a symptom and toward the psychological and behavioral disturbances that underlie the sleep disorder.

To date, only anecdotal information exists to support the efficacy of intensive psychotherapy for insomnia. Available information on the psychological characteristics and pathology of patients with insomnia, coupled with the clinical experience of therapists who are accustomed to seeing such patients, suggests that this method is efficacious for properly selected patients. A clear demonstration of its relative merits in comparison to other treatment forms awaits further study.

There is no question that a substantial number of individuals will not be suited to insight-oriented, intensive psychotherapy. Nevertheless, such patients can be managed effectively with a more supportive, reality-oriented psychotherapy approach. The ongoing availability and support of the therapist may provide many individuals with the degree of reassurance and practical guidance necessary for adequate control of the problem. Ongoing discussion of sleep hygiene, behavioral complications, and day-to-day stresses that contribute to the sleep disturbance can, over time, give rise to significant change, particularly when coupled with other techniques such as behavioral therapy.

TREATMENT OF DISORDERS OF THE SLEEP-WAKE CYCLE

In recent years, disorders of the sleep-wake cycle have been accorded an increasing amount of attention. This is, in part, due to the developments in chronobiology, which have facilitated a more sophisticated understanding of these disorders and their importance in sleep disorders medicine. Among the diagnoses that are subsumed under this heading in the official ASDC nosology, the delayed sleep phase syndrome (DSPS) has been a subject of particular interest.

The delayed sleep phase syndrome is characterized by an inability to fall asleep at the desired time coupled with difficulty awakening in the morning. Individuals with DSPS do not have difficulty maintaining sleep, once established. Their sleep is simply "misplaced" or delayed with respect to the conventional timing of sleep-wake rhythm. As a result, such individuals may suffer significant social and occupational impairment. In subjects presenting to sleep disorders centers with a complaint of insomnia, studies have demonstrated the frequency of DSPS to range from seven percent (Weitzman et al, 1979) to ten percent (Dement et al, 1975). The syndrome is undoubtedly often misdiagnosed by general practitioners as difficulty initiating sleep, presumably of psychological or psychophysiological origin. As a result, many of these patients are inappropriately treated with hypnotics, often on a chronic basis.

An effective nonpharmacological treatment approach for DSPS has been described by Czeisler et al (1981). It is hypothesized that individuals with DSPS have an impaired ability to phase advance: that is, to move their sleep times ahead to earlier, more conventional hours. Therefore, chronotherapy for this disorder entails a phase delay of approximately three hours on each consecutive day. Thus, over a five- to six-day period, the affected individual is able to achieve the desired sleep-wake schedule (Weitzman et al, 1981). However, it must be stressed that this progressive phase delay is not easy to accomplish and requires close supervision. Having established a normal sleep-wake schedule, the next task is to maintain it. Because of their limited ability to phase advance, DSPS patients must adhere to a rigid schedule. "Late nights," followed by delayed morning awakening, will result in a recurrence of the original disorder. Some patients will find it necessary to repeat the progressive phase delay routine periodically (Weitzman et al, 1981).

In addition to the delayed sleep phase syndrome, a variety of other disorders of the sleep-wake cycle are clinically relevant. The non-24-hour sleep-wake syndrome is manifested by an inability to maintain a 24-hour sleep-wake cycle, resulting in a desynchronization with the customary day-night pattern of wakefulness and sleep. The observed cycle length of such individuals has, thus far, always proven to be significantly greater than 24 hours, sometimes as long as 35 to 40 hours, suggesting that this disorder may be a more extreme form of DSPS (Weitzman, 1981). Although no significant data exist regarding treatment of these patients, it is theoretically possible that those whose sleep-wake cycle lengths do not greatly exceed 24 hours might respond to treatment similar to that described for DSPS.

The advanced sleep syndrome has not been clearly described as a clinical entity, although reported cases do exist (Cleghorn et al, 1983). A tendency toward phase advancement may be, in part, a result of aging (Weitzman, 1981). This would certainly account for the not uncommon observation that many older individuals demonstrate a tendency to awaken earlier and retire earlier in the evening. Chronotherapy, which consists of progressive phase advancement to the desired schedule, could presumably benefit such persons.

The most common varieties of sleep-wake cycle disturbance are the "jet lag" syndrome (rapid time zone change) and those related to shift work. The difficulties that arise from "jet lag" or frequent shift changes will generally be transient, whereas those occurring in association with frequently changing shift work may be persistent. In all cases, a desynchronization between the sleep-wake cycle and other circadian rhythms is induced. Insomnia, daytime fatigue, poor concentration, and sleepiness at inappropriate times may result. Clearly the optimal (but, for many people, impossible) solution is regularization of the sleep-wake schedule. Short of this, attempts to minimize the number of shift changes may ameliorate the condition. Careful observance of sleep hygiene issues for such individuals is vital, if only to avoid secondary behavioral complications. Some individuals will inherently tolerate shift changes better than others, sleeping and functioning reasonably well in spite of the disruption, while others will have poor tolerance for such changes. A natural selection process occurs, to some extent, with respect to those who remain in shift work for any length of time. Age may play a role, as well, in that the capacity to tolerate the repetitive upheavals in schedule may be compromised as one gets older.

TREATMENT OF INSOMNIA IN CHILDREN

Some children suffer from insomnias secondary to organic disorders, such as nocturnal asthma, nocturnal epilepsy, sleep apnea, or pain (Rabe, 1974). Other childhood insomnias relate to psychiatric problems such as a pathological interaction between parent and child, childhood neurosis, or excessive stress. These problems need to be addressed by a competent pediatrician or child psychiatrist. However, most chronic sleep problems during childhood are behavioral, related to inappropriate management and to the reinforcement of an occasional temporary sleep disturbance. This is especially true of the preschool child (Battle, 1970). Adolescents, on the other hand, may often show disturbances in the sleep-wake cycle more like those seen in adults.

The goal of behavioral treatment is to have children go to bed without complaint, fall asleep easily, and sleep throughout the night in their own bed. Research has shown, however, that it is quite natural for children and adults to awaken a few times each night. Most of us easily fall asleep again and never remember awakening. However, if something memorable occurs during these awakenings, such as an anxiety-provoking thought or some fear-provoking stimulus, the short awakenings expand into highly disturbing events. Parents tread a fine line between showing adequate concern for the child's problem during such an awakening and not reinforcing the sleep-disturbing behavior.

The process of growing up involves different tasks that are to be mastered at certain ages (Ferber and Rivinus, 1979). For example, one- to three-year-olds need to explore separateness from parents, test the limits of their own will, find out how safe they are alone in a given environment, and become comfortable in the dark when they are occasionally unable to sleep. Children aged four through six enter the sometimes frightening world of consciously remembered dreams, and they need to learn the difference between sleeping and dying. Mastering these tasks is not always easy.

Sleep can only occur when one is relaxed. Thus, the time surrounding sleep is *not* the time to begin setting limits or to explore how it feels to be alone. Rather, these issues need to be worked through during alert wakefulness. Similarly, fear of the dark or of monsters may be worked through during wakefulness by parents interacting with their children as the room gets gradually darker, or by sitting with the child in a dark room watching what happens down in the well-lit street.

Young children have a great need for attention. If parents are busy, nighttime is often seen as an opportune time to force parental attention, because the threat of screaming or crying and thereby waking others makes parents especially malleable. For parents, it seems much better to satisfy that need during the day. For example, one might cook a special breakfast for the child after a silent night and still save time rather than spending time in the middle of the night quieting the child. The goal is not simply to eliminate the undesired nighttime activity, but rather to be sensitive to what the child's needs are during alert wakefulness.

Parents may unwittingly contribute to nighttime disturbances (Ferber and Boyle, 1983a). Assume that an adult were trained to fall asleep in a certain situation; for example, in his own bed. Assume then that this adult now suddenly awakens in the middle of the night (as we all do) to find himself lying on a sunny beach or in a hospital bed. Such a situation would cause immediate arousal and concern and would make it impossible to return to sleep. Nevertheless, this is exactly what we ask our children to do if we establish a bedtime routine of their being rocked to sleep in the mother's arms or falling asleep while nursing. The totally new situation in which that child then finds himself when awakening in the middle of the night may be frightening, and the child understandably takes all necessary steps to re-establish the familiar situation as it was when he or she fell asleep. We are creatures of habit. If we learn to fall asleep in mother's arms, we have trouble falling asleep alone in the crib.

As an aside, there is evidence that large fluid intake in itself may cause frequent awakenings. While parents may think that the bottle is needed to have the child fall asleep, drinking may actually awaken the child unnecessarily a few hours later and cause insomnia (Ferber and Boyle, 1983b).

Gradual approximations may be necessary for the younger child. Instead of rocking the child to sleep in one's arms, one might first rock him in his own crib. Later one may keep the hand lightly on his back, later remain in the room without touching him, then sit outside the room with an open door, etc. Each step will be objected to with some crying, but if this crying does not result in a return to the old situation, it will soon stop.

With older children, one can discuss the matter verbally and then institute a drastic change from which one does not relent. For example, if the child has a habit of getting out of his own bed in the middle of the night and climbing into the parents' bed, a chain lock might have to be applied to the door. This will result in much protest for the first few nights, but if it is ignored, while proper reinforcement is used for the desired behavior, improvement is likely. Proper precautions need to be taken to carry the plan to its conclusion because a retreat reinforces the old pattern. If one of the parents feels unable to stand the pain of hearing the child cry for 30 minutes, that parent might have to sleep at a friend's house for the first few nights. If one lives with neighbors close by, one might start this treatment when they are out of town, or at least one might notify them of it. One might remove dangerous objects from the child's room to be confident that nothing terrible is happening in there. One rewards appropriate behavior by giving at least the same amount of positive attention to the child during the next day as it had taken in the past to settle the issues during the night.

As with adults, children vary in their sleep patterns. Some may be sound sleepers, others light sleepers. Some "settle" (sleep through the night) before the age of three months, some rarely sleep through the night before they are 12 months old for purely biological reasons (Guilleminault and Anders, 1976). Thus, having a child with a sleep problem should not necessarily reflect badly on the parents; some of them have a much more difficult task than others.

In the development of a treatment plan, parents need to be heavily involved, because only they know how far they are able to go. The program has to make sense to them, and they need to be reassured that they are not doing any harm by carrying it out. They should be required to chart the progress; for example, to measure the length of crying each night as the program is instituted. Often, what seems like no change over the course of a week can be shown to be gradual improvement when the problem is charted. Also, at least in difficult cases, a daily follow-up call from the therapist to the parents may be necessary to reward them in this difficult endeavor.

SUMMARY

The treatment of chronic insomnia and disorders of the sleep-wake schedule is a challenging task, requiring ingenuity and patience on the part of the clinician. The etiologies and secondary complications of the disorders are numerous. While the current state of knowledge in this area contributes important information to help guide the course of diagnosis and treatment, it does not provide clear answers to the many questions that arise. It is only by means of a careful assessment of psychological, behavioral, and physiological factors, and a treatment plan that is tailored to address the relative contributions from each of these areas, that success can be achieved. Flexibility, a willingness to modify the treatment approach, and establishment of realistic, limited goals will serve the clinician well.

REFERENCES

Ascher LM, Efran JS: Use of paradoxical intention in a behavioral program for sleep onset insomnia. J Consult Clin Psychol 46:547-550, 1978

Ascher LM, Turner RM: A comparison of two methods for the administration of paradoxical intention. Behav Res Ther 18:121-126, 1980

Aschoff J, Hoffman K, Pohl H, et al: Reentrainment of circadian rhythms after phase-shifts of the zeitgeber. Chronobiologia 2:23-78, 1975

Battle CU: Sleep and sleep disturbances in young children: sensible management depends upon understanding. Clin Pediatr 9:675-682, 1970

Bootzin RR, Nicassio PN: Behavioral treatments for insomnia, in Progress in Behavior Modification. Edited by Hersen M, Eisler R, Miller P. New York, Academic Press, 1978

Borkovec TD: Insomnia. J Consult Clin Psychol 50:880-895, 1982

Borkovec TD, Weerts TC: Effects of progressive relaxation on sleep disturbance: an electroencephalographic evaluation. Psychosom Med 38:173-180, 1976

Borkovec TD, Grayson JB, O'Brien GT, et al: Relaxation treatment of pseudoinsomnia and idiopathic insomnia: an electroencephalographic evaluation. J Appl Behav Analysis 12:37-54, 1979

Borkovec TD, Lane TW, VanOot PH: Phenomenology of sleep among insomniacs and good sleepers: wakefulness experience when cortically asleep. J Abnorm Psychol 90:607-60, 1981

Browman C, Tepas D: The effects of presleep activity on all-night sleep. Psychophysiology 13:536-540, 1976

Carey WB: Night waking and temperament in infancy. J Pediatr 84:756-758, 1974

Cleghorn JM, Bellissimo A, Kaplan RD, et al: Insomnia: II. Assessment and treatment of chronic insomnia. Can J Psychiatry 28:347-353, 1983

Coates TJ, Thoresen CE: Treating arousals during sleep using behavioral self-management. J Consult Clin Psychol 47:603-605, 1979

Coursey RD, Buchsbaum M, Frankel BL: Personality measures and evoked responses in chronic insomniacs. J Abnorm Psychol 84:239-249, 1975

Coursey RD, Frankel BL, Gaarder KR, et al: A comparison of relaxation techniques with electrosleep therapy for chronic, sleep-onset insomnia, a sleep-EEG study. Biofeedback and Self-Regulation 5:57-73, 1980

Czeisler CA, Richardson GS, Coleman RM, et al: Chronotherapy: resetting the circadian clocks of patients with delayed sleep phase insomnia. Sleep 4:1-21, 1981

Dement WC, et al: The pathologies of sleep: a case series approach, in The Nervous System, Vol 2. Edited by Tower DB. New York, Raven Press, 1975

Downing RW and Rickels K: Coffee consumption, cigarette smoking, and reporting of drowsiness in anxious patients treated with benzodiazepines or placebo. Acta Psychiatr Scand 64:398-408, 1981

Dudukgian E: Acupuncture treatment of insomnia. Am J Acupuncture 2:175-179, 1974

Fara JW, Rubinstein EH, Sonnenschein RR: Visceral and behavioral responses to intra-duodenal fat. Science 166:110-111, 1969

Ferber R, Boyle MP: Sleeplessness in infants and toddlers: sleep initiation difficulty masquerading as a sleep maintenance insomnia. Sleep Research 12:240, 1983a

Ferber R, Boyle MP: Nocturnal fluid intake: a cause of, not treatment for, sleep disruption in infants and toddlers. Sleep Research 12:243, 1983b

Ferber R, Rivinus TM: Practical approaches to sleep disorders of childhood. Medical Times 107:71-80, 1979

Frankel BL, Buchbinder R, Coursey R, et al: Sleep patterns and psychological test characteristics of chronic primary insomniacs. Sleep Research 2:149, 1973

Freedman RR, Sattler HL: Physiological and psychological factors in sleep-onset insomnia. J Abnorm Psychol 91:380-389, 1982

Geer HJ, Katkin ES: Treatment of insomnia using a variant of systematic desensitization: a case report. J Abnorm Psychol 71:161-164, 1966

Globus G, Friedmann J, Cohen H, et al: The effects of aircraft noise on sleep electrophysiology as recorded in the home, in Proceedings of the International Congress on Noise as a Public Health Problem. Edited by Ward WD. Washington, DC, US Environmental Protection Agency, 1974

Good R: Frontalis muscle tension and sleep latency. Psychophysiology 12:465-467, 1975

Griffin, SJ, Trinder, J: Physical fitness, exercise and human sleep. Social Psychophysiological Research 15(5):447-450, 1978

Guilleminault C, Anders TF: Sleep disorders in children, part II, in Advances in Pediatrics, vol 22. Edited by Schulman I. Chicago, Year Book Medical Publishers, 1976

Hauri P: The influence of evening activity on the onset of sleep. Psychophysiology 5:426-430, 1969

Hauri P: Treating psychophysiologic insomnia with biofeedback. Arch Gen Psychiatry 38:752-758, 1981

Hauri P, Olmstead E: What is the moment of sleep onset for insomniacs? Sleep 6:10-15, 1983

Hauri PJ, Percy L, Hellekson C, et al: The treatment of psychophysiologic insomnia with biofeedback: a replication study. Biofeedback and Self-Regulation 7:223-235, 1982

Haynes SN, Follingstad DR, McGowan WT: Insomnia: sleep patterns and anxiety level. J Psychosom Res 18:69-74, 1974

Haynes SN, Price MG, Simons JB: Stimulus control treatment of insomnia. J Behav Ther Exp Psychiatry 6:279-282, 1975

Haynes SN, Adams A, Franzen M: The effects of presleep stress on sleep-onset insomnia. J Abnorm Psychol 90:601-606, 1981

Iijima S, Sugita Y, Teshima Y, et al: A new and safe device of electrosleep for insomniacs. Sleep Research 12:339, 1983

Johns MW, Gay TJA, Marston JP, et al: Relationship between sleep habits, adrenocortical activity and personality. Psychosom Med 33:499-508, 1971

Jordan JB, Hauri P, Phelps PJ: The sensorimotor rhythm (SMR) in insomnia. Sleep Research 5:175, 1976

Kales A, Kales JD, Bixler EO: Insomnia: an approach to management and treatment. Psychiatric Annals 4:28-43, 1974

Kales A, Caldwell AB, Preston TA, et al: Personality patterns in insomnia. Arch Gen Psychiatry 33:1128-1134, 1976

Kales A, Kales J, Soldatos CR: Insomnia and other sleep disorders. Med Clin North Am 66:971-991, 1982

Kales A, Caldwell AB, Soldatos CR, et al: Biopsychobehavioral correlates of insomnia. II. Pattern specificity and consistency with the Minnesota Multiphasic Personality Inventory. Psychosom Med 45:341-356, 1983

Karacan I, Thornby JI, Anch AM, et al: Dose-related sleep disturbances induced by coffee and caffeine. Clin Pharmacol Ther 20:682-689, 1976

Karasu TB: Psychotherapy with the somatically ill patient, in Psychotherapeutics in Medicine. Edited by Karasu TB, Steinmuller RI. New York, Grune and Stratton, 1978

Lacks, P, Bertelson AD, Sugerman J, et al: The treatment of sleep-maintenance insomnia with stimulus-control techniques. Behav Res Ther 21:291-295, 1983

Lichstein K, Rosenthal T: Insomniac's perceptions of cognitive versus somatic determinants of sleep disturbance. J Abnorm Psychol 89:105-107, 1980

Lindsley JG: A "chunking" intervention for pre-sleep intrusive cognitions: theoretical considerations. Sleep (in press)

Marchini EJ, Coates TJ, Magistad JG, et al: What do insomniacs do, think, and feel during the day? A preliminary study. Sleep 6:147-155, 1983

Monroe L: Psychological and physiological differences between good and poor sleepers. J Abnorm Psychol 72:255-264, 1967

Nemiah JC, Sifneos PE: Affect and fantasy in patients with psychosomatic disorders, in Modern Trends in Psychosomatic Medicine, vol 2. Edited by Hill OW. London, Butterworths, 1970

Nemiah JC, et al: Alexithymia: a view of the psychosomatic process, in Modern Trends in Psychosomatic Medicine, vol 3. Edited by Hill OW. London, Butterworths, 1976

Nicassio P, Gil E: Individualized, multifaceted behavior therapy for insomnia. Paper presented at the twelfth annual convention of the Association for the Advancement of Behavior Therapy, 1978

Nicassio PN, Boylan MB, McCabe TG: Progressive relaxation, EMG biofeedback and biofeedback placebo in the treatment of sleep-onset insomnia. Br J Med Psychol 55:159-166, 1982

Paterson DC: Hypnosis: an alternate approach to insomnia. Can Fam Physician 28:768-770, 1982.

Porter JM, Horne JA: Bed-time food supplements and sleep: effects of different carbohydrate levels. Electroencephalogr Clin Neurophysiol 51:426-433, 1981

Rabe EF: Recurrent paroxysmal nonepileptic disorders, in Current Problems in Pediatrics, vol 4, no 8. Edited by Gluck L, Cone TE Jr, Dodge PR, et al. Chicago, Year Book Medical Publishers, 1974

Rechtschaffen A, Monroe LJ: Laboratory studies in insomnia, in Sleep: Physiology and Pathology. Edited by Kales A. Philadelphia, Lippincott, 1969

Relinger H, Bornstein PH: Treatment of sleep onset insomnia by paradoxical instruction. Behav Mod 3:203-222, 1979

Roth T, Kramer M, Lutz T: The nature of insomnia: a descriptive summary of a sleep clinic population. Comp Psychiatry 17:217-220, 1976

Rundell OH, Lester BK, Griffiths WJ, et al: Alcohol and sleep in young adults. Psychopharmacologia 26:201-218, 1972

Schmidt-Kessen W, Kendel K: Einfluss der Raumtemperatur auf den Nachtschlaf. Res Exp Med (Berlin) 160:220-233, 1973

Sifneos PE: The prevalence of "alexithymic" characteristics in psychosomatic patients, in Topics of Psychosomatic Research. Basel, Switzerland, Karger, 1972

Soldatos CR, Kales A, Kales JD: Management of insomnia. Ann Rev Med 30:301-312, 1979

Soldatos CR, Kales JD, Scharf MB, et al: Cigarette smoking associated with sleep difficulty. Science 207:551-553, 1980

Southwell PR, Evans CR, Hunt JN: Effect of a hot milk drink on movements during sleep. Br Med J 2:429-431, 1972

Spielman AJ, Saskin P, Thorpy MJ: Sleep restriction: a new treatment of insomnia. Sleep Research 12:286, 1983

Spinwveber CL: Pre-sleep AEP procedures reduce sleep latency in poor sleepers. Sleep Research 12:287, 1983

Sterman MB, MacDonald LR: Effects of central corticol EEG feedback training on incidence of poorly controlled seizures. Epilepsia 19:207-222, 1978

Thoresen CE, Coates TJ, Kirmil-Gray K, et al: Behavioral self-management in treating sleep-maintenance insomnia. J Behav Med 4:41-52, 1981

Turner RM, Ascher LM: A within-subject analysis of stimulus control therapy with severe sleep-onset insomnia. Behav Res Ther 17:107-112, 1979

Walker JI: Sleep disorders. Part III: Insomnias and parasomnias. North Carolina Medical Journal 43:26-29, 1982

Webb WB, Agnew HW Jr: Sleep onset facilitation by tones. Sleep 1:281-286, 1979

Weitzman ED, et al: Delayed sleep phase syndrome: a biological rhythm disorder. Sleep Research 8:221, 1979

Weitzman ED, Czeisler CA, Coleman RM, et al: Delayed sleep phase syndrome: a chronobiological disorder with sleep-onset insomnia. Arch Gen Psychiatry 38:737-746, 1981

Williams RL, Ware JC, Ilaria RL, et al: Disturbed sleep and anxiety, in Phenomenology and Treatment of Anxiety. Edited by Fann WE et al. New York, Spectrum Publications, 1979

Woolfolk RL, Carr-Kaffashan L, McNulty TF, et al: Meditation training as a treatment for insomnia. Behav Ther 7:359-365, 1976

Ziegler AJ: Dream emotions in relation to room temperature, in Physiology, Biochemistry, Psychology, Pharmacology, Clinical Applications. Edited by Koella WP, Levin P. Basel, Switzerland, First European Congress on Sleep Research, 1972

Chapter 20

Pharmacological Treatment of Insomnia

by Wallace B. Mendelson, M.D.

About 35 percent of the American population complains of difficulty going to sleep or maintaining sleep, and perhaps half of this group considers it a major problem (Mellinger and Balter, 1983). As a consequence, many persons consult a physician, and 4.3 percent receive a prescription medication for sleep each year. (About 60 percent of these receive a traditional hypnotic, and the remainder obtain anxiolytics and antidepressants.) About three-fourths of these individuals take medication for less than two weeks, while 11 percent receive medication nightly for sleep for over one year. Although the use of hypnotics is widespread, total numbers of prescriptions are declining. Since careful data were first collected in 1964, the number of prescriptions rose from 32.5 million to a peak of 42 million in 1971, and gradually declined to 21 million in 1982.

The National Prescription Audit indicates that in 1982 about two-thirds of hypnotic prescriptions were for a single benzodiazepine compound, flurazepam. Barbiturates comprised nine percent, and the remaining 25 percent were non-benzodiazepine, non-barbiturate hypnotics (Mellinger and Balter, 1983). A survey of more than 4,000 physicians indicates that they found a complaint of insomnia in about 17 percent of their patients; the specialists to whom such complaints were most common were psychiatrists, who reported insomnia in 32.4 percent of their patients (Bixler et al, 1979).

When the indications for prescribing hypnotics are examined, it appears that physicians usually see themselves as treating insomnia in the context of some other disturbance. Data from the National Disease and Therapeutic Index indicate that in 1982 only 12 percent of prescriptions were for insomnia alone; about one-third were for insomnia in patients seen as having a mental disorder; and the remainder were for patients with various medical disorders (Mellinger and Balter, 1983).

This chapter will examine the role of hypnotics in the treatment of sleep disturbance. After a few comments on some aspects of insomnia and the pharmacology of these agents, possible benefits of hypnotic use and possible undesirable consequences will be considered. Among the latter are issues of residual daytime effects, reliance, effects on respiration, and special problems of the elderly.

ASPECTS OF INSOMNIA

Perhaps the major movement in sleep research in the last decade has been the growing recognition that insomnia may be a manifestation of a variety of disor-

This chapter was written by Dr. Wallace B. Mendelson in his private capacity. No official support or endorsement by the USPHS or by NIMH in intended or should be inferred.

ders. This viewpoint culminated in a systematic nosology of sleep disorders (Association of Sleep Disorders Centers, 1979), which describes a variety of pathophysiologic and psychologic conditions that result in the sensation of disturbed sleep. For many of these conditions, relatively specific treatments are available: for example, tricyclic antidepressants for patients with sleep disturbance due to affective disorders, or surgical procedures for obstructive sleep apnea. In most of these cases, hypnotics are unlikely to help and in some conditions may conceivably be dangerous, as in patients with sleep apnea (Mendelson et al, 1981). With a few special exceptions, then, it seems reasonable to suggest that hypnotic use be confined to those disorders in which no major pathophysiology has been found. In terms of the current nosology, many of these cases fall into categories such as persistent psychophysiological disorders of initiating and maintaining sleep (DIMS) (A.1.b.), subjective DIMS complaint without objective findings (A.9.b.), and not otherwise specified complaints (A.9.c.). Possible exceptions to this rule of thumb might be the adjunctive use of hypnotics in major affective disorders, the benefits of which have not been well established; and use of hypnotics after acute phase shifts of the sleep-waking cycle, an area currently under active investigation.

PHARMACOLOGY OF HYPNOTICS

Prescription hypnotics may conveniently be classed into three groups, the pharmacology of which has been reviewed in detail elsewhere (Mendelson, 1980).

Barbiturates

From the time that Veronal was introduced by Fischer and Von Mering in 1903, these compounds were widely used as sedatives and hypnotics, declining only after the introduction of the benzodiazepines in the early 1960s. In 1982 barbiturates represented only nine percent of hypnotic prescriptions. However, there may be continuing concern about lethality in acute overdose (generally about ten therapeutic doses), abuse potential, interaction with alcohol, and stimulation of hepatic microsomal oxidizing systems responsible for metabolizing a variety of drugs. The barbiturates most often used as hypnotics are secobarbital, amobarbital, and pentobarbital, which are considered short- to intermediate-acting, with plasma half-lives of 14 to 48 hours. They are rapidly distributed in body tissues, inactivated primarily by hepatic metabolism, and excreted as conjugated hydroxyl compounds in the urine.

Benzodiazepines

These compounds were introduced as the anxiolytics chlordiazepoxide and diazepam in the 1960s, and flurazepam was marketed as a hypnotic in 1970. The use of flurazepam has risen dramatically over the years and was estimated to represent 66 percent of all hypnotic prescriptions in 1982. More recently, short-acting benzodiazepines recommended for anxiety (lorazepam) and sleep (temazepam) have become available, as has the triazolobenzodiazepine hypnotic triazolam. Benzodiazepines are relatively benign compared to other drug classes when taken alone in acute overdose. Although at low doses and with relatively subtle measures, there may be no interaction (or even antagonism) of alcohol effects; toxicity is clearly potentiated by alcohol in clinical overdose. There has been virtually no development of traditional drug abuse with these agents, in contrast to other classes of hypnotics. On the other hand, at least one study suggests that patients are as likely to develop reliance (prolonged use of prescribed doses) with benzodiazepines as with barbiturates (Clift, 1975).

Benzodiazepines are not thought to stimulate hepatic microsomal oxidizing systems, but their own metabolism may be altered by drugs that do affect hepatic function. Flurazepam is absorbed relatively rapidly; it is, however, a relatively long-acting agent, the active metabolite (desalkylflurazepam) having a plasma half-life of 47 to 100 hours. After hepatic transformation, metabolites are excreted primarily in the urine, where approximately 81 percent can be found after 98 hours (Schwartz and Postma, 1970). Among the short-acting benzodiazepines, temazepam decreases in the plasma in a biphasic manner with half-lives of 0.6 and nine hours. Perhaps due to its current pharmaceutical preparation, absorption is delayed, and peak levels are not achieved for two to three hours. Triazolam and lorazepam, with half-lives of 1.5 to five and 10 to 20 hours, respectively, have peak blood levels in one to two hours. In contrast to long-acting benzodiazepines such as flurazepam, all are metabolized to inactive compounds before excretion.

Non-barbiturate, Non-benzodiazepine Hypnotics

These include compounds from a variety of pharmacological classes, including chloral hydrate, methaqualone, the piperidinedione compounds glutethimide and methyprylon, ethchlorvynol, and ethinamate. In 1982, these agents were thought to comprise about 25 percent of hypnotic prescriptions. Because of the heterogeneity of this group, generalizations are difficult. Most are very toxic in acute overdose, have enhanced toxicity when combined with alcohol, and are associated with varying degrees of abuse potential. With the possible exception of ethchlorvynol, they tend to stimulate hepatic microsomal oxidizing systems.

EFFICACY

The issue of how best to assess the efficacy of hypnotics is a complex subject in its own right. Insofar as the ultimate goal is the patient's sense of having slept well, non-laboratory studies of subjective response are important. On the other hand, EEG studies provide objective measures and guard against the possibility that patients prefer a particular agent for some other property than sleep induction; for example, euphoriant qualities. Thus, at this time it seems wise to assess hypnotics by both means. Some of the issues in hypnotic testing have recently been reviewed (Mendelson et al, 1981), and basic standards for studies have been discussed by a number of authors, including Kay et al (1976). The following section discusses only efficacy studies of flurazepam, insofar as it is the most commonly prescribed hypnotic, and some of the newer short-acting benzodiazepines. A review of the literature since 1980 suggests that few, if any, efficacy studies of barbiturates or other nonbenzodiazepine hypnotics have been conducted since that time; studies of these agents have been summarized in detail by Mendelson (1980).

Flurazepam

SUBJECTIVE. One study in geriatric outpatients (Reeves, 1977) and one in younger insomniacs (Dement et al, 1978) found that 30 mg flurazepam was helpful in sleep induction over 28 nights. A variety of studies summarized by Mendelson (1980), as well as recent studies by Hartmann (1983), Fillingim (1982), and Roehrs et al (1982) indicate clear benefits with administration of a week or less. Little difference in benefit between 15 and 30 mg was brought out by these various subjective reports. In the Boston Collaborative Drug Surveillance Program (1972), physicians who made a judgment about efficacy felt that 85.7 percent of patients receiving 15 mg and 91.4 percent taking 30 mg flurazepam had a "satisfactory" response.

EEG STUDIES. Reports of one (Hartmann, 1968), four (Vogel et al, 1976), five (Kales et al, 1971), and seven (Roehrs et al, 1982) nights' flurazepam administration have demonstrated increased total sleep time as well as decreased sleep latency and intermittent wakefulness. In the latter study, the latency to persistent sleep reached statistical significance only on the first drug night. Four studies involved administration for 28 nights. Kales et al (1975) administered 30 mg flurazepam to four subjects and reported that total sleep time rose by six to eight percent, while intermittent waking decreased by 14 to 17 minutes. Sleep latency was significantly decreased only on nights 11 through 13 in this study; when these data were later combined with those from shorter-term studies (Kales et al, 1976), sleep latency was decreased starting on the second night. Dement et al (1978) administered 30 mg flurazepam to five insomniacs and reported that total sleep time was increased by roughly one to two hours over the 28 nights; decreases in sleep latency and intermittent waking time did not reach statistical significance. Mendelson and colleagues (1982) gave 30 mg flurazepam to ten insomniacs and found total sleep to be increased by over an hour during the second and fourth weeks. Both sleep latency and intermittent waking time tended to decrease but did not reach statistical significance. Kales and colleagues (1982) reported that in six insomniacs given 30 mg flurazepam for 28 nights, there was improvement in percent sleep time throughout the study. Improvement in sleep latency was no longer evident by the fourth week.

Temazepam

SUBJECTIVE. Fowler (1977) reported that of 147 general practice outpatients who had already responded well to temazepan for one week, 90 percent reported a "good" or "very good" response over 12 weeks. A study of eight psychiatric patients by Maggini et al (1969) described patient reports of quieter and more restful sleep. Bixler et al (1978), in a 28-night study of 30 mg temazepam in six insomniacs, found consistent benefits only in terms of decreased number of awakenings. Mitler et al (1975) gave 30 mg temazepam for 35 nights to seven insomniacs and reported an estimated increase in total sleep but no change in sleep latency.

EEG STUDIES. In the Maggini et al (1969) study, temazepam decreased sleep latency and increased total sleep. Bixler et al (1978) found no effects on sleep latency or percentage sleep. The number of waking episodes was decreased, however. Mitler et al (1975) found no effect on sleep latency but did report decreased intermittent waking time and increased total sleep. In summary, there is some evidence of benefit from temazepam, but the results are mixed.

Triazolam

SUBJECTIVE. A variety of studies have compared triazolam to flurazepam (Nair and Schwartz, 1978; Fabre et al, 1977; Reeves et al, 1977; Sunshine, 1975; Vogel et al, 1976; Leibowitz and Sunshine, 1978), nitrazepam (Ellingsen, 1983), secobarbital and placebo (Rickels et al, 1975), or placebo (Kales et al, 1976; Vogel et al, 1975) in various patient groups. In most cases, 0.5 mg triazolam was preferred by patients (or in some manner showed better ratings) than 30 mg flurazepam, 5 mg nitrazepam, or 100 mg secobarbital. (In the Vogel et al [1976] study and in the 12-week study of Leibowitz and Sunshine [1978], ratings of the two drugs were roughly comparable.) When 0.4 and 0.8 mg triazolam were studied, only 0.8 mg was consistently better than placebo in a study by Sunshine (1975). Roth et al (1977), however, found dosage-dependent benefits of 0.25 and 0.5 mg in comparison to placebo. In the Reeves et al (1977) study, 0.25 mg triazolam was rated during 28 nights and found to be better than placebo but different from 15 mg flurazepam on only one of six measures (duration of sleep). Similarly, Okawa (1978) found that among elderly insomniacs, triazolam 0.5 mg was of benefit on several measures but was considered more effective than 15 mg flurazepam on only one out of five scales. In summary, a variety of studies have documented benefits of triazolam, which are substantially more evident for the 0.5 mg dose.

EEG STUDIES.   Kales et al (1976), in a two-week study of 0.5 mg triazolam in insomniacs, found increased percentage of sleep and decreased waking time in the first week. Sleep latency tended to decrease, but this change did not reach statistical significance. A two-week study of 0.5 mg by Roth et al (1976) found decreased sleep latency and awake time. In a comparison of 0.5 mg triazolam and 30 mg flurazepam for four nights, Vogel et al (1976) found both drugs comparably effective and better than placebo on a variety of measures. In a seven-night dose-response study, Vogel et al (1975) found that 0.5 mg triazolam decreased sleep latency, increased total sleep time, and decreased waking time, while 0.25 mg had relatively less effect. A six-night study of poor sleepers found that 0.5 mg triazolam reduced sleep latency and increased total sleep time and sleep efficiency (Spinweber and Johnson, 1982). Thus, most EEG studies have documented a variety of benefits of triazolam in studies of up to two weeks, but again largely at the 0.5 mg dose.

RESIDUAL DAYTIME EFFECTS

General Issues

At least two different target symptoms may lead to the prescription of hypnotics. One of these, which has just been discussed, is, of course, better sleep at night. The second is improved daytime functioning. The distinction between these goals is important because the relative efficacy of hypnotics is very different in the two situations. While most prescription hypnotics appear to improve some aspects of nocturnal sleep (at least in the short-term), evidence for improvement by day is slight. Detailed reviews by Mendelson (1980) and Johnson and Chernik (1982) described a host of studies documenting decrements in daytime performance in subjects taking a variety of hypnotics, the best results often being a lack of effect. (A review of the literature since that time has found only one possible exception, which will be described later.) Several studies suggest that daytime decrements in performance are not merely of academic interest. Linnoila (1978), for instance, in a study in Finland, found diazepam in blood samples from five percent of injured drivers, compared to two percent of controls. Binnie (1983) points out that among patients in a general practice in Britain, those taking benzodiazepines had a higher incidence of automobile accidents while on medication but not when they were off medication. (Patients taking antidepressants or phenothiazines, incidentally, did not have increased accidents.) While these data are associational and do not necessarily imply causality, other studies seem to suggest that the drugs may be responsible for this effect. Betts and Birtle (1982) had 12 female volunteers drive a Datsun through a test course on the morning after taking 15 mg flurazepam, 20 mg temazepam, or placebo. On a test in which the cars had to be driven on a weaving course, drivers who had previously taken flurazepam significantly more often hit the ballards that defined the course. On a task involving driving through a narrow gap, drivers hit the side more often after having taken either drug, compared to placebo. A variety of other studies have documented such effects in the laboratory, both in terms of motor performance and cognitive function.

It has sometimes been argued that although decrements in daytime performance are well described in normals, such findings do not necessarily apply to insomniacs, in whom the benefits from a good night's sleep will outweigh any detrimental pharmacological effects. This does not seem to be the case, for several reasons. The first concern with this viewpoint is that although the sense of discomfort of the insomniac is apparent, actual deficits in daytime performance are subtle and probably only in narrow, specific areas. Church and Johnson (1979) found no difference in performance between insomniacs and good sleepers on such tasks as digit-symbol substitution, choice reaction time, and digit span. Linnoila et al (1980), studying patients chosen by history but without confirmatory EEG studies, found greater variability in performance measures over time and some decrements in tracking and reaction time. Mendelson et al (in press) compared insomniacs and controls on a wide variety of tasks, including tracking tasks thought to have some relevance to driving skills. Deficits were found on only one measure, the quantitative Romberg task. Weingartner et al (in press) and Mendelson et al (in press) also found that although insomniacs did not differ from controls on a variety of performance measures such as a pegboard task, finger tapping rate, and letter cancellation, some difficulties with semantic memory could be found. The impression from the literature at this point seems to be that although a few subtle deficits have been described (and clearly need further exploration), by and large the few performance decrements of insomniacs are small compared to the host of drug-induced deficits.

The second point is that a large number of studies, described in the reviews mentioned above, have documented hypnotic-induced residual daytime effects in insomniacs. Mendelson et al (1982), for instance, found that when insomniacs took 30 mg flurazepam for 28 nights, there were very potent detrimental effects on cognitive performance during the first few days, with scores comparable to related studies of subjects taking alcohol or scopolamine.

Perhaps one last point that should be considered in evaluating studies of sedative-hypnotics on performance is that they occasionally do bring small improvements in performance in normals when given by day, probably by reducing anxiety. Linnoila et al (1974), for instance, showed that chronic diazepam administration improved reaction time and slightly improved coordination on a simulated driving task when performed at a fixed speed. On the other hand, subjects taking diazepam "drove" faster and made more errors when they were allowed to set the speed themselves. Thus, improvements in performance after daytime administration are usually selective. It has been suggested that such effects are most noticeably manifest in untrained subjects, in whom anxiety may be playing a relatively larger role and that this confounding effect may be minimized by using well-trained subjects (Linnoila, 1978).

Performance Data

Studies of daytime effects of hypnotics since 1980 have focused on the short-acting benzodiazepines. Ogura et al (1980) examined EEGs of normal volunteers kept in bed for 24 hours after administration of 0.25 and 0.5 mg triazolam, 15 and 30 mg flurazepam, and 5 and 10 mg nitrazepam. Daytime effects (usually in terms of percentage sleep time or sleep latency) were noted with doses of both flurazepam and nitrazepam; the only major effect of triazolam was some decrement in sleep latency in the morning recording. Spinweber and Johnson (1982) gave 0.5 mg triazolam for six nights to 20 men who were poor sleepers. Morning testing 8.25 hours post-drug showed no decrements on a variety of mood and performance measures, although there was a small decrement on morning six in terms of long-term memory assessed by a recognition task. Pishkin et al (1980) gave a single nighttime dose of 30 mg temazepam, 30 mg flurazepam, or 200 mg secobarbital/amobarbital to 50 normal male volunteers. On a variety of motor and cognitive tasks, the barbiturate and (to a lesser degree) flurazepam induced decrements; there was no decreased performance on the morning after temazepam administration.

The one notable exception to the various studies showing drug-induced deficits is a series of studies of triazolam from Stanford University. Using the multiple sleep latency test (MSLT) as a measure of daytime alertness, Dement et al (1982) showed that 0.5 mg triazolam increased, and 30 mg flurazepam decreased alertness in normals; they found similar results in a multi-laboratory study of insomniacs. Interestingly, in the normal group, these alterations occurred without changes in nocturnal sleep. Carskadon et al (1982) found similar results of 0.25 mg triazolam and 15 mg flurazepam on the MSLT of elderly insomniacs. Again, there were only minor nonsignificant correlations of daytime wakefulness and nocturnal sleep. If these studies are confirmed (there is some disagreement with the work of Ogura et al [1980] mentioned above), this will be the first evidence of objective daytime benefits of hypnotics. One other possible daytime effect of 0.5 mg triazolam which has been raised, however, is enhanced daytime anxiety (Morgan and Oswald, 1982). Other authors such as Carskadon et al (1982) have described relative absence of mood changes after 0.25 mg triazolam in elderly insomniacs. Certainly the issue deserves further clarification.

THE ELDERLY

Sleep disturbances in the elderly present a number of special issues. The incidence of complaints of poor sleep rises with age. Interestingly, sleep disturbance and disruptive behavior at night among elderly invalids may be the most common reason cited by relatives for bringing them for chronic care in institutions (Sanford, 1975). As was mentioned earlier, hypnotics are prescribed to older persons greatly out of proportion to their numbers. In 1975, for instance, 20 to 45 percent of hypnotic prescriptions were given to persons over 60, although they comprised only about 14 percent of the population (Cooper, 1977). In nursing homes, usage is much greater still, ranging in different studies from 26 percent (Martilla et al, 1977) to 100 percent (Derbez and Grauer, 1967).

This finding takes on a greater significance in light of the increased incidence of adverse side effects of virtually all classes of drugs in the elderly. In but one example, Hurwitz (1969) found that persons over 60 were 2.5 times more likely to experience drug reactions while in the hospital as compared to younger individuals. The reasons are probably due to a combination of factors, including altered drug kinetics and possible changes in nervous system sensitivity. In terms of kinetics, the half-life ($t_{1/2}$) of many psychotropic drugs increases with age, leading to the possible increased accumulation of drug. It is often assumed that this may be due to decreased hepatic clearance. It turns out that each drug must be considered separately in this regard. For diazepam, for instance, half-life increases with age, but clearance is unaltered (Klotz et al, 1975), at least in women (Greenblatt et al, 1980). Other factors include decreased serum albumin concentrations in the elderly (Greenblatt, 1979), which can lead to larger amounts of unbound drug free to enter tissues. Sometimes the increased $t_{1/2}$ reflects an increasing volume of distribution with age. Interestingly, for flurazepam 15 mg, half-life may increase with age in men but not women (Greenblatt et al, 1981). Although the reasons are complex, the end result of enhanced side effects of flurazepam in the elderly seems real. Estimates of the degree have varied. In a study of hospitalized medical patients in Boston, adverse reactions from flurazepam occurred in 1.9 percent of patients under 60 and rose to 7.1 percent in those over 60. Of patients over 70 who received 30 mg, 39 percent experienced adverse reactions (Greenblatt and Shader, 1977). In a study of five nursing facilities, Martilla et al (1977) found adverse reactions such as ataxia, confusion, and hallucinations in 26 percent of patients studied.

The second issue of great concern about use of hypnotics in the elderly is the substantially higher incidence of sleep apnea and nocturnal myoclonus. In elderly subjects who do not complain about poor sleep, a significant degree of apneas or hypopneas (greater than five per hour) have been found in 44 to 67 percent in several studies (Smallwood et al, 1983; Ancoli-Israel et al, 1981; Krieger et al, 1980; Block et al, 1979; Carskadon and Dement, 1981). Among those who complain of poor sleep, primary sleep pathologies (sleep apnea or nocturnal myoclonus) may occur in 87 percent (Dement, 1980). In another study, six out of seven elderly patients complaining of poor sleep had a primary pathology of sleep such as sleep apnea or narcolepsy (Reynolds et al, 1980). The concern here is that prescribing hypnotics would not only be unhelpful if one of these disorders is overlooked, but it might be dangerous in the case of undiagnosed sleep apnea. This possibility emphasizes the need for careful evaluation of sleep disorders in the elderly, as well as consideration of nonpharmacologic means of treatment. In those patients in whom sleep pathophysiology has been ruled out, it is also reasonable to consider moderate use of wine. Mishara and Kastenbaum (1974), in a study of long-term geriatric patients in a psychiatric hospital, found that when wine was made available, there were major decreases in chloral hydrate use.

BENZODIAZEPINES AND RESPIRATION

In the preceding section, the concern was raised that hypnotic use in patients with undiagnosed sleep apnea might result in significant respiratory suppression or arrest. While this has long been a concern with barbiturates and other hypnotics, evidence is appearing that benzodiazepines may (to a lesser degree) also have significant effects on respiration in susceptible individuals. Nitrazepam, for instance, has been reported to cause increased pCO_2 and decreased respiratory drive in patients with chronic bronchitis (Rudolf et al, 1978) and obstructive lung disease (Model, 1973), and diazepam is known to induce respiratory suppression during endoscopy (Rao et al, 1973). Therapeutic doses of chlordiazepoxide have also been shown to increase mixed venous carbon dioxide tension in chronic bronchitis patients (Model and Berry, 1974).

There is some evidence that this process is not confined to patients with known lung disease. Mendelson et al (1981) described a 38-year-old insomnia patient who had two to 18 apneas on placebo nights (well below the usual definition of sleep apnea syndrome), whose apneas rose to 100 on the second night of 30 mg flurazepam treatment, and returned to basal levels when the drug was discontinued. In subsequent studies, Carskadon et al (1982) found no effect of a lower dose (15 mg) of flurazepam on elderly insomniacs, who had previously been screened to eliminate those with apnea. On the other hand, Dolly and Block (1982) found that the number of apneas almost doubled in 20 normal volunteers (mean age 49) given 30 mg flurazepam. Kripke and Garfinkel (1984) approached this problem using data from the American Cancer Society's 1959 health survey, which had shown that persons who use hypnotics (in this case, usually barbiturates) had a 50 percent increased risk of dying. Since sleep apnea is one of the most common causes of excessive sleepiness, they studied time of death in persons who reported relatively long (nine hour) sleep times. In this group, which might be more likely to contain many persons with undiagnosed apnea, persons taking hypnotics were much more likely to die during the hours of sleep than those who did not. Although the data from this particular study are associational and not necessarily causal, the weight of the several studies described here suggests that the potential for respiratory suppression is real and should be considered when prescribing all hypnotics, including benzodiazepines.

In passing, it should be also mentioned that 0.5 mg triazolam and 30 mg flurazepam have been associated with increased heart rate during sleep (Muzet et al, 1982), but it is not clear that this finding has clinical significance.

RELIANCE AND DEPENDENCE

Overt abuse of hypnotics has been well described and is put in good historical perspective by Allgulander (1978). Of more recent concern are the twin issues of reliance (a continuing need for recommended doses) and dependence (the occurrence of a withdrawal syndrome). As mentioned earlier, a recent study suggests that perhaps 11 percent of persons currently taking sleeping pills have been on them for at least a year (Mellinger and Balter, 1983). Although the differences in drug classes have been well described in terms of liability for overt abuse, it is not clear whether there are major differences in terms of reliance. A study by Clift (1975) of a British general practice group suggests that patients started on nitrazepam or amobarbital are equally likely to be taking their medication six weeks later. After two years, despite encouragement to discontinue medications, eight percent had been on hypnotics continuously and seven percent more were currently taking them after some drug-free period. Although the extent of reliance (and degree of liability for any one drug) needs to be much more carefully studied, it is clear that one consequence of starting patients on hypnotics is that a certain small percentage will continue to use them for prolonged periods.

The last few years have seen growing concern about possible withdrawal disturbances from recommended doses of hypnotics. This has long been recognized as a problem with barbiturates and non-barbiturate, non-benzodiazepine hypnotics (for example, Kales et al, 1974) and has recently been raised with regard to the newer short-acting benzodiazepines (Kales and Kales, 1983). Although the claim has been made that long-acting benzodiazepines such as flurazepam do not have this difficulty (Kales et al, 1982), evidence is appearing that withdrawal sleep disturbance or daytime dysphoria do indeed occur, albeit after several days and perhaps somewhat more mildly in degree. Berlin and Conell (1983), for instance, described initial insomnia, dizziness, blurred vision, and other symptoms three days after a 37-year-old man was changed from 30 mg flurazepam to 30 mg temazepam. Mendelson et al (1982) described patient reports of poor sleep and dysphoria by the sixth day of withdrawal from flurazepam. A variety of withdrawal symptoms plus even hallucinations and psychosis have been described after withdrawal from therapeutic doses of diazepam (Greenblatt and Shader, 1978; Haskell, 1975). Such data have led several groups, including the authors of The Medical Letter (1981) and an NIMH Consensus Development Conference (1983), to conclude that all benzodiazepines may induce withdrawal reactions, albeit somewhat more mildly with long-acting agents.

CLINICAL RECOMMENDATIONS

With these conclusions and caveats from controlled studies in mind, what considerations should guide the clinician treating a patient suffering from a sleep disorder? Perhaps the most widely disseminated guidelines are the conclusions from the NIMH Consensus Development Conference on "Drugs and Insomnia:

The Use of Medications to Promote Sleep" (1983), referred to in the previous section. It must be emphasized, however, that insomnia is a complaint that can result from a variety of disorders, such as nocturnal myoclonus and sleep apnea, among others. The fundamental approach to the patient with insomnia should be first to look for such illnesses and, when they are found, to provide specific treatment. In those patients in whom such processes are not found, one may consider psychological and pharmacological therapies. The selection of a specific hypnotic should be based on its pharmacological properties in conjunction with the clinical situation and needs of the patient. Physicians should educate their patients about use of the drug and should monitor them to evaluate and reduce the risks of dependence, side effects,and possible withdrawal difficulties.

If a benzodiazepine is selected for an individual patient, pharmocologic factors to be considered include: therapeutic index, dose, rate of absorption, lipophilicity, rate of tissue distribution, elimination half-life, presence or absence of active metabolites, presence or absence of drug interactions, and various pharmacodynamic characteristics that mediate drug effect. Although low lethality gives the physician considerable leeway in individualizing the dose for each patient, the principle of using the lowest effective dose that achieves the desired result is still a good guide in avoiding unwanted side effects. This recommendation applies especially to the elderly. The most common risk associated with the use of benzodiazepines is diminished daytime performance as a result of carryover effects from the previous evening's medication. This problem can be reduced by using lower doses or more rapidly eliminated drugs.

For transient insomnia related to minor situational stress, lasting usually only a few days (for example, hospitalization, jet lag), drug treatment may or may not be necessary. Where elected, the treatment should be a small dose of a rapidly eliminated hypnotic, usually a benzodiazepine; treatment should last only a few nights.

In short-term insomnia lasting only a few weeks (such as that usually related to stress associated with work and/or family life) the problem may, in part, be ameliorated by educating the patient on the habits of good sleep hygiene. If drug treatment is also required, the smallest effective dose should be used, with titration of dose if necessary, and for a treatment period usually of not more than three weeks. The drug may be used intermittently, with the patient skipping the nightly dosage after one or two nights of good sleep. Therapy should be discontinued gradually.

The use of medication for long-term insomnia lasting several months or more remains an area of controversy, since this problem may be related to underlying psychiatric conditions, chronic drug/alcohol dependence, or medical conditions such as nocturnal myoclonus or sleep apnea. Insomnia patients who have failed to respond to non-drug strategies and for whom major psychiatric and medical disorders have been ruled out are appropriate for referral to a sleep disorders center. Usually, long-term insomnia not attributable to medical and psychiatric disorders, and such specific sleep disturbances as sleep apnea, may be treated with the use of principles of sleep hygiene and behaviorally oriented therapeutic techniques, with possible adjunctive use of hypnotics. Although not well documented by formal studies, the clinical impression of many physicians is that occasional intermittent use may be appropriate in this situation. If benzodiazepines are not appropriate for the individual patient, the physician may consider a sedative antidepressant such as amitriptyline 25-100 mg at bedtime. For patients who respond to this program, therapy should be discontinued gradually after three to four months.

CONCLUSIONS

In summary, hypnotics continue to be used widely, although in somewhat decreasing amounts. A small but persistent group of patients is likely to continue taking them for prolonged periods. In the last decade the benzodiazepines have come to be the predominant agents prescribed for sleep, and in recent years the interest in short-acting agents has increased. Several of them may have certain advantages in terms of lack of drug accumulation but, because of slightly less reliable absorption, they might well be taken somewhat earlier than bedtime.

There are many issues to consider in evaluating efficacy of hypnotics, and at this point it seems wise to consider different aspects of data from both subjective and EEG studies. In general, most prescription hypnotics have been shown to have some benefits for nocturnal sleep for a few weeks, with very little data being available for nightly use longer than four weeks. In contrast, with only the exception of one short-acting benzodiazepine, studies of hypnotics have not shown benefits to daytime mood, functioning, or alertness. (These daytime changes, incidentally, do not necessarily correlate with drug-induced alterations in the previous night's sleep.) On the contrary, many agents may adversely affect daytime cognition and performance in such crucial areas as driving skills. There is little evidence to suggest that such performance decrements are somehow compensated for by the benefit of improved sleep for insomniacs; data to date suggest only a few, very selective, decrements in the daytime functioning of unmedicated insomniacs.

The elderly have a higher incidence of complaints of poor sleep and use hypnotics in disproportionately large numbers. Prescribing hypnotics for persons over 60 should be done with caution, both because of a higher likelihood of side effects and a higher incidence of primary sleep disorders such as sleep apnea syndrome. All hypnotics are respiratory suppressants, and the benzodiazepines are no exception. Withdrawal sleep disturbance and daytime dysphoria are apparent for virtually all hypnotics, including perhaps slightly more mild disruptions from long-acting benzodiazepines.

REFERENCES

Allgulander C: Dependence on sedative and hypnotic drugs—a comparative clinical and social study. Acta Psychiatr Scand Suppl 270:1-102, 1978

Ancoli-Israel S, Kripke DF, Mason W, et al: Sleep apnea and nocturnal myoclonus in a senior population. Sleep 4:349-58, 1981

Association of Sleep Disorders Centers Diagnostic Classification of Sleep and Arousal Disorders. Sleep 2:1-137, 1979

Berlin RM, Conell LJ: Withdrawal symptoms after long-term treatment with therapeutic doses of flurazepam: a case report. Am J Psychiatry 140:488-489, 1983

Betts TA, Birtle J: Effect of two hypnotic drugs on actual driving performance next morning. Br Med J 285:852, 1982

Binnie GAC: Psychotropic drugs and accidents in a general practice. Br Med J 287:1349-1350, 1983

Bixler EO, Soldatos CR, Scarone S, et al: Similarities of nocturnal myoclonic activity in insomniac patients and normal subjects. Sleep Research 7:213, 1978

Bixler EO, Kales A, Soldatos CR: Sleep disorders encountered in medical practice. Behavioral Medicine, 2:13-21, 1979

Block AJ, Boysen PG, Wynne JW, et al: Sleep apnea, hypopnea and oxygen desaturation in normal subjects. A strong predominance. N Engl J Med 300:513-517, 1979

Boston Collaborative Drug Surveillance Program: A clinical evaluation of flurazepam. J Clin Pharmacol 12:217-220 May-June 1972

Carskadon MA, Dement WC: Respiration during sleep in the aged human. J Gerontol 36:420-3, 1981

Carskadon MA, Seidel WF, Greenblatt DJ, et al: Daytime carryover of triazolam and flurazepam in elderly insomniacs. Sleep 5:361-371, 1982

Church MW, Johnson LC: Mood and performance of poor sleepers during repeated use of flurazepam. Psychopharmacology 61:309-316, 1979

Clift AD: Prediction of the dependence-prone patient: a general practice investigation, in Sleep Disturbances and Hypnotic Drug Dependence. Edited by Clift AD. Excerpta Medica, Amsterdam, 1975

Cooper JR: Sedative-hypnotic drugs: risks and benefits. Bethesda, Maryland, National Institute on Drug Abuse, US Department of Health, Education and Welfare, 1977

Dement WC: Sedative/hypnotics and sleep apnea. Presentation to Project Sleep, July 1980

Dement WC, Carskadon MA, Mitler MM, et al: Prolonged use of flurazepam: a sleep laboratory study. Behavioral Medicine 1:25-31, October 1978

Dement WC, Seidel W, Carskadon MA: Daytime alertness, insomnia and benzodiazepines. Sleep 5:528-545, 1982

Derbez R, Grauer H: A sleep study and investigation of a new hypnotic compound in a geriatric population. Can Med Assoc J 97:1388-1393, 1967

Dolly RF, Block JA: Effect of flurazepam on sleep-disordered breathing and nocturnal oxygen desaturation in asymptomatic subjects. Am J Med 73:239-243, 1982

Ellingsen AP: Double-blind trial of triazolam 0.5 mg vs nitrazepam 5 mg in outpatients. J Acta Psychiatr Scand 67:154-158, 1983

Fabre LF, Cross L, Pasigajen V, et al: Multiclinic double-blind comparison of triazolam and flurazepam for seven nights in outpatients with insomnia. J Clin Pharmacol 17:402-409, 1977

Fillingim JM: Double-blind evaluation of temazepam, flurazepam, and placebo in geriatric insomnia. Clin Ther 4:396-380, 1982

Fowler LK: Temazepam (Euphypnos) as a hypnotic: a twelve-week trial in general practice. J Int Med Res 5:295-296, 1977

Greenblatt DJ: Reduced serum albumin concentration in the elderly: a report from the Boston collaborative drug surveillance program. J Am Geriatr Soc, 27:20-22, 1979

Greenblatt DJ, Shader RI: Nonprescription psychotropic drugs, in Pharmacology in the Practice of Medicine. Edited by Jarvik ME. New York, Appleton-Century-Crofts, 1977

Greenblatt DJ, Shader RI: Dependence, tolerance and addiction to benzodiazepines: clinical and pharmacokinetic considerations. Drug Metab Rev 8:13-28, 1978

Greenblatt DJ, Allen MD, Harmatz JS, et al: Diazepam disposition determinants. Clinical Pharmacology and Therapeutics 27:301-312, 1980

Greenblatt DJ, Divoll M, Harmatz JS, et al: Kinetics and clinical effects of flurazepam in young and elderly non-insomniacs. Clinical Pharmacology Research, 30:475-486, 1981

Hartmann E: The effect of four drugs on sleep patterns in man. Psychopharmacologia 12:346-353, 1968

Hartmann E: Chronic insomnia: effects of tryptophan, flurazepam, secobarbitol and placebo. Psychopharmacol Bull 80:138-142, 1983

Haskell D: Letter: withdrawal from diazepam. JAMA 233:135, 1975

Hurwitz N: Predisposing factors in adverse reactions to drugs. Br Med J 1:536, 1969

Johnson LC, Chernik DA: Sedative-hypnotics and human performance. Psychopharmacology 76:101-113, 1982

Kales A, Bixler EO, Tan T, et al: Chronic hypnotic-drug use: ineffectiveness, drug-withdrawal insomnia, and dependence. JAMA 227:513-517, 1974

Kales A, Kales JD, Bixler EO, et al: Effectiveness of hypnotic drugs with prolonged use: flurazepam and pentobarbital. Clinical Pharmacology and Therapeutics 18:356-363, 1975

Kales A, Kales J, Bixler E, et al: Hypnotic efficacy of triazolam: sleep laboratory evaluation of intermediate, term effectiveness. J Clin Pharmacol 16:399-406, 1976

Kales A, Bixler, EO, Soldatos CR, et al: Quazepam and flurazepam: long-term use and extended withdrawal. Clinical Pharmacology and Therapeutics 32:781-788, 1982

Kales A, Kales JD: Sleep laboratory studies of hypnotic drugs: efficacy and withdrawal effects. J Clin Psychopharmacol 3:140-149, 1983

Kales J, Lakes A, Bixler EO, et al: Effects of placebo and flurazepam on sleep patterns in insomniac subjects. Clinical Pharmacology and Therapeutics 12:691-697, 1971

Kay DC, Blackburn AB, Buckingham JA, et al: Human pharmacology of sleep, in Pharmacology of Sleep. Edited by Williams RL, Karacan I. New York, John Wiley & Sons, 1965

Kay DC, Jarinski DR, Eisenstein RB, et al: Quantified human sleep after pentobarbital. Clin Pharmacol Ther 13:221-231, 1972

Klotz U, Avant GR, Hoyumpa A, et al: The effects of age and liver disease on the disposition and elimination of diazepam in adult man. J Clin Invest 55:347-359, 1975

Krieger J, Mangin P, Kurtz D: Les modifications respiratories au cours sommeil du sujet age normal. Rev EEG Neurophysiol 10:177-185, 1980

Kripke DF, Garfinkel L: Excess nocturnal deaths related to sleeping pill and tranquilizer use. Lancet Jan 14, 1(8368):99, 1984

Leibowitz M, Sunshine A: Long-term hypnotic efficacy and safety of triazolam and flurazepam. J Clin Pharmacol 18:302-309, 1978

Linnoila M: Psychomotor effects of drugs and alcohol on healthy volunteers and psychiatric patients, in Advances in Pharmacology and Therapeutics, Vol 8. Edited by Olive G. New York, Pergamon Press, 1978

Linnoila M, Otterstrom S, Mattila M: Serum chlordiazepoxide, diazepam, and thioridazine concentrations after the simultaneous ingestion of alcohol or placebo drink. Ann Clin Res 6:4-6, 1974

Linnoila M, Erwin CW, Logue PE: Efficacy and side effects of flurazepam and a combination of amobarbital and secobarbital in insomniac patients. J Clin Pharmacol 20:117-123, 1980

Maggini C, Murri M, Sacchatti G: Evaluation of the effectiveness of temazepam on the insomnia of patients with neurosis and endogenous depression. Arzneimittelforsch 19:1647-1652, 1969

Martilla JK, Hammel RJ, Alexander B, et al: Potential untoward effects of long-term use of flurazepam in geriatric patients. Journal of the American Pharmaceutical Association 17:692-695, 1977

Medical Letter: "Choice of Benzodiazepines," 23:41-42, 1981

Mellinger GD, Balter MB: Prevalence of insomnia and drug treatment. Abstract at NIMH Consensus Development Conference "Drugs and Insomnia," Nov 15-17, 1983, Bethesda, Maryland

Mendelson WB: The Use and Misuse of Sleeping Pills, New York, Plenum Press, 1980

Mendelson WB, Garnett D, Gillin JC: Flurazepam-induced sleep apnea syndrome in a patient with insomnia and mild sleep-related respiratory changes. J Nerv Ment Dis, 169:261-264, 1981

Mendelson WB, Weingartner H, Greenblatt DJ, et al: A clinical study of flurazepam. Sleep 5:350-360, 1982

Mendelson W, Garnett D, Linnoila M: Do insomniacs have impaired daytime functioning? Biol Psychiatry (in press)

Mishara BL, Kastenbaum R: Wine in the treatment of long-term geriatric patients in mental institutions. J Am Geriatr Soc 22:88-94, 1974

Mitler M, Phillips RL, Billiard M, et al: Long-term effectiveness of temazepam 30 mg HS on chronic insomniacs. Sleep Res 4:109, 1975

Model DG: Nitrazepam-induced respiratory depression in chronic obstructive lung disease. Br J Dis Chest 67:128-130, 1973

Model DG, Berry DJ: Effects of chlordiazepoxide in respiratory failure due to chronic bronchitis. Lancet 2:869-870, 1974

Morgan K, Oswald I: Anxiety caused by a short-life hypnotic. Br Med J, 284:942, 1982

Muzet A, Johnson LC, Spinweber CI: Benzodiazepine hypnotics increase heart rate during sleep. Sleep 5:256-261, 1982

Nair NPV, Schwartz G: Triazolam in insomnia: a standard-controlled trial. Current Therapeutic Research, Clinical and Experimental 23:388-392, 1978

NIMH Consensus Development Conference on Drugs and Insomnia, Bethesda, Maryland, Nov 15-17, 1983

Okawa KK: Comparison of triazolam .25 mg and flurazepam 15 mg in treating geriatric insomniacs. Current Therapeutic Research, Clinical and Experimental 23:381-387, 1978

Ogura C, Nakayawa K, Majima K, et al: Residual effects of hypnotics: triazolam, flurazepam and nitrazepam. Psychopharmacology 68:61-65, 1980

Pishkin V, Lowallo WR, Fishkin SM, et al: Residual effects of temazepam and other hypnotic compounds on cognitive function. J Clin Psychiatry 41:358-364, 1980

Rao S, Sherbaniuk RW, Prosad K, et al: Cardiopulmonary effects of diazepam. Clin Pharmacol Ther 14:182-189, 1973

Reeves RL: Comparison of triazolam, flurazepam, and placebo as hypnotics in geriatric patients with insomnia. J Clin Pharmacol 17:319-323, 1977

Reynolds CF, Coble P, Black R, et al: Sleep disturbances in a series of elderly patients: polysomnographic findings. J Am Geriatr Soc 28:164-170, 1980

Rickels K, Gingrich R, Morris R, et al: Triazolam in insomniac family practice patients. Clin Pharmacol Ther 18:315-324, 1975

Roehrs T, Zouck F, Kaffeman M, et al: Flurazepam for short-term treatment of complaints of insomnia. J Clin Pharmacol 22:290-296, 1982

Roth T, Kramer M, Lutz T: Intermediate use of triazolam: a sleep laboratory study. J Int Med Res 4:59-63, 1976

Roth T, Kramer M, Lutz T: The effects of hypnotics on sleep, performance, and subjective state. Drugs and Experimental Clinical Research 1:279-287, 1977

Rudolf M, Geddis DM, Turner JA McM, et al: Depression of central respiratory drive by nitrazepam. Thorax 33:97-100, 1978

Sanford JRA: Tolerance of debility in elderly dependents by supporters at home: its significance for hospital practice. Br Med J 3:471-473, 1975

Schwartz MA, Postma E: Metabolism of flurazepam, a benzodiazepine, in man and dog. J Pharm Sci 59:1800-1806, 1970

Smallwood RF, Vitiello MV, Giblin EC, et al: Sleep apnea: relationship to age, sex, and Alzheimer's dementia. Sleep 6:16-22, 1983

Spinweber CL, Johnson LC: Effects of triazolam (0.5 mg) on sleep, performance, memory and arousal threshold. Psychopharmacology 76:5-12, 1982

Sunshine A: Comparison of the hypnotic activity of triazolam, flurazepam hydrochloride, and placebo. J Clin Pharmacol Ther 5:17, 573-577, 1975

Vogel GW, Thurmond A, Gibbons P, et al: The effects of triazolam on the sleep of insomniacs. J Psychopharmacologia 41:65-69, 1975

Vogel GW, Barker K, Gibbons P, et al: A comparison of the effects of flurazepam 30 mg and triazolam 0.5 mg on the sleep of insomniacs. J Psychopharmacologia 47:81-86, 1976

Weingartner H, Mendelson W, Garnett D, et al: Cognitive processes in chronic insomnia patients. Sleep Research 12 (in press)

Afterword

by David J. Kupfer, M.D.

Despite the extensive strides made in the last ten years, there is much that remains to be learned about sleep and sleep disorders. Our present lack of knowledge falls roughly into two categories. The first encompasses those areas that deal directly with the treatment of patients with sleep disorders. In many instances, researchers and clinicians are now working to fill these knowledge gaps. Some of them are obvious. The reader should recognize from the omissions in the previous seven chapters, for example, that we still know little about sleep disorders in children and adolescents. In fact, there is even a lot about the normal sleep of individuals in these groups that remains to be learned. This brings us to the second area of our insufficient knowledge about sleep—questions of basic sleep physiology for which the answers have thus far eluded us. However, much of this preclinical work is well underway, and many of the clues that guide our search relate to the ontogeny of biological rhythms; for the sleep-wake cycle is one of the basic cycles of living. For example, researchers have recently studied the development of various bodily rhythms in newborn animals and have identified developmental stages at which certain of these rhythms appear. Once we know how the rhythms develop and when they assume a given pattern, it will be possible to plot that pattern over developmental time in both animals and humans and explore their underlying mechanisms (Davis, 1981). This baseline will then allow the assessment of variations and deviations from it.

Questions of both types also remain to be answered about the sleep changes that we know occur as individuals approach the far end of the age spectrum. Most work in the elderly has been with clinical populations. We have yet to learn all we need to know about how sleep architecture changes with increasing age, and how the changes that occur naturally with the aging process interact with those that accompany pathology. These areas need further investigation.

We now have refined, efficacious treatments for only a few of the sleep disorders that have been described and defined in our nosological systems. And while it is important to disseminate the message to patients and the public that treatments for selected sleep disorders are available, the next frontier of sleep research should be the understanding of the disorders for which no treatments yet exist, and the creation of better treatments in those instances in which the therapy creates problems of its own. For instance, although narcolepsy has been treated with some success with stimulant medications, these drugs are subject to tolerance and are less than ideal over the long run.

There is an entire catalogue of sleep puzzles that have yet to be solved. We know very little about the incidence and prevalence of sleep disorders within the population as a whole, since we tend to study only those people who come to us with complaints. How many individuals have disorders, perhaps of equal severity, who have not sought treatment or were unaware that treatment was available? Do these people ever mention these sleep problems to their family physicians, and how do they describe them? What treatments do the family doctors prescribe for these complaints? For those insomniacs who do not seek treatment, we need to know how many attempt self-treatment with over-the-counter medications, alcohol, or even warm milk before bedtime. We also do not know how these untreated individuals tolerate their problems and what deficits in functioning, if any, they endure. What are the costs in somatic, psychological, social, and economic terms?

It is only by creating profiles of the various categories of sleep disorders and patients' responses to interventions that we can develop effective and safe treatments. And it is only through a broad public education effort about what can be done for individuals with insomnia, hypersomnia, or any of the other problems that interfere with sleep, that we can fully apply our current body of knowledge. Sleep continues to confront us with many mysteries; but we have not yet tired of the search for answers.

REFERENCES

Davis FC: Ontogeny of circadian rhythms, in Handbook of Behavioral Neurobiology 4 (Biological Rhythms). Edited by Aschoff J. New York, Plenum Press, 1981

IV
Eating Disorders

Contents

Eating Disorders
Introduction
by Joel Yager, M.D., Section Editor

Clinical descriptions of conditions similar to those we currently classify as eating disorders have appeared for hundreds of years. Cases that closely resemble anorexia nervosa were reported at least as early as the 1600s (Dally and Gomez, 1979); and a condition of ravenous hunger called "boolmot" in Hebrew (bulimy in Greek) was described in the Talmud, together with recommendations that it be treated with such sweet foods as honey (Kaplan and Garfinkel, 1984). Obesity and its behavioral concomitants such as gluttony have, of course, been recognized since ancient times.

In spite of the antiquity of these conditions, only recently has serious systematic attention been focused on their research and treatment. A great deal of public awareness has emerged regarding anorexia nervosa and bulimia within the past few years: anorexia nervosa has been described as the syndrome of the '70s, and bulimia as the syndrome of the '80s. The field spawned its own journal in 1981, the *International Journal of Eating Disorders*. As will be evident from the following chapters, the prevalence of eating disorders appears to have increased dramatically during the last several decades, and this does not appear to be due simply to better case finding and diagnosis. Eating disorders clinics and treatment units have been springing up at a rapid rate, presumably in response to an increased demand for services. Bulimia was not even recognized as a separate syndrome in its own right until the 1960s. What, then, can account for such an explosion in the appearance of bulimia and other eating disorders?

Disorders have a way of coming and going throughout history with a cycle of their own, influenced by forces not always understood by those who live through the epidemics. We can point to several in psychiatry and medicine that have emerged, flourished, and then waned. Consider peptic ulcer and even coronary artery disease, both of which currently appear to be decreasing in incidence. Are the causes genetic? viral? related to changing modes of diet, stress and exercise? Is it possible that the recent rise in reports of eating disorders in the past few decades represents new phenotypic expressions, perhaps in large measure culturally shaped, for the manifestation of those amorphous miasmas that previously appeared as grand hysteria and neurasthenia?

It is possible that anthropologists can help us to understand the rapid growth of eating disorders. In all westernized countries cultural pressure for thinness in women has increased in a palpable and quantifiable manner; stress is placed on slimness as a prerequisite for beauty. Instead of using footbinding and tight whalebone corsets, women are encouraged to shrink their entire bodies into slim designer jeans in order to feel good about themselves and be attractive to contemporary men. Can this relatively recent cultural pressure be related to eating disorders? In a recent article in *Glamour* magazine, Drs. Wayne and Susan Wooley described the responses of 33,000 women who completed a brief survey in August, 1983 (*Glamour*, February 1984). The results were striking: 75 percent of the respondents felt "too fat" although according to even conservative height-weight tables only one quarter would actually be considered overweight; 45 percent of the underweight women felt too fat; and only 6 percent felt unequivocally positive about their bodies. Only 12 percent had never used moderate calorie restriction, and only 5 percent had never used exercise to control their weight. Large percentages of the women indicated that they sometimes or often used severe forms of weight control/reduction methods: liquid formula diets—27 percent; diet pills—50 percent; laxatives—18 percent; fasting/starving—45 percent; and self-induced vomiting—15 percent. While these women do not represent a randomly selected community sample (and they certainly did not all have diagnosable eating disorders), they do illustrate the emphasis upon weight preoccupation, body dissatisfaction and self-abuse in the service of weight reduction among young American women.

Given our relatively recent attention to these disorders, it is not surprising that many areas of uncertainty regarding diagnosis still exist. Kennedy and Garfinkel, and Mitchell et al, consider some of the diagnostic uncertainties concerning anorexia nervosa and bulimia, respectively. Many European and Canadian clinicians would not accept the stringent weight criterion of weight loss of at least 25 percent below starting weight set forth in *DSM-III* for the diagnosis of anorexia nervosa. Moreover, they might include the presence of amenorrhea, not a diagnostic criterion in *DSM-III*. Furthermore, a substantial proportion of women with so-called normal weight bulimia have periods of amenorrhea and oligomenorrhea. Might some of these women, who fall within normal ranges according to standard weight tables, nevertheless be "underweight" in relation to their own presumed set points? This is discussed by Stunkard in chapter 22. At the present time, these are unresolved issues.

Another diagnostic question that will be evident to the reader throughout this section is the confused relationship between anorexia nervosa and bulimia. Although *DSM-III* has chosen to define anorexia nervosa and bulimia as distinct disorders, most authorities would argue that this distinction is artificial and invalid. No doubt, *DSM-IV* will correct this and portray the two as being more closely related. While current evidence would suggest that some useful distinction might be made between restricting and bulimic anorexia nervosa patients as described in the chapters by Kennedy and Garfinkel and Garner and Isaacs, a strong case can be made that a continuum exists between bulimic anorexia nervosa and normal weight bulimia. This continuum is most striking to the clinician who evaluates large numbers of supposedly normal weight bulimic patients whose overt goal in coming for treatment is to stop binge eating, but whose covert goal is to continue to eat very little. In other words, some normal weight bulimics seem bent on becoming better at achieving a restricted type of anorexia nervosa! They want to remain unnaturally thin. The question becomes, then, the dimensions along which *all* patients with eating disorders should be evaluated.

In evaluating patients with eating disorders, two principles must be kept in mind. First, for the patient with anorexia nervosa (and possibly for those with normal weight bulimia who force themselves into thinner bodies than they're meant to have), virtually all physical and laboratory abnormalities seem to be sequelae rather than antecedents of the starvation and maladaptive behaviors. Moreover, as demonstrated in the classic experiments by Keys and associates (described in Chapter 23), healthy conscientious objectors who are starved to 25 percent below initial body weight begin to manifest psychological sequelae that resemble features of both anorexia nervosa and bulimia: food preoccupation, gorging when food is available, irritability, depression, mood lability, and so forth. Even starved rats begin to hoard food, a behavior that is seen in anorexia nervosa and usually attributed to psychopathology.

The second basic principle is that anorexia nervosa, bulimia, and obesity are all heterogenous conditions. Accordingly, the assessment of these patients requires attention to a number of dimensions, each of which may have important implications for treatment and prognosis. Patients with bulimia, for example, may vary as widely as do patients who smoke or who abuse alcohol: For some, bulimia is the principal manifestation of emotional disorder; for others, a bulimic syndrome may be only the tip of the iceberg in an impulse ridden character disorder.

The following areas require particular attention in the assessment of each eating disorder patient:

THE EATING DISORDER PER SE: age of onset of the various psychological and behavioral components; current eating practices and rituals; extent and nature of normal eating; detailed accounts of binging and purging behaviors; a statement of the patient's desired weight, often a telling single indicator of body image distortion.

WEIGHT AND FEEDING HISTORY: infancy, childhood, latency, adolescence, as well as weight history for the entire family.

PHYSICAL STATUS: comprehensive medical history and physical examination, and laboratory tests as described in the following chapters, particularly for the underweight patient who is at greatest risk for serious physical morbidity and mortality.

AFFECTIVE DISTURBANCE IN PATIENT AND FAMILY: depressive symptoms may occur in the wake of eating disorder syndromes and remit with proper rehabilitation; a clear picture of how the affective and eating disorder symptoms are temporally related may have implications for treatment.

PERSONALITY DIMENSIONS: predominant cognitive and coping styles of the patient enter into treatment planning, particularly rigidity and obsessionality or, conversely, impulsivity and inability to modulate tension. These factors are critical with respect to planning psychotherapy and also in pharmacotherapy in certain cases.

SUBSTANCE ABUSE: simultaneous abuse of other substances such as alcohol, amphetamines, and cocaine. Setting treatment priorities may require that initial attention be directed toward these problems before or during treatment of the eating disorder.

THE FAMILY AND CULTURAL CONTEXT: the extent to which peers and family contribute to the maintenance of pathogenic attitudes, the extent to which significant others are hostile and destructive toward the patient.

This brief preview of the salient dimensions should quickly alert the clinician to the need for a comprehensive perspective about eating disorders, with regard both to pathogenesis and to treatment. The fact is that no single point of view—biological, psychological, interpersonal, or cultural—can currently claim primacy. To best understand and treat these disorders, the clinician must step beyond the narrow confines of any single school of thought to grasp the potential influences and potential "therapeutic receptor sites" in any given patient. The chapters in this section reflect this point of view.

Chapter 21 offers an account of the physiological mechanisms that underlie hunger and satiety. James Gibbs and Gerard P. Smith review aspects of the peripheral and central nervous system, neurohumoral and hormonal systems, and gastrointestinal system that have been studied in relation to feeding and its disorders. Although many of these processes and structures undoubtedly mediate some elements of the eating disorders, it is far from clear which, if any, of these are of primary importance in their etiology. Nevertheless, familiarity with the physiological mechanisms involved in hunger, feeding, satiety, fasting, taste, bloating, vomiting, and possibly in some of the related subjective experiences of the patients, is useful. The search for rational therapies for certain aspects of the eating disorders—for example, the use of domperidone for gastric emptying in some patients—should be based on a firm knowledge of this physiology.

Chapter 22 considers obesity. Albert J. Stunkard cogently summarizes an enormous amount of research that has appeared about this disorder, involving studies from most of the basic biological sciences and from internal medicine, pediatrics, surgery, public health and psychiatry. As previously mentioned, psychological aspects of obesity appear for the most part to be largely secondary, appearing as consequences of negative social pressure and ostracism with resulting shame in the severely obese in our society. As has been demonstrated in many community surveys, weight preoccupation is a major pastime of Americans, and millions if not billions of dollars are spent each year in weight reduction efforts. The accumulated data on proper treatment strategies currently available for persons with different severities of obesity is analyzed and discussed.

In Chapter 23 Sidney Kennedy and Paul E. Garfinkel provide a comprehensive clinical description of anorexia nervosa. These authors stress the multifactorial hypotheses of pathogenesis, describe the epidemiology of this disorder suggesting strong cultural contributions, and thoroughly review its signs and symptoms and its variable clinical course. Their delineation of the restricter and bulimic subtypes of anorexia nervosa supports the view that this disorder does not constitute a single disease entity. Their discussion of management highlights the need for individualized treatment planning, the substantial morbidity of these disorders, and the importance of multidimensional treatment. A humane, compassionate, yet firm and active approach to these patients seems the most sensible position to take. The seriousness of the disorder is underscored by the fact that full recovery can be expected to occur in fewer than half the patients.

In Chapter 24, James E. Mitchell, Richard L. Pyle and Elke D. Eckert review currently available information regarding bulimia. The reader will note that the majority of references cited have been published within the past half dozen years, further evidence for the extremely recent interest in this group of disorders. In addition to delineating the clinical pictures, these authors discuss the known linkages of bulimia to other psychiatric syndromes. The need for comprehensive evaluation and treatment planning is evident. Active debate is now flourishing as to the proper indications for various treatment strategies, including individual and group psychotherapy, medications and hospitalization. Studies suggesting that each of these modalities may be very effective for some patients have emerged, and the process of sorting out which therapy is best for which patient is underway.

Chapter 25 presents a review of family aspects of the eating disorders, by Michael Strober and myself. As we point out, these disorders have naturally drawn the attention of clinicians and researchers interested in both psychological and biological perspectives on pathogenesis and treatment. The diversity of observed family patterns and current formulations regarding specific patterns of family interaction are critically analyzed. Of note is emerging evidence that the extent to which the families are hostile and critical constitutes an important negative prognostic indicator for anorexia nervosa. A strategy for assessment and treatment is provided. The available systematic information on family aspects of bulimia is discussed, and family aspects in the appearance and treatment of obesity are also considered.

In Chapter 26, David M. Garner and Paul Isaacs review psychological issues in pathogenesis and treatment. These authors survey a variety of theories, including formulations based primarily on early life experiences and those which focus on later issues in development. They stress the ways in which multiple complex formulations, including those derived from object relations, self psychology, Piagetian development and others, may be partially integrated; and how the extent to which each element is salient varies from patient to patient. Many similarities between anorexia nervosa and bulimic patients are apparent from clinical observations and psychometric assessment. Here again, the diversity of these syndromes is evident, for example in the nature and extent of personality disturbance. In regard to treatment, these authors describe the prevalent distortions in attitudes and self concepts seen in eating disorder patients, and emphasize the potential utility of a "two track" approach which attends to both the complicated psychological issues *and* to the eating behaviors themselves. Both psychodynamic and behavioral approaches are couched in an empathetic, nurturing and active relationship.

To help the interested reader learn more about these disorders through independent study, several key references in each chapter have been asterisked. These references will provide additional detailed information about the various topics. Finally, in an afterword, I have summarized a few of the many remaining questions and difficulties that face clinicians and researchers alike. It should be clear that what is presented in this section constitutes our best available information, not the best information that will ever be.

REFERENCES

Dally P, Gomez J: Anorexia Nervosa. London, Wm. Heinemann, 1979

Kaplan AS, Garfinkel PE: Bulimia in the Talmud. Am J Psychiatry 141:721, 1984

Wooley W, Wooley S: Feeling fat in a thin society: 33,000 women tell how they feel about their bodies. Glamour Magazine 198–252, February, 1984

Chapter 21

The Physiology of Hunger and Satiety

by James Gibbs, M.D. and Gerard P. Smith, M.D.

Research on the physiological mechanisms controlling hunger and satiety has a long history, and has resulted in the gathering of impressive techniques. A great number of facts and observations at analytical levels ranging from the cellular to the behavioral have been accumulated. Facts have been organized and reorganized into a mix of broad theories. Nevertheless, a compelling case cannot be made for any one of these theories. We do not understand how body weight is regulated normally, nor how it becomes distorted in obesity or anorexia nervosa.

This chapter cannot attempt to be comprehensive, particularly in regard to the complexities of long-term energy balance. Encyclopedic reviews already exist (Lytle, 1977). Instead, we have selected the individual meal as our focus. The functional unit of eating is the meal (Richter, 1922). All mammals eat in intermittent bouts. If we can understand the biological regulation of this pervasive phenomenon, we should be in the position to ask incisive questions about the more complex biological regulation of body weight. In addition, we hope to show that research employing this strategy already shows promise of delivering benefits in the clinic.

MEAL INITIATION (HUNGER): A REVIEW OF RESEARCH

Gastric Contractions

In 1912, Walter Cannon published a paper entitled "An explanation of hunger" (Cannon and Washburn, 1912). In this study, Cannon reported a good temporal correlation in one human subject between periods of increased gastric motility (recorded via an inflated gastric balloon) and the subjective sense of hunger; it may have been significant for the results that this subject was coached by Cannon to recognize and respond to hunger sensations. Based on the temporal correlation he found, Cannon referred to these periods of increased motility as "hunger contractions." Using similar techniques, Carlson apparently confirmed these results in a large number of subjects (Carlson, 1913). It seemed that solid experimental evidence in support of a traditional speculation about the necessary stimulus for hunger had been produced. But the evidence was less solid than it seemed: First, it became clear that gastrectomized patients clearly experienced hunger (Inglefinger, 1944); thus, the observed gastric motility changes could not be the only antecedent of hunger. Second, Stunkard and Fox (1971) showed that when subjects were not coached in advance to associate hunger with increased gastric motility, the apparently robust correlation disappeared. We now know that gastric contractions are not reliably associated with hunger sensations in humans or with the onset of a meal in animals.

Glucoprivation

Another theory to account for the beginning of meals soon replaced the gastric contraction hypothesis. This theory explained eating in terms of changes in cellular metabolism. The initial event was thought to be a decrease in levels of circulating glucose or, alternatively, a decrease in the glucose which could be utilized by cells (glucoprivation); such a decrease was postulated to occur as a result of a period of nonfeeding. Thus, the initiation of a meal was seen as a response to a metabolic deficit which accrued between meals (Mayer, 1953). This new theory had intuitive appeal: We eat in response to a need, and that need is a deficit in the availability of a prime fuel, glucose, for cellular use. When Silverstone and Besser showed that insulin-induced hypoglycemia could elicit the subjective experience of hunger and the initiation of eating in humans (Silverstone and Besser, 1971), this demonstration increased the credibility of the theory.

The question of the way this experimentally induced eating related to the spontaneous eating we experience each day remained unanswered. It was apparent that frank hypoglycemia, such as that seen after exogenous insulin administration, never occurred in normal animals or humans, and could not account for the onset of any meal. Some very subtle shift in circulating glucose levels which might provoke the beginning of each meal has been proposed (Le Magnen, 1980) but not rigorously tested. Furthermore, attempts to prevent meal taking by infusing glucose have usually been unsuccessful (for example, see Strubbe and Steffens, 1977).

Nevertheless, it was thought that a decrease in intracellular glucose utilization rate, perhaps even by some specialized set of inaccessible neurons, was the critical event which led to feeding behavior. A new pharmacological tool, 2-deoxy-D-glucose (or 2-DG), was brought to bear on this possibility. This glucose analogue crosses cell membranes and competitively inhibits the enzyme involved in glycolysis, thus depriving the cell of energy. Like insulin, it also elicits the subjective experience of hunger and the initiating of eating in humans (Thompson and Campbell, 1977).

However, 2-DG-induced glucoprivation can also lead to a "metabolic emergency" (Smith, 1982), as evidenced by an adrenal-mediated epinephrine discharge, hepatic glycogenolysis, and a hyperglycemia intended to counteract the intracellular energy deficit. This emergency situation clearly does not occur at mealtime, in humans or animals. These two characteristics of the drug led to a clear test of the glucostatic hypothesis: Could a dose of 2-DG be found that would decrease food intake in animals *without* producing an abnormal metabolic state, as evidenced by hyperglycemia? Such a dose could not be found, in spite of extensive tests in rats and rhesus monkeys—feeding could not be elicited without causing a metabolic emergency (Smith et al, 1972). The results mean one of two things: Either the 2-DG model is inadequate for the glucoprivation postulated to occur before eating—in that case there is no adequate model, and the glucostatic theory for meal taking is faith, not fact—or, glucoprivation has little or no role in the initiation of spontaneous feeding.

Neurochemistry

The classic demonstrations of large changes in body weight and food intake following electrolytic lesions of the hypothalamus in animals, and of similar changes in humans with hypothalamic tumors (Reeves and Plum, 1969), have been enormously influential. In 1939, Hetherington and Ranson found that bilateral lesions in the ventromedial hypothalamus made rats markedly obese. Brobeck et al (1943) demonstrated that overeating played a major role in this experimental obesity. In contrast, more lateral lesions in the hypothalamus produced the opposite picture of marked aphagia and gross weight loss (Anand and Brobeck, 1951).

These dramatically different results gave rise to the notion of dual and opposing centers controlling feeding behavior—a "satiety center" in the medial hypothalamus, a "hunger center" in the lateral hypothalamus. This simple and widespread interpretation of the two syndromes has been considerably weakened by the realization that the lesions are nonspecific. A variety of behaviors besides feeding are affected. Furthermore, studies in animals have shown that deficits in satiety per se (that is, the decrease in eating produced as a consequence of the food ingested at an individual meal) are not a consequence of obesity-producing hypothalamic lesions (McHugh et al, 1975). These findings mean that the dramatic behavioral consequences of ventromedial or lateral hypothalamic damage can best be viewed as *syndromes*. These syndromes remain interesting problems. They must certainly be important clues as to how the long-term regulation of body weight is achieved so precisely in animals and humans; but up to this point they have not led us to a neurology of hunger and satiety.

The discovery of these syndromes has led to intensive experimentation in many areas. One of these areas is the exploitation of the chemistry of these brain regions.

Studies in rats have shown that the direct application of adrenergic agents to different regions of the hypothalamus can produce changes in food intake (Grossman, 1960; Leibowitz, 1970; Margules, 1970). The direction of these changes depends on the specific anatomical site which is stimulated. Of particular interest in relation to the problem of meal onset is the fact that norepinephrine, a known hypothalamic neurotransmitter, can elicit robust and relatively short-lived increases in food intake when it is injected in apparently small doses in the medial hypothalamus. In this area, the paraventricular nucleus is an especially sensitive site (Leibowitz, 1978). It has been suggested, but not proven, that norepinephrine stimulates feeding because it acts at this site to inhibit a function of the ventromedial hypothalamus (Hoebel, 1984). Pharmacological studies indicate that an alpha-adrenergic receptor is the mechanism for this effect (Leibowitz, 1975; Leibowitz, 1978). Whether this stimulatory effect of exogenous norepinephrine delivered to the medial hypothalamus actually reflects activation of some of the physiological mechanisms involved in initiating a normal meal remains to be answered.

In 1977, Grandison and Guidotti showed that intrahypothalamic injections of β-endorphin stimulated feeding. Shortly thereafter, Margules and his collaborators (1978) reported that genetically obese mice and rats had higher levels of brain β-endorphins and were more sensitive to the feeding inhibitory effects of opiate antagonists than were their lean littermates. These intriguing observations have stimulated many investigations in animals and humans. In animals, it has shown that enkephalins as well as $^\beta$-endorphins stimulate food intake. One endogenous opioid peptide which contains leucine enkephalin is dynorphin, and Morley and Levine (1981) have shown that dynorphin is a potent stimulant of feeding in rats when it is injected into the central nervous system. Naloxone, an opiate antagonist which may act centrally (Jones and Richter, 1981) has been shown in some studies to decrease food intake in obese subjects (Atkinson, 1982) and in patients suffering from the Prader-Willi syndrome (Kyriakides et al, 1980). These last observations raise the hope that opiate antagonists will be shown to reduce body weight in obese humans.

Learned Cues

The idea that the initiation of feeding is not adequately explained by purely internal biological cues is appealing. We all believe that we occasionally (or even frequently) eat, not because we are consciously hungry, but because external signals tell us to—"It is lunch-time." If our beliefs are true, such eating might significantly influence caloric intake over time.

Though this might seem unpromising ground for experimentation, it has been tested in an interesting way in animals. Weingarten (1983) has shown that rats can be trained to associate the brief appearance of a palatable food with light and sound stimuli. That is, they will learn to eat the proferred food when the stimuli appear. Then, in the second phase of the study, the palatable food is always present. Even though the animals keep themselves sated on the food, they will still eat more when the previously associated light and sound stimuli appear. They not only eat more, they eat a lot more—up to 20 percent of their daily food intake when the stimuli appear. Furthermore, these normal, lean rats compensate for their learned episodes of eating by consuming less at other times of the day. That is, their total daily food intake on test days remains equal to their total intake on nontest days. It will be of interest to determine whether obese animals, or those genetically predisposed to obesity, fail to compensate under similar circumstances and gain weight. At any rate, this study demonstrates that environmental cues can initiate meal-taking in the absence of metabolic deficits or physiological needs.

MEAL MAINTENANCE (REWARD)

Dopamine

It seems reasonable to assume that the rewarding properties of food must play an important role in sustaining feeding during a meal. Pleasant taste is certainly one of these rewarding properties, but other, less obvious ones may exist beyond the palate—for example, some positive post-ingestive feedback from the upper gastrointestinal tract. The brain neurotransmitter dopamine has been implicated in motivational or reinforcement processes (Wise et al, 1978; Fibiger and Phillips, 1979). Wise (1982) has suggested that the blockade of normal dopamine function (for example, by neuroleptic drugs) decreases the reward value of various stimuli, including food. In keeping with this prediction, Xenakis and Sclafani (1981) showed that the dopamine receptor antagonist pimozide, a drug with actions similar to those of haloperidol, would decrease the intake of a highly palatable sweet solution by rats, in the same way that simply diluting the solution would do. To get at the question of whether pimozide was blocking a reward produced by the sweet taste of the solution or a reward produced by a post-ingestive effect of the solution, Geary and colleagues tested the effects of pimozide on sham-feeding—that is, in a situation in which all of a palatable fluid was removed from the stomach as it was ingested by rats. The results were the same as in real feeding: Pimozide decreased intake just as dilution of the sweet solution did (Geary et al, 1983). These findings are consistent with the hypothesis that central dopaminergic synaptic activity mediates the rewarding effects of sweet taste. Once again, the question of whether these basic findings can be success-fully and safely exploited to treat syndromes such as bulimia, in which humans engage in extended binges of highly palatable foods, awaits testing.

MEAL TERMINATION (SATIETY)

Where Does Food Act to Produce Satiety?

Since we experience satiety before large amounts of food can be digested and absorbed, ingested food must produce the necessary signals at one or more sites along the surface of the upper gastrointestinal tract. In order to determine whether these powerful signals arise from oral, gastric, or intestinal sites—or from all three—simple surgical techniques have been tested in animals. When chronic cannulas or catheters are placed in the esophagus or stomach so that they can be temporarily opened during a test to allow drainage and recovery of an ingested food (sham feeding), all species overeat (Janowitz and Grossman, 1949; James, 1963; Young et al, 1974; Davis and Campbell, 1973). These observations demon-strate that food stimuli in the mouth are not sufficient to exert a normal satiety reaction. Meal termination cannot be totally controlled by past experience and the learning associated with the taste and texture of food. Furthermore, if these results, obtained in several animal species under a variety of conditions, have any relevance to human feeding, meal termination cannot be primarily controlled by the scheduling of meals enforced by social customs.

The results of this kind of behavioral testing in animals can be more dramatic and more interesting: When total recovery of an ingested liquid food is achieved in sham feeding rhesus monkeys, satiety is *absent* (see Figure 1). These results mean that the accumulation of food in the stomach and/or the entry of food into the intestine is necessary for satiety. We investigated this problem further by asking whether food infused directly into the small intestine would reduce sham feeding in rhesus monkeys. Small amounts of intestinal food produced a highly significant, dose-related suppression of sham feeding (Gibbs et al, 1981). Similar results have been obtained in rats (Liebling et al, 1975; Reidelberger et al, 1983). These findings were important on several counts. First, the potency of the small intestine in inhibiting food intake was clear. Second, intestinal food did not require the presence of gastric distention to inhibit feeding, since gastric disten-tion cannot occur when gastric cannulas are open. Third, intestinal food not only inhibited food intake, but it elicited the other behaviors normally seen in

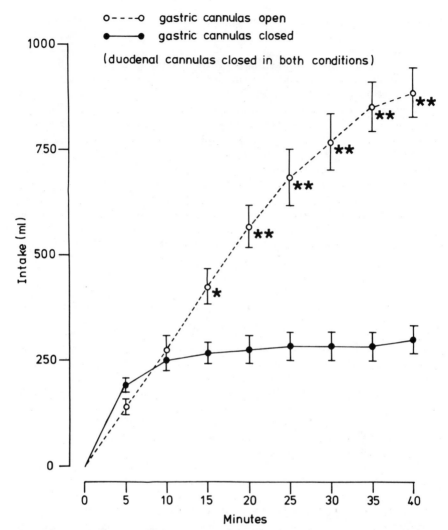

Figure 1. When no food accumulates in the stomach or small intestine, satiety disappears. The figure shows the mean cumulative liquid food intakes (in mean ± SEM milliliters) by four rhesus monkeys during tests under two different conditions: on days when gastric fistulas were closed (filled circles) and all ingested food remained within the gastrointestinal tract; and on days when gastric fistulas were open (open circles). All tests were carried out after overnight food deprivation. Under both conditions, food was smelled, tasted, and swallowed normally, but when fistulas were open, and no food remained in the gut, feeding was continuous. Liquid food was a high carbohydrate preparation with a density of 1 kcal/ml. *$p<.05$; **$p<.01$, statistical differences from results when cannulas were closed. Reprinted by permission from *Journal of Comparative and Physiological Psychology* 95:1003–1015, 1981; copyright © 1981, American Psychological Association. (See Gibbs et al, 1981, for details.)

animals when a meal ends: grooming, exploration, and apparent sleep. This was good evidence that natural satiety, not discomfort or some other artifact, had occurred.

It is of special interest to note that an early instance of human sham feeding (the result of a chronic fistula following a traumatic penetrating wound of the upper intestine) has been recorded. In this report, the victim's physician noted ". . . It is not easy to imagine the intense hunger and greed with which the patient consumed colossal amounts of food . . . without reaching the feeling of satiation . . ." (Busch, 1858). The experimental studies and the clinical case converge to indicate that the intestine (or possibly an early postabsorptive event) plays an important role in ending meals.

Is the role of the intestine a necessary component of satiety? This question has been experimentally addressed by artificially preventing the normally rapid initial emptying of ingested food from stomach into intestine. This can be achieved by using a noose device (Kraly and Smith, 1978) or an inflatable cuff (Deutsch et al, 1978) at the pylorus to inhibit gastric emptying temporarily. Whatever the technique, the results are the same: rats do not overeat when food is restricted to the stomach. They display normal satiety. Thus, the stomach, as well as the intestine, is the source of at least one satiety signal.

How Does Food Act to Produce Satiety?

It is widely thought that the abdominal vagus is the primary avenue of satiety traffic produced by food in the stomach; but we found that vagotomized rats, in which ingested food was limited to the stomach by a pyloric noose, were no different from similar sham-operated rats in the amount of food they ate at a test meal (Kraly and Gibbs, 1980). Gastric satiety did not require vagal innervation of the stomach or of the abdomen. Koopmans (1981) extended this finding. Using an inbred strain, he transplanted an extra stomach from donor rats into recipient rats. The transplanted stomach opened into the small intestine of each recipient rat, but passage of experimentally injected food into the intestine during a test could be prevented by the use of a pyloric noose. Injections of food into the transplanted stomach had a strikingly accurate satiety effect, even though the transplanted stomach had no extrinsic neural connections.

These results suggested that the gastric satiety signal might be hormonal. Since gastrin, the classic gastric peptide, had no effect on food intake even in huge doses (Lorenz et al, 1979), we turned our attention to bombesin, a recently discovered peptide. Bombesin, or a peptide closely resembling bombesin, is present in large amounts in the gastrointestinal tract, and at particularly high concentrations in the stomach. Systemic injections of bombesin produced a potent and dose-related inhibition of normal feeding (Gibbs et al, 1979; see Figure 2), a similar effect on sham feeding, and it elicited the natural behavioral sequence of satiety in rats (Martin and Gibbs, 1980). Recently bombesin was shown to reduce food intake significantly at a test meal in normal-weight human volunteers (Muurahainen et al, 1983). Obese subjects have not been tested yet.

In a parallel effort, we attempted to decipher the code for intestinal satiety. Once again, hormones appear important. Cholecystokinin (CCK) is an intestinal peptide which is released into blood in proportion to the amount of food which enters the duodenum, and which has several established gut functions. Systemic

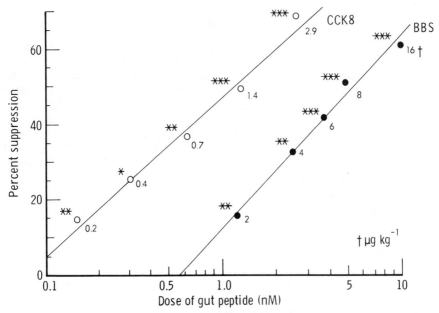

Figure 2. As doses of cholecystokinin (CCK) and bombesin (BBS) increase, the resulting suppressions of food intake increase. The figure shows the suppressions of liquid food intakes in 11 rats during the first 15 minutes after intraperitoneal injections of various doses of the synthetic C-terminal octapeptide of CCK (CCK-8, open circles) and of BBS (filled circles). Suppressions are expressed as mean percent suppressions compared with intakes on control tests (vehicle injections of 0.15 M NaCl). Numbers along regression lines indicate doses of peptide in µg/kg. Doses of the two peptides on the abscissa are arranged along a nanomolar logarithmic scale. Liquid food was 25 percent EC116 (GIBCO). Control intakes ranged from 13.7 to 20.5 ml. $*p<.05$; $**p<.01$; $***p<.001$, statistical differences from results in respective 0.15 M NaCl control tests. Correlation coefficients (Pearson product-moment): for CCK-8, $r=0.97$ ($p<.005$); for BBS, $r=0.91$ ($p<.025$). Slopes of regression lines were not significantly different ($t=.22$, $p>.05$). Reprinted by permission from *Nature* 282:208–210; copyright © 1979, MacMillan Journals Limited. (See Gibbs et al, 1979, for further details.)

injections of CCK produce potent dose-related suppressions of feeding (see Figure 2) in a wide variety of animals, including rhesus monkeys. This effect is chemically and behaviorally specific. Like food in the intestine, cholecystokinin (CCK) suppresses sham feeding in rats and rhesus monkeys. Like food in the intestine, CCK elicits a sequential display of satiety-related behaviors. (For review of the satiety actions of CCK in experimental animals, see Gibbs and Smith, 1984). Finally, in humans, the acute intravenous infusion of this peptide reduces food intake at a test meal in lean (Kissileff et al, 1981; Stacher et al, 1982) and in obese (Pi-Sunyer et al, 1982) subjects. Whether the chronic administration of CCK will reduce body weight in obese humans has not been studied, but CCK did produce weight loss in genetically obese rats (Campbell and Smith, 1983).

How Do Gut Signals Reach the Brain?

In no case is the mechanism of action for a putative satiety signal understood. It has been assumed that CCK must first act somewhere in the periphery, because it is unlikely to cross the blood-brain barrier to have a direct central effect. Consistent with this assumption, Moran and McHugh (1982) have good evidence to support their suggestion that the satiety action of CCK is indirect, depending on its well-known inhibition of gastric emptying. What is clear is that the satiety action of systemically administered exogenous CCK is critically dependent on the integrity of the abdominal vagus nerve, and specifically on its gastric branches (Smith et al, 1981). Furthermore, the vagal afferent fibers are the ones necessary for CCK's satiety function (Smith et al, 1983). The requirements are quite different for bombesin; its satiating effect is not blocked by a total abdominal vagotomy or by a high spinal cord section, but only by a combination of these two procedures (Stuckey et al, 1984).

One can see that clear distinctions between these two putative signals are emerging: They have different anatomical sites of origin, they are blocked by different neural lesions, and they must consequently have different mechanisms of action.

Two other major candidates as satiety signals are pancreatic glucagon (Stunkard et al, 1955; VanderWeele et al, 1979; Geary and Smith, 1982) and somatostatin (Lotter et al, 1981; Levine and Morley, 1982). These substances are also gastrointestinal peptides released by ingested food, and they each show interesting similarities to, and differences from, CCK and bombesin.

These characteristics are displayed in Table 1. They show that the differences between these signals are quite distinct. The comparisons strongly suggest that the seeming unitary state we experience regularly after meals may actually be the complex summation of a mosaic of neuroendocrine messages, each responding to different features of ingested food, each with a different mediating mechanism which allows privileged entry into brain tissue, and each interacting in intricate ways with other members of the group. Further research will determine whether this suggestion has merit. Further research will no doubt reveal other candidate signals and should also tell us whether a functional excess or deficit of one of these peptide messages plays a role in the psychopathology of anorexia nervosa, bulimia, or obesity.

CONCLUSION

This chapter has concentrated almost exclusively on basic studies dealing with the individual meal. The power of research adopting this focus (rather than one based on energy balance or body weight regulation) is that it concentrates attention around the only identified stimulus we know—food. Ingested food produces rapid and dramatic changes in behavior. Many of the biological studies we have reviewed used this close temporal association to advantage, asking how the information released by food cascades from gut to brain.

Are there suggestions here for clinical research? We believe there are. The measurement of hormonal and neuroendocrine responses to ingested food in the eating disorders are obvious possibilities. But food also produces rapid and dramatic changes in *experience*. It is likely that patients suffering from anorexia nervosa, bulimia, and obesity have important and interesting pathology to report concerning their subjective reactions to ingested food. Unfortunately, there are

Table 1. Characteristics of four putative satiety signals

Peptide	Inhibition of Feeding	Inhibition of Sham Feeding	Means of Blockade	Interaction With	Effect in Human
Cholecystokinin (CCK)	Yes	Yes	Gastric vagotomy	• Pregastric food • Gastric load • Exogenous BBS	Yes
Bombesin (BBS)	Yes	Yes	Visceral disconnection	Exogenous CCK	Yes
Pancreatic glucagon	Yes	No	• Hepatic vagotomy • Glucagon antibody	—	Yes
Somatostatin	Yes	—	Subdiaphragmatic vagotomy	—	—

Dashes indicate no study has been published.

few studies in which these patients have been interviewed in this regard (Garfinkel, 1974).

What does food do? The biological, behavioral, and experiential answers to this question will surely provide insights into the clinical disorders of eating and body weight.

REFERENCES

Anand BK, Brobeck JR: Hypothalamic control of food intake. Yale J Biol Med 24:123–140, 1951

Atkinson RL: Naloxone decreases food intake in obese humans. J Clin Endocrinol Metab 55:196–198, 1982

Brobeck JR, Tepperman J, Long CNH: Experimental hypothalamic hyperphagia in the albino rat. Yale J Biol Med 15:831–853, 1943

Busch W: Contribution to the physiology of the digestive organs. Archiv für Pathologische Anatomie und Physiologie und für Klinische Medizin 14:140–186, 1858

Campbell RG, Smith GP: CCK-8 decreases body weight in Zucker rats. Society for Neurosciences Abstracts 9:902, 1983

Cannon WB, Washburn AL: An explanation of hunger. Am J Physiol 29:441–454, 1912

Carlson AJ: Contributions to the physiology of the stomach. II. The relation between the contractions of the empty stomach and the sensation of hunger. Am J Physiol 31:175–192, 1913

Davis JD, Campbell CS: Peripheral control of meal size in the rat: Effect of sham feeding on meal size and drinking rate. J Comp Physiol Psychol 83:379–387, 1973

Deutsch JA, Young WG, Kalogeris TJ: The stomach signals satiety. Science 201:165–167, 1978

Fibiger HC, Phillips AG: Dopamine and the neural mechanisms of reinforcement, in The Neurobiology of Dopamine. Edited by Horn AS, Korf J, Westerink BHC. London, Academic Press, 1979

Garfinkel PE: Perception of hunger and satiety in anorexia nervosa. Psychol Med 4:309–315, 1974

Geary N, Smith GP: Pancreatic glucagon and postprandial satiety in the rat. Physiol Behav 28:313–322,1982

Geary N, Lange D, Smith GP: Pimozide decreases sham feeding of sucrose as an inverse function of sucrose concentration. Proceedings of the Eastern Psychological Association 54:94, 1983

Gibbs J, Fauser DJ, Rowe EA, et al: Bombesin suppresses feeding in rats. Nature 282:208–210, 1979

Gibbs J, Maddison SP, Rolls ET: Satiety role of the small intestine examined in sham-feeding rhesus monkeys. J Comp Physiol Psychol 95:1003–1015, 1981

Gibbs J, Smith GP: The neuroendocrinology of postprandial satiety, in Frontiers in Neuroendocrinology. Edited by Martini L, Ganong WF. New York, Raven Press, 1984

Grandison L, Guidotti A: Stimulation of food intake by muscimol and beta-endorphin. Neuropharmacology 16:533–536, 1977

Grossman SP: Eating or drinking elicited by direct adrenergic or cholinergic stimulation of hypothalamic mechanisms. Science 132:301–302, 1960

Hetherington AW, Ranson SW: Experimental hypothalamo-hypophyseal obesity in the rat. Proc Soc Exper Biol Med 41:465–466, 1939

Hoebel BG: Neurotransmitters in the control of feeding and its rewards: monamines, opiates, and brain-gut peptides, in Eating and Its Disorders (Association for Research in Nervous and Mental Disease) vol 62. Edited by Stunkard AJ, Stellar E. New York, Raven Press, 1984

Inglefinger FJ: The late effects of total and subtotal gastrectomy. New Engl J Med 231:321–327, 1944

James WT: An analysis of esophageal feeding as a form of operant reinforcement in the dog. Psychol Rep 12:31–39, 1963

Janowitz HD, Grossman MI: Some factors affecting the food intake of normal dogs and dogs with esophagostomy and gastric fistula. Am J Physiol 159:143–148, 1949

Jones JG, Richter JA: The site of action of naloxone in suppressing food and water intake in rats. Life Sci 28:2055–2064, 1981

Kissileff HR, Pi-Sunyer FX, Thornton J, Smith GP: Cholecystokinin-octapeptide (CCK-8) decreases food intake in man. Am J Clin Nutr 34:154–160, 1981

Koopmans HS: The role of the gastrointestinal tract in the satiation of hunger, in The Body Weight Regulatory System: Normal and Disturbed Mechanisms. Edited by Cioffi LA, James WPT, van Itallie TB. New York, Raven Press, 1981

Kraly FS, Gibbs J: Vagotomy fails to block the satiating effect of food in the stomach. Physiol Behav 24:1007–1010, 1980

Kraly FS, Smith GP: Combined pregastric and gastric stimulation by food is sufficient for normal meal size. Physiol Behav 21:405–408, 1978

Kyriakides M, Silverstone T, Jeffcoate W, et al: Effect of naloxone on hyperphagia in Prader-Willi syndrome. Lancet I:876–877, 1980

Leibowitz, SF: Hypothalamic β-adrenergic "satiety" system antagonizes an L-adrenergic "hunger" system in the rat. Nature (Lond) 226:963–964, 1970

Leibowitz SF: Ingestion in the satiated rat: Role of alpha and beta receptors in mediating effects of hypothalamic adrenergic stimulation. Physiol Behav 14:743–754, 1975

Leibowitz SF: Paraventricular nucleus: A primary site mediating adrenergic stimulation of feeding and drinking. Pharmacol Biochem Behav 8:163–175, 1978

LeMagnen J: The body energy regulation: the role of three brain responses to glucopenia. Neurosci Biobehav Rev 4:Suppl 1, 65–72, 1980

Levine AS, Morley JE: Peripherally administered somatostatin reduces feeding by a vagally mediated mechanism. Pharmacol Biochem Behav 16:897–902, 1982

Liebling DS, Eisner JD, Gibbs J, et al: Intestinal satiety in rats. J Comp Physiol Psychol 89:955–965, 1975

Lorenz DN, Kreielsheimer G, Smith GP: Effect of cholecystokinin, gastrin, secretin and GIP on sham feeding in the rat. Physiol Behav 23:1065–1072, 1979

Lotter EC, Krinsky R, McKay JM, et al: Somatostatin decreases food intake of rats and baboons. J Comp Physiol Psychol 95:278–287, 1981

Lytle LD: Control of eating behavior, in Nutrition and the Brain, Vol 2. Edited by Wurtman RJ, Wurtman JJ. New York, Raven Press, 1977

Margules DL: Alpha-adrenergic receptors in hypothalamus for the suppression of feeding behavior by satiety. J Comp Physiol Psychol 73:1–12, 1970

Margules DL, Moisset B, Lewis M, et al: Beta-endorphin is associated with overeating in genetically obese mice (ob/ob) and rats (fa/fa). Science 202:988–991, 1978

Mayer J: Glucostatic mechanisms in regulation of food intake. New Engl J Med 249:13–16, 1953

Martin CF, Gibbs J: Bombesin elicits satiety in sham feeding rats. Peptides 1:131–134, 1980

McHugh PR, Gibbs J, Falasco JD, et al: Inhibitions on feeding examined in rhesus monkeys with hypothalamic disconnexions. Brain 98:441–454, 1975

Moran TH, McHugh PR: Cholecystokinin suppresses food intake by inhibiting gastric emptying. Am J Physiol 242:R491–R497, 1982

Morley JE, Levine AS: Dynorphin-(1-13) induces spontaneous feeding in rats. Life Sci 29:1901–1903, 1981

Muurahainen NE, Kissileff HR, Thornton J, et al: Bombesin: another peptide that inhibits feeding in man. Society for Neuroscience Abstracts 9:183, 1983

Palkovits M, Kiss JZ, Beinfeld MC, et al: Cholecystokinin in the nucleus of the solitary tract of the rat. Brain Res 252:386–390, 1982

Pi-Sunyer X, Kissileff HR, Thornton J, et al: C-terminal octapeptide of cholecystokinin decreases food intake in obese men. Physiol Behav 29:627–630, 1982

Reeves AG, Plum F: Hyperphagia, rage, and dementia accompanying a ventromedial hypothalamic neoplasm. Arch Neurol 20:616-624, 1969

Reidelberger RD, Kalogeris TJ, Leung PMB, et al: Postgastric satiety in the sham-feeding rat. Am J Physiol 244:R872–R881, 1983

Richter C: A behavioristic study of the activity of the rat. Comparative Psychology Monographs 1: No 2, 1922

Silverstone JT, Besser M: Insulin, blood sugar and hunger. Postgrad Med J 47:427–429, 1971

Smith GP: The physiology of the meal, in Drugs and Appetite, Edited by Silverstone T. New York, Academic Press, 1982

Smith GP, Gibbs, Strohmayer AJ, et al: Threshold does of 2-deoxy-D-glucose for hypoglycemia and feeding in rats and monkeys. Am J Physiol 222:77-81, 1972

Smith GP, Jerome C, Cushin BJ, et al: Abdominal vagotomy blocks the satiety effect of cholecystokinin in the rat. Science 213:1036–1037, 1981

Smith GP, Jerome C, Norgren R: Vagal afferent axons mediate the satiety effect of CCK-8. Society for Neuroscience Abstr 9:902, 1983

Stacher G, Steinringer H, Schmierer G, et al: Cholecystokinin octapeptide decreases intake of solid food in man. Peptides 3:133–136, 1982

Strubbe JM, Steffens AB. Blood glucose levels in portal and peripheral circulation and their relation to food intake in the rat. Physiol Behav 19:303-307, 1977

Stuckey J, Gibbs J, Smith GP: Neural disconnection of the gastrointestinal tract from the brain blocks the effect of bombesin on meal size but not intermeal interval. Proceedings of the Eastern Psychological Association 55:88, 1984

Stunkard AJ, Fox S: The relationship of gastric motility and hunger. Psychosom Med 33:123-134, 1971

Stunkard AJ, Van Itallie ITB, Reis BB: The mechanism of satiety: effect of glucagon on gastric hunger contractions in man. Proc Soc Exper Biol Med 89:258, 1955

Thompson DA, Campbell RG: Hunger in man induced by 2-deoxy-D-glucose: glucoprivic control of taste preference and food intake. Science 198:1065–1068, 1977

VanderWeele DA, Geiselman PJ, Novin D: Pancreatic glucagon, food deprivation and feeding in intact and vagotomized rabbits. Physiol Behav 23:155–158, 1979

Weingarten HP: Conditioned cues elicit feeding in sated rats: A role for learning in meal initiation. Science 220:431–433, 1983

Wise RA: Neuroleptics and operant behavior: The anhedonia hypothesis. Behavioral and Brain Sciences 5:39–87, 1982

Wise RA, Spindler J, deWit H, Gerber GJ: Neuroleptic-induced "anhedonia" in rats: pimozide blocks reward quality of food. Science 201:262–264, 1978

Xenakis S, Sclafani A: The effects of pimozide on the consumption of a palatable saccharin-glucose solution in the rat. Pharmacol Biochem Behav 15:435–442, 1981

Young RC, Gibbs J, Antin J, et al: Absence of satiety during sham feeding in the rat. J Comp Physiol Psychol 87:795–800, 1974

Zarbin MA, Wamsley JK, Innis RB, et al: Cholecystokinin receptors: presence and axonal flow in the rat vagus nerve. Life Sci 29:697–705, 1981

Chapter 22

Obesity

by Albert J. Stunkard, M.D.

HISTORICAL BACKGROUND

Obesity has long been a topic of interest to psychiatrists, and the relationship between emotions and obesity has occupied a prominent place in the psychiatric literature. Our understanding of this relationship, however, has changed dramatically.

Forty years ago the crusading zeal of the psychoanalytic movement claimed a large part of obesity for the domain of the mind. While conceding the existence of occasional "organic" types of the disorder, analytic theorists found in obesity the very model of a pregenital conversion. Overeating was the logical manifestation of the orality which they saw as the defining characteristic of obese persons. An apparently irrefutable formula became popular: Obesity arises as a result of food intake in excess of that required for physiological needs. If the needs are not physiological, they can only be psychological. And a psychological need that leads to such maladaptive consequences is precisely what is meant by neurosis. The cause of obesity seemed clear—psychogenesis. Psychopathology caused obesity.

Forty years later this formulation has been turned on its head. No longer is psychopathology viewed as a cause of obesity. Instead, it is seen as a consequence of obesity, either directly (via societal discrimination against obese people) or indirectly (from the dieting that is a response to this discrimination).

Today we are far more modest about our understanding of the causes of obesity. We know more and claim less. The old psychologic/organic dichotomy has broken down and the search for *the* cause of obesity has been abandoned. Psychologic and organic elements are present in every case of obesity. Extensive animal experimentation suggests that obesity is a multiply determined disorder with a number of different clinical manifestations. Genetic predisposition must surely interact with early feeding opportunities; and the ready availability of highly palatable food must surely interact with labor-saving devices to influence everyone in an affluent society.

Today we also view the goals of treatment in a more modest way. In the old days, we didn't fool around: The goal was to *cure* obesity. You were supposed to resolve the underlying neurosis so that the fat went away and never came back. It was clearly a difficult task and it was not apparent that anyone had ever actually accomplished it. But it was an inspiring adventure, particularly when compared to today's modest goal of helping obese people to adhere to weight reducing regimens.

What have been the effects on the clinician of this reassessment of the relationship between emotions and obesity? Has it shrunk the domain of treatment to the purely mechanical and pharmacologic? The answer, surprisingly, is "no."

Psychological factors seem as important in the treatment of obesity as they ever were. Lowering our sights has not lessened the importance of these factors; we now take a more accurate aim at the target. Let us define this target.

DEFINITION

Obesity is a condition characterized by excessive accumulation of fat in the body. Unlike many "real" diseases (and like hypertension) obesity represents one arm of a distribution curve with no sharp cut-off point. As a result, the conventional criterion is as reasonable as any: a body weight that exceeds by 20 percent the standard weight listed in the usual height/weight tables. This measure of obesity is only an approximate one at lesser degrees of overweight, but a more precise definition is not particularly useful. For most clinical purposes the eyeball test is perfectly adequate: If a person looks fat, he is fat.

EPIDEMIOLOGY

The prevalence of obesity is usually stated to be 35 percent of the male and 40 percent of the female population, but the criterion used to determine these figures is rarely given. More valid figures have been reported in 1983 by the National Center for Health Statistics, which utilized two criteria—"overweight" relative to an ideal weight and "obesity" as determined by skinfold thickness (Abraham, 1983). Relative to ideal weight, 23 percent of men and 30 percent of women were classified as overweight, while 19 percent of men and 28 percent of women were classified as obese.

Three demographic factors are closely associated with obesity and, in fact, help to determine it. The first is gender: Obesity is far more common among women than among men (Abraham, 1983).

The second major influence on obesity is age. There is a steady increase in the prevalence of obesity from childhood to age 50, with a two- to three-fold increase between the ages of 20 and 64.

The third major influence on obesity is social factors. Social factors determine the prevalence of obesity in both affluent and developing societies, but the direction of the influence differs markedly. In developing societies only the upper classes can afford enough food to become obese, and only they are obese. In affluent societies, the distribution of obesity by social class is reversed. Persons of lower socioeconomic status can afford to become obese and they do. For reasons that are not at all apparent, the upper classes can afford to become obese, but they do not. In fact, among women, the higher the social class, the greater the prevalence of thinness, a finding surely bearing upon the higher prevalence of anorexia nervosa among upper class women.

A striking example of the influence of social factors on the prevalence of obesity is illustrated in Figure 1, which shows that obesity is six times more common among women of lower socioeconomic status than among those of high status (Goldblatt et al, 1965). Furthermore, this relationship is far more than a simple association: it is a causal one. Socioeconomic status of origin was linked to the prevalence of obesity almost as strongly as was the subject's own social class. Although obesity may influence one's own social class, it can hardly

Obesity by socioeconomic status (women)

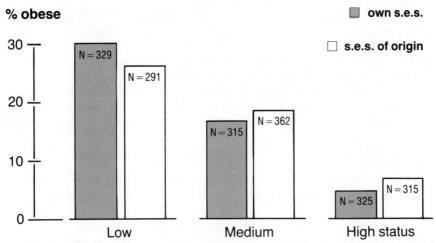

Figure 1. Decreasing prevalence of obesity with increasing socioeconomic status (S.E.S.) among women in a large American city. Socioeconomic status of origin is almost as strongly linked to obesity as is the person's own socioeconomic status. From "Social Factors in Obesity," by P.B. Goldblatt et al, JAMA 192: 1039, 1965. Copyright © 1965 by the American Medical Association. Reprinted by permission of the American Medical Association.

have influenced the social class of one's parents. The social class must have influenced the obesity!

CLINICAL CHARACTERISTICS

Physical Problems

Controversy has been aroused in recent years by suggestions that the ill effects of milder degrees of obesity have been overestimated. The life expectancy of persons who are as much as 25 percent overweight may well be as great or greater than that of thinner persons (Andres, 1980). However this controversy is eventually resolved, there is no debate about the ill effects of greater degrees of obesity. As one example, young men who are 100 percent overweight have 10 times the mortality rate of their nonobese peers (Drenick, 1980). Furthermore, even milder degrees of obesity often precipitate latent tendencies toward hypertension, diabetes, and hyperlipidemias. All three disorders are problems in their own right, and they make a major contribution to cardiovascular disease, the cause of more than half of the deaths in this country. Fortunately, the ill effects of obesity are reversed by weight reduction, which adds a sound medical argument to the usual cosmetic reasons for the treatment of obesity.

Emotional Problems

The old view that obese persons have a specific personality profile is no longer held, and population studies of obese people show that they differ little, if at all, from nonobese people in overall levels of psychopathology (Stunkard, 1976). Certain subgroups of obese persons, however, are at high risk for emotional disturbance. Young, upper class women head the list.

Three types of emotional disturbance seem specific to obesity—overeating, the complications of dieting, and disparagement of the body image.Obesity is evidence of overeating in the sense that, at some time in the person's past, he consumed more calories than he expended. It is not, however, evidence that he is doing so at the present time or even that he consumed more calories than a nonobese peer in the past. Paradoxical as it may seem, there is little evidence that most obese people overeat. But a few do and their overeating is closely linked to emotional problems. Bulimia and night-eating are the clinical manifestations.

OVEREATING. The first form of overeating, bulimia, when it occurs among obese persons, is much like that which occurs among nonobese persons and anorexics, with one significant exception: Most obese bulimics do not vomit after binging. As a result, they do not obtain the relief that often accompanies vomiting, and the burden of an unwanted food intake is added to the depressed mood and self-deprecatory thoughts that regularly follow an eating binge. Obese bulimic persons (as well as bulimics of milder degrees of overweight) sometimes lose large amounts of weight by radically restrictive diets, but such efforts are almost always interrupted by a resumption of eating binges. Indeed, dieting may play a role in bulimia among obese persons as well as among those of normal weight. About five percent of obese persons may be bulimic.

Another form of overeating is the night-eating syndrome, characterized by morning anorexia, evening hyperphagia, and insomnia (Stunkard, 1976). The syndrome, which afflicts primarily women, appears to be precipitated by stressful life circumstances and may represent a form of depression. Attempts at weight reduction in persons suffering from night-eating appear to have a poor outcome and may even precipitate more severe psychological disturbance. About ten percent of obese persons may be night eaters.

COMPLICATIONS OF DIETING. The second form of emotional disturbance specific to obese persons is the complications of dieting. As many as half of all patients treated for obesity by family physicians experience mild anxiety and depression (Stunkard and Rush, 1974). Such emotional disturbances may arise from precisely the same mechanism as in the case of a normal-weight person who tries to lose weight—starvation. If this is the case, it would be their proneness to dieting, not their proneness to emotional disturbance, that would distinguish emotionally disturbed persons. This interpretation finds support in the view, discussed below, that obese persons may have an elevated body weight set point. Reducing below this set point may leave them biologically underweight even while they remain statistically overweight.

DISPARAGEMENT OF THE BODY IMAGE. The third form of emotional disturbance specific to obese persons is a disparagement of the body image (Stunkard and Mendelson, 1967). Obese persons with this disturbance characteristically feel that their bodies are grotesque and loathesome and that others view them with hostility and contempt. This feeling is closely associated with self-consciousness and impaired social functioning. One might suppose that all obese persons have derogatory feelings about their bodies, but such is not the case. Emotionally healthy obese persons have no body image disturbances; in fact, only a minority of neurotic obese persons have such disturbances. The disorder is confined to those who have been obese since childhood; even among these juvenile-onset obese persons, fewer than half suffer from it. In the group with body image disparagement, however, neurosis is closely related to obesity, and this group contains a majority of obese persons with bulimia and night-eating.

ETIOLOGY AND PATHOGENESIS

The Regulation of Body Weight

In one sense the cause of obesity is quite simple: Fat accumulates when more calories are consumed as food than are expended as energy. In another sense, the answer is elusive, hidden in the mystery of the regulation of body weight.

The idea that body weight is regulated has achieved rapid acceptance (Keesey, 1984). Part of this acceptance springs from the strong evidence for regulation of body weight among experimental animals. Not only animals of normal weight, but also obese animals, maintain a remarkably constant weight even in the face of severe challenges. The reason for their obesity is that there is an elevation of the level, or set point, about which their body weight is regulated.

Humans of normal weight, as well as animals, seem to be able to regulate their body weight with considerable accuracy. Lifetime weight histories of *obese* persons, however, suggest that they do not. Here is a curious phenomenon: Obese people seem to be the only mammals that fail to regulate their body weight! One explanation of this failure may be that it is only an apparent failure. Obese people may well have the capacity to regulate their body weight. The set point about which their weight would be regulated if subject only to biological pressures, however, is higher than that approved by society. As a result of this societal pressure, obese people diet and reduce their weight below what is biologically normal for them. The consequence is the paradox noted above, of a person who is at the same time biologically underweight (starved) while remaining statistically overweight (Nisbett, 1972).

Two types of evidence support this theory. First, dieters (whether obese or not) share certain psychological characteristics that distinguish them from people who are not dieting. These characteristics may well derive from a body weight that is below set point (Nisbett, 1972). Second, the demonstration of elevated numbers of fat cells among some obese persons provides a plausible mechanism for an elevated set point (Sjostrom, 1980).

If body weight is indeed regulated, this fact has profound implications for the treatment of obesity. The clinician already knows how difficult it is for patients to lose weight and to maintain their weight losses. The regulation of body weight provides an explanation for this difficulty, for it means that efforts to lose weight are opposed by powerful biological systems, and the treatment of obesity may mean that the physician must help patients to exercise cognitive controls over biological systems. For some patients, it may mean learning to live in a semi-starved manner.

Determinants of Obesity

There are at least five determinants of obesity. Social determinants have been discussed under "Epidemiology," and emotional determinants under "Clinical Characteristics." The other three are heredity, development, and physical inactivity.

GENETIC DETERMINANTS. There is evidence that human obesity "runs in families." Eighty percent of the offspring of two obese parents are obese, compared to 40 percent of the offspring of one obese parent, and only ten percent of the offspring of lean parents. However, because most humans obtain their genes and their eating patterns from the same people, family studies cannot disentangle the respective contributions of heredity and environment. Twin studies and a recent adoption study, however, suggest that there is a large genetic component to human obesity (Foch and McClearn, 1980).

DEVELOPMENTAL DETERMINANTS. Some obese persons have an increased number of fat cells—so-called "hyperplastic obesity." Others have an increase in the size of their fat cells—"hypertrophic obesity." A large number of obese persons, and most severely obese ones, have an increase in both number *and* size—"hyperplastic-hypertrophic obesity." Whereas the size of fat cells can be increased at any time in life, the number of fat cells appears to be determined early, perhaps through an interaction between genetic predisposition and overfeeding (Sjostrom, 1980). Once formed, fat cells persist indefinitely. Consequently, when obese persons lose weight, it is solely by a decrease in the size of their fat cells. The number of their fat cells does not change. Such persons can thus reduce to a statistically normal body weight only by reducing the lipid content of their individual fat cells to abnormally low levels. It seems quite likely that these circumstances are signalled to the central regulatory processes, initiating the powerful counter-regulation designed to restore body weight to its usual level. These special characteristics of adipose tissue thus provide a cellular locus for the elevated set point that may play such an important part in obesity.

PHYSICAL ACTIVITY. Obesity is a rarity in most underdeveloped nations, and not solely because of malnutrition. In some areas, high levels of physical activity are also important in preventing obesity. The marked decrease in physical activity in affluent societies must surely contribute to the recent increase in the prevalence of obesity.

Experiments with genetically obese animals shed further light on the role of physical inactivity in promoting obesity, and the role of activity in controlling it (Stern, 1984). When the tendency towards obesity is strong, as in the obese hyperglycemic mouse (*ob/ob*), the obese Zucker rat (*fa/fa*), and animals with large lesions in the ventromedial hypothalamus, exercise can lessen, although it cannot prevent, the development of obesity. When the tendency towards obesity is weaker, as in the yellow obese mouse (*Ay/a*) and in animals with small lesions in the ventromedial hypothalamus, exercise can often actually prevent the development of obesity.

Physical activity controls obesity by three mechanisms (Stern, 1984). First, physical activity increases caloric expenditure. Although the caloric expenditure produced by most forms of activity is small, the cumulative effects of continued activity are not negligible. Second, physical activity may actually *decrease* food intake among sedentary persons. Third, physical activity may affect obesity by increasing metabolic rate. One of the major effects of caloric restriction is a fall in basal metabolic rate. Physical activity can prevent or lessen this fall in metabolic rate, thereby obviating a major problem of dieting.

TREATMENT

Classification of Obesity

The treatment of obesity by weight reduction should be simple; it involves nothing more than the establishment of an energy deficit by reducing caloric intake below caloric output. All of the many treatments of obesity share this common goal. How they pursue it, however, varies greatly. Perhaps the large number of women who try to reduce without medical assistance, with the help of diets and advice from the women's magazines, are reasonably successful. But most persons who come to the doctor's office find obesity to be a remarkably stubborn condition, resistant to treatment and prone to relapse.

In medicine, treatment ideally follows diagnosis, which specifies the precise form that the treatment should take. Although it is generally believed that obesity is not a single entity, but a multiply determined disorder, there is no system of diagnosis or classification based upon etiology and pathogenesis. Recently, however, a classification of obesity based simply on the severity of the disorder has proven surprisingly useful in specifying the nature of the treatment (Garrow, 1982; Stunkard, 1984). The classification is a simple three-fold one, of mild, moderate, and severe obesity, characterized by body weights that are, respectively, 20 to 40 percent overweight, 41 to 100 percent overweight, and more than 100 percent overweight. Table 1 shows that the percentage of obese women falling into these three categories is, respectively, 90.5 percent, nine percent and 0.5 percent (Abraham, 1983). It should be emphasized that these are percentages of the *female obese* population, not of the total population. Data for men are similar.

Table 1 shows the nature of the treatment that is indicated for each of the three categories of obesity. Severe obesity is most effectively treated by surgical measures. Moderate obesity is probably best treated by diet and behavior modification under medical auspices. For mild obesity, diet and behavior modification under lay auspices are indicated.

Severe Obesity

The prevalence of severe obesity is no more than 0.5 percent of the *obese* population. This percentage, however, means that more than 200,000 persons in the United States suffer from severe obesity and psychiatrists will encounter them in practice. It is, accordingly, important for them to recognize that the condition is both dangerous and potentially treatable. Severe obesity is the one form of obesity which presents medical complications in almost every person who suffers from it. Many of these complications are reversed and even abolished by weight reduction; and weight reduction has become a reasonable possibility in recent years through the development of new surgical techniques (Mason, 1981).

The first widely used surgical treatment of obesity, intestinal bypass, has been

Table 1. Classification and Treatment of Obesity

Type	Mild	Moderate	Severe
Percentage overweight	20–40 percent	41–100 percent	> 100 percent
Prevalence (among obese women)	90.5 percent	9.0 percent	0.5 percent
Pathology	Hypertrophic	Hypertrophic, hyperplastic	Hypertrophic, hyperplastic
Complications	Uncertain	Conditional	Severe
Treatment	Behavior therapy (lay)	Diet and behavior therapy (medical)	Surgical

From "The Current Status of Treatment for Obesity in Adults," in Eating and Its Disorders. Edited by A. J. Stunkard and E. Stellar. Copyright © 1984 by Raven Press. Reprinted by permission of Raven Press.

supplanted by gastric restriction procedures designed to radically reduce the volume of the stomach to as little as 50 ml, and the passageway from this restricted stomach to no more than 1.2 cm in diameter. These operations are associated with the usual complications of major surgery, and are not to be performed casually or solely for cosmetic purposes. Nevertheless, for appropriately selected patients, they may provide major health benefits. Weight losses of 40 to 60 kg (about 90 to 130 pounds) are achieved in the course of two years with relatively little difficulty, and they tend to be well maintained. Health benefits include marked alleviation of hypertension, diabetes, hyperlipidemia, and, in fact, all of the complications attributable to severe obesity.

The benefits to physical health resulting from surgical treatment of severe obesity are paralleled by the benefits to mental health. These benefits were first described by Solow et al (1974) in their report on the benign social and emotional course of many severely obese persons following the now-discontinued intestinal bypass surgery. This landmark report noted improvement in mood, self-esteem, interpersonal and vocational effectiveness, body image, and level of physical activity. Almost all subsequent accounts agree on this benign emotional course, irrespective of the type of surgery. The early studies, however, underestimated the benefits of this surgery, for in assessing the emotional sequelae of surgery, they used an inappropriate control period—the time just before the surgery. The appropriate control period is previous times when the patient was losing weight by non-surgical treatments and, as we have noted above, such times are often marked by complications of dieting. The more severe the obesity, the more severe the complications. In one study of severely obese persons, 15 percent reported severe depressive reactions during dieting and another 26 percent reported moderately severe depression (Halmi et al, 1980). Only a minority had not experienced some degree of depression and even fewer reported no anxiety, irritability, or preoccupation with food.

The emotional response of these same patients to gastric bypass surgery was far more benign, even though they lost far more weight. Half of them reported "much less" dysphoric mood following bypass surgery, and another five to 15 percent reported "less" dysphoria. The benefits of gastric bypass surgery extended also to an increase in positive emotions. Half of the patients reported "much more" elation and self confidence and 75 percent reported "much more" feelings of well-being (Halmi et al, 1980).

Surgery also improved the body image disparagement which had afflicted 70 percent of the patients. After surgery, no more than four percent reported severe disparagement and nearly half were symptom-free. This result is particularly striking since it occurred before the patients had lost more than a small amount of weight, and when they still appeared to others as grossly obese.

A striking change in another form of behavior following gastric bypass surgery affected a patient's food likes and dislikes (Halmi et al, 1981). Fifty percent of the patients reported that high density fats and high density carbohydrates were no longer enjoyable, and smaller percentages also reported a lack of enjoyment of breads, high fat meats, high calorie beverages, eggs, cheese and peanut butter. Not only did the patients develop a dislike of these foods, but they also ate less of them.

Improvement in eating habits had been found earlier in the now-discontinued intestinal surgery (Bray et al, 1980; Mills and Stunkard, 1976). Most patients reported chaotic patterns of excessive food intake before surgery. After surgery, there was a marked decrease in binge-eating, night-eating, excessive snacking and difficulty in stopping eating. One finding of this study was particularly interesting. Before surgery, a very large percentage of these severely obese patients—as is true of such persons—ate no breakfast. Following surgery, and even while they were rapidly losing weight, these patients began to eat breakfast!

These changes in eating patterns were not only extensive but they occurred without voluntary effort on the part of the patients. Clearly this surgery must do far more than simply alter the functioning of the gastrointestinal tract; it must produce major changes in the biology of the organism. A parsimonious explanation of these changes is that surgery lowers the set point about which body weight is regulated (Halmi et al, 1980). Such an explanation helps to explain the infrequency of dysphoric reactions to weight loss, the normalization of eating patterns, and the minimal effort that suffices to ensure weight loss. With a lowered body weight set point, patients need no longer struggle against biological pressures to support a higher weight and can easily limit their food intake until a new, lower set point is reached.

Moderate Obesity

Moderate obesity, from 40 to 100 percent overweight, afflicts about nine percent of the obese population. The adipose tissue of these persons is usually of the hypertrophic type and may be, in addition, hyperplastic. Complications depend upon the presence of conditions which can be precipitated or aggravated by obesity—hypertension, diabetes, etc.

Paradoxically, treatment of moderate obesity is probably less successful than that of either severe or mild obesity, and the most effective type of treatment is still a matter of debate. Basically, treatment is of two types—diet and behavior modification. Both are best conducted under medical auspices.

DIET.   The primary goal of dietary treatment of moderate obesity is the most rapid weight loss that the patient can tolerate with safety and comfort. Fasting produces rapid weight losses but is limited in safety and comfort. The more conventional diets are both safe and comfortable, but they produce such slow weight loss that they are not really practical for persons who are 30 to 50 kg (66 to 100 pounds) overweight. The "very-low-calorie diet" (Wadden et al, 1983) is a promising compromise between these extremes.

Also called the "protein-sparing-modified fast," this diet provides from 400 to 700 calories, largely or exclusively protein, in the form of either formula or natural foods such as fish, fowl or lean meat. They appear to be safe when administered under careful medical supervision for periods of up to three months. And weight losses achieved by these diets are striking. Patients lose 1.5 to 2.3 kg (3.3 to 5.1 pounds) a week, the extent of weight loss depending upon the initial amount of excess weight.

The big question in all dietary treatment of obesity is how well the weight losses are maintained. Unfortunately, extensive experience with these diets makes it clear that weight losses are poorly maintained (Wadden et al, 1983).

BEHAVIOR MODIFICATION.   The second type of treatment of moderate obesity is behavior modification (Stuart, 1978). The starting point for the behavioral treatment of obesity is an applied behavioral analysis that considers in great detail the *behavior* to be changed, its *antecedents* and its *consequences*. The primary *behavior* to be changed is eating, and a number of exercises are designed to slow the rate of eating and allow the physiological mechanisms of satiety to exert their effect. An even greater focus is placed upon the *antecedents* of eating behavior. Efforts extend from the control of relatively remote antecedents, such as shopping for food, to more proximate ones, such as the ready availability of high calorie food. Patients are helped to remove from their environments any stimuli that might elicit eating, to plan strategies to control eating when such stimuli are present, and to avoid television and reading materials that might distract their attention from efforts at stimulus control. The third element in applied behavioral analysis is the *consequences* of behavior, with rewards for carrying out the various prescribed behaviors, primarily those involving stimulus control.

In addition to this basic behavioral analysis, behavioral treatment of obesity includes four other elements:

Self-monitoring, or the recording in exquisite detail of a large number of the behaviors to be modified. This kind of careful record-keeping makes it possible to determine which aspects of behavior should be modified, to develop programs to modify them, to monitor the effectiveness of these programs, and to use this information to make necessary corrections.

Nutrition education. It is not possible to make sensible choices among foods without a clear idea of their nutritional value, and simple didactic exercises comprise an important part of behavioral programs.

A program to increase physical activity is a key element of behavioral programs, for the various reasons noted above.

Cognitive restructuring, to overcome the self-defeating and maladaptive attitudes of so many obese persons towards weight reduction and towards themselves.

A major strength of behavioral treatment of obesity is that the weight losses that it produces tend to be relatively well maintained. The weakness of the treatment is that these losses tend to be small and often of no clinical significance. Traditional behavioral treatments usually produce weight losses of no more than 4.5 kg (10 pounds) (Wing and Jeffrey, 1979). Although a recent, more aggressive behavioral treatment achieved losses of 10.9 kg (24 pounds) (Craighead et al, 1981), even this achievement is too limited for persons who are 30 to 50 kg (66 to 110 pounds) overweight.

At the present time the treatment of moderate obesity is on the horns of a dilemma: Either use diets that produce good weight loss but poor maintenance, or use behavior modification that produces good maintenance but poor weight loss. The ideal may be a treatment that combines the two modalities; a recent study by Wadden et al (1984) suggests that this is so.

COMBINATION TREATMENT. Wadden et al (1984) treated 17 moderately obese (87.5 percent overweight) women for six months with a combination of very-low-calorie diet (400 to 500 calories) and behavior modification designed to assist maintenance of weight loss. After an introductory month of treatment, patients received the very-low-calorie diet for no more than two months, following which they received three more months of training in weight loss maintenance. Figure 2 shows that patients lost 20.5 kg (45.1 pounds) during a treatment which produced also a significant improvement in psychological functioning. Furthermore, this weight loss was well maintained. During the year after treatment, patients regained no more than 2.1 kg (4.6 pounds).

APPETITE SUPPRESSANT MEDICATION. Figure 2 also presents data from an earlier study that provided a strong argument against the use of appetite suppressant medication (Craighead et al, 1981). This study was undertaken to determine whether combining such medication with behavior modification might increase weight loss. Figure 2 shows that this goal was achieved: Patients receiving combined treatment lost 15.0 kg (33 pounds) compared to the 10.9 kg (24 pounds) lost by patients receiving behavior modification alone. During the year after treatment, patients who had received the combined treatment regained far more weight than those who had received only behavior modification.

One interpretation of these findings is that the medication acted by lowering a body weight set point, which made it easier for patients to control their food intake (Stunkard, 1982). The medication did indeed suppress appetite, but this suppression of appetite was secondary to the lowering of a body weight set point. These findings, plus evidence from animal experiments, suggest that any benefits derived from starting medication are lost when the medication is stopped. If this is so, it suggests a radical revision in current prescribing practices for appetite suppressant medication: Such medication should be used indefinitely or not at all.

Mild Obesity

Mild obesity, from 20 to 40 percent overweight, is by far the most common form of the disorder, afflicting more than 90 percent of obese persons. The adipose

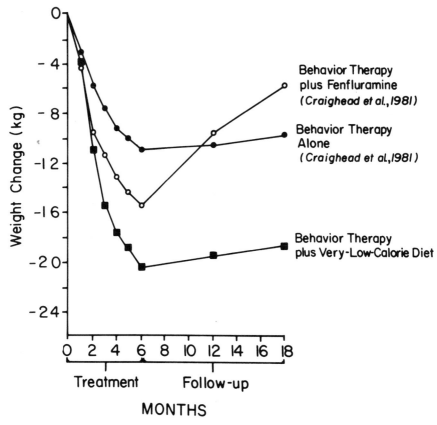

Figure 2. Weight loss (in kg) at the end of six months of treatment and one-year follow-up of patients treated with behavior therapy plus very-low-calorie diet. These results are contrasted with those obtained in an earlier study comparing the results of behavior therapy alone and behavior therapy plus fenfluramine. From "Treatment of moderate obesity by behavior therapy and very-low-calorie diet: a pilot investigation," by T.A. Wadden et al. Journal of Consulting and Clinical Psychology, in press. Copyright © 1984 by the American Psychological Association. Reprinted by permission of the author.

tissue of mildly obese persons is usually hypertrophic and it is hyperplastic only in persons who maintain a lowered body weight by constantly dieting. The two types of treatment are the same as those for moderate obesity—diet and behavior modification—but with significant differences. The diet is far more moderate and the behavior modification is delivered by lay-led groups.

DIET. The very-low-calorie diet is *not* indicated for mildly obese persons. Instead they can choose from among a wide variety of diets. And there is a wide variety!

There are diets high in protein and low in protein, high in fat and low in fat, high in carbohydrates and low in carbohydrates, and, recently, a special diet from Beverly Hills that is high in papayas and mangos. A discussion of dietary treatment could easily fill this volume without exhausting the topic, but the general principal is simple—any diet that reduces calorie intake below caloric expenditure will produce weight loss. In this sense all treatments for obesity are dietary. But diets today have become far more than simply a means of producing a calorie deficit. They have acquired all manner of magical properties in the minds of the lay public; just consider the categories of diets listed above! How does one make a rational choice?

Perhaps one should not choose; the whole idea of dieting for mildly over-weight persons may be unwise. *Going on* a diet implies *going off* it and resuming old eating habits. For this reason the most effective diet may not be a diet at all but rather a gradual change in eating habits and a shift to foods that the patient can continue to eat indefinitely. This means increasing the intake of complex carbohydrates, particularly fruits, vegetables, and cereals, and decreasing the intake of fats and concentrated carbohydrates. This course of action probably gives the best chance of maintaining the weight that is lost, and it is an eminently safe one. A diet that consists primarily of sensible eating habits does not require medical monitoring and is particularly well suited to use by the lay organizations that are assuming the dominant role in the treatment of mild obesity.

BEHAVIOR MODIFICATION. Behavior modification programs such as that described above were developed for the treatment of mildly obese persons, and they are admirably suited to this purpose. Furthermore, the key elements of behavior modification are easy to specify and therefore easy to learn. Many of them are readily packaged in easy-to-use treatment manuals. As a result, behavior modification has been administered by persons with progressively less formal training, even by those with no professional background. Behavior modification provides a technology that can promise modest weight losses at minimal risk. Although it is being applied by professional therapists, particularly psychologists, by far the largest number of obese persons is being treated under the auspices of lay-led groups (Stuart, 1977).

TREATMENT VEHICLES—LAY-LED GROUPS. Lay-led groups for obesity antedate the development of behavioral weight control by several years. Prominent among them are TOPS (Take Off Pounds Sensibly), the largest of the non-profit groups, and Weight Watchers, the largest commercial group. TOPS, founded in 1948, was the first self-help group for obesity, and it now enrolls more than 300,000 persons (Levitz and Stunkard, 1974). The key elements of TOPS are weekly meetings that provide group support, weigh-ins that are high points of the meeting, and policy supervision from the national headquarters. The membership of TOPS is almost exclusively female, middle-aged and of lower-middle socioeconomic status; the average member is 60 percent overweight. This group's effectiveness is difficult to assess, however, because of the very high drop-out rates.

Commercial weight loss organizations appeal to much the same clientele as do the non-profit ones, and with somewhat greater success—500,000 persons a week attend just one such organization, Weight Watchers (Stuart, 1974). The commercial organizations have added three important elements to the programs pioneered by the non-profit groups—behavior modification, inspirational lecturers drawn from successful members, and a carefully designed nutritional program. They are readily available to persons with even a casual interest in weight reduction. But they too suffer from high attrition rates: 50 percent of the members of one such group dropped out in six weeks and 70 percent in 12 weeks (Volkmar et al, 1981). Drop-out rates of this magnitude make it difficult to assess reports of weight lost by the survivors.

Despite these problems, the low cost and ready availability of lay-led groups makes them an important resource for the control of mild obesity. Large numbers of persons can be reached by these groups, and their very low costs mean a favorable ratio of cost to effectiveness. For example, it costs far more to lose comparable amounts of weight in an exemplary university clinic than in a neighboring commercial program, even with its high drop-out rate (Yates, 1978). For the well-motivated person with mild obesity, commercial weight loss programs are probably the treatment of choice.

TREATMENT OF OBESE CHILDREN. Until recently, weight reduction programs for children have been characterized by modest losses, poor maintenance of these losses, untoward emotional reactions, and high attrition rates (Coates and Thoresen, 1978). The introduction of behavioral principles into the treatment of obese children has changed this gloomy picture, and a small number of recent studies suggest that behavioral weight reduction of children may be at least as effective as behavioral weight reduction of adults. The most promising of these studies was that recently reported by Brownell et al (1983).

Forty-two children (33 girls and nine boys) between the ages of 12 and 16 were treated for four months for moderately severe obesity, averaging 55.7 percent overweight. Treatment was modelled on traditional behavioral principles, carried out in groups that met for periods of about an hour. All children received the same treatment, with the exception of the type of parental involvement. In one treatment condition the mother and child were treated separately (Mother-Child Separately); in the second, mother and child were treated together (Mother-Child Together); and in the third the child was treated alone, without parental involvement (Child Alone). The difference between the first two conditions was that children and their mothers were either seen in groups together, or were seen in separate groups which met at the same time, but in different rooms.

Weight losses were as large as any reported in the pediatric literature. Children in the Mother-Child Separately condition lost 8.4 kg (18.5 pounds), compared to 5.3 kg (11.7 pounds) and 3.3 kg (7.0 pounds) for the Mother-Child Together and the Child Alone conditions, respectively. The superiority of the Mother-Child Separately condition was maintained at the one-year follow-up, when children in this condition still showed a loss of 7.7 kg (17.0 pounds), compared with a gain of 3 kg in the other two conditions. Even the children in the latter two conditions, however, maintained the decrease in their degree of obesity, despite their gain in weight. Figure 3 shows that there was no change in percentage overweight of any of the groups, since increases in weight were offset by increases in height.

The surprisingly large weight losses and the excellent maintenance of these weight losses in the Mother-Child Separately condition may herald a new era in the treatment of childhood obesity. The fact that these results were obtained so early in the application of behavioral principles to the treatment of childhood obesity is grounds for optimism about even further progress.

PSYCHOANALYSIS. The results of a recent large-scale study of psychoanalysis suggest that this modality may be of more value in the treatment of obesity

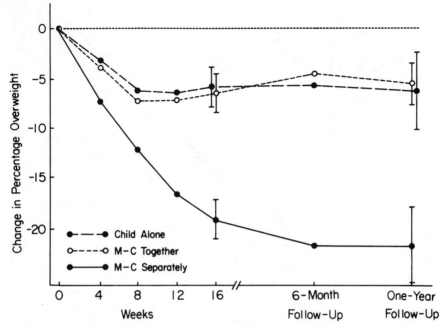

Figure 3. Mean changes in weight for three treatment conditions (Child Alone, Mother-Child Together, Mother-Child Separately) during treatment and one-year maintenance period. From "Treatment of obese children with and without their mothers: changes in weight and blood pressure," by KD Brownell et al. Pediatrics 71:515-523, 1983. Copyright American Academy of Pediatrics 1983. Reprinted by permission of the American Academy of Pediatrics.

than we had believed (Rand and Stunkard, 1983). The study involved 84 obese men and women treated by 72 psychoanalysts over a period of several years. Weight losses compared favorably with those achieved by other conservative measures. After a median duration of 33 months of treatment, weight losses averaged 4.5 kg (9.9 pounds). At an 18-month follow-up, weight loss had increased to 9.5 kg (20.9 pounds); and at a four-year follow-up it had increased still further, to 11.6 kg (25.5 pounds).

Not only were significant amounts of weight lost during treatment, but these weight losses were well-maintained at follow-up of as much as four years duration. This good maintenance is well illustrated in Figure 4, which plots individual weight changes of the 30 patients who had terminated treatment at least one year before this assessment. Duration of treatment had been 40 months (range 29 to 60 months) and patients were assessed 28 months (range 12 to 36 months) after termination. Figure 4 shows that the weight of 40 percent of the obese patients fell along the main diagonal, indicating that their weight was approximately the same at follow-up as it had been at the end of treatment. Thirty-three percent of the patients had continued to lose weight following treatment, and 27 percent had regained some weight. These results are similar to those of one-year follow-up studies of obese patients treated with behavior therapy (Craighead et al, 1981).

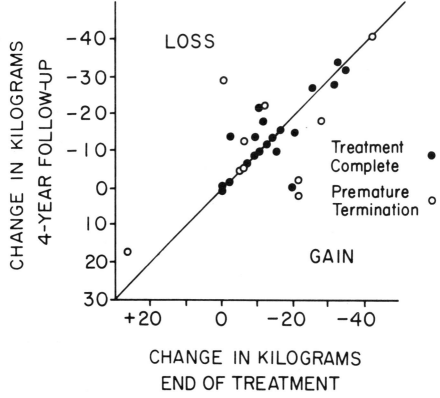

Figure 4. Weight changes of 30 obese patients from the end of treatment to the four-year follow-up. Weight loss during treatment is plotted on the horizontal axis and net weight loss (from the end of treatment to the four-year follow-up) is plotted on the vertical axis. Further weight loss after the end of treatment results in data points above the main diagonal; weight gain results in data points below the main diagonal. From "Obesity and psychoanalysis: treatment and four-year follow-up," by CSW Rand and AJ Stunkard, American Journal of Psychiatry 140:1140-1144, 1983. Copyright © 1983, the American Psychiatric Association. Reprinted by permission.

In addition to these unexpected results of the psychoanalysis of obese persons, there were other, less surprising, ones. Notable among them was a marked reduction in the prevalence of severe body image disparagement. At the beginning of treatment 39 percent of patients reported severe disparagement of the body image; this percentage had fallen to 18 percent at follow-up.

Since this study may reawaken interest in the psychoanalytic psychotherapy of obese persons, some cautions should be noted. There is no evidence that uncovering putative unconscious causes of overeating can alter the symptom choice of obese people who overeat in response to stress. Years after successful psychotherapy and successful weight reduction, persons who overeat under stress continue to do so. Furthermore, many obese people seem inordinately vulnerable to the overdependency on the therapist and to the severe regression that can occur in psychoanalytic therapy. Bruch (1973) has provided excellent descriptions of ways to minimize such regression, and to increase the patient's often seriously inadequate sense of personal effectiveness.

Psychoanalysis is clearly not the first choice among therapies for obesity, if for no other reason than its expense. It may, however, be a reasonable option for persons with sufficient time, money, and interest, particularly if they suffer from disparagement of the body image. Psychoanalysis and psychoanalytic therapy may be indicated also for treatment of bulimia, among obese as well as among nonobese persons. Furthermore, many obese persons seek psychotherapy for reasons other than their obesity; helping them to cope with their obesity may help them to resolve other problems. Many obese people overeat under stress. If psychotherapy helps them live less stressful and more satisfying lives, they are less likely to overeat. As a result, they may reduce and stay reduced. These benefits are not less significant for being nonspecific results of treatment.

CONCLUSION

Obesity is a common disorder, afflicting 25 percent of the adult population, and is seen somewhat more frequently among women than among men. The old view of the relationship between psychopathology and obesity has been reversed in the last 40 years. Psychopathology is no longer viewed as a cause of obesity but, rather, as a consequence either of the societal discrimination against obese people, or of the dieting that is a response to this discrimination. Discrimination contributes to the body image disparagement that afflicts a significant minority of obese persons, while dieting may lead directly to anxiety and depression and, indirectly, to bulimia.

A classification of obesity based upon severity provides a guide to treatment. Severe obesity (more than 100 percent overweight), which afflicts 0.5 percent of the adult population, is most effectively treated by surgical procedures that reduce the size of the stomach. Mild (20 to 40 percent overweight) and moderate (41 to 100 percent overweight) obesity are best managed by a combination of behavior modification and diet. The relatively strict diets used with moderate obesity usually require medical supervision. The treatment of mild obesity, on the other hand, which afflicts 90 percent of the population, is largely managed by commercial and nonprofit lay-led groups.

Behavioral treatment of obesity in children has recently been introduced, and the results are sufficiently encouraging that wider application is expected. Psychoanalysis produces psychological benefits *and* weight losses that compare favorably with other treatments, but the costs of psychotherapy relative to other modalities will probably restrict its application to a small minority of obese persons.

REFERENCES

Abraham S: Obese and overweight adults in the United States. National Center for Health Statistics, Vital and Health Statistics Series 11, No 230. DHHS Pub No 83–1680. Public Health Service. Washington, US Government Printing Office, January 1983

Andres R: Effect of obesity on total mortality. Int J Obes 4:381–386, 1980

Bray GA, Dahms WT, Atkinson RL, et al: Factors controlling food intake: a comparison of dieting and intestinal bypass. Am J Clin Nutr 33:376–382, 1980

Brownell KD, Kelman JH, Stunkard AJ: Treatment of obese children with and without their mothers: changes in weight and blood pressure. Pediatrics 71:515–523, 1983

Bruch H: Eating Disorders: Obesity, Anorexia and the Person Within. New York, Basic Books, 1973

Coates TJ, Thoresen CE: Treating obesity in children and adolescents: a review. Am J Public Health 68:143–151, 1978

Craighead LW, Stunkard AJ, O'Brien R: Behavior therapy and pharmacotherapy of obesity. Arch Gen Psychiatry 38:763–768, 1981

Drenick EJ, Bale GS, Seltzer F, et al: Excessive mortality and causes of death in morbidly obese men. JAMA 243:443–445, 1980

Foch TT, McClearn GE: Genetics, body weight and obesity, in Obesity. Edited by Stunkard A. Philadelphia, W.B. Saunders Company, 1980

Garrow JS: Treat Obesity Seriously: A Clinical Manual. London and New York, Churchill Livingston, 1982

Goldblatt PB, Moore ME, Stunkard AJ: Social factors in obesity. JAMA 192:1039–1044, 1965

Halmi KA, Stunkard AJ, Mason EE: Emotional responses to weight reduction by three methods: diet, jejunoileal bypass, and gastric bypass. Am J Clin Nutr 33:446, 1980

Halmi KA, Mason EE, Falk J, et al: Appetitive behavior after gastric bypass for obesity. Int J Obes 5:457–464, 1981

Keesey R: Defense of the body weight set point: metabolic contributions, in Eating and its Disorders. Edited by Stunkard AJ, Stellar E. New York, Raven Press, 1984

Levitz LS, Stunkard AJ: A therapeutic coalition for obesity: behavior modification and patient self-help. Am J Psychiatry 131:423–427, 1974

Mason EE: Surgical Treatment of Obesity. Philadelphia, W.B. Saunders Company, 1981

Mills MJ, Stunkard AJ: Behavioral changes following surgery for obesity. Am J Psychiatry 133:527–531, 1976

Nisbett R: Hunger, obesity and the ventromedial hypothalamus. Psychol Rev 79:433–453, 1972

Rand SW, Stunkard AJ: Obesity and psychoanalysis: treatment and four-year follow-up. Am J Psychiatry 140:1140–1144, 1983

Sjostrom L: Fat cells and body weight, in Obesity. Edited by Stunkard AJ. Philadelphia, W.B. Saunders Company, 1980

Solow C, Silberfarb PM, Swift K: Psychosocial effects of intestinal bypass surgery for severe obesity. New Eng J Med 290:300–304, 1974

Stern J: Is obesity a disease of inactivity, in Eating and Its Disorders. Edited by Stunkard AJ, Stellar E. New York, Raven Press, 1984

Stuart RB: Self-help for self-management, in Behavioral Self-Management. Edited by Stuart RB. New York, Brunner/Mazel, 1977

Stuart RB: Act Thin, Stay Thin. New York, William Norton, 1978

Stunkard AJ: The Pain of Obesity. Palo Alto, Bull Publishing Company, 1976

Stunkard AJ: Anorectic agents lower body weight set point. Life Sciences 30:2043–2055, 1982

Stunkard AJ: The current status of treatment for obesity in adults, in Eating and Its Disorders. Edited by Stunkard AJ, Stellar E. New York. Raven Press, 1984

Stunkard AJ, Mendelson M: Obesity and the body image. I. Characteristics of disturbance in the body image of some obese persons. Am J Psychiatry 123:1296–1300, 1967

Stunkard AJ, Rush AJ: Dieting and depression reexamined: a critical review of reports of untoward responses during weight reduction for obesity. Ann Intern Med 81:526–533, 1974

Volkmar FR, Stunkard AJ, Woolston J, et al: High attrition rates in commercial weight reduction programs. Arch Intern Med 141:426–428, 1981

Wadden TA, Stunkard AJ, Brownell KD: Very low calorie diets: their efficacy, safety and future. Ann Intern Med 99:675–684, 1983

Wadden TA, Stunkard AJ, Brownell KD, et al: Treatment of moderate obesity by behavior therapy and very low calorie diet: a pilot investigation. J Clin Consult Psychol 52:692-694, 1984

Wing RR, Jeffrey RW: Outpatient treatments of obesity: a comparison of methodological and clinical results. Int J Obes 3:261–272, 1979

Yates BT: Improving the cost-effectiveness of obesity programs: three basic strategies for reducing the cost per pound. Int J Obes 2:249–266, 1978

Chapter 23

Anorexia Nervosa

by Sidney Kennedy, M.B., B.Ch.
and Paul E. Garfinkel, M.D.

It is now more than a century since Gull (1868) and Lasegue (1873) independently described anorexia nervosa. Since their initial descriptions of the illness, there have been a variety of different conceptions of it. At times it has been subsumed as a primary endocrine disorder (pituitary insufficiency) (Simmonds 1914) and it has also been thought of as a variant of other psychiatric disorders—in particular, hysteria (Hobhouse, 1938), affective disorder (Cantwell, 1977), schizophrenia (Nicolle, 1939) and compulsive disorder (Palmer and Jones, 1939). Only within the past two decades has it reemerged, by consensus, as a separate clinical syndrome. This recognition, together with its increasing frequency and resistance to treatment, have served as stimuli for diverse areas of study including physiological and neuroendocrine aspects, individual and family psychopathology, and treatment.

DIAGNOSTIC ISSUES

Russell (1970) proposed three operational criteria for any psychiatric syndrome: constancy of association of various clinical features; similarity in course and outcome of illness; and the elucidation of a clear-cut etiology. He argued that anorexia nervosa, like most psychiatric disorders, satisfies the first two requirements.

While many diagnostic criteria have been proposed for anorexia nervosa, they all have in common the emphasis on the individual's desire for a smaller body size and avoidance of weight gain or fat to the point where it interferes with the individual's daily living. Crisp (1965a) suggested the term "weight phobia" to describe the anorexic's avoidance of normal weight.

Primary and secondary forms of the disorder were proposed by King (1963) and supported by others (Bruch, 1965; Russell, 1970). Bruch distinguished the primary group by their "relentless pursuit of thinness" in association with disturbances in body image, disturbances in recognition of internal perceptions, and a sense of personal ineffectiveness. In the secondary group, weight loss occurs but other criteria are variable, and they probably represent various emotional disorders (Garfinkel and Garner, 1982), which should be described by their Axis I diagnoses rather than as variants of anorexia nervosa.

Beyond the basic desire for thinness, various other criteria have been required for the diagnosis. Feighner et al (1972) defined criteria for anorexia nervosa which allowed comparative research to become established. While these criteria ensured that patients who were described in various clinical investigations were definite cases of the illness, and thus comparable, some of their criteria are overly restrictive in clinical practice (Garfinkel and Garner, 1982): Not all patients are under 25 at the onset; weight loss may not be as much as 25 percent of original body weight; and true anorexia is unlikely to be present until late in the illness; in fact, appetite is usually increased but strongly resisted. Because of these requirements many people with the disorder are excluded using the Feighner criteria.

Much more clinically useful are the *DSM-III* criteria for anorexia nervosa which are as follows (American Psychiatric Association, 1980):

A. Intense fear of becoming obese, which does not diminish as weight loss progresses.
B. Disturbance of body image; for example, claiming to "feel fat" even when emaciated.
C. Weight loss of at least 25 percent of original body weight; or, if under 18 years of age, weight loss from original body weight plus projected weight gain expected from growth charts may be combined to make 25 percent.
D. Refusal to maintain body weight over a minimal weight for age and height.
E. No known physical illness that would account for the weight loss.

These criteria represent an acknowledgement that true anorexia and amenorrhoea are not essential for the diagnosis of anorexia nervosa, although primary or secondary amenorrhoea remain prominent symptoms of the disorder.

A further question regarding diagnosis relates to whether anorexia nervosa represents a distinct diagnostic entity, or simply an extreme point on a weight continuum. Nylander (1971) originally proposed this "continuum" hypothesis when he found that the majority of female high school students in Sweden felt fat and that nearly ten percent reported at least three symptoms found in anorexia nervosa and in association with weight loss. Others have also reported that many individuals display some of the symptoms of the illness without meeting accepted diagnostic standards: They have been called by such different names as "partial syndrome" (Szmuckler, 1983), "subclinical" anorexia nervosa (Button and Whitehouse, 1981), or anorexic behavior (Garfinkel and Garner, 1982). While this group lends support to the idea that anorexia nervosa represents one end of a continuum, others have argued that the essential psychopathology differentiates anorexics from the more mild expressions of the syndrome (Bruch, 1973; Crisp, 1970; Selvini-Palazzoli, 1974). In a recent study of anorexic and extremely weight preoccupied and non-weight preoccupied women, Garner et al (1983) demonstrated support for fundamental differences in the psychopathology of the anorexic, while at the same time finding that some of the features do exist on a continuum. While such issues as perfectionism and dissatisfaction with one's body can be viewed as being on a continuum, the anorexics' scores on measures of ineffectiveness, interoceptive awareness, and interpersonal distrust differentiated them clearly from weight preoccupied nonanorexics. Anorexia nervosa cannot be viewed simply as the extreme of dieting concerns.

Differential Diagnosis

Three aspects will be considered in relation to differential diagnosis: medical conditions; other psychiatric disorders; and the presence or absence of bulimic symptoms in anorexic patients.

MEDICAL CONDITIONS.   Brain tumors, particularly of the hypothalamus or third ventricle; endocrine disorders such as hyperthyroidism, panhypopituitarism, Addison's disease, and diabetes mellitus; and gastrointestinal disorders—inflammatory bowel disease, bowel tumors, and peptic ulcer—should all be considered. In these instances patients do not display the active pursuit of thinness and distortion of body image common to anorexics. Patients with these illnesses will display appropriate concern for the weight loss and efforts to regain weight, as well as other signs and symptoms of the primary metabolic disorder.

PSYCHIATRIC DISORDERS.   With the current awareness of anorexia nervosa the risk of underdiagnosis is clearly lessened. However, other functional disorders which can present with weight loss may be overlooked (Garfinkel et al, 1983). Conversion disorder is perhaps the hardest to distinguish and represents what was previously described as "atypical anorexia nervosa." Here, weight loss and food avoidance are more likely to represent a conflict and a means of controlling others, but there is no primary intent to lose weight. Major depression and anorexia nervosa are not mutually exclusive, but dysphoric mood and other "depressive symptomatology" are often the result of starvation. When distinguishing a major depression, the extent to which self-esteem and other symptoms are tied to weight change and physical appearance should help in clarifying the diagnosis. Occasionally a schizophrenic patient may experience food related delusions and lose weight, but the presence of more generalized thought disorder should separate this from the drive for thinness and associated weight loss of anorexia nervosa.

RESTRICTING VS. BULIMIC FORMS.   Among patients having anorexia nervosa, the most clinically relevant question to emerge recently has been whether the low body weight is reached and maintained by restriction of food intake only, or alternately varies with periods of gross overeating or bulimia. This distinction will be discussed in the clinical section.

EPIDEMIOLOGY

Despite concerns about the denial and ambivalence of patients with anorexia nervosa to come forward for treatment, two findings appear consistent: first, that the prevalance has increased; and second, that the disorder remains much more common in women. Measures of incidence have relied mainly on established case registers. Theander (1970) surveyed hospital records of departments of psychiatry, internal medicine, pediatrics, and gynecology at two university hospitals in southern Sweden between 1931 and 1960. He reported an incidence of 0.24 cases per 100,000 with the rate for the last decade studied being considerably higher (0.45 per 100,000). Several authors have reported on surveys based on the Monroe County, New York, Case register. Kendell et al (1973) found an incidence of 0.37 per 100,000 for the period 1960 to 1969. Jones et al (1980) extended their search to psychiatric and other hospital records in Monroe County, and noted a dramatic increase in white females (15 to 24) from 0.55 per 100,000 per year during 1960 to 1969 to 3.26 per 100,000 per year during 1970 to 1976. Overall, the incidence doubled during the period under study. These studies all required the individual to have been diagnosed as suffering from anorexia nervosa.

Several prevalence studies have surveyed large groups of young women or teenage girls. Nylander (1971) concluded that anorexia nervosa was present in severe form in about 1 in 150 adolescent girls in Sweden. Crisp, Palmer, and Kalucy (1976) studied populations of schoolgirls in both private and state schools in England. Overall they found one serious new case for every 250 girls aged 16 and over. The illness was much more common in the private schools. Ballot (1981) determined the prevalence in South African school girls to be three percent, with the same additional finding as Crisp—that those girls from the higher socioeconomic backgrounds were more at risk. Szmuckler (1983) found a prevalence of one in 90 females over age 16 in a survey in England more recently. Pope et al (1984) surveyed over 300 shoppers in the United States and found 0.7 percent had anorexia nervosa at some point in their lives. The age of onset varies but has a bimodal distribution at ages 14 and 18 years. Although most patients have developed the illness by age 25, five percent in our series first had overt symptoms after this age. Isolated reports of postmenopausal anorexia nervosa exist (Kellet et al, 1976).

Others have also found that the highest social classes are at greatest risk, and this dates back 100 years (Fenwick, 1880). Theander (1970) suggested that the overrepresentation in upper classes is related to superior case detection in these groups. However, Jones et al (1980) studied the incidence over a period in which two community health centers providing services to the lower classes were opened, and noted no increase in case detection. They concluded that the expression of anorexia nervosa is related to the socioeconomic class itself rather than to differential utilization of psychiatric care. Garfinkel and Garner (1982) have more recently proposed that this social class distribution of the illness may have been eroded in the 1970s.

CLINICAL CHARACTERISTICS

Individuals are traditionally reluctant to initiate referral of their own accord; more often a concerned relative will have been responsible for the initial clinical contact. While previous medical consultations may have been obtained (for example, gynecological or gastrointestinal), they may not have focused on dietary habits and attitude to weight; and the patient is unlikely to volunteer such information herself. Symptoms and signs occur as a result of the intertwined effects of a relentless drive for thinness and the manifestations of starvation.

Symptoms

The most prominent symptom is the drive for thinness (Bruch, 1970; Garfinkel and Garner, 1982). This goes far beyond "normal" dieting and may involve a variety of techniques to maintain the phobic avoidance of weight gain. Losing weight or maintaining low weight to achieve "the look" are closely bound to the quest for self-control and an improvement in low self-esteem. In understanding this adaptation, Bruch (1962) described three areas of psychological disturbance that are clinically relevant. The first area is disturbance in body image: This can be recognized clinically by the patient's lack of recognition of the degree of her weight loss; by her preoccupation that a particular body part is still too large; and by the degree of loathing the patient experiences about her body. The second area is faulty perception of inner sensations, including such visceral sensations as hunger and satiety but extending to affective states. This is often mixed with the effects of starvation. For example, patients who are being nourished and are starting to take responsibility for their own diet experience great difficulty sensing what is "enough" at meal times. This is true for other starving persons who often feel hungrier after they have eaten (Keys et al, 1950) and may be further confounded by a strong subjective sense of bloating or early fullness. Recently, objective measures have demonstrated delayed gastric emptying in emaciated patients with anorexia nervosa (Russell et al, 1983). Patients often describe a lack of awareness of other feelings, including fatigue, sexual excitement, and affective states. The third area of disturbance involves a pervasive sense of personal ineffectiveness. Anorexia nervosa represents the individual's attempt to achieve a sense of mastery or personal control.

Cognitive distortions have been identified, particularly a dichotomous or all-or-nothing form of reasoning (Garner and Bemis, 1982). This can prevail in every aspect of the individual's life, not just in relation to eating and weight (for example, "if I'm not the top A student, then I'll undoubtedly fail"). Anorexics do not see in-betweens in any areas of their lives; this includes their sense of self-worth and assessment of others, who tend to be either idealized or villified. Other cognitive distortions include their personalizing of many situations, over-generalization, and a superstitious style of thinking. (Garfinkel and Garner, 1982). These features are discussed at greater length in the chapter by Garner and Isaacs.

Even though they are starving, anorexics often experience excess energy. Many will exercise rigorously, engaging in exact amounts of self-prescribed calisthenics or daily running. Most patients channel their energy into the restricted activities of exercise and school work, while other activities are neglected. Social relationships are curtailed and the individual may become secretive and irritable. Life within the family becomes strained, with increasing pressure directed toward the person to eat, to no avail.

The relationship between anorexia nervosa and depressed mood is complex. When self-esteem is intimately linked to weight and appearance, even minimal weight gain may result in a sense of self-loathing and depression. Depressed mood may also be a physiological effect of starvation. The nonanorexic male volunteers who completed the Minnesota starvation studies (Keys et al, 1950) experienced depressed mood, decreased libido, restricted interests, and impaired concentration, which resolved on refeeding. Disturbed sleep patterns have also been reported in conjunction with starvation (Crisp et al, 1971). Depressive symptoms may be present and persist in a subgroup of anorexic patients during and after weight gain. This is likely to represent a depressive syndrome which may benefit from specific treatment. Using RDC criteria, Piran et al (1983) have shown evidence of a depressive syndrome in 80 percent of patients, while 50 percent showed anxiety and phobic symptoms.

Physical symptoms commonly reported include constipation, abdominal pain, and cold intolerance. As weight loss progresses, the initial capacity to sustain demanding exercise schedules gives way to feelings of weakness and lethargy. Amenorrhea, although not essential for the diagnosis, occurs in virtually 100 percent of cases. Weight loss generally precedes loss of menses, supporting the belief that a critical weight or critical body fat is required to trigger ovulation. (Frisch, 1977; Frisch and McArthur, 1974; Richardson et al, 1977). However, in about 20 percent of cases, loss of menstruation is said to predate weight loss (Russell, 1970). Both exercise and emotional stress may play a role in such a circumstance. Other physical symptoms depend on the complications from starvation and are described further in the section on complications.

RESTRICTIVE VS. BULIMIA. There are consistent differences between the group of anorexic patients who achieve and maintain their low weight purely by restricting intake of food (restricters) and those who alternate between starvation and engorgement (bulimics). Bulimia is recognized in *DSM-III* (APA, 1980) as a distinct syndrome, although these criteria require the absence of anorexia nervosa. There is some evidence to suggest that this dichotomy between bulimics with and without anorexia nervosa may be false (Garner et al, in press). Several studies (Garfinkel et al, 1980) have reported that about 50 percent of patients meeting criteria for anorexia nervosa also suffer from bulimia, and this appears to represent a dramatic increase in the prevalence of bulimia over the past 20 years. Different authors have used various terms to describe this syndrome: bulimarexia (Boskind-Lodahl, 1976), dietary chaos syndrome (Palmer, 1979), and bulimia nervosa (Russell, 1979).

We recently reviewed the differences in various measures between restrictive and bulimic patients who met criteria for anorexia nervosa and who were seen at the Clarke Institute and Toronto General Hospital between 1970 and 1983. Patients with bulimia but with no history of weight loss were excluded for the purposes of this comparison. There were significant differences in the frequency of vomiting, laxative abuse, and diuretic abuse (see Table 1). The bulimic subgroup were significantly heavier premorbidly both in absolute terms and when considered against percentages of standardized weights for age and height. They had also reached a significantly higher maximum ever weight (see Table 2) and tended to come from families with more frequent obesity. Behaviors characterized by low impulse control (see Table 3), such as street drug use, stealing, selfmutilation, and suicide attempts, were significantly more common among the bulimic group. Bulimics also tend to be more socially outgoing and engage in

Table 1. Differences in Weight Control Methods Between Two Groups of Anorexia Nervosa Patients

	% Vomiting	% Laxative Abuse	% Diuretic Abuse	% Exercise
Restricting (N = 170)	20	27	4	70
Bulimic (N = 156)	70[++]	55[++]	14[+]	65

[+]p<.005
[++]p<.0001

Table 2. Differences in Weight Measures Between Two Groups of Anorexia Nervosa Patients

	Maximum Weight (Kg)	% of ave.	Minimum Weight (Kg)	% of ave.	Weight at Consultation	Height cms
Restricting	56	96	37	63	39	162
Bulimic	62[++]	106[++]	39[+]	67[++]	44[++]	163*

*NS
[+]p<.001
[++]p<.0001

Table 3. Differences in Impulse Related Behavior Between Two Groups of Anorexia Nervosa Patients

	% Street Drug Use	% Alcohol Use Weekly	% Stealing	% Self-mutilation	% Suicide Attempts
Restricting (N = 170)	16	8	4	5	10
Bulimic (N = 156)	32[+]	14	20[+++]	15[+]	25[++]

[+]p<.005
[++]p<.001
[+++]p<.0001

sexual relationships, which are often perceived by the individual as unsatisfying and degrading.

Signs

The "classic" signs of anorexia nervosa that appear upon physical examination are a direct effect of starvation. The typical patient will look emaciated and wear loose-fitting and often excessive clothing that she will retain during interview rather than emphasize the degree of wasting and weight loss. In a series of 100 patients, Silverman (1983) reported skin changes in 83 percent, commonly a dry cracking skin, with yellowish discoloration (thought to be due to increased carotene deposition) and a fine downy hair or lanugo which may cover extremities, face, and trunk. Pubic and axillary hair remain unchanged (Beck and Brochner-Mortensen, 1954) but scalp hair may be lost. A perioral dermatitis may be a sign of the repeated irritating effects of vomiting. There may be callous formation on the dorsum of the hand as a result of repeated friction of fingers pressing against the teeth while vomiting (Russell, 1979). Hypotension and bradycardia occur in up to 50 percent of reported cases (Garfinkel and Garner, 1982; Silverman, 1983). Peripheral edema can be seen on initial evaluation and may recur during the refeeding process. This is rarely a sign of renal or cardiac failure and may be related, in part, to the excessive standing or salt ingestion of some patients. Dental problems are common, particularly in patients who vomit (Hurst, Lacey, and Crisp, 1977).

NEUROENDOCRINE CHANGES. A great deal of attention has been devoted to neuroendocrine abnormalities in anorexia nervosa. At times anorexia nervosa has been confused with hypopituitarism but, beside such obvious clinical differences as lack of desire for thinness and little weight loss in the hypopituitary group, major hormonal differences between pituitary hypofunction and anorexia nervosa involve ACTH, growth hormone (GH) and prolactin.

Hypothalamic-pituitary-gonadal axis. Amenorrhea in anorexia nervosa is due to low plasma gonadotrophin (LH and FSH) levels (Beumont 1973, Hurd et al, 1977) which correlate with low body weight (Brown et al, 1977) and return to normal with weight restoration (Wakeling, 1977; Sherman and Halmi, 1977). With significant weight loss the normal circadian pulsatile pattern of LH production is also lost, leaving a prepubertal pattern (Boyar et al, 1974). Release of LH and FSH is controlled by luteinizing hormone releasing hormone (LHRH), which has been artificially synthesized and has been used to study pituitary responses to its systemic injection in anorexic patients. While both LH and FSH responses to LHRH are reduced (Jeuniewic et al, 1978), it appears that FSH responses are normalized with weight gain earlier than LH (Warren et al, 1975).

Other studies have examined the effect of clomiphine on LH (Marshall and Fraser, 1971). At normal weight it releases LH by blocking the negative feedback of estrogens at the hypothalamic level, but in the underweight anorexic the response is blunted (Beumont et al 1973, Brown et al, 1977).

The sequence of return of these hormonal responses has been noted to parallel the earlier maturation process through puberty (Donovan and Ven der Werfften Bosch, 1965).

Hypothalamic-pituitary-adrenal axis. Elevated morning cortisol has been reported by a series of authors (Boyar et al, 1977; Brown et al, 1977; Walsh et al, 1978) with a flattening of the circadian rhythm (Garfinkel et al, 1975). There is incomplete suppression of cortisol after oral dexamethasone administration in some, but not all, anorexic patients (Walsh, 1978; Gerner and Gwirtsman, 1981). This has been compared to the nonsuppression of cortisol in some patients with major depression, although it is unclear whether this represents only a weight-related phenomenon. Other changes are the result of the effects of starvation on the thyroid gland and include a prolongation of the half life of cortisol in plasma and a delay in its metabolic clearance (Weiner, 1983).

Hypothalamic-pituitary-thyroid axis. Thyroxine (T4) levels are usually at the low end of the normal range (Lundberg et al, 1972; Brown et al, 1977) but triiodothyronine (T3) is significantly reduced, while reverse T3 is elevated. This represents the body's adaptive response to starvation and, in particular, to carbohydrate deprivation, aimed at reducing the metabolic rate (Chopra and Smith, 1975). Clearly there is no role for thyroid replacement to correct the abnormal laboratory values under such circumstances. Thyroid stimulating hormone (TSH) levels are normal and the TSH response to thyrotropin-releasing hormone (TRH) is reported to be of normal magnitude, but may be delayed (Lundberg et al, 1972; Miyai et al, 1975). Wakeling et al (1979) reported a normalization of the TRH response with weight gain.

Other hormonal variations. TRH is also responsible for the stimulation of prolactin from the anterior pituitary. However, elevated prolactin levels, common in other causes of secondary amenorrhea (Bohnet et al, 1976), do not appear in anorexia nervosa. Rather, basal levels of prolactin are normal and their responses to dopamine blocking agents are also of a normal increase. The one abnormality of prolactin secretion is a flattening of the nocturnal rhythm; this is very likely related to dietary intake (Darby et al, 1983).

Growth hormone (GH) is characteristically elevated in starvation and returns to normal on refeeding (Garfinkel et al, 1975; Frankel and Jenkins, 1975). Para-doxical GH responses to glucose loading in some anorexic patients have been reported (Van der Laan et al, 1970; Casper et al, 1977) as well as to insulin-induced hypoglycemia. These revert to normal with weight restoration.

Amines and Peptides

Three-methoxy, 4 hydroxy-phenylglycol (MHPG) is one of the end products of norepinephrine (NE) metabolism and is believed to represent, at least in part, central nervous system catecholamine metabolism. Plasma NE concentrations and urinary excretion of the catecholamine metabolites MHPG and HVA are low in untreated patients with anorexia nervosa (Gross et al, 1979), suggesting reduced activity in both central and peripheral sympathetic nervous systems. The lowered levels of MHPG appear to be influenced by such factors as diet and exercise, and to be most closely related to levels of body fat (Johnson et al, in press). The reduced heart rate blood pressure, metabolic rate, and core body temperature may all partially relate to these abnormalities in sympathetic activity.

Plasma tryptophan is one of the factors regulating brain serotonin synthesis (Garfinkel and Coscina, 1982). Plasma tryptophan levels have been found to be lowered in anorexia nervosa by Coppen et al (1976). Recently Johnson et al (in press) confirmed this reduction and observed elevated plasma valine which would further reduce both brain tryptophan availability and serotonin synthesis.

Endogenous opiates are known to be increased in non-specific stress (Amir et al, 1980) and in starvation (Mandenhoff et al, 1982). It has been suggested that opiates may promote obesity in animals by both stimulating appetite and decreasing metabolic rate, and by lowering the set point for body temperature (Mandenhoff et al, 1982; Margules, 1979). Higher levels of endorphins might be expected in anorexia nervosa, and be weight related, as has been reported by Kaye et al (1982). This finding may be of some clinical relevance as it may be responsible for the intense hunger, food preoccupations and other food related behavior seen in anorexic and other starving people.

Defects in control of arginine vasopressin (AVP) secretion subsequent to star-vation may play a further role in some of the symptoms induced by starvation, especially those related to memory. Gold et al (1983) reported that emaciated anorexics had normal levels of AVP but that this hormone was being secreted independently of saline injections, and AVP levels were elevated in CSF relative to plasma.

PATHOGENESIS

There is no persuasive evidence that a single pathway leads to anorexia nervosa: A current view is of a multidimensional interactional model involving risk factors within the individual, the family, and the culture (Garfinkel and Garner, 1982).

Individual Predispositions

Psychodynamic theories may be considered as evolving through three historical phases. Initially Freud believed that impairment of the nutritional instinct depended on the individual's failure to master sexual excitation. Waller and colleagues (1940) modified this to suggest that the conflict represented "a wish to be impregnated through the mouth," with consequent starvation or compulsive eating. Clinical and research work has not borne out these findings. More recent developmental theorists have focused on various aspects of the mother-child relationship.

Bruch (1973) has been foremost in proposing defects in ego development during the first years of life that impair cognitive functioning. This may result in later difficulties in achieving personal autonomy and identity. Selvini-Palazzoli (1978) has taken a similar viewpoint and emphasized developmental problems based on faulty interaction with the mother. This has been further developed by Rizutto (1981), who has described "a disturbance in the sense of self . . . the beginning (of which is) located at the level of the mirroring phase, within which the mother is unable to see and reflect the child as itself." These theoretical concepts involving disturbances of self perception and personal helplessness correlate well to experimental measures of body image disturbance and psychopathology (see Chapter 26 of this volume, and Garfinkel, 1981, for a review).

Within the individual, theories of primary hypothalamic dysfunction, linked to neurotransmitter abnormalities, have been proposed (Barry and Klawans, 1976; Mawson 1974) but not substantiated.

Premorbid obesity may be a risk factor with biological, psychological, and sociocultural implications. It has been proposed that body weight is maintained around a "set point" or a regulated level and that this is under hypothalamic control (Nisbett, 1972). Bulimic patients have been shown to be premorbidly obese when compared to the general population or to restrictive anorexics (Garfinkel et al, 1980). This has prompted the theory of excess restraint and counter-regulation (Wardle, 1980; Herman and Polivy, 1975) to explain why some individuals who stray excessively from their "set weight" may rebound into bulimia. In addition, obesity may be associated with cultural undesirability and a personal sense of humiliation and failure, particularly in relation to psychosexual maturity.

The notion of a distinct personality type which predisposes to anorexia nervosa has been disputed by some (Morgan and Russell, 1975), while others (Bruch, 1973; Crisp, 1965; Halmi et al, 1977) have emphasized the compliant, perfectionist, dependent characteristics of many patients. For many people there seems to be an excessive reliance on external phenomena for maintaining their sense of self-worth. This makes them very vulnerable to familial, peer, and cultural influences. Different traits have been emphasized among patients in whom bulimia is also present (Russell, 1979; Garfinkel et al, 1980).

Familial Predispositions

There is limited evidence of a genetic factor increasing the risk of developing anorexia nervosa, based on the higher incidence among siblings and a four-to-five-fold difference in concordance rates between monozygotic and dizygotic twins (Askevold and Heiberg, 1979; Garfinkel and Garner, 1982). Others have reported a high incidence of affective disorder, phobic disorder, and alcohol abuse in these families (Cantwell, 1977; Kalucy, 1977; Piran et al, 1983).

Several others (in particular Minuchin et al, 1978, and Selvini-Palazzoli, 1970) have considered anorexia nervosa to be an expression of familial dysfunction, whereby pathological interactions may interfere with the development of autonomy. Garfinkel et al (1983) recently compared families with an anorexic member in Ireland and Canada, together with a nonanorexic matched control group of families. They found in both countries that families with an anorexic member perceived more problems in areas of performance expectations, role adaptability, style of communication, and expression of feelings. As with other studies in this area, it is impossible to conclude whether these effects relate to pathogenesis or whether they represent the sequelae of long-term illness in a family. These issues are more fully reviewed in Chapter 25, and by Rakoff (1983).

Cultural Predisposition

There is some evidence to link two cultural factors to the pathogenesis. These are: (1) the idealization of the thin female form and (2) pressures on women to achieve, often for others rather than for themselves. Garner and Garfinkel (1980) hypothesized that if pressure to be slim was a risk factor of the illness, anorexia nervosa would be more common in women who had to be slim because of career choice. They found an increased prevalence of the disorder in dance and modelling students. Moreover, the frequency of anorexia nervosa developing within dance settings varied greatly; anorexia nervosa was almost twice as common in those dance settings which were intensely achievement- and performance-oriented.

Factors which predispose an individual to the illness may be quite different from those which precipitate it or sustain it. Precipitating factors are varied and non-specific (Garfinkel and Garner, 1982). Generally they have in common the need for the individual to adapt to new circumstances and the resulting threats that these new circumstances produce. Factors that perpetuate the illness may vary widely. Common sustaining factors include the presence of the starvation syndrome, relying on vomiting as a means of controlling weight, the familial relationships that change with the illness, the person's social and vocational skills, and the failure to resolve the predisposing psychosocial conflicts.

ANOREXIA NERVOSA IN MALES

A number of studies have reported that five to ten percent of all cases of anorexia nervosa occur in males (Dally, 1969; Crisp and Toms, 1972; Hogan et al, 1974). This may represent an underestimate because of subjects' reluctance to come forward, and also because physicians are less likely to be aware of the condition in males. Following reports of increasing incidence of anorexia nervosa and bulimia in women, the occurrence of bulimia has also been noted recently in men (Gwirtsman et al, 1984).

In our series of 326 patients, 29 males were referred for evaluation between 1970 and 1983. Only 16 met *DSM-III* criteria (American Psychiatric Association, 1980) for anorexia nervosa: In six, the disorder was confined to caloric restriction, while ten also met *DSM-III* criteria for bulimia. The small sample size prevents direct comparison with the female group but, in the males, as with females, differences in frequency of vomiting, laxative abuse and premorbid obesity were seen in a comparison with bulimic and restrictive subgroups.

As with female subjects, most endocrine abnormalities occur secondary to weight loss, and include decreased gonadotrophins and testosterone levels (Beumont, 1972). Crisp et al (1982) and Andersen (1982) have reported that these hormones return to normal values with weight restoration, although such a rise may not always be complete (NcNab and Hawton 1981). Gender identity disturbances may occur in up to 50 percent of cases (Dally, 1969). There is also likely to be an association with affective disorder (Crisp and Toms, 1972). Reports that males are a more difficult group to treat, and carry a poorer prognosis, probably only reflect the relative lack of familiarity that even established eating disorder units have in the treatment of male patients. It will be of considerable interest to observe whether or not the current cultural emphasis on pursuit of fitness and weight control among men as well as women is followed by an increase in anorexia nervosa and bulimia among males.

MANAGEMENT

While individual treatment strategies may differ, there is general agreement among authors that weight restoration and establishment of normal eating patterns must accompany other interventions (Garfinkel and Garner, 1982). Admission to the hospital has the advantage of providing a supportive, controlled environment which at times may be life saving. On the other hand, it reinforces the view that the individual has to give up (at least temporarily) the control she has been trying to achieve. We will largely confine our discussion to inpatient therapies, since outpatient psychotherapies are covered more fully in Chapter 26.

Hospitalization

Less than 50 percent of our patients are admitted to hospitals. The indications for hospitalization of the anorexic patient include one or more of the following: rapid weight loss of greater than 30 percent within a six-month period; signs of severe loss of energy; evidence of marked electrolyte imbalance—hypokalemia less than 3.0 mEq/L or EKG changes, in spite of potassium supplements; a cycle of binge eating, vomiting, and restriction which cannot otherwise be broken.

A preadmission interview involving the patient and at times other family members is valuable. It emphasizes a team approach to treatment, allows for discussion of the program or any anticipated problems, and avoids daily negotiations about each and every detail of treatment. Naturally, the preadmission interview can be scheduled only for elective admissions. However, the team approach is useful, for all patients.

Following routine admission procedures, bedrest with supervised meals is instigated. During the first week a detailed assessment of the patient's psychological state and eating problems is completed; weight is recorded three times weekly. After this a program is presented where reinforcement may be contingent on weight gain, or eating behavior, or both.

A target weight is established, based primarily on the individual's own premorbid weight, except where it is apparent that such a weight was never reached. Patients start with bedrest activities of their choice. A consultation is obtained from the occupational therapist and patients may be involved in such activities as reading, craft work, or writing. Nursing staff are active in monitoring physical health, mental status, and supervising meals and encouraging the elimination of anorexia nervosa-related activities such as attempts to exercise, vomiting, or laxative or diuretic abuse. They also provide emotional support and encourage the appropriate expression of affect, rather than allowing the patient to deal with unpleasant feelings through behavior. The dietitian's role is to encourage a normal eating pattern by providing a balanced diet as recommended by Canada's Food Guide. The avoidance of refined and staple carbohydrates such as breads, cereals, and potatoes and red meats is considered part of anorexic restriction and is not permitted. While some programs have recommended a substantial calorie intake—4,000-5,000 calories per day right from the start (Dally and Gomez, 1979)—we favor a more gradual increase, starting at 1,500 calories per day and increasing in increments of 300 calories as required (Garfinkel and Garner, 1982; Lucas et al, 1976). Weight gain of 1–2 kg weekly is considered adequate, and attempts to gain weight more rapidly as a way of bringing forward the discharge time generally represents poor motivation for subsequent psychological change.

PSYCHOLOGICAL MANAGEMENT. Opinions are divided about the role of behavioral strategies. Bruch (1974) considered them "potentially . . . dangerous methods" while others have claimed more rapid weight gain where operant conditioning is compared to psychotherapy (Wulliemier et al, 1975). Garfinkel and Garner (1982) concluded that "most patients gain weight with this treatment (behavioral methods) and that while not proving harmful, there is no evidence to suggest that it is superior to other conventional therapies in the long run." Most treatment programs utilize some principles of behavior modification, for example by rewarding weight gain with time out of bed. However, these may be preferred to more formal behavioral programs with contracts, as endless time can be spent negotiating every detail of the reward system, to the detriment of other psychological treatment. In the majority of patients a reward system based on increasing activities with weight gain works well. In a minority, however, these are not reinforcers of behavioral change. The patient may be profoundly depressed and need specific antidepressant treatment before further changes are possible.

Individual psychotherapy may be more appropriately supportive in some instances and interpretive in others, depending on the individual's ego strength, self-reflective capacities and interest in psychotherapeutic work. Individual psychotherapy may be started in the hospital and continue following discharge. Recurrent themes deal with separation—individuation and the search for a healthy autonomy. Important issues frequently relate to recognition and appropriate expression of affects and enhancement of self-esteem independent of appearance (Bruch, 1973; Garfinkel and Garner, 1982). Principles of cognitive therapies are also valuable when incorporated into the psychotherapy of anorexia nervosa as described elsewhere in detail (Garner and Bemis, 1982). This area is more extensively reviewed in Chapter 26 of this volume.

In a younger patient population (16 or less and living at home), family therapy using a "systems" approach has been considered the treatment of choice (Minuchin et al, 1978; Selvini-Palazzoli, 1978). Work with the family is initiated during hospitalization, but continues as part of ongoing treatment following discharge. In older patients, family therapy may be an integral part of treatments involving marital therapy as well as therapy with the family of origin. The principles stated by Hedblom et al (1982), though not restricted to anorexia nervosa families, are worth restating: "Approach families in a nonblaming way; assume families have done their best; recognize that families are tired from stress; assume families want help." Family therapy is described in greater detail in Chapter 25 of this volume.

Some patients benefit from group therapy. This should be instituted where the starvation symptoms have begun to be reduced (Hedblom et al, 1982). Group therapies are best considered as an adjunct to individual and family therapies (Polivy, 1981) and should deal with practical issues related to improving interpersonal skills. Groups of inpatients, outpatients, and some which combine both have been utilized. The danger of fostering the "anorexic identity" in group settings must be avoided.

The behavioral, individual, family, and group psychotherapy aspects of treatment are often combined during both hospital and outpatient treatment. How they are combined, and the relationship of the various personnel involved in the treatment, varies from center to center. In some settings, a single clinician conducts, or at least coordinates, all aspects of care. In others, various aspects of the treatment plan are delegated to colleagues whose training provides the additional expertise not always available in a single clinician. Which options are selected and how they are combined depends upon the specifics of the case, and the patient's and family's own attitudes—their cooperativeness and ability to participate in various forms of treatment are of paramount importance. Whenever a large number of therapists are involved in treatment, it is essential that coordinated treatment planning occur and that frequent communication take place among those involved, so that splitting by the patient, and operations at crossed purposes by professionals, are minimized.

On an inpatient unit special difficulties may arise. These may relate to the psychological problems of the individual patient, the family, or to staff attitudes. These have been described in detail elsewhere (Garfinkel et al, in press).

PHARMACOTHERAPIES. While a series of drug treatments have been advocated in recent years, there is no established pharmacotherapy for anorexia nervosa. Most reports are of small case series or uncontrolled trials. Although appetite is generally not reduced (Garfinkel, 1974), insulin was formerly recommended in view of its appetite stimulant properties (Wall, 1959). Its use is not warranted. Chlorpromazine was advocated as a mainstay of hospital treatment (Dally and Sargant, 1960; Crisp, 1965), both because of its tranquilizing and appetite enhancing effects. Other neuroleptics have been used. Riding and Munro (1975) reported specific indications for pimozide in treating hypochondriacal monosymptomatic psychosis. This led others (Plantey, 1977; Hoes, 1980) to compare the apparent clinical similarities of anorexia nervosa to this syndrome, and to report on individual responses of anorexic patients to pimozide, which was also considered to have a role in the treatment of anorexia nervosa on neurochemical grounds. Barry and Klawans (1976) postulated that an overactive dopaminergic system could account for major symptoms in anorexia nervosa. Pimozide is thought to act as a selective dopamine blockade (Pinder et al, 1976). Vandereycken and Pierloot (1983) reported in a double blind placebo controlled study that pimozide had a modest effect on weight gain and attitudinal dimensions. Bromocriptine, in contrast, is a dopaminergic agent which was used by Harrower (1978) in an uncontrolled study, on the basis that it would reduce elevated prolactin production. No significant improvement was reported. Cyproheptadine, also an appetite stimulant and a 5-HT antagonist, has been evaluated in a multicenter, multitreatment trial involving the drug and placebo, with and without behavior therapy (Goldberg et al, 1979). Again, results showed only modest benefit in inducing weight gain.

Antiepileptic drugs have also been tried. Green and Rau (1974) initially reported clinical improvement in nine out of ten severe binge eaters on diphenylhydantoin (Phenytoin). This led to the hypothesis that a subgroup of anorexics may have abnormal EEG findings and has more recently been extended to include a trial of carbamazepine for patients with bulimia (Kaplan et al, 1983). The exact role of antiseizure medications has not yet been clarified.

For brief periods of treatment on an inpatient unit, anxiolytics have several advantages over neuroleptics. They have anticonvulsant properties rather than the effect of lowering the seizure threshold. They are less hypotensive and do not aggravate hypothermia. Their disadvantage is the risk of dependency, which may be of most concern in patients who are bulimic. When severe anxiety symptoms limit further treatment progress, we have found it beneficial to prescribe small amounts of short acting benzodiazepines (for example, oxazepam 15 mg or alprazolam 0.25 mg) before meals.

In view of the similarities described between anorexia nervosa and affective disorder, it is not surprising that antidepressant drugs have been advocated. Needleman and Waber (1976) reported weight gain and mood improvement with amitriptyline in six pediatric patients. Paykel et al (1973) have, however, noted carbohydrate craving with this drug in a nonanorexic population, so that there may be a significant risk of precipitating bulimia in some anorexics. Lacey and Crisp (1980) reported on a double blind controlled trial of clomipramine, but the dose was limited to 50 mg per day.

Whereas the use of antidepressant medication for some patients with bulimia has received some support (see Chapter 24, by Drs. James Mitchell, Richard Pyle, and Elke Eckert, in this volume), the contribution that such medication can make to the treatment of patients with bulimia in the context of anorexia nervosa is still uncertain.

Following the rationale that weight gain occurs as a side effect of lithium carbonate in nonanorexic patients, Gross et al (1981) reported on a double blind controlled study of 16 anorexic patients in which significant weight gain occurred. However, there are severe risks of lithium intoxication in this population where dieting, vomiting, laxative misuse, and sodium restriction may occur. A recent report (Moore et al 1981) suggests naloxone, an endorphin antagonist, may produce weight gain in anorexic patients by virtue of its antilipolytic effect.

MANAGEMENT AFTER DISCHARGE FROM HOSPITAL

It is probably most appropriate to consider hospitalization as one intervention along the road to recovery and not, in itself, a means of recovery. Provided this is clearly explained during inpatient treatment, subsequent alarm and disappointment may be avoided if setbacks occur after discharge.

Some form of individual psychotherapy is generally regarded as the mainstay of longer-term treatment of anorexia nervosa (Crisp, 1965; Dally and Gomez, 1979; Garfinkel and Garner, 1982), although outcome studies involving controlled comparisons of different treatment regimens have not yet been reported.

While there is a need for the therapist to be flexible in his therapeutic approach, certain general principles can be applied. First, weight- and food-related issues should not be divorced entirely from psychological aspects of therapy. Some therapists address this issue by having a colleague assume responsibility for physical care. We prefer a single therapy in which both aspects of treatment are acknowledged. It is unlikely that the patient will feel entirely comfortable with either her weight or the dietary regimen she followed while in the hospital. She may only be partially aware of cues such as hunger or satiety, and this realization may trigger earlier feelings of losing control, becoming "fat" and "failing totally." A realistic approach is to recognize these issues while urging that, for now at least, she should follow the external cues for meal planning and eating; her fear that uncontrollable weight gain will follow should be challenged. This is possible when a successful therapeutic alliance has been established. The therapist should agree that, if weight gain beyond the target range occurs, treatment involving dietary counselling will be instigated in the same way as when weight loss occurred. Reassurance can be given that individuals who have not been premorbidly obese rarely overshoot their restored weight. As the relationship between patient and therapist develops, the temptation to settle for a lower target weight should be avoided. Such compromise may well result in a breakdown in therapeutic confidence, a repetition of the parental struggles, and relapse of the illness.

The second principle relates to the underlying belief held by many anorexics that the therapist is only interested in the battle for control of attitudes to weight and dieting. Although weight gain has taken place in the hospital, return of menses may occur as an outpatient. This is often symbolically a critical time. One patient recently commented, in a state of distress at this time, "I'm not the child I was before and I don't feel like the woman I'm supposed to be." Such issues allow the therapist to demonstrate an interest in the patient which goes beyond weight gain and thus challenges the inner sense of worthlessness. Arieti's model for depressed patients (Arieti 1962) may be similarly applied in the therapeutic relationship with an anorexic patient. The patient has previously lived and sought approval from an external source, "the dominant other," or by struggling to achieve the "dominant goal"—body control through starvation. This has inevitably produced a sense of failure and worthlessness that may be addressed by the therapist in assuming the position of a "dominant third"—

that is, an important figure who no longer permits such a struggle for acceptance. During therapy this role becomes more of a "significant third" who supports the development of a healthy autonomous individual.

The third, and perhaps most difficult, aspect of long-term treatment relates to alternatives to anorexia nervosa. Not all patients in treatment have decided to give up the "anorexic solution" to conflicts and interpersonal difficulties. For such individuals, it is often necessary to clarify that treatment can only be supportive and crisis oriented. For those who are committed to the abandonment of anorexia nervosa, affective symptoms may more appropriately be experienced. These can be frightening if not appropriately recognized and may, in rare cases, be followed by self-harm as a mark of feeling out of control.

If weight and food preoccupations no longer occupy the majority of an individual's waking hours, what fills the vacuum? Apart from weight loss, anorexic patients can recall few sources of pleasure. Previous hobbies or activities have often been abandoned because of the inability to achieve total perfection. A return to such nonanorexic activities should be encouraged. The artist who returns to painting after several years of inactivity may be following a successful course. For others, the development of new hobbies and career goals may be essential. Activities that provide support for anorexic behavior may no longer be possible—for example, recovering anorexics should not return to such jobs as aerobics teachers or models.

Recent reports suggest benefits from combining individual, behavioral, family, and drug therapies (Geller, 1975; Parker et al, 1977; Hersen and Detre, 1980), and this makes empirical sense. This can be extended to include couple therapy where the patient is involved in a significant relationship, as well as other forms of group therapy, which on an outpatient basis may include self-help and relative support groups (Polivy and Garfinkel, 1984).

For some individuals, a first hospitalization may have been unsuccessful or only partially successful. Discharge may have been precipitous, or the individual may have eaten merely to reach a target weight. In such cases outpatient therapy may be an essential preparation for readmission. We have seen many individuals realize the benefits of earlier hospitalizations only after several admissions and dedicated and persistent outpatient management. If this is borne in mind, the patient may avoid strong feelings of "letting the therapist down" and being "a failure yet again," should relapse occur.

MEDICAL COMPLICATIONS

Despite advances in the understanding of anorexia nervosa, the condition is still associated with significant morbidity and mortality (Garfinkel and Garner, 1982). The most common medical complications involve disturbance of electrolyte balance and cardiac and gastrointestinal functions, although abnormalities may occur in virtually every system in the body.

Electrolyte Disturbances

Potassium depletion is the most frequent serious problem, occurring in up to one-third of patients where vomiting also occurs (Elkington and Huth, 1959). This danger intensifies when patients use several methods simultaneously to reduce weight, such as starvation, vomiting, and diuretic or laxative misuse. When death occurs, it is most likely to be due to cardiac arrest. Cardiac arrhythmia and tetany may also occur (Garfinkel and Garner, 1982).

When potassium supplements are given to maintain the plasma level above 3.0 mEq/liter, especially on an out patient basis, care must be taken that the patient does not "forget" for several days and then "overdose" on the day of testing. Recently, Russell et al (1983) have reported on total body potassium and nitrogen depletion in anorexic patients, which appears to be related to impaired skeletal muscle function.

Cardiac Irregularities

Electrocardiographic changes have been reported in up to 60 percent of patients (Garfinkel and Garner, 1982). These include sinus bradycardia, low amplitude, T wave inversion, and atrioventricular block, and are similar to the findings reported in nonanorexic starvation (Keys et al, 1950). A small number of patients regularly ingest emetine-containing emetics (such as Ipecac) to induce vomiting after eating. Emetine is a muscle poison. This practice may result in a peripheral or cardiomyopathy and has on occasion proved fatal (Brotman et al, 1981).

Gastrointestinal Problems

Gastrointestinal disturbances are common and may limit weight gain. The subjective sensation of early satiety and gastric discomfort has been correlated with objective measures of delayed gastric emptying (Holt et al, 1981) and has prompted the evaluation of domperidone, a drug with gastrokinetic properties, in treating this aspect of the disorder (Russell et al, 1983). Gastric dilatation and perforation have been reported (Browning, 1977) following rapid refeeding of starving patients, and may be avoided by gradual and controlled calorie increases. In rare cases a paralytic ileus may develop, particularly when phenothiazines are used in high doses. A nonpainful enlargement of the parotid glands occurs commonly in bulimia and is associated with elevations of the serum amylase.

Other Medical Complications

Reduced glomerular filtration rates occur in anorexia nervosa and in obese individuals who fast (Edgren and Wester, 1971). Neurological complications include: convulsions, peripheral neuropathy, and cerebral atrophy. Hematological abnormalities include: normochromic, normocytic anemia, and bone marrow hypoplasia, together with a leukopenia and thrombocytopenia. The most encouraging aspect of these complications is that, with careful refeeding, they virtually all disappear.

COURSE AND OUTCOME

Recent reviews (Hsu et al, 1980; Schwartz and Thompson, 1981; Garfinkel and Garner, 1982) have emphasized serious methodological problems which have limited the value of outcome studies that have been conducted to date. Nevertheless, there is consistency in the findings that have been reported from different centers. These studies have documented the extremely variable course of the disorder. Overall, about 40 percent of patients are asymptomatic at follow-up about 5.8 years later, while 30 percent are significantly improved. However, about 20 percent remain actively symptomatic and about nine percent have died. Several recent larger studies have shown a reduced mortality to about 5 percent (Morgan and Russell, 1975; Hsu et al, 1980).

Two studies have examined the patient's mental state at follow-up: Cantwell et al (1977) reported the presence of primary affective disorder in over 40 percent of their patients; Stonehill and Crisp (1977) noted that biologically recovered anorexics were, as a group, more socially phobic four years later.

The duration of follow-up from time of treatment may account for significant differences in outcome. Vandereycken and Pierloot (1983) noted substantial improvements in the group followed for more than two years as compared to those followed for less than two years. The duration of illness in those who do eventually recover can be quite variable. While weight stabilization can occur relatively soon after weight gain, it may take several years for all symptoms to abate. Some patients stabilize in weight and eating habits but have a recurrence one or more years later. Theander (1970) reported this in 11 out of 94 patients in a long term follow-up.

A series of factors related to prognosis have been described (Crisp et al, 1977; Bemis, 1978). Earlier age of onset (less than 17 years) is associated with a higher rate of recovery (Theander, 1970; Morgan and Russell, 1975). Some clinical features are associated with a poor outcome: premorbid obesity, bulimia, vomiting, and laxative misuse (Garfinkel and Garner, 1982). The patient's educational, vocational, and social adjustment premorbidly are also important (Garfinkel et al, 1977). Some marriages may carry a bad prognosis in that they may represent an attempt to meet "the powerful neurotic needs of both partners" (Hsu et al, 1979; Crisp et al, 1977).

CONCLUSION

Anorexia nervosa is a complex, multidimensional group of disorders whose origins are incompletely understood. While social and cultural pressures have been implicated in explaining the increasing prevalence of these disorders, contributions to pathogenesis from individual and family psychopathology and from biological factors, as well, appear to be important. Treatment requires attention to the state of nutrition, often in a hospital setting, and to the individual's psychological and family factors that may sustain the disorder. No specific treatments, either psychological or biological, have yet been described that conclusively benefit long-term prognosis.

REFERENCES

American Psychiatric Association: Diagnostic and Statistical Manual of Mental Disorders, 3rd ed. Washington, D.C., American Psychiatric Association, 1980

Amir S, Brown ZW, Amit A: The role of endorphins in stress: evidence and speculations. Neurosci Biobehav Rev 4:77–91, 1980

Andersen AE, Wirth JB, Stralilam ER: Reversible weight-related increase in plasma testosterone during treatment of male and female patients with anorexia nervosa. International Journal of Eating Disorders 1:74–83, 1982

Arieti S: The psychotherapeutic approach to depression. Am J Psychother 16:397–406, 1962

Askevold F, Heiberg A: Anorexia nervosa—two cases in discordant MZ twins. Psychother Psychosom 32:223–228, 1979

Ballot NS, Delaney NE, Erskine PJ, et al: Anorexia nervosa—a prevalence study. South African Medical Journal 59:992–993, 1981

Barry VC, Klawans HL: On the role of dopamine in the pathophysiology of anorexia nervosa. J Neural Transm 38:107–122, 1976

Beck JC, Brochner-Mortensen K: Observations on the prognosis in anorexia nervosa. Acta Med Scand 149:409–430, 1954

Bemis KM: Current approaches to the etiology and treatment of anorexia nervosa. Psychol Bull 85:593–617, 1978

Beumont PJV, Beardwood CF, Russell GFM: The occurrence of the syndrome of anorexia nervosa in male subjects. Psychol Med 2:216–231, 1972

Beumont PJV, Carr PJ, Gelder MG: Plasma levels of luteinizing hormone and of immunoreactive oestrogens (oestradiol) in anorexia nervosa: response to clomiphene citrate. Psychol Med 3:495–501, 1973

Bohnet HG, Dahlen HG, Wuttke W, et al: Hyperprolactinemic anovulatory syndrome. J Clin Endocrinol Metab 42:132–143, 1976

Boskind-Lodahl M: Cinderella's stepsisters: a feminist perspective on anorexia nervosa and bulimia. Signs: Journal of Women in Culture and Society 2:342–356, 1976

Boyar RM, Katz J, Finkelstein JW, et al: Anorexia nervosa: immaturity of the 24-hour luteinizing hormone secretory pattern. N Engl J Med 291:861–865, 1974

Boyar RM, Hellman LD, Roffwarg H, et al: Cortisol secretion and metabolism in anorexia nervosa. N Engl J Med 296:190–193, 1977

Brincat M, Parsons V, Studd J: Anorexia nervosa. Br Med J 287:1306, 1983

Brown GM, Garfinkel PE, Jeuniewic N, et al: Endocrine profiles in anorexia nervosa, in Anorexia Nervosa. Edited by Vigersky R. New York, Raven Press, 1977

Browning CH: Anorexia nervosa: complications of somatic therapy. Compr Psychiatry 18:399–403, 1977

Brotman MC, Forbath N, Garfinkel PE, et al: Ipecac syrup poisoning in anorexia nervosa. Can Med Assoc J 125:453–454, 1981

Bruch H: Perceptual and conceptual disturbances in anorexia nervosa. Psychosom Med 24:187–194, 1962

Bruch H: The psychiatric differential diagnosis of anorexia nervosa, in Symposium on anorexia nervosa, Gottingen. Edited by Meyer JE, Feldmann H. Stuttgart, Thieme Verlag, 1965

Bruch H: Changing approaches to anorexia nervosa, in Anorexia and Obesity. Edited by Rowland C. Boston, Little, Brown & Co., 1970a

Bruch H: Instinct and interpersonal experience. Compr Psychiatry II:495-506, 1970b

Bruch H: Eating Disorders. New York, Basic Books, 1973

Bruch H: Perils of behavior modification in treatment of anorexia nervosa. JAMA 230:1419–1422, 1974

Button EJ, Whitehouse A: Subclinical anorexia nervosa. Psychol Med II:509–516, 1981

Cantwell, DP, Sturzenberger S, Burroughs J, et al: Anorexia nervosa: an affective disorder? Arch Gen Psychiatry 34:1087–1093, 1977

Casper RC, Davis JM, Ghanshyam NP: The effect of the nutritional status and weight changes on hypothalamic function tests in anorexia nervosa, in Anorexia Nervosa. Edited by Vigersky RA. New York, Raven Press, 1977

Chopra IJ, Smith SR: Circulating thyroid hormones and thyrotropin in adult patients with protein-calorie malnutrition. J Clin Endocrinol Metab 40:221–227, 1975

Coppen AM, Gupta RK, Eccleston ZG, et al: (Letter) Plasma tryptophan in anorexia nervosa. Lancet 1:961, 1976

Crilly RG, Francis RM, Nordin BEC: Steroid hormones, ageing and bone. Clin Endocrinol Metab 10:115–139, 1981

Crisp AH: Clinical and therapeutic aspects of anorexia nervosa: a study of 30 cases. J Psychosom Res 9:67–68, 1965a

Crisp AH: A treatment of anorexia nervosa. Br J Psychiatry 112:505–512, 1965b

Crisp AH: Anorexia nervosa: "feeding disorder," "nervous malnutrition," or "weight phobia?" Review of Nutrition and Dietetics 12:452–504, 1970

Crisp AH, Stonehill E: Aspects of the relationship between psychiatric status, sleep, nocturnal motility and nutrition. J Psychosom Res 15:501–509, 1971

Crisp AH, Toms DA: Primary anorexia nervosa or weight phobia in the male: report on 13 cases. Br Med J 1:334–338, 1972

Crisp AH, Stonehill E, Fenton GW: The relationship between sleep, nutrition, and mood: a study of patients with anorexia nervosa. Postgrad Med J 47:207–213, 1971

Crisp AH, Palmer RL, Kalucy RS: How common is anorexia nervosa? Br J Psychiatry 128:549–554, 1976

Crisp AH, Kalucy RS, Lacey JH, et al: The long-term prognosis in anorexia nervosa: some factors predictive of outcome, in Anorexia Nervosa. Edited by Vigersky R. New York, Raven Press, 1977

Crisp AH, Hsu LKG, Chen CN: Reproductive hormone profiles in male anorexia nervosa, before, during and after weight restoration of body weight to normal: a study of twelve patients. International Journal of Eating Disorders 1:3–9, 1982

Dally P: Anorexia Nervosa. New York, Grune and Stratton, 1969

Dally P, Sargant W: A new treatment of anorexia nervosa. Br Med J 1:1770–1773, 1960

Dally P, Gomez J: Anorexia Nervosa. London, Heinemann Medical Books, 1979

Darby PL, Brown GM, Garfinkel PE: Circadian patterning of prolactin in anorexia nervosa, in Anorexia Nervosa: Recent Developments in Research. Edited by Darby PL, Garfinkel PE, Garner DM, et al. New York, 65–82, 1983

Donovan BT, Van Der Werfften Bosch JJ: Physiology of Puberty: Monographs of the Physiological Society. London, Edward Arnold, 1965

Edgren B, Wester PO: Impairment of glomerular filtration in fasting or obesity. Acta Med Scand 190:389–393, 1971

Elkington JR, Huth EJ: Body fluid abnormalities in anorexia nervosa and undernutrition. Metabolism 8:376–403, 1959

Feighner JP, Robins E, Guze SB, et al: Diagnostic criteria for use in psychiatric research. Arch Gen Psychiatry 26:57–63, 1972

Fenwick S: On atrophy of the stomach and on the nervous affections of the digestive organs. London, Churchill, 1880

Frankel RJ, Jenkins JS: Hypothalamic pituitary function anorexia nervosa. Acta Endocrinologica (Copenh) 78:209–221, 1975

Frisch RE: Food intake, fatness and reproductive ability, in Anorexia Nervosa. Edited by Vigersky RA. New York, Raven Press, 1977

Frisch RE, McArthur JW: Menstrual cycles: fatness as a determinant of minimum weight for height necessary for their maintenance for onset. Science 185:949–951, 1974

Garfinkel PE: Perception of hunger and satiety in anorexia nervosa. Psychol Med 4:309–315, 1974

Garfinkel PE, Coscina DV: The biology and psychology of hunger and satiety, in Eating, Sleeping and Sexuality: Treatment for Disorders of Basic Functions. Edited by Zales MR. New York, Brunner/Mazel, 1982

Garfinkel PE, Garner DM: Anorexia Nervosa, a Multidimensional Perspective. New York, Brunner/Mazel, 1982

Garfinkel PE, Brown GM, Stancer HC, et al: Hypothalamic pituitary function in anorexia nervosa. Arch Gen Psychiatry 32:739–744, 1975

Garfinkel PE, Moldofsky H, Garner DM: The outcome of anorexia nervosa: significance of clinical features, body image and behavior modification, in Anorexia Nervosa. Edited by Vigersky R. New York, Raven Press, 1977

Garfinkel PE, Moldofsky H, Garner DM: The heterogeneity of anorexia nervosa: bulimia as a distinct subgroup. Arch Gen Psychiatry 37:1036–1040, 1980

Garfinkel PE, Garner DM, Rose J, et al: A comparison of characteristics in families of patients with anorexia nervosa and normal controls. Psychol Med 13:821–828, 1983a

Garfinkel PE, Garner DM, Kaplan NAS, et al: Differential diagnosis of emotional disorders that cause weight loss. Can Med Assoc J 129:939–945, 1983b

Garfinkel PE, Garner DM, Kennedy S: Special problems in in-patient management, in Handbook for Treatment of Anorexia Nervosa and Bulimia. Edited by Garner DM and Garfinkel PE. New York, Guilford Press, in press

Garner DM, Bemis K: A cognitive-behavioral approach to anorexia nervosa. Cognitive Therapy and Research 6:1–27, 1982

Garner DM, Garfinkel PE: Sociocultural factors in the development of anorexia nervosa. Psychol Med 10:647–656, 1980

Garner DM, Garfinkel PE: Body image in anorexia nervosa: measurement, theory and clinical implications. In J Psychiatry Med II:263–284, 1981

Garner DM, Olmsted MP, Garfinkel PE: Does anorexia nervosa occur on a continuum? Subgroup of weight-preoccupied women and their relationship to anorexia nervosa. International Journal of Eating Disorders 2:11–20, 1983

Garner DM, Garfinkel PE, O'Shaughnessy M: Validity of the distinction between bulimia with and without anorexia nervosa. Am J Psychiatry, in press

Geller JL: Treatment of anorexia nervosa by the integration of behaviour therapy and psychotherapy. Psychother Psychosom 26:167–179, 1975

Gerner RH, Gwirtsman HE: Abnormalities of dexamethasone suppression test and urinary MHPG in anorexia nervosa. Am J Psychiatry 138:650–653, 1981

Gold PW, Kaye W, Robertson GL, et al: Abnormalities in plasma and cerebral spinal–fluid arginine vasopressin in patients with anorexia nervosa. N Eng J Med 308:1117–1123, 1983

Goldberg SC, Halmi KA, Eckert E, et al: Cyproheptadine in anorexia nervosa. Br J Psychiatry 134:67–70, 1979

Green RS, Rau JH: Treatment of compulsive eating disturbances with anticonvulsant medication. Am J Psychiatry 131:428–432, 1974

Gross HA, Lake CR, Ebert MH, et al: Catecholamine metabolism in primary anorexia nervosa. J Clin Endocrinol Metab 49:805–809, 1979

Gross HA, Ebert MH, et al: A double blind controlled trial of lithium carbonate in primary anorexia nervosa. J Clin Psychopharmacol 1:376–381, 1981

Gull WW: Anorexia nervosa. Transactions of the Clinical Society (London) 7:22–28, 1874. Reprinted in Anorexia Nervosa: a Paradigm. Edited by Kaufman RM and Heiman M. New York, International Universities Press, 1964

Gwirtsman HE, Roy-Byrne P, Lerner L, et al: Bulimia in men: report of three cases with neuroendocrine findings. J Clin Psychiatry 45:78–81, 1984

Halmi KA, Goldberg SC, Eckert E, et al: Pretreatment evaluation in anorexia nervosa, in Anorexia Nervosa. Edited by Vigersky R. New York, Raven Press, 1977

Harrower ADB: Bromocriptine in anorexia nervosa. Br J Hosp Med 672–675, 1978

Hedblom JE, Hubbard FA, Andersen AE: Anorexia nervosa: multidisciplinary treatment program for patient and family. Social Work in Health Care 7:67–83, 1982

Herman CP, Polivy J: Anxiety, restraint and eating behaviour. J Personality 84:666–672, 1975

Hersen M, Detre T: The behavioural psychotherapy of anorexia nervosa, in Specialized

Techniques in Individual Psychotherapy. Edited by Karasu TB and Bellak L. New York, Brunner/Mazel, 1980

Hobhouse N: Discussion of paper by Grace Nicolle on prepsychotic anorexia. Proceedings of the Royal Society of Medicine 32:153–162, 1938

Hoes MJ: Copper sulfate and pimozide for anorexia nervosa. Journal of Orthomolecular Psychiatry 9:48–51, 1980

Hogan WM, Huerta E, Lucas AR: Diagnosing anorexia nervosa in males. Psychosomatics 15:122–126, 1974

Holt S, Ford MJ, Grant S, et al: Abnormal gastric emptying in primary anorexia nervosa. Br J Psychiatry 139:550–552, 1982

Hsu LKG: Outcome of anorexia nervosa: a review of the literature (1954–1978). Arch Gen Psychiatry 37:1041–1046, 1980

Hsu LKG, Crisp AH, Harding B: Outcome of anorexia nervosa. Lancet 1:61–65, 1979

Hurd HP, Palumbo PJ, Gharid H: Hypothalamic-endocrine dysfunction in anorexia nervosa. Mayo Clin Proc 52:711–716, 1977

Hurst PS, Lacey JH, Crisp AH: Teeth, vomiting and diet: a study of the dental characteristics of seventeen anorexia nervosa patients. Postgrad Med J 53:298–305, 1977

Jeuniewic H, Brown GM, Garfinkel P, et al: Hypothalamic function as related to body weight and body fat in anorexia nervosa. Psychosom Med 40:187–198, 1978

Johnson JL, Lieter LA, Burrow GN, et al: Excretion of urinary catecholamines in anorexia nervosa: effects of body composition and energy intake. Am J Clin Nutr, in press

Jones DJ, Fox MM, Babigian HM, et al: Epidemiology of anorexia nervosa in Monroe County, New York, 1960–1976. Psychosom Med 42:551–558, 1980

Kalucy RS, Crisp AH, Harding B: A study of 56 families with anorexia nervosa. Br J Med Psychol 50:381–395, 1977

Kaplan AS, Garfinkel PE, Darby PL, et al: Carbamazepine in the treatment of bulimia. Am J Psychiatry 140:1225–1227, 1983

Kaye WH, Pickar D, Naber D, et al: Cerebral spinal fluid opioid activity in anorexia nervosa. Am J Psychiatry 139:643–645, 1982

Kellet J, Trimble M, Thorley A: Anorexia nervosa after the menopause. Br J Psychiatry 128:555–558, 1976

Kendell, RE, Hall DJ, Hailey A, et al: The epidemiology of anorexia nervosa. Psychol Med 3:200–203, 1973

Keys A, Brozek J, Henschel A, et al: The Biology of Human Starvation. Minneapolis, University of Minnesota Press, 1950

King A: Primary and secondary anorexia nervosa syndrome. Br J Psychiatry 109:470–474, 1963

Lacey JH, Crisp AH: Hunger, food and weight: the impact of clomipramine on refeeding an anorexia nervosa population. Postgrad Med J 56:79–85 Suppl 1, 1980

Lesègue C: De l'anorexic hysterique. Arch Gen de Med 385, 1873. Reprinted in Evolution of Psychosomatic Concepts. Anorexia Nervosa: A Paradigm. Edited by Kaufman RM and Heiman M. New York, International Universities Press, 1964

Lucas AR, Duncan JW, Piens V: The treatment of anorexia nervosa. Am J Psychiatry 133:1034–1038, 1976

Lundberg PO, Walinder J, Werner I, et al: Effects of thyrotropin-releasing hormone on plasma levels of TSH, FSH, LH and GH in anorexia nervosa. Eur J Clin Invest 2:150–153, 1972

McNab D, Hawton K: Disturbances of sex hormones in anorexia nervosa in the male. Postgrad Med J 57:254–256, 1981

Mandenhoff A, Fumeron F, Apfelbaum M, et al: Endogenous opiates and energy balance. Science 215:1536–1538, 1982

Margules DL: Beta-endorphin and endoloxone: hormones of the autonomic nervous system for the conservation of expenditure of bodily resources and energy in anticipation of famine or feast. Neurosci Biobehav Rev 3:155–162, 1979

Marshall JC, Fraser TR: Amenorrhoea in anorexia nervosa: assessment and treatment with clomiphene citrate. Br Med J 4:590–592, 1971

Mawson AR: Anorexia nervosa and the regulation of intake: a review. Psychol Med 4:289–308, 1974

Minuchin S, Baker L, Rossman BL, et al: Arch Gen Psychiatry 32:1031–1038, 1975

Minuchin S, Rosman BL, Baker L: Psychosomatic families: anorexia nervosa in context. Cambridge, Harvard University Press, 1978

Miyai K, Yamamoto T, Azukizawa M, et al: Serum thyroid hormones and thyrotropin in anorexia nervosa. J Clin Endocrinol Metab 40:334–338, 1975

Morgan HG, Russell GFM: Value of family background and clinical features as predictors of long term outcome in anorexia nervosa: four-year follow up of 41 patients. Psychol Med 5:355–371, 1975

Moore R, Mills IH, Forster A: Naloxone in the treatment of anorexia nervosa: effect on weight gain and lipolysis. Journal of the Royal Society of Medicine 74:129–131, 1981

Needleman HL, Waber D (Letter): Amitriptyline therapy in patients with anorexia nervosa. Lancet 2:580, 1976

Nicolle G: Prepsychotic anorexia. Proceedings of the Royal Society of Medicine 32:153–162, 1939

Nylander I: The feeling of being fat and dieting in a school population: an epidemiologic interview investigation. Acta Socio-medica Scandinavica 3:17–26, 1971

Nisbett RE: Hunger, obesity and the venteromedial hypothalamus. Psychol Rev 79:433–453, 1972

Palmer HD, Jones MS: Anorexia nervosa as a manifestation of compulsive neurosis. Archives of Neurology and Psychopathology 41:856–860, 1939

Palmer RL: The dietary chaos syndrome: a useful new term? Br J Med Psychol 52:187–190, 1979

Parker JB, Blazer D, Wyrick L: Anorexia nervosa: a combined therapeutic approach. Southern Medical Journal 70:448–52, 1977

Parsons V, Szmukler G, Brown SJ: Fracturing osteoporosis in young women with anorexia nervosa. Calcif Tissue Int 35:Suppl A 72, 1983

Paykel ES, Mueller PS, De La Vergne P: Amitriptyline, weight gain and carbohydrate craving: a side effect. Br J Psychiatry 123:501–507, 1973

Pinder RN, Brogden RN, Sawyer PR, et al: Pimozide: a review of its pharmacological properties and therapeutic uses in psychiatry. Drugs 12:1–40, 1976

Piran, N, Kennedy S, Owens M, et al: The presence of affective disorder in patients with anorexia nervosa and bulimia. Abstr 97:133–134, presented at the 33rd Annual Meeting of the Canadian Psychiatric Association, Ottawa, September 1983

Plantey F (Letter): Pimozide in treatment of anorexia nervosa. Lancet 1:1105, 1977

Polivy J: Group therapy for anorexia nervosa. J Psychiatr Res 3:279–283, 1981

Polivy J, Garfinkel PE: Anorexia Nervosa: Helping Patients and Their Families Cope With Medical Problems. Edited by Roback HB. San Francisco, Jossey Bass, 1984

Pope HG Jr, Hudson JI, Yurgelun-Todd D: Anorexia nervosa and bulimia among 300 suburban women shoppers. Am J Psychiatry 141:292–294, 1984

Rakoff V: Multiple determinants of family dynamics in anorexia nervosa, in Anorexia Nervosa: Recent Developments in Research. Edited by Darby PL, Garfinkel PE, et al. New York, Alan R Liss Inc, 1983

Richardson BD, Pieters L: Menarche and growth. Am J Clin Nutr 30:288–20–91, 1977

Riding J, Munro A: Pimozide in the treatment of monosymptomatic hypochondriacal psychosis. Acta Psychiatr Scan 52:23–30, 1975

Rizzuto AM, Peterson RK, Reed M: The pathological sense of self in anorexia nervosa. Psychiatric Clinics of North America 4:471–487, 1981

Russell DM, Freedman ML, Feighlin DHI, et al: Delayed gastric emptying in anorexia nervosa: improvement with domperidone. Am J Psychiatry 140:1235–1236, 1983a

Russell DM, Prendergast PJ, Jeejeebhoy IN, et al: A comparison between muscle function and body composition in anorexia nervosa: the effect of refeeding. Am J Clin Nutr 38: 229–237, 1983b

Russell GFM: Anorexia nervosa, its identity as an illness and its treatment, in Modern Trends in Psychological Medicine, 2nd Edition. Edited by Price JH, London, Butterworth, 1970

Russell GFM: Bulimia nervosa: an ominous variant of anorexia nervosa. Psychol Med 9:429–448, 1979

Schwartz DM, Thompson MG: Do anorectics get well? Current research and future needs. Am J Psychiatry 138:319–323, 1981

Selvini-Palazzoli M: Anorexia nervosa, in the World Biennial of Psychiatry and Psychotherapy, vol 1. Edited by Arieti S. New York, Basic Books, 1970

Selvini-Palazzoli MP: Self-starvation. London, Chaucer Publishing Co, 1974

Selvini-Palazzoli MP: Self-starvation: From Individual to Family Therapy, in The Treatment of Anorexia Nervosa, 2nd Edition. New York, Jason Aronson, 1978

Sherman BM, Halmi KA: Effect of nutritional rehabilitation on hypothalamic-pituitary function in anorexia nervosa, in Anorexia Nervosa. Edited by Vigersky RS. New York, Raven Press, 1977

Silverman JA: Medical consequences of starvation: the malnutrition of anorexia nervosa: caveat medicus, in Anorexia Nervosa: Recent Developments in Research. Edited by Darby PL, Garfinkel PE, et al. New York, Alan R Liss Inc, 1983

Simmonds M: Ueber embolische prozesse in des hypophysis. Arch F Path. Anat 217:226–239, 1914

Stonehill E, Crisp AH: Psychoneurotic characteristics of patients with anorexia nervosa before and after treatment and at follow-up 4-7 years later. J Psychosom Res 21:189–193, 1977

Szmuckler G: Weight and food preoccupation in a population of English schoolgirls, in Understanding Anorexia Nervosa and Bulimia. Columbus, Ohio, Ross Laboratories, 1983

Theander S: Anorexia nervosa: a psychiatric investigation of 94 female patients. Acta Psychiatr Scand Supplement 214, 1970

Vandereycken W, Pierloot R: Combining drugs and behavior therapy in anorexia nervosa: a double-blind placebo/pimozide study, in Anorexia Nervosa: Recent Developments in Research. Edited by Darby PL, Garfinkel PE, et al. New York, Alan R Liss Inc, 1983a

Vandereycken W, Pierloot R: Long-term outcome research in anorexia nervosa: the problem of patient selection and follow-up duration. International Journal of Eating Disorders 2:237–242, 1983b

Van der Laan WP, Parker DC, Rossman LC, et al: Implications of growth hormone release in sleep. Metabolism 19:891–897, 1970

Wakeling A, deSousa V, Beardwood CJ: Effects of administered estrogen on luteinizing hormone release in subjects with anorexia nervosa in acute and recovery stages, in Anorexia Nervosa. Edited by Vigersky RA. New York, Raven Press, 1977

Wakeling A, deSousa VFA, Gore MBR, et al: Amenorrhoea, body weight and serum hormone concentrations, with particular reference to prolactin and thyroid hormones in anorexia nervosa. Psychol Med 9:265–272, 1979

Wall JH: Diagnosis, treatment and results in anorexia nervosa. Am J Psychiatry 115:997–1001, 1959

Waller JV, Kaufman MR, Deutsch F: Anorexia nervosa: a psychosomatic entity. Psychosom Med 2:3–16, 1940

Waller JV, Kaufman MR, Deutsch F: Anorexia nervosa: a psychosomatic entity, in Evolution of Psychosomatic Concepts. Edited by Kaufman MR, Heiman M. New York, International Universities Press, 1964

Walsh BT, Katz JL, Levin J, et al: Adrenal activity in anorexia nervosa. Psychosom Med 40:499–506, 1978

Wardle J: Dietary restraint and binge eating. Behavioral Analysis and Modification 4:201–209, 1980

Warren MP, Jewelewicz R, Dyrenfurth I, et al: The significance of weight loss in the evaluation of pituitary response to Lh-Rh in women with secondary amenorrhoea. J Clin Endocrinol Metab 40:601–611, 1975

Weiner H: Abiding problems in the psychoendocrinology of anorexia nervosa, in Understanding Anorexia Nervosa and Bulimia. Columbus, Ohio, Ross Laboratories, 1983

Wulliemier F: Anorexia nervosa: gauging treatment effectiveness. Psychosomatics 19:497–499, 1975

Chapter 24

Bulimia

*by James E. Mitchell, M.D., Richard
L. Pyle, M.D. and Elke D. Eckert, M.D.*

Patients with the eating disorder bulimia demonstrate a markedly abnormal eating pattern characterized by binge-eating episodes alternating with periods of little or no food intake. The binge-eating behavior is pursued in isolation and usually is followed by depressive feelings and low self-esteem. Patients with this problem also frequently either self-induce vomiting or abuse laxatives in an attempt to prevent weight gain or promote weight loss. Most are chronically concerned about their weight.

This chapter will begin by reviewing the terminology and the systems which are used to diagnose bulimia and disorders closely related to it. Subsequent sections will consider the epidemiology of the disorder, the clinical characteristics of bulimia, the pathogenesis of the disorder, management and treatment techniques, and what is known about the longitudinal course of the illness. As will become abundantly clear in the pages ahead, we know far less about this disorder than we know about anorexia nervosa and obesity. However, much has been learned in the last few years, and we are beginning to move beyond simple description of the problem to experimentation with treatment techniques.

DIAGNOSTIC AND DEFINITIONAL CONSIDERATIONS

There is currently considerable debate concerning the diagnosis of this disorder. There are two main diagnostic systems which are in wide usage, neither of which is without problems and both of which will probably be revised. These two systems will be discussed separately and then contrasted.

The clinical syndrome originally delineated by Russell in 1979, and subsequently discussed at length by Fairburn (1982, 1982a) was termed bulimia nervosa. Russell's use of the term bulimia nervosa stressed the relationship between this disorder and anorexia nervosa. He considered the former a variant of the latter. The inclusion criteria included the following: The patient suffers from powerful and intractable urges to overeat; the patient seeks to avoid the "fattening" effects of food by inducing vomiting or abusing purgatives or both; the patient has a morbid fear of becoming obese.

DSM-III assumed a slightly different approach to the problem, the focus being on the binge-eating behavior itself. *DSM-III* offers the following criteria for bulimia:

1. Recurrent episodes of binge-eating (rapid consumption of a large amount of food in a discrete period of time, usually less than two hours at a time).
2. At least three of the following: consumption of high caloric, easily ingested food during a binge; inconspicuous eating during a binge; termination of

such eating episodes by abdominal pain, sleep, social interruption, or self-induced vomiting; repeated attempts to lose weight by severely restricted diet, self-induced vomiting or use of cathartics and/or diuretics; frequent weight fluctuations greater than 10 pounds due to alternating binges and fasts.
3. Awareness that the eating pattern is abnormal and fear of not being able to stop eating voluntarily.
4. Depressed mood and self-deprecating thoughts following eating binges.
5. Bulimic episodes are not due to anorexia nervosa or any known physical disorder. (American Psychiatric Association, 1980)

This system was proposed before much research on nonanorectic bulimia had actually been published. Although the criteria have proven quite useful, their lack of specificity has generated much concern in the research community. Of particular concern is the lack of frequency parameters, since it has been demonstrated that many bulimic-type behaviors, such as binge-eating and self-induced vomiting, are not uncommon in populations of college age women (Halmi et al, 1981; Pyle et al, 1983).

In considering Russell's and *DSM-III's* criteria certain points can be made. In the criteria for bulimia nervosa, the inclusion of a criterion requiring vomiting or laxative abuse suggests the delineation of a smaller, more highly characterized group of patients, since these behaviors are much less common in the general population than binge-eating. By contrast, the *DSM-III* criteria, built around the central problem of binge-eating, may identify many more people in the "normal" population, depending upon how broadly the criteria are interpreted (Pyle et al, 1983). A second consideration in examining the criteria is the issue of weight. It is well established that bulimic symptoms can be seen in a subgroup of patients with anorexia nervosa (Casper et al, 1980) and the *DSM-III* specifically excludes these patients (they are described in Chapter 23 of this volume). However, *DSM-III* provides no differentiation of normal weight bulimia (where the problems of self-induced vomiting or laxative abuse are very common) from the binge-eating seen in patients who are overweight, and are much less likely to self-induce vomiting or abuse laxatives. This latter group of overweight binge-eaters is less likely to be identified by the bulimia nervosa criteria because of the absence of purging behavior.

Several other terms have been suggested to describe clinical syndromes similar to that of bulimia including "bulimarexia" (Boskind-Lodahl and White, 1978) and the dietary chaos syndrome (Palmer, 1979). These disorders appear to have considerable overlap with what we describe clinically as bulimia. In this chapter we use the term bulimia to imply the *DSM-III* diagnosis of the syndrome of bulimia. Any other usage of the term bulimia, such as the use of the term to indicate the act of binge-eating itself, will be so indicated.

EPIDEMIOLOGY

Several recent epidemiological investigations have attempted to determine the frequency of bulimia in the general population. Before discussing the results of these investigations, it is best to consider that these studies have been hindered by several problems. Most obvious is the diagnostic confusion already discussed. This problem has been paralleled by difficulty in defining the problem behaviors when designing questionnaires. For example, researchers frequently differ as to how to define binge-eating episodes. Because of this lack of agreement it is difficult to compare studies. A third problem is that most of this research has been limited to samples of college students. While this age group appears to be at particular risk and while college samples are often available to investigators, our knowledge of these problems in other groups is very limited. Finally, the inherent limitation of questionnaire studies must be considered. However, what is known suggests that bulimia is a common disorder.

Stangler and Printz (1980) first suggested the magnitude of the problem. They reported that 3.8 percent of a consecutive series of 500 students being seen at a student health service for emotional disturbance had received a diagnosis of bulimia. Subsequent studies which have appeared in the literature have been summarized in Table 1. The study by Hawkins and Clement (1980) involved a questionnaire survey of 247 psychology students. Although the majority admitted to binge-eating behavior, less than ten percent admitted to self-inducing vomiting. The subsequent study by Halmi and associates (1981) of 355 students again showed that the majority of subjects admitted to binge-eating episodes. Halmi and associates (1981) found that 13 percent of those surveyed (19 percent of females and 6.1 percent of the males) would have met all the major criteria for bulimia as defined by *DSM-III*, although only 1.7 percent admitted to self-induced vomiting at least once a week as part of their eating problem. Sinoway (1982) attempted to rigorously define binge-eating and reported that although 47 percent of a surveyed sample of 1,172 female college students admitted to binge-eating episodes, only 25 percent were felt to have true binge-eating episodes after an examination of clarification questions. 13.7 percent were thought to meet the diagnostic criteria for bulimarexia (Boskind-Lodahl and White, 1978).

Our group completed a questionnaire survey of 1,355 college students and again found a high percentage of subjects who admitted to binge-eating episodes (57.4 percent of females, 41 percent of males) (Pyle et al, 1983). Our results indicated that 7.8 percent of the females and 1.4 percent of the males would probably have met the *DSM-III* criteria for bulimia based upon their responses. However, we found that if we applied more rigid criteria, such as a minimum of weekly binge-eating combined with either weekly self-induced vomiting or weekly laxative abuse, only one percent would have met criteria. However, these same more rigid criteria correctly identified 91.9 percent of a series of 37 patients who had been seen in our clinic and diagnosed by *DSM-III* criteria as having bulimia. This suggested to us that the more rigid criteria would select individuals in the population who most resemble patients seeking treatment for this problem.

Two recent studies from England (Cooper and Fairburn, 1983; Clark and Palmer, 1983) have provided additional information relative to the question of the rigidity of criteria. Both surveys found high rates of self-reported binge-eating behavior. However, the percentage of women reporting at least weekly binge-eating was 7.1 percent in the Clark and Palmer study (1983) and 7.3 percent in the Cooper and Fairburn study (1983). The percentages of women

Table 1. Epidemiology of Bulimia and Related Disorders

Population	Hawkins and Clement 1980	Halmi and associates 1981	Sinoway 1982	Pyle and associates 1983	Cooper and Fairburn 1983	Clarke and Palmer 1983	Johnson and associates 1983
	College Students	College Students	College Students	College Students	Clinic Patients	College Students	High School Students
N	247	355	1,172	1,355	369	206	1,268
% female	73.7%	87%	100%	42.4%	100%	100%	100%
% male	26.3%	13%	0%	57.6%	0%	0%	0%
% response	100%	66%	65%	98.3%	96.1%	76%	100%
Binge-eat							
Female	79%	68.1%	47% (25%)[1]	57.4%	26.4%[2]	46.2%[3]	57%
Male	49%	60.2%	—	41%	—	—	—
Bulimia							
Female		19% (1.7%)[4]	13.7%[5]	7.8% (1.1%)[6]	1.9%[7]	—	8%
Male		6.1%	—	1.4%	—	—	—

[1] 47% binge-eat; 25% "true" binge-eaters using clarification question
[2] 20.9% current; 7.3% at least weekly
[3] 30.2% current; 7.1% at least weekly
[4] 1.7% vomit at least once/week
[5] Bulimarexia rather than bulimia
[6] 1% binge-eat at least once/week and also self-induce vomiting and use laxatives once/week
[7] Bulimia nervosa

reporting at least weekly self-induced vomiting were 0 percent and 1.1 percent respectively.

Taken together, the available epidemiological studies suggest that binge-eating episodes, as losely defined in most questionnaire studies, are relatively common in both young men and women. It would appear, however, that this behavior does not necessarily indicate a significant eating disorder. Studies also indicate that between eight percent and 20 percent of young women meet *DSM-III* criteria for bulimia based upon their responses to questionnaires. However, if one is attempting to ascertain the prevalence of bulimia as a significant eating disorder, the vagueness of *DSM-III* criteria may yield a prevalence rate that is too high. When more rigid criteria are used, such as those that will correctly identify most patients seen clinically for bulimia, the prevalence drops to around one percent, a figure considerably more conservative, yet one which still indicates that bulimia is a common disorder.

CLINICAL CHARACTERISTICS

Several series of patients with bulimia or bulimia nervosa have been reported in the literature. These are summarized in Table 2. As can be seen from an examination of this table, the usual age of onset of these disorders is the late teenage years, and most patients have problems for several years before seeking treatment when they are in their early to mid-twenties. Although patients beyond the age of 40 have been reported, the vast majority of patients reported in the literature have been young. Less than five percent of the reported cases have been males.

The prevalence and frequency of various abnormal eating related behaviors such as binge-eating, self-induced vomiting, and laxative abuse are also summarized in Table 2. In a series of identified patients with bulimia or bulimia nervosa, patients usually are binge-eating at least once a day and are also self-inducing vomiting at least once a day. Between 20 percent and 40 percent of patients also abuse laxatives at least once a week for weight control purposes. A smaller percentage use diuretics for weight control purposes.

A history of anorexia nervosa is not uncommon in these patients. This rate varies from about 30 percent to 80 percent in a series of identified patients, again suggesting a close relationship between the two disorders.

As mentioned previously, in the *DSM-III* criteria the critical behavior is binge-eating. The term binge-eating has unfortunately been interpreted in various ways by different authors. The *DSM-III* criteria suggest that binge-eating involves ingestion of large amounts of food in a short period of time, and indeed most patients with bulimia do ingest abnormally large amounts of food during an eating binge. However the size of binge-eating episodes varies considerably. Russell originally reported that some patients consumed as many as 5,000 to 20,000 calories in binge-eating episodes (1979). Other research groups substantiated this finding (Johnson and Larson, 1982; Mitchell et al, 1981). However, not all patients ingest large amounts of food during a binge. During binge-eating, patients tend to consume high carbohydrate or high fat foods which are easy to ingest and which do not require much preparation or chewing (Mitchell et al, 1981). Commonly ingested items include ice cream, bread, toast, candy,

Table 2. Reported Series of Patients with Bulimia, Bulimia Nervosa and Bulimarexia

	Russell 1979	Fairburn 1980	Pyle and Associates 1981	Abraham and Beumont 1982	Fairburn and Cooper 1982	Johnson and Associates 1982	Herzog 1982	Mitchell and Associates 1983
Total N	30	11	34	32	499	316	30	168
Female	28	11	34	30	499	316	29	164
Male	2	0	0	2	0	0	1	4
Source	Patients	Patients	Patients	Patients	Advertisement	Wrote clinic	Patients	Patients
Diagnosis	Bulimia Nervosa	Bulimia Nervosa	Bulimia	Binge-Eaters	Bulimia Nervosa	Bulimia	Bulimia	Bulimia
Age (mean)			24[1]	24	23.8	23.7	24.6	24
Age onset Eating Disorder	18.8	16.1	18[1]	17	18.4	18.1	18.4	20
Binge-eat once/day or more			56% ⎫	100%	27.2%	51.5%		63.8%
Binge-eat once/week or several times/week			44.1% ⎭		32.6%	41.8%		26.7%
Vomit once/day or more			47.1% ⎫	53%	56.1%	59.2%		56.6%
Vomit once/week or several times/week			41.2% ⎭		17.5%	28.6%		23.2%
Laxative abuse once/day or more			2.9%			24.5%		7.9%
Laxative abuse once/week or several times/week			11.8%		18.8%	30.2%		17.8%

[1]Median

and donuts (Mitchell et al, 1981). A characteristic which seems to underlie much of the current thinking regarding binge-eating is that patients who binge-eat experience a distressing sense of loss of control over their eating. Other characteristics of binge-eating include the secretive nature of the episodes, the fact that the episodes are frequently precipitated by stressful events, and that individuals with bulimia can easily differentiate a binge-eating episode from other eating behavior.

The individual episodes of binge-eating may be precipitated by stress. An examination of the emotional status of the patients immediately prior to binge-eating episodes has proven useful. Patients have frequently reported feeling anxious or tense (Abraham and Beumont, 1982), craving certain foods (Pyle et al, 1981), or being unhappy (Pyle et al, 1981). For some patients, any food intake may trigger a binge-eating episode. Most bulimic individuals binge-eat late in the day, particularly when they return home from work or school. They report that they eat very rapidly when they binge-eat and many state that they don't really taste the food. They may watch TV, read, or think about other things. The duration of the typical binge-eating episode is usually two hours or less as described by *DSM-III* but can last as long as eight hours or more (Abraham and Beumont, 1982).

It also should be remembered that most patients with bulimia do not eat normally when they are not binge-eating. Many fast for prolonged periods to compensate for the presumed excess caloric intake during the binge. Patients with bulimia also report frequent weight swings (Fairburn, 1982a) and tend to be very sensitive about their weight. It has also been suggested that patients with this problem may have a faulty perception of their body image, a problem also described in patients with anorexia nervosa (Fairburn and Cooper, 1982).

A variety of other problems have been described in association with bulimia. Most commonly described has been depression (Russell, 1979; Pyle et al, 1981). Patients with bulimia are frequently noted to be depressed when first seen for evaluation. This high prevalence of depressive symptoms has led several authors to speculate about the association between bulimia and affective disorders, and to suggest that many cases of bulimia may represent variants of primary affective disorder. For example, Hudson and associates (1983) found that fully 80 percent of a series of 70 patients with bulimia met *DSM-III* criteria for major affective disorder, using the NIMH diagnostic interview schedule. Several other lines of evidence suggest a relationship between bulimia and affective disorders, including an increased incidence of affective disorders in the relatives of these patients (Hudson et al, 1982; Hudson et al, 1983a), a high rate of nonsuppression on the DST in patients with bulimia (Hudson et al, 1983b), and the apparent utility of antidepressants in the treatment of patients with bulimia. This latter point will be discussed in more detail below. How commonly the depression seen in patients with bulimia represents a primary depression as opposed to being secondary to the physical and psychosocial sequelae of the illness is at this point unclear. However, there is a strong link between the two problems, suggesting that this area requires vigorous investigation.

Several other problems have been described in association with bulimia, including problems with impulse control (Fairburn and Cooper, 1982) and a higher than expected rate of chemical abuse problems (Pyle et al, 1981). Our group reported that of 34 patients seen with bulimia, eight had previously completed chemical dependency treatment and one was thought to merit a diagnosis of alcoholism. Herzog (1982) subsequently reported that ten of the 30 bulimic patients in his series reported alcoholism in at least one first-degree family member. Furthermore, the abuse of food seen in bulimia and the abuse of alcohol or other drugs seen in patients with drug abuse problems have certain features in common, including loss of control over the use of the substance, an intense preoccupation with the substance, the secretiveness of the behavior, and the social isolation which accompanies the behavior (Hatsukami et al, 1982). It would appear that patients at risk for one type of substance abuse may be at higher risk for another.

Unfortunately, very little is known about the psychological adjustment prior to the illness of patients who later develop bulimia. Several lines of evidence suggest impairment when patients are seen for bulimia. MMPI studies have shown that the profiles in bulimic women and women with alcohol and drug abuse problems are quite similar, evidencing elevation on the scales for depression, impulsivity, anger, anxiety, and social withdrawal (Hatsukami et al, 1983; Norman and Herzog, 1983). Weiss and Ebert (1983) compared a sample of normal weight female bulimics with a sample of normal weight female controls. The two groups were matched for age, socioeconomic status, and IQ. The bulimia patients demonstrated higher levels of psychopathology and impulsive behavior, and a history of more suicide attempts, psychiatric hospitalizations, episodes of stealing, and problems with drug usage. They also consistently rated themselves as sicker on all psychometric scales employed.

The available studies, taken together, suggest that as a group bulimic patients tend to be impulsive and depressed, and appear to be at high risk for drug abuse problems. However, clinical experience also reveals that patients with a variety of personality types seem to develop this disorder.

Bulimia can be associated with a variety of physical complications. Patients with these disorders frequently complain of lethargy, impaired concentration, and abdominal pain. They also can develop a variety of more severe medical complications. Studies using screening laboratory tests indicate that some of these patients have elevated serum blood urea nitrogen (BUNs), indicating probable dehydration. They also frequently demonstrate fluid and electrolyte abnormalities. Russell (1979) originally reported hypokalemia in 13 of the 24 subjects in his original series of bulimia nervosa patients. Our group (Mitchell et al, 1983) subsequently reported that 82 of 168 patients with bulimia or atypical eating disorder demonstrated some type of electrolyte abnormality, the various abnormalities including metabolic alkalosis (27.4 percent), hypochloremia (23.8 percent) and hypokalemia (13.7 percent). Patients who reported that they self-induced vomiting at least daily were significantly more likely to manifest alkalosis than patients reporting less frequent self-induced vomiting behavior. In rare cases, patients also demonstrated metabolic acidosis, presumably related to fasting or secondary to acute diarrhea from laxative abuse.

Another medical complication of considerable concern is that of gastric rupture. In a review of this problem, Saul and associates (1981) reported the case of a normal weight individual with a history of anorexia nervosa who excessively overate and appears in retrospect to meet criteria for bulimia. The patient developed infarction and perforation of the stomach. In Saul's review of 66 cases of spontaneous rupture of the stomach, approximately half of the cases appeared to be related to ingestion of large amounts of food and/or acute gastric dilatation. Eleven of the cases had been diagnosed as having anorexia nervosa and most of these were undergoing refeeding. We previously reported a case of gastric dilatation in a normal weight person with bulimia which was successfully managed medically (Mitchell et al, 1982). It would appear that gastric dilatation and infarction are possible complications of bulimia as well as of anorexia nervosa.

Salivary gland swelling has been demonstrated in patients with bulimia (Levin et al, 1980). The clinical picture is one of painless swelling of a salivary gland, the parotid gland being most frequently involved. Biopsy findings have usually revealed normal tissue or asymptomatic noninflammatory salivary gland enlargement. The pathophysiology of this problem is unclear but has been variously attributed to high carbohydrate intake, alkalosis or malnutrition.

Problems of dentition are also quite common in patients with bulimia or in anorexia nervosa patients who vomit. Decalcification of the lingual, palatal and posterior occlusal surfaces of the teeth have been described. The clinical appearance is one of erosion of the enamel and dentin with rounded contours and absence of staining on dental surfaces. This subject has been recently reviewed (Stege et al, 1982).

There has also been some concern about the possibility of EEG abnormalities in patients with eating disorders. Part of this concern stems from clinical reports documenting primary neurological problems which have presented as abnormal eating patterns (Rau and Green, 1975). In a series of studies, Rau, Green, and their colleagues have described certain EEG abnormalities in patients with "compulsive eating disorders" (Rau et al, 1979). However, the clinical significance of the EEG patterns described are unclear and there remains some question whether these EEG abnormalities are actually associated with any behavioral abnormality (Maulsby, 1979).

Available studies also indicate that there are certain neuroendocrine abnormalities in patients with bulimia, although the clinical significance of most of these abnormalities are at this point unclear. Blunted TSH responsiveness to TRH administration (Gwirtsman et al, 1983), increase in growth hormone following TRH or glucose administration (Gwirtsman et al, 1983; Mitchell and Bantle, 1983), and elevated basal serum prolactin (Mitchell and Bantle, 1983) have been described. As mentioned previously, the rate of dexamethasone nonsuppression has been found to be fairly high in patients with bulimia.

ETIOLOGY AND PATHOGENESIS

How does this problem start? The disorder frequently starts following a period of dieting behavior (Abraham and Beumont, 1982; Johnson et al, 1983). However, many patients with bulimia have been chronically concerned about their weight and may be dieting off and on most of the time. Some patients also tend to link bulimia to traumatic events, particularly a history of loss or separation (Pyle et al, 1981). There is also some evidence that patients who develop bulimia may have had prior periods of being overweight (Halmi et al, 1981; Johnson et al, 1983). Regardless of the initiating event, the symptoms of bulimia appear to assume an independence of their own and to become a regular institutionalized pattern of behavior in the individual's life. In considering the treatment of this condition, this quality of habit must be considered.

One can speculate that certain individuals may be more at risk for developing these disorders. Those who are quite concerned about their weight, perhaps those who have had problems with being overweight when younger, and those individuals who are more impulsive may be at greater risk. Whether depression is a predisposing factor as well as a sequelae to the illness is unclear. Both patterns more than likely typify subgroups of patients with bulimia.

The etiology of this disorder also must be considered in the cultural context. Our culture provides an abundance of food at the same time it insists on thinness as a model of attractiveness for young people. Perhaps because of this preoccupation with thinness, perhaps for other reasons, our culture seems to predispose to bulimia. When viewing this problem in a cultural context and given the knowledge that many young women experiment with bulimic behaviors, the question then becomes: Why does this behavioral pattern escalate out of control in some people? This is the crucial question which we cannot yet answer.

MANAGEMENT AND TREATMENT

The first step in the management of patients with bulimia is to carefully delineate the particular problems for the individual patient so that an appropriate treatment plan can be devised. This involves careful inquiry into several areas related to eating patterns and weight as well as psychological health or dysfunction. It is important to determine the presence or absence of eating-related behaviors such as binge-eating, laxative abuse, diuretic abuse, the use of diet pills, the use of enemas, and whether or not the patient chews and spits out food without swallowing it. All of these behaviors can occur in patients with bulimia. The examining physician must determine the frequencies of these behaviors if they are present and, if laxative or diuretic abuse is an issue, the frequency and amount as well as maximum doses used. One cannot assume that these behaviors are not present if they are not mentioned spontaneously.

The second step in the management of a patient with bulimia is to insure medical stability. Physiological sequelae of bulimia, particularly fluid and electrolyte abnormalities, may prove serious if undetected. Because of this, patients generally require laboratory assessment as part of the evaluation process. A careful medical history and physical examination should be included. Particular attention should be paid to the state of hydration, oral hygiene, cardiac functioning, and vital signs. Careful neurological assessment is also indicated to rule out any primary neurological problem which might be presenting as a disordered eating pattern. Routine laboratory screening should include, at minimum: plasma glucose, electrolytes, and renal function tests. A more complete battery including CBC, liver function tests, and thyroid functions may prove useful. If the history is atypical or if the physical examination or laboratory work reveals unexpected findings, a more careful medical/neurological evaluation is indicated, which will include skull films combined with visual fields or, as an alternative, a CT scan. Some patients may require ongoing monitoring of their physical status, particularly their electrolytes, during the course of therapy.

Some discussion needs to be given to the appropriateness of different treatment settings, with the assumption that a patient is found to be medically stable. Both inpatient and outpatient treatment programs have been described, and at this point it is unclear whether patients fare better in any particular treatment setting. One advantage of hospitalization, assuming a proper ward environment, is that a hospital stay can provide an interruption of the binge-eating/purging cycle. However, this necessitates taking the control of eating behavior away from the patient, which can only be a temporary solution. Indications for hospitalizing patients with normal weight bulimia include marked medical instability, severe depression with suicidality, failure to improve with adequate outpatient treatment (Fairburn 1982a), and the need to initiate medication trials where monitoring of medical aspects and of adherance in the outpatient setting is problematic. Outpatient treatment programs offer the advantage of keeping the responsibility for eating behavior with the patient, but present a bigger problem in terms of interrupting the binge-eating/purging cycle. Different authors have employed different approaches to solve this problem, including seeing patients more frequently—as often as several times a week or even daily during the early part of therapy—to provide the necessary support (Fairburn, 1982a; Mitchell et al, in press).

There are several situations in which hospitalization may be necessary. When a patient is in medical danger because of her behavior, hospitalization may be called for. The most common indication would be severe fluid and electrolyte disturbances. A second indication would be severe depression, particularly if the patient is suicidal. The third relative indication for hospitalization is severe laxative abuse. In our experience, patients with this complication have a great deal of difficulty withdrawing from laxatives when out of the hospital and may require inpatient supervision.

Reports in the literature have favored one of two general treatment approaches, the first being psychotherapeutic and the second being pharmacological. As will be seen, there is a growing literature to support the utility of both approaches, which of course may be combined in some therapeutic situations.

We will discuss the psychotherapy approaches first. Most of the programs that have been described have used behavioral approaches to modify eating behavior. Both individual and group formats have been suggested. Fairburn has described the use of an individual cognitive behavioral approach to the treatment of bulimia (Fairburn, 1981). Treatment was divided into two phases. During the initial phase, the patients were seen frequently, usually twice or three times a week in order to interrupt the binge-eating and vomiting cycle. This phase of treatment focused on education about the illness, the use of self-monitoring techniques, the development of alternative behaviors, and the use of goal-setting. In the second part of therapy, increasing emphasis was placed on the development of improved coping skills, the use of behavioral problem-solving techniques, and an examination of irrational concerns. The patients were also encouraged to reintroduce feared foods into their diet. Several other authors have reported behaviorally based treatment programs utilizing an individual therapy format (Long and Cordle, 1982; Rosen and Leitenberg, 1982; Grinc, 1982; Mizes and Lohr, 1983).

Several group approaches have also been described (Boskind-Lodahl and White,

1978; White and Boskind-White, 1981; Dixon and Kiecolt-Glaser, 1981; Lacey, 1983; Johnson et al, 1983; Mitchell et al, in press). While using a variety of strategies, these groups generally have favored a structured, time-limited, closed group approach.

Most of the psychotherapy approaches that have been described, whether group or individual, have certain basic features in common. One such element is the need for patient education. Several authors have commented on the need to educate patients about their disorder and its consequences. Most programs employ the use of self-monitoring techniques, acknowledging that if patients are made aware of their eating behavior they will be better able to change it. In addition, most programs include an examination of behavioral antecedents and consequences of bulimic behaviors. It is well known that a variety of antecedents can precede binge-eating episodes, including situational factors, social factors, emotional factors, physiological factors, and cognitive factors. If patients can come to understand what factors trigger binge-eating episodes they will better be able to avoid or to modify them. As a corollary, most programs also stress the need to develop alternative or competing behaviors for patients when they have an urge to binge-eat. Most programs attempt to improve the adaptive skills of patients with bulimia. This may involve employing specific strategies such as assertiveness training, behavioral problem-solving, and relaxation training. Lastly, most stress the need for cognitive restructuring. Patients with bulimia frequently have distorted ideas about their own self-worth, the role of food in their lives, and their body image. A cognitive approach which examines and challenges these beliefs appears to be indicated.

In the last few years, there has been a growing interest in the pharmacological treatment of bulimia, and several studies have suggested that pharmacotherapy can be quite helpful for many patients. Interest has centered around two types of agents: anticonvulsants and antidepressants. The anticonvulsants were the first drugs employed. Much of the research in this area has been done by Rau, Green, and their colleagues (1979). This work originally grew out of a demonstrated association between abnormal eating behaviors and neurological dysfunctions, such as partial complex seizures (Rau and Green, 1975). Rau, Green, and their colleagues attempted to delineate electroencephalographic and soft neurological signs which might be associated with abnormal eating patterns. Recently, these authors summarized their experience with phenytoin in the treatment of compulsive eating (Rau et al, 1979). A total of 47 patients were felt to have had adequate trials with the drug. The authors' analysis indicated a high percentage of EEG abnormalities among compulsive eaters and concluded that patients with abnormal EEGs were more likely to respond to the drugs. Blood levels were not correlated with response. The protocols employed by this group have been nonblind in design, with the exception of treatment protocols for a few patients. A subsequent placebo-controlled, double-blind trial by Wermuth and associates (1977) attempted to solve some of these methodological problems. Nineteen bulimic women, one of whom was also anorectic, were evaluated in this six-week crossover trial. Three subjects had definitely abnormal EEGs and four had questionably abnormal EEGs. There was no significant relationship between drug response and EEG abnormality. Overall, phenytoin treatment was associated with fewer binge-eating episodes, and eight patients were felt to show "marked" improvement. In the phenytoin to placebo sequence the number of binge-eating episodes decreased during drug treatment; however, the improvement continued when the subjects were placed on placebo. This finding confounded the results. There have been additional case reports of phenytoin treatment for bulimia, most of which have been negative (Greenway et al, 1977; Weiss and Levitz, 1976; Moore and Rakes, 1982).

Kaplan and associates (1983) recently reported a double-blind, crossover trial with carbamazepine in a series of six bulimic patients. One patient, who had a history suggestive of bipolar affective disorder, responded dramatically to the medication while the other five showed equivocal or no response to the drug. The authors concluded that there might be a subgroup of patients with bulimia and mood instability who might respond to this compound.

A number of recent reports from several groups of investigators have indicated that antidepressant therapy may be helpful for patients with bulimia. Pope and Hudson (1982) first reported on the utility of tricyclic antidepressants in a series of eight patients. These patients had received a variety of antidepressants in usual therapeutic doses, imipramine being the most commonly employed agent. Six patients obtained moderate or marked reduction in binge-eating frequency which persisted for from two to seven months. Pope and associates (1983) subsequently reported a placebo-controlled, double-blind trial of imipramine versus placebo in 19 chronically bulimic patients. Subjects on active drug demonstrated a 70 percent reduction in binge-eating after six weeks of therapy compared to virtually no change in the control group. Imipramine was also associated with significant decrease in intensity of binges and decreased preoccupation with food. Sabin and associates (1983) reported a randomized, placebo-controlled, double-blind trial of mianserin in a series of 50 patients with bulimia nervosa. Subjects initially received 30 mg with a subsequent increase to 60 mg a day after one week of therapy. The trial lasted eight weeks. There were no significant differences between the two groups in the amount of change in the various instruments used for rating depression or eating attitudes. The number of days each week the subjects reported binging, vomiting, or purging did not change throughout the eight-week trial. Mitchell and Groat (1984) recently completed a placebo-controlled, double-blind trial of amitriptyline in a series of 32 female outpatients with bulimia. The results indicated that the drug had a significant antidepressant effect. Patients in both the placebo and active drug groups also received a minimal behavior therapy program, and both groups demonstrated considerable overall improvement in their eating behavior. It should be noted that the use of the drug was not associated with weight gain or carbohydrate craving. Pope and associates (1984) subsequently summarized their results in a large series of patients they have treated with a variety of antidepressants or antidepressant combinations.

An important question regarding the use of antidepressants in bulimia concerns their mechanism of action. A recent report by Brotman and associates (1984) described a retrospective analysis of 22 patients with bulimia treated with antidepressants. The authors concluded that the medication might have separate effects on binge-eating behavior and depression in different patients, and that improvement in one type of symptom did not necessarily predict improvement in the other. However, the analysis by Mitchell and Groat (1984) indicated a significant correlation between antidepressant effect and improvement in eating behavior in the subgroup of depressed patients receiving antidepressants. Further work is needed in this area.

An additional report suggested the utility of monoamine oxidase inhibitors in patients with bulimia. Walsh and associates (1982) reported a series of six patients who received phenelzine in doses of 60 to 90 mg a day. All experienced prompt improvement in eating behavior and mood.

Taken together, the pharmacological studies suggest that some patients do appear to respond to phenytoin. Additional studies are needed to establish whether or not this therapy is efficacious for typical patients with bulimia, since it is not clear that the EEG abnormalities are effective predictors of response. Of the three controlled trials using antidepressants, the two using traditional tricyclic antidepressants both favored active drug as being effective in treatment. Whether this is a primary effect against bulimic behaviors or whether the effect is mainly on the depression remains a matter of debate. However, available information indicates that antidepressants should be considered as therapeutic agents in patients with bulimia, particularly where affective symptoms are prominent.

COURSE AND OUTCOME

Very little is known about the longitudinal course of this illness. Patients report markedly different patterns over time. Some indicate that the problem waxes and wanes, and that at times they are able to assume control of their eating behavior for weeks or months. Other patients indicate that the illness is continuous and progressive in that the frequency of the bulimic behaviors increase over time. The results of epidemiological investigations suggest that some patients may develop a bulimic pattern and, without treatment, revert to more normal eating. How commonly this happens is unknown.

Fairburn (1982a) reported that many patients experience an initial loss of weight when beginning bulimic symptomatology, which may tend to reinforce the behavior. A typical patient then seems to reach a nadir of weight at approximately 12 months, before beginning to gain weight. In our experience, this may be accounted for by changes in the binge-eating episodes themselves. As patients progress in the course of the illness, the frequency of the binge-eating episodes and the amount of food eaten while binge-eating seem to increase. However, a small percentage of patients with bulimia eventually cease binge-eating yet continue to self-induce vomiting. The patterns vary dramatically among patients. Most patients have been ill for several years before seeking treatment and many report that the bulimic behaviors have increasingly come to dominate their lives. A typical pattern would be one of increasing social disruption including problems with relationships, occasional occupational problems, and a lowering of self-esteem.

CONCLUSIONS

In examining our knowledge about the various facets of the bulimia syndrome, it quickly becomes apparent that we know little and that nearly everything we have learned about this condition has been reported in the last six years. Many important questions remain to be answered. Why do bulimic behaviors, which are so common in the general population, escalate out of control in certain people? What are the cultural determinants of this disorder? What exactly are the relationships among bulimia, affective disorders, and other substance abuse problems? What happens to these patients with and without treatment?

Clinicians and researchers are encountering important challenges in dealing with bulimia. We are faced with a serious psychiatric syndrome which is already quite common and which by consensus appears to be increasing in incidence. Clearly much effort will be required by innovative researchers and therapists if this problem is to be effectively confronted.

REFERENCES

Abraham SF, Beumont PJV: How patients describe bulimia or binge-eating. Psychol Med 12:625-635, 1982

American Psychiatric Association: Diagnostic and Statistical Manual of Mental Disorders. Third edition. Washington, DC, the American Psychiatric Association, 1980

Boskind-Lodahl M, White WC: The definition and treatment of bulimarexia in college women: a pilot study. Journal of the American College Health Association 27:84-86, 1978

Brotman AW, Herzog DB, Woods SW: Antidepressant treatment of bulimia: the relationship between bingeing and depressive symptomatology. J Clin Psychiatry 45:7-9, 1984

Casper RC, Eckert ED, Halmi K, et al: Bulimia—its incidence and clinical importance in patients with anorexia nervosa. Arch Gen Psychiatry 37:1030-1040, 1980

Clark MG, Palmer RL: Eating attitudes and neurotic symptoms in university students. Br J Psychiatry 142:299-304, 1983

Cooper PJ, Fairburn CG: Binge-eating and self-induced vomiting in the community—a preliminary study. Br J Psychiatry 142:139-144, 1983

Dixon KN, Kiecolt-Glaser J: Group therapy for bulimia. Presented at the American Psychiatric Association Meeting, New Orleans, May 15, 1981

Fairburn CG: A cognitive behavioral approach to the treatment of bulimia. Psychol Med 11:707, 1981

Fairburn CG: Binge-eating and bulimia nervosa. S.K. and F. Publications 1:1-20, 1982

Fairburn CG: Binge-eating and its management. Br J Psychiatry 141:631-633, 1982a

Fairburn CG, Cooper JP: Self-induced vomiting and bulimia nervosa: an undetected problem. Br Med J 284:1153-1155, 1982

Greenway FL, Dahms WT, Brag DA: Phenytoin as a treatment of obesity associated with compulsive eating. Current Therapeutic Research 21:338-342, 1977

Grinc GA: A cognitive-behavioral model for the treatment of chronic vomiting. J Behav Med 5:135-141, 1982

Gwirtsman HE, Roy-Byrne P, Yager J, et al: Neuroendocrine abnormalities in bulimia. Am J Psychiatry 140:559-563, 1983

Halmi KA, Falk JR, Schwartz E: Binge-eating and vomiting: a survey of a college population. Psychol Med 11:697-706, 1981

Hatsukami D, Owen P, Pyle R, et al: Similarities and differences on the MMPI between women with bulimia and women with alcohol or drug abuse problems. Addictive Behaviors 7:435-439, 1982

Hawkins II, Clement PF: Development and construct validation of a self-report measure of binge eating tendencies. Addictive Behaviors 5:219-226, 1980

Herzog DB: Bulimia: the secretive syndrome. Psychosomatics 23:481-487, 1982

Hudson JI, Laffer PS, Pope HG: Bulimia related to affective disorder by family history and response to the dexamethasone suppression test. Am J Psychiatry 139:685-687, 1982

Hudson JI, Pope HG, Jonas JM: Bulimia: a form of affective disorder? Paper presented at the American Psychiatric Association Meeting, New York, May 1983

Hudson JI, Pope HG, Jonas JM, et al: Family history study of anorexia nervosa and bulimia. Br J Psychiatry 142:133-138, 1983a

Hudson JI, Pope HG, Jonas JM, et al: Hypothalamic-pituitary-adrenal axis: hyperactivity in bulimia. Psychiatry Res 8:111-117, 1983b

Johnson C, Larson R: Bulimia: an analysis of moods and behavior. Psychosom Med 44:341-351, 1982

Johnson CL, Stuckey MK, Lewis LD, et al: Bulimia: a descriptive survey of 316 cases. International Journal of Eating Disorders 2:3-16, 1982

Johnson CL, Connors M, Stuckey M: Short-term group treatment of bulimia: a preliminary report. International Journal of Eating Disorders 2:199-208, 1983a

Johnson CL, Lewis C, Love S, et al: A descriptive survey of dieting and bulimic behavior in a female high school population, in Understanding Anorexia Nervosa and Bulimia. Columbus, Ohio, Ross Laboratories, 1983b

Kaplan AS, Garfinkel PE, Darby PL, et al: Carbamazepine in the treatment of bulimia. Am J Psychiatry 140:225-226, 1983

Lacey JH: Bulimia nervosa, binge-eating and psychogenic vomiting: a controlled treatment study and long-term outcome. Br Med J 286:1609-1613, 1983

Levin PA, Falko JM, Dixon K, et al: Benign parotid enlargement in bulimia. Ann Intern Med 93:827-829, 1980

Long CG, Cordle CJ: Psychological treatment of binge-eating and self-induced vomiting. J Med Psychol 55:139-145, 1982

Maulsby RL: EEG patterns of uncertain diagnostic significance, in Current Practice of Clinical Electroencephalography. Edited by Klass DW, Daly DD. New York, Raven Press, 1979

Mitchell JE, Bantle JP: Metabolic and endocrine investigations in women of normal weight with the bulimia syndrome. Biol Psychiatry 18:355-365, 1983

Mitchell JE, Groat R: A double-blind placebo controlled trial of amitriptyline in bulimia. J Clin Psychopharmacology 4:186-193, 1984

Mitchell JE, Pyle RL, Eckert ED: Frequency and duration of binge-eating episodes in patients with bulimia. Am J Psychiatry 138:835-836, 1981

Mitchell JE, Pyle RL, Miner RA: Gastric dilatation as a complication of bulimia. Psychosomatics 23:96-97, 1982

Mitchell JE, Pyle RL, Eckert ED, et al: Electrolyte and other physiological abnormalities in patients with bulimia. Psychol Med 13:273-278, 1983

Mitchell JE, Hatsukami D, Goff G, et al: An intensive outpatient group treatment program for patients with bulimia, in A Handbook for the Treatment of Anorexia Nervosa and Bulimia. Edited by Garner D, Garfinkel P. New York, Guilford Press, in press

Mizes JS, Lohr SM: The treatment of bulimia (binge-eating and self-induced vomiting). International Journal of Eating Disorders 2:59-60, 1983

Moore SL, Rakes SM: Binge eating—therapeutic response to diphenylhydantoin: case report. J Clin Psychiatry 43:385-386, 1982

Norman DK, Herzog DB: Bulimia, anorexia nervosa, and anorexia nervosa with bulimia: a comparative analysis of MMPI profiles. International Journal of Eating Disorders 2:43-52, 1983

Palmer RL: The dietary chaos syndrome: a useful new term? Br J Med Psychol 52:187-190, 1979

Pope HG, Hudson JI: Treatment of bulimia with antidepressants. Psychopharmacology 78:176-179, 1982

Pope HG, Hudson JI, Jonas JM, et al: Bulimia treated with imipramine: a placebo-controlled double-blind study. Am J Psychiatry 140:554-558, 1983

Pope HG, Hudson JI, Jonas JM: Antidepressant treatment of bulimia: preliminary experience and practical recommendations. J Clin Psychopharmacol 3:274-281, 1984

Pyle RL, Mitchell JE, Eckert ED: Bulimia: a report of 34 cases. J Clin Psychiatry 42:60-64, 1981

Pyle RL, Mitchell JE, Eckert ED, et al: The incidence of bulimia in freshman college students. International Journal of Eating Disorders 2:75-85, 1983

Rau JH, Green RS: Compulsive eating: a neuropsychologic approach to certain eating disorders. Compr Psychiatry 16:223-231, 1975

Rau JH, Struve FA, Green RS: Electroencephalographic correlates of compulsive eating. Clin Electroencephalogr 10:180-189, 1979

Rosen JC, Leitenberg H: Bulimia nervosa: treatment with exposure and response prevention. Behavior Therapy 13:117-124, 1982

Russell G: Bulimia nervosa: an ominous variant of anorexia nervosa. Psychol Med 9:429-448, 1979

Sabin EJ, Yonace A, Farrington AJ, et al: Bulimia nervosa: a placebo controlled double-blind therapeutic trial of mianserin. Br J Clin Pharmacol 15:1955-2025, 1983

Saul SH, Dekker A, Watson CG: Acute gastric dilatation with infarction and perforation. Gut 22:978-983, 1981

Sinoway CG: The incidence and characteristics of bulimarexia in Penn State students. Paper presented at the American Psychological Association Meeting, Washington, DC, 1982

Stege P, Visco-Dangler L, Rye L: Anorexia nervosa: review including oral and dental manifestations. Journal of the American Dental Association 104:648-652, 1982

Stangler RS, Printz AM: DSM-III: psychiatric diagnosis in a university population. Am J Psychiatry 137:937-940, 1980

Walsh BT, Stewart JW, Wright L, et al: Treatment of bulimia with monoamine oxidase inhibitors. Am J Psychiatry 139:1629-1630, 1982

Weiss SR, Ebert MH: Psychological and behavioral characteristics of normal-weight bulimics and normal-weight controls. Psychosom Med 45:293-303, 1983

Weiss T, Levitz L: Diphenylhydantoin treatment of bulimia. Am J Psychiatry 133:1093, 1976

Wermuth BM, Davis KL, Hollister LE, et al: Phenytoin treatment of the binge-eating syndrome. Am J Psychiatry 134:1249-1253, 1977

White WC, Boskind-White M: An experiential-behavioral approach to the treatment of bulimarexia. Psychotherapy: Theory, Research and Practice 18:501-507, 1981

Chapter 25

Family Aspects of Eating Disorders

by Joel Yager, M.D. and Michael Strober, Ph.D.

Eating disorders have attracted considerable attention from clinicians and researchers interested in psychological and biological perspectives of the family. It is natural for eating disorders to come under scrutiny. In the clinical setting it is often a family member rather than the patient herself who first seeks professional help. In some instances an entire family appears agitated while trying to contend with a troubled eating disorder patient. Many of the patients are adolescents and young adults who are still living with or just leaving their families of origin. These families have provided veritable laboratories for family systems researchers who have sought psychopathogenetic mechanisms in maladaptive family process and structures, poor communication patterns, and destructive relationships. Large numbers of these families have been well-to-do and relatively intact; their verbal capacities, attention to psychological issues, and interest in participating in psychotherapeutic investigation and treatment have been, in general, as good as or better than other psychiatric populations. Biologically-minded clinicians and researchers have sought explanations of the individual's psychopathology and clues to treatment in presumed biological vulnerabilities transmitted through the family. Both the family systems and biological levels of inquiry have produced exciting observations and hypotheses, the meanings and implications of which are by no means fully understood.

Since most work in eating disorders has focused on anorexia nervosa, a large part of this chapter will deal with this syndrome. Bulimia, much more recently delineated as a syndrome, has been less well examined from a family perspective; thus, our comments will be more limited. Finally, we will briefly mention family aspects of obesity.

ANOREXIA NERVOSA

The earliest reports of anorexia nervosa noted that families interact with the patients in ways usually believed to be detrimental to the patients. Subsequent authorities have differed widely in their views about the role of the family in its pathogenesis.

To put the role of the family into a comprehensive perspective, we will consider the following issues: the transmission of anorexia nervosa in families; family stress response patterns; family systems formulations; the prognostic importance of family characteristics; and family therapy.

The stereotypic anorexia nervosa family has been portrayed as upper-middle-class and achievement oriented, in which parents and siblings are very weight and exercise conscious. The family is, according to this model, very concerned with external appearances and diligently puts up a congenial facade; but below the surface lurks the parents' lack of fulfillment as a couple. One parent may be particularly insecure while the other is aloof. The family communicates along narrow lines and fearfully avoids overt anger, at the cost of clarity and honesty. Parental stresses are deflected toward the children, and one parent, often the mother, becomes overinvested in and overdirective toward them, leading to a situation in which a vulnerable daughter (most often) becomes preoccupied with obtaining external parental approval. Furthermore, the parents inadequately acknowledge or encourage the child's autonomy so that her sense of self is poor. She feels ineffective and lacks areas for meaningful self control, and she tries to fill her inner void by pleasing her parents. At a point of minor upheaval during her adolescence, anorexia nervosa begins: This may be related to parental friction, the illness or death of a relative, an academic difficulty, a peer or sexual situation, or a mother's increased fearfulness about her daughter's growing up and away from her. The anorexia nervosa may start in the guise of an ordinary diet to "just lose a few pounds," and is often accompanied by the well-intentioned encouragement of family and friends.

This sketch fuses descriptions provided by Bruch (1973, 1978), Crisp and colleagues (1980), Minuchin and colleagues (1978) and Selvini-Palazzoli (1978) among others, and a growing number of popular books and television programs. However, as with most clinical problems, there are no universal patterns and this stereotype often falls short. Similar stereotypes portraying bulimic patients as impulsive, promiscuous and prone to substance abuse are also frequently inaccurate. At this stage, the physician would be wiser to avoid pat, narrow formulas to explain anorexia nervosa or bulimia primarily in family, or any other terms. An attitude of guarded skepticism, while we await additional information to support, modify, or refute the myriad of current hypotheses, is recommended. Given the wide diversity in the syndromes of anorexia nervosa, it is difficult to see how any of the current hypotheses could explain them all. Patients differ widely with respect to age of onset and clinical features. Personality varies enormously so that dysthymic, obsessional, histrionic, borderline, avoidant, and other personality patterns are seen. Patients differ with respect to ego strength, psychosexual development and experience, academic and social striving, and social competence. A *spectrum* of anorexia nervosa and bulimia syndromes may exist analogous to the schizophrenia syndromes, and many subclinical "anorexoids" are encountered (Yager et al, 1983). The range of family psychopathology is wide, too, and in many respects lacks specificity to the condition (Crisp et al, 1974, Kalucy et al, 1977, Dally and Gomez, 1979).

Serious methodological shortcomings beset the literature on family studies, as was true with the early work on the families of schizophrenics. Much of the eating disorder family literature is impressionistic and speculative; few reliable, well-validated techniques have been available to precisely delineate the wide array of family patterns described by insightful clinicians; and family processes have been observed only following the onset of the condition, so that cause is not easily separated from consequence. Observer biases in researchers, retrospective distortion in family members, differences in sample selection, diagnostic criteria, socioeconomic status, among other things, make comparison difficult among different series in the literature (Yager, 1982).

With these cautions in mind we will examine the following questions about the possible role of the family in the pathogenesis of anorexia nervosa and bulimia:

1. What characterizes the family in which a member exhibits an eating disorder rather than another mode of breakdown?
2. Can we distinguish *necessary* preconditions in the family from those that are simply permissive but nonessential in promoting an eating disorder in a vulnerable person? As a corollary, to what extent are family patterns described in relation to eating disorders found in the general nonafflicted population (for example, food faddisms, parental overcontrol, enmeshment)?
3. To what extent may the "typical" family patterns represent stress reactions in the wake of eating disorders ("states") rather than preexisting and enduring family patterns ("traits")?
4. What family factors are conducive to maintaining the syndrome and influencing prognosis?

While some preliminary answers have been tentatively suggested, most of these issues remain confused.

FAMILIAL TRANSMISSION

The Transmission of Eating Disorders

Anorexia nervosa is a relatively uncommon disorder, but its incidence among members of afflicted families is much higher than in the general population. In a careful but preliminary study, Gershon et al (1983) found that eating disorders occurred in 6.4 percent of the first degree relatives of anorexia nervosa patients, as compared to 1.3 percent of control relatives. Similarly, Strober (1983) found eating disorders to aggregate more in the relatives of anorexic probands than among affective disorder probands. About half of the 25 monozygotic twin pairs reported with anorexia nervosa are concordant for the disorders, but controversy exists and as yet no strong genetic case for anorexia nervosa can be made (Nowlin, 1983; Vandereycken and Pierloot, 1981). Kalucy et al (1977) studied 56 families, and found an explicit history of significantly low adolescent weight, anorexia nervosa or weight phobias in 27 percent of mothers and 16 percent of fathers. Crisp et al (1980) have reported "probable" anorexia nervosa to have been present in a first degree relative in 29 percent of 102 consecutive cases. The estimated prevalence of anorexia nervosa among mothers and sisters of anorexia nervosa patients in other studies is between three and ten percent (Morgan and Russell, 1975; Dally and Gomez, 1979; Theander, 1970; Garfinkel et al, 1980; Beumont et al, 1978). The incidence of anorexia nervosa in the children of women who themselves have had anorexia nervosa is unknown.

Such findings cannot be simplisticly attributed to genetic causes, and further research using adoptive and half sibling studies will be necessary to separate possible genetic contributions. In this regard, Crisp (1980) provides us with a particularly instructive case in which the *adopted* daughter of a man with chronic anorexia nervosa developed the disorder.

The importance of determining whether genetic and other biological factors contribute to the syndrome is directly relevant to family therapy. The guilt that parents feel is ubiquitous, and the ambiguity of pathogenesis leads many parents to blame themselves severely. While the parents of diabetic children, too, feel guilty about their children's illnesses, their guilt may be easier to bear: Somehow biology "can't be helped," whereas psychogenesis is viewed as being controllable.

Although weight pathology has been studied in these families, too few studies have included appropriate comparison groups, so that the significance of the findings cannot be adequately evaluated. For example, Kalucy et al (1977) found 23 percent of mothers and 20 percent of fathers to be overweight, and 16 percent of mothers and nine percent of fathers to be underweight; 11 percent of mothers and seven percent of fathers had "weight fluctuation"; 27 percent of mothers and 16 percent of fathers had "dieting behavior"; 25 percent of patients had an obese sibling; and 14 percent had some other obese family member, almost always the maternal grandmother. But, in a carefully controlled investigation, Halmi et al (1978) found that parents of anorexia nervosa patients did not differ from control parents with respect to either average weight or variations in weight. In comparing parental weights of 68 anorexia nervosa patients who experienced bulimia with those of 73 patients who did not ("restricters"), Garfinkel et al (1980) reported the mothers of the bulimics to have a significantly higher prevalence of obesity than those of restricters (48 percent vs. 28 percent). The fathers did not differ (18 percent in each case). Strober (1981) found no significant differences in the history of maternal or paternal obesity between the two groups. Clearly, this area deserves further study.

Transmission of Psychiatric and Psychosomatic Disorders

Emotional disturbances have been reported in 21 to 66 percent of the parents of patients with anorexia nervosa but descriptions differ widely (Beumont et al, 1978; Dally, 1969; Kay and Leigh, 1954). Studies have reported affective disorders in 13 to 33 percent of first degree relatives of patients with anorexia nervosa, in each series substantially higher than among control relatives (Cantwell et al, 1977; Winokur et al, 1980; Hudson et al, 1983). Kalucy et al (1977) found marked phobic avoidance in 33 percent of mothers and 11 percent of fathers, depression in 33 percent of mothers and nine percent of fathers, and manic-depressive psychosis in 14 percent of fathers, an unusually high prevalence not observed in other series. In a careful case controlled study Gershon et al (1983) found a lifetime prevalence for unipolar depression among first degree relatives of anorexia nervosa patients vs. controls of 13.3 percent vs. 5.8 percent and of bipolar illness of 8.3 percent vs. 1.0 percent. Strober (1983) also found the prevalence of affective disorder among first degree relatives of depressed anorexia nervosa patients to be nearly twice that of nondepressed anorexia nervosa patients (24 percent vs. 12 percent). It should be noted that neither Gershon nor Strober found increased eating disorders among the first degree relatives of affective disorders probands, arguing against the straight genetic hypothesis that these types of disorders are merely alternative expressions of the same dispositions. Schizophrenia is rarely reported in relatives of anorexia nervosa patients.

Several studies have found higher prevalences of psychiatric disturbance, particularly depression and alcoholism, among parents of anorexia nervosa patients with bulimia as compared with parents of restricters (Garfinkel et al, 1980; Strober et al, 1982).

In one survey only 12 percent of 746 respondents with mixed eating disorders reported neither parent to have an emotional or weight problem (Yager et al, 1983). The underlying issue may be that these are all emotionally vulnerable families, and that such families are more likely to be breeding grounds for eating disorders than are sturdier families. Dally and Gomez (1979), who found that 24 percent of patients had parents who required psychiatric treatment, concluded that the incidence of neurosis or psychosis in first degree relatives of anorexia nervosa patients is similar to that found in groups of other "neurotic" patients.

Psychosomatic disturbances have been reported in 16 to 50 percent of first degree relatives of patients with anorexia nervosa (Halmi et al, 1977; Kalucy et al, 1977; Kay and Leigh, 1954). Halmi et al (1977) found peptic ulcer in 16 percent, gastritis in 32 percent and irritable colon in 23 percent, while Kalucy et al (1978) reported that 30 percent of their patients' mothers suffered from migraine, a figure they believed to exceed that in the general population.

PERSONALITY CHARACTERISTICS OF PARENTS

"Typical" personalities among parents of anorexia nervosa patients have been suggested. Cobb (1943) described the typical home situation to consist of a robust, nagging mother and passive father; subsequent investigators have by no means agreed. Kalucy et al (1977) found marked obsessionality in 29 percent of fathers and 14 percent of mothers, and Wold (1973) stressed that rigidity and compulsivity in fathers was potentially important in pathogenesis. Dally (1969) found great diversity. In 21 percent of families, mothers were forceful and robust while fathers were weak and remote; in 17 percent, mothers were tense, neurotic, and forceful, and fathers were passive; in three percent, a normal mother was forced into a dominant role due to the early death of a husband; in five percent, a domineering, aggressive, constantly quarreling father was found; in eight percent, the father was domineering but not aggressive; in four percent, the father was psychopathic, unreliable, and inconsistantly domineering; and so on. In other words, there is little consistency at this level of observation. One begins to suspect that if common personality patterns are to be found in these families, they will have to be at more subtle levels. Few systematic observational studies of parental personality characteristics apart from their families have been conducted. Goldstein (1981) described that when they were tested on the WAIS, parents of anorexia nervosa patients demonstrated far more dependency and insecurity in relation to the examiner than did parents of other disturbed adolescents. But Garfinkel et al (1983) found that neither mothers nor fathers of anorexia nervosa patients differed from controls on the HSCL, Beck Depression Inventory, or 16 Personality Factor (16 PF) tests, except that on the 16 PF fathers of anorexia nervosa patients displayed higher degrees of conscientiousness than controls.

Parent-Child Interactions

Considerable variation also marks available descriptions of parent-child interactions in anorexia nervosa.

On the basis of careful family interviews, Morgan and Russell (1975), found that relations between family and patient were disturbed in 54 percent of their patients prior to the onset of illness. In other series, oversolicitous mothers with "very" attached daughters are reported to occur in from 31 to 39 percent, ambivalent relationships between mother and daughter in about one-third, mothers who are strict disciplinarians in about 12 percent, and overly rejecting mothers in one to 11 percent (Kay and Leigh, 1954, Dalley 1969, Kalucy et al, 1977, Beumont et al, 1978). A gamut of father-daughter relationships are also seen: Some fathers are lenient/kind/affectionate, others are cool and antagonistic, others overtly hostile, and so forth. In some families both parents hold similar attitudes toward the child, whereas in others parents hold opposite attitudes. In some instances the daughter with anorexia nervosa appears to be overprotective toward one or another of the parents, most often the mother. This is thought to represent projective identification as a component of the daughter's defenses. It should be noted that satisfactory or "normal" relationships between parents and their children are also reported to be present in 11 to 25 percent of anorexia nervosa families.

Several studies have attempted to investigate parent-child interactions with precise methods. A study by Hall and Brown (1983) using a semantic differential found no difference in the extent to which the mothers of anorexia nervosa patients were more likely than mothers of controls to misinterpret or misunderstand their daughters' fears of growing up or to overvalue thinness, attitudes which were shared alike by the anorexia nervosa patients and control adolescent girls. Crisp and Kalucy (1974) used a standardized measure of body width estimation and found some families in which the parents seemed to prefer an anorectic body size for their daughters. Goldstein and colleagues (1981) studied 42 intact families, each of which had an adolescent daughter being treated psychiatrically as an inpatient or outpatient, among whom were ten hospitalized anorectics. While no single pattern was found, mothers of patients with anorexia nervosa were generally found to be more highly directive of their children's behavior than were the fathers or the mothers of the outpatient groups, but not more projective than the latter groups. Fathers were varied in their responses; some were directly involved but others were indirect and intrusive with high projection patterns. The conclusions of this study are very tentative but are consistent with hypotheses derived from the work of Minuchin et al to be discussed below.

FAMILY STRESS RESPONSE PATTERNS

Stress response syndromes have been well studied in individuals, but not in whole family systems. Following major catastrophes, families experience transient adjustment responses and demonstrate disturbed behavior that may not be typical for them. Under stress, exaggerated responses show family members' defensive operations in bold relief, whereas during calmer times such families may not appear to be so pathological.

Parents face a willfully starving child and a potentially fatal situation; they confront the problem at every meal. Given the etiological ambiguity, parental guilt (and/or denial and projection of guilt) is virtually inescapable. Parents recall every one of their behaviors that might have "caused" the anorexia nervosa—their own "neuroses," misguided ignorance, or unavoidable misfortunes. They wonder how much the other parent is to blame, or if they are all still acting in a harmful way. They find few agreed-upon guidelines regarding how to proceed. How can they know when to force their daughter to eat and when not to? Threaten or not threaten? Be vigilant or ignore?

Cognitive styles and stress response patterns vary in individuals as well as in families. Some are predominantly minimizers or deniers, others are hypervigilant worriers, and others are adaptive information seekers and action-oriented copers (Lazarus et al, 1974). Some parents appear exceedingly neurotic and disorganized when the anorexia nervosa patient first presents, yet rapidly reintegrate and demonstrate unexpected resources with the child's recovery; others are not so seriously disturbed upon admission but manifest serious adjustment problems as the child improves (Crisp et al, 1974; Kalucy et al, 1977). Dally (1969) described five types of mother/daughter interactions with anorexia nervosa, essentially an exaggeration of all possible patterns of usual adolescent-parent conflicts: (1). Mother meets daughter halfway, and the two live amicably together sharing household functions, somewhat like sisters. (2). Mother and daughter are highly competitive, particularly if mother and father are on bad terms. Mother may break down, go to work, or leave in some other way. (3). Mother withstands daughter's attempts to take her place. Then the daughter retreats and is extruded from the home. (4). Mother beats off daughter's attacks, but daughter is unable to leave home and regresses instead into virtual isolation and solitariness in the house. (5). Daughter regresses to a baby-like state, shows no initiative and becomes totally dependent on her mother (or a substitute).

Just as individual responses to stress change over time, a family system's defense patterns may shift in the wake of catastrophe (Kaplan et al, 1973). The initial display of parental depression, enmeshment, or directiveness may partly reflect how serious and "out of control" they perceive the child's illness to be. Somewhat telescoped, mother and/or father may minimize or deny at first, and then go through high emotional arousal, perhaps followed by apathy after chronic defeat with regard to changing their child's behavior. Each family member's shifting states of adjustment affects others, resulting in widely varying family interaction characteristics over time. Thus, although a family may appear to be very enmeshed during an acute crisis (perhaps in part reflecting attempts to increase family cohesion), it may later appear "burned out" and disengaged. Such characteristics require study over time to see how enduring they are once acute stress is alleviated. Reductions in family enmeshment that have been attributed to family therapy may in part represent natural phasic resolutions of family stress response patterns.

FAMILY SYSTEMS

An intriguing approach to eating disorders has been proposed by family systems theorists who have formulated pathogenic and treatment models that relate family structure and processes to these disorders (Minuchin et al, 1978; Selvini-Palazzoli, 1978; Crisp, 1980). The family is viewed as a self-regulating, constantly evolving system with characteristic structures, transactions, and subsystems composed of the various members aligned by age, role, and other parameters. Family systems can be characterized by communication rules, the clarity and expressiveness of ideas and feelings, power structures, role flexibility, closeness, family and individual boundaries, myths, and secrets. Family systems can also be described by its efficacy as a problem-solving unit to accomplish the dual tasks of helping individuals to have a sense of belonging to the family while at the same time developing their autonomy. Communications may be clear or diffuse, roles may be complementary or symmetrical, and so on. In this perspective the patient's symptoms can be thought of as being evoked, supported, and reinforced by certain transactions in the system, and as playing a part in the family's entire psychological economy. The reader is referred to Hoffman (1981) and to Nichols (1984) for excellent overviews of these concepts. In general, families of many anorexia nervosa patients fall into the dysfunctional but not chaotic group, stable with respect to dominance and submission roles. These families are often characterized by powerful coalitions that may be more important than the bond between the parents, for example between a submissive parent and a child or between a parent and a grandparent.

Such concepts about anorexia nervosa families have been detailed by Minuchin et al (1978). Employing standardized assessment measures, these researchers have identified characteristics that they believe typify the "psychosomatic families" of patients with juvenile onset diabetes mellitus, bronchial asthma, and anorexia nervosa. One such characteristic is *enmeshment*, in which family members are overinvolved with one another, each may answer for any other, and family members intrude on each other's thoughts and feelings; this is said to result in family members developing poorly differentiated perceptions of one another and of themselves. Other characteristics include *overprotectiveness*, in which parents and children may be highly protective of one another; *rigidity*, expressed as needs to maintain "appearances" and conventional social roles; and a tendency to avoid overt conflict within the family, with consequent lack of conflict resolution. The child may be forced to side with one parent against the other, sometimes shifting from one to the other, and sometimes more permanently aligning with one parent. Or, the parents may suppress their own conflicts and focus on the child, often requiring the child to reassure them about their own parenting.

Chronic discord in these relatively stable marriages are common, and although pre-illness parental separation has been reported in high percentages of families (Kalucy et al, 1977), Dally and Gomez (1979) found broken homes among only 18 percent of patients who developed anorexia nervosa before the age of 15, which they estimated to be less than in other populations. Therefore, it has been postulated that the distraction of a sick child helps diffuse the conflict, the child's symptoms are rewarded and sustained, and the symptoms become embedded in the family organization. But in spite of such theorizing, as Dally and Gomez point out, "anorexia nervosa does not result in greater marital harmony and cessation of open warfare" (1979).

Some experimental support for the idea that the patient's symptoms help to regulate and keep the family together was offered by Crisp et al (1974), who found parents, especially those with poor marriages, to be more anxious and depressed when their child with anorexia nervosa was improving and gaining weight than when the child initially entered the hospital. Although one might conclude that parental symptoms increase at this point because the child no longer serves as a focus for family conflict, an alternative interpretation is that such families become more anxious in the face of the impending discharge from hospital of the still emotionally precarious patient.

Similar family systems difficulties in anorexia nervosa are described by Selvini-Palazzoli (1978). She reports that family members commonly reject messages sent by others; parents are reluctant to assume responsibility and each parent blames his or her decisions on the other; family members never attribute their actions to their own personal preferences, but to other member's needs, so that all decisions are for someone else's "good"; blame is shifted all around, and although mothers tend to overblame themselves, they attribute their behavior to their devotion to the children. Each parent feels particularly victimized, as if she or he is making great sacrifices for the family.

Crisp et al (1974) have also postulated that anorexia nervosa is more likely to develop in families with "neurotic constellations" that prohibit adolescent maturation (or at least fail to prepare the patient to cope with puberty and adolescence). A wide variety of immediate pre-illness events that threaten family homeostasis can precipitate the illness. But, for the most part, these are the universal problems of troubled families with their adolescent children, so the question remains, why anorexia nervosa?

The studies reviewed above have examined family systems primarily through clinical interviews. Some studies have used standardized psychological tests and questionnaires to take semiquantitative snapshots of the family at one or two points in time. Many of the family test measures are as yet of unproven validity (Miller et al, 1982), and all have of necessity been administered after the family has been in the throes of wrestling with anorexia nervosa. However, they offer a potentially useful approach to family assessment. For example, Sours (1980) reported that MMPIs support the impression that the families strive to look perfect and present a caricature of normality while at the same time showing signs of withdrawal and isolation—the MMPIs yield low F–K scores ("fake good") and high SC scores. Strober (1981) administered two family measures in his study of parents of bulimic and restricter anorexia nervosa patients. Each set of parents jointly completed the Moos Family Environment Scale (FES) with a view toward describing family patterns that antedated their daughter's illness, and parents also completed the Lock Wallace short marital adjustment test. On the FES, bulimic families were characterized by significantly higher levels of conflictual interactions and expressions of negativity among members; restricter families were more strongly associated with greater cohesiveness (that is, mutual support and concern among family members) and organization (that is, clarity of structure and rules, and division of responsibilities). With regard to marital adjustment ratings, considerable disharmony was evident in both groups, but significantly higher levels were reported by parents of anorexia nervosa bulimics as compared to restricters. This finding is supported by studies of Garner et al (1983) and Garfinkel et al (1983) who used the Family Assessment Measure (FAM), a self-report instrument which obtains perceptions of the family's function in various areas including task accomplishment, role performance, communication, and affective expression. Families of anorexia nervosa patients reported more difficulty for all of these subscales than did controls. Such difficulty is *not* specific to anorexia nervosa, and is found in other families with chronic dysfunction as well. However, when responses of normal weight bulimics, anorexia nervosa bulimics, and anorexia nervosa restricters were compared, the first two groups were found to be comparable and indicating disturbed function, whereas the families of anorexia nervosa restricters were described as significantly less disturbed.

To summarize this point, we cannot generalize any of the current family systems formulations to all anorexia nervosa families because a diverse number of patterns have been found (the anorexia nervosa syndrome is heterogenous at least regarding restricters and bulimics), and even those patterns which are typically associated with anorexia nervosa are specific neither for anorexia nervosa nor for only what Minuchin et al have chosen to call "psychosomatic families". This is one reason why clinicians who have had little experience with anorexia nervosa find these concepts intuitively familiar. While such family systems formulations may help to explain how symptoms can be provoked and sustained once they appear, they do not explain the appearance of anorexia nervosa rather than any other illness. They don't account for the intermediate mechanisms that bring about the desire for thinness, early amenorrhea, behavioral hyperactivity, and other clinical features of the syndrome.

Kalucy et al (1977) attempt to explain some of the specificity for anorexia nervosa by suggesting that concerns about eating, body shape, and weight can become major content vehicles for maladaptive family interaction and communication processes. They reported deviant eating patterns in 23 percent of their families; for example, one person always eating separately, restrictions against conversations at meals, and so on. In dysfunctional weight-preoccupied families, concerns about food and physical appearance may constitute some of the few available communication channels. Food preoccupations help emphasize dependency and may be used to defend against aggressive, sexual, and autonomous strivings. Similarly, Dally and Gomez (1979) found that food was given special prominence in 25 percent of families: vegetarian diets, avoidance of red meat, devotion to "natural foods", and so forth. Nevertheless, such food idiosyncracies are undoubtedly more common among contemporary families than is anorexia nervosa, and these authors believe that strong family food eccentricities are associated with eating disorders *only* when associated with parental discord; that is, a "two factor" theory. But, does this mean such food prominence is *not* a factor in the other 75 percent of anorexia nervosa families? All of these writers clearly point out that such primary abnormalities in the family surrounding eating are not characteristics of all anorexia nervosa families. For example, Garfinkel et al (1983) found that compared to control parents, parents of anorexia nervosa patients did *not* have undue preoccupation with dieting, weight control, or other symptoms of anorexia nervosa, and did not report dissatisfaction with their bodies, overestimate their body sizes or idealize thinness. So, all would agree that within family systems formulations for anorexia nervosa much room exists for considering the intrapsychic and biological vulnerabilities of the individual child.

Furthermore, in the last decade the field of family theory has been mushrooming, and many of the newer concepts, dimensions, and measurement instruments are just now beginning to be applied to eating disorders. To name but a few, concerns about high negative expressed emotion in families, a characteristic found so important in schizophrenia, are now being considered in anorexia nervosa families (Szmuckler, 1983). Concepts that merit further study in relation to these families include those regarding consensus-sensitive vs. environment-sensitive families (Reiss, 1981), living systems theory (Miller and Miller, 1983) and several new structural and process typologies that provide a more complex conception of the family than has hitherto been available (see, for example, Beavers and Voller, 1983; Kantor and Lehr, 1975; Kog et al, 1983; Olson et al, 1983; Werthheim, 1973). The dimensions and typologies they suggest promise to further modify, and build on the family systems hypotheses currently available, and we can certainly rest assured that many more ways of looking at families are yet to come.

THE RELATIONSHIP OF FAMILY PATHOLOGY TO PATIENT PROGNOSIS

As with many psychiatric disorders, the sickest patients usually come from the sickest families. Several authors have reported parental conflict and dominant, rejecting, or neurotic parents to be related to poor outcome (Dally & Gomez, 1979, Crisp 1980, Morgan et al, 1983). For example, Crisp et al (1974) found mothers of poor outcome patients to have been more depressed than mothers of good outcome patients, but others have not found this relationship (Theander, 1970, Pierloot et al, 1975). Crisp (1980) also found poor outcome to be predicted by disturbed parental relationship, disturbed relationship of patients to parents prior to the illness, fixed rigid attitudes, denial of problems in the parents, and lower social class. Morgan et al (1983) found poorer prognosis if the family was hostile to the patient, and when there was a "disturbed relation between patient and family," strikingly similar to the relationship between high negative expressed emotion in families to poor outcome in schizophrenia. Studies examining the prognostic and treatment implications of negative expressed emotion in anorexia nervosa families are now underway (Szmuckler, 1983).

FAMILY THERAPY

In the minds of most contemporary clinicians, anorexia nervosa and family therapy are so linked that the question is not *should* family therapy be undertaken, but in what ways and to what extent should the family be involved in a particular case (Vandereycken and Meerman, 1984). At the same time, most clinicians would agree that family therapy represents only one component of a comprehensive treatment program that should include individual therapy, medical management, and hospitalization as needed. Most major centers have incorporated family therapy into inpatient and outpatient programs (Anderson et al, 1983; Dare, 1983; Garfinkel and Garner, 1982; Sargent, 1983; Stern et al, 1981). Yet great diversity exists among these programs. Some rely heavily on brief medical hospitalizations with intensive family therapy started immediately (Dare, 1983; Sargent, 1983). Others employ a variable type and period of separation of the family from the hospitalized patient, perhaps only to restrict visiting at mealtimes, to limit the numbers of hours of visits and phone calls during the week, or to institute an initial period of extremely limited contact (for example, during therapy sessions only)—a modified "parentectomy" (Harper, 1983). This points out that even within family therapy circles little uniformity of approach exists, and that in spite of increasingly sophisticated conceptualizations there is still plenty of room for both art and controversy.

The extremes of family therapy include the timid therapist, who is fearful of saying anything harsh or afraid of offending nonpatient family members who might precipitously pull the patient out of treatment; the therapist who allies with the patient in an antagonistic struggle against the rest of the family, intending to perform a rescue operation; and the therapist who attacks the family system structure, sometimes deftly, and sometimes with the subtlety of a sledgehammer, in dazzling displays of therapeutic bravado designed to shake up, confuse, and provoke change.

There are dangers and limitations—as well as theoretical gains to be had—from each approach. While the timid therapist may keep the family in therapy and together, nothing much may happen to effect change. The family may never fulfill its potential for differentiation and evolution.

The therapist who allies with the patient *may* help separate a child from her parents, but will more often lose a tug of war since the family has greater influence, and since parents and child somehow all know that if separated prematurely the child will wither rather than ripen.

The therapist who focuses exclusively on the family system, peppering it with directives to provoke structural changes or with paradoxes to induce oppositional rebounds into healthier interactional processes, may do just that. Or, failing to appreciate the limiting constraints in the families' subsystems (for example, problems *within* the patient) such therapists may stir up a frenzy of family arousal that nevertheless has little chance of effecting change in the patient, while it is likely to create additional ill will. By analogy, after a family member has had a cerebrovascular accident—apoplexy blamed on family strife—no amount of change in the family system will undo the neurological damage and assure complete recovery. A better family environment will no doubt contribute to optimum rehabilitation, and this is as true for anorexia nervosa as for a stroke, so that family therapy is *still* important. But, the issue here is setting realistic goals based on accurate appraisal of *all* parts of the family system, including its various individual subsystems.

Our position regarding family therapy in eating disorders should be clear at the outset. In spite of the plethora of theoretical family systems constructs, the available literature fails to demonstrate the superiority of any one type of family therapy. Moreover, we are unaware of any systematic study that has yet convincingly demonstrated that *any* carefully described family therapy in and of itself or in combination with other therapies has significantly altered the long-term outcome in any controlled series of cases of anorexia nervosa.

But, as clinicians, we find family therapy to be intuitively appealing and clinically useful. The blend of tactics we employ reflects no one "school" and varies from case to case depending on the specifics of patient and family. We are highly attentive to the "nonspecific" factors in therapy, and attempt to be empirically pragmatic. In our work, family therapy is but one facet, albeit an important one, of comprehensive treatment. Since we remain skeptical about the *universality* of available family formulations, therapy varies with the assessment of the individual case.

Rationale for Family Therapy

Many of the observations and formulations described above may provide a rationale for family therapy. To the extent that family operations such as enmeshment, overprotectiveness, rigidity, avoidance of conflict, weight preoccupation, and so forth are thought to be pathogenic or merely sustaining of symptoms, a determined attempt to alter these phenomena either directly or by working through their psychopathological underpinnings might promise therapeutic benefit. Family therapy can alter the "ruts" in which a family system finds itself, and can have both positive nonspecific effects as well as specific effects. A high intensity family therapy intervention may serve to boost a family's morale and reduce hopelessness (nonspecific effect), and at the same time theoretically provide the energy of activation required to upset pathological family equilibria and permit the establishment and testing of new patterns; that is, a specific effect—a transformation of structure and process. In the latter case pressure may be diverted away from the child toward the parents, and family problems may be rechannelled to be worked out between the parents.

Even if family factors played no role at all in pathogenesis, family therapy may help reduce the illness sustaining factors, thereby facilitating "natural" remission. Rational therapy must be directed at all accessible "therapeutic receptor sites" where one can gain leverage, even if these sites seem removed from proximal levels of cause in the disorder.

Goals of Family Therapy

Goals for family therapy have been implied in much of the previous discussion. A primary concern is to maintain each person's self-esteem, and to help each person to deal with issues of worry, panic, and shame that derive from the impact of the disorder on the family. In general, family therapy strives to help each family member, including the patient, to become more autonomous and less enmeshed, to communicate more directly and precisely, to strengthen appropriate coalitions, and to enable family members to resolve conflicts at their proper locus, usually within generation boundaries. Such therapy will attend to *each* family members' concerns and anxieties, those antedating as well as those consequent to the appearance of anorexia nervosa. Some therapists attempt to alter borderline personality organizations in the family. This is a most ambitious and optimistic goal, at best exceedingly difficult to do, and often an exercise in utter futility dedicated to a theoretical outcome that to our knowledge has never been convincingly documented.

Therapeutic goals vary with the patient's developmental status and with the family's stage in its life cycle. Therapy for younger adolescents who remain at home should strive to increase parental effectiveness and control, strengthen the parental coalition, and resolve their conflicts. With older adolescent patients, the family should be helped to allow the adolescent to individuate and become independent. With the young adult patient already out of the home, the family may be ambivalent or inconsistent about keeping the patient out, and the capacity for sustained independence during periods of regression must be addressed. For the older anorexia nervosa patient in a marriage or a serious relationship, the important (and workable) family may be the "family of insertion" rather than the family of origin. In some cases, the goals may be to get the family to accept the patient's limitations and chronicity. In some cases, a family may be so "toxic"—so permeated with unremitting hostility and abuse toward the patient—that the therapist's best intervention may be to severely limit the patient's contact with the family. But, while a certain number of patients and families are virtually intractable, the majority are not. Careful assessment and reassessment over time are required, and in general at *least* modest improvements are achievable in most cases.

With the family as a whole, the clinician should do the following:

1. Educate: The therapist should provide everyone with whatever information is available and not side-step direct questions regarding the patient's condition. This promotes direct coping on the part of the family. Books for the laity, self-help groups, and so forth, are all useful. Multiple family groups are especially well received, permit sharing of experiences and coping strategies, and may be vehicles for more fundamental change (Vandereycken and Meerman, 1984).

2. Investigate and alleviate blame and guilt: It is cruel and counterproductive to simply allow parents, siblings, and patients to believe that they "created" the situation. Each person simultaneously blames himself or herself and feels blamed by others. An early task of the therapist is to clear the air regarding these issues. For example, after each person recites a list of indictments directed toward self or others, the therapist may review the facts that not enough is known about the causes of anorexia nervosa to be able to definitely assign "blame," that each person no doubt did the best of which he or she was capable at the time, that each person's behavior was itself the result of complicated forces beyond anyone's control, and that blaming or feeling guilty has little payoff in terms of correcting the situation for the future.

   Sometimes explorations of guilt reveal additional hidden assumptions that need to be unravelled, as in the following example: Both parents of a daughter with anorexia nervosa were concentration camp survivors. The father was berating himself pitilessly for having caused his daughter's illness. "After all, I must have been crazy about food and eating! I must have made her crazy in the same way!" After listening to the father at length, the therapist said: "It's all well and good that you want to take the blame—or the credit—for your daughter's condition. But nothing that we know about the causes of anorexia nervosa would make me certain that you're the cause." Rather than to reassure or console him, these remarks seemed only to further agitate the father, who began to pound the desk, saying, "It *must* be my fault! It *must* be my fault!" After a moment's hesitation, the therapist asked the father, "Why is it so important that it be your fault?" The father immediately started to cry freely, slumping in his chair. "Because if it's my fault, then there should be something I could do different to make it better."

3. Address primary concerns: Common themes include the need of the family

to believe that the problems are entirely physical and glandular (often evidenced by doctor shopping); the need of the family to have the child hospitalized for long periods of time ("until she's all better, so we don't have to worry about her at home"); the need of the family to use the therapist as a threat ("tell her that if she doesn't eat you'll do such and such"); the needs of the family to blame the patient (for being "willful, spiteful, and wanting to kill me by how she behaves").

4. Clarify communications: In dealing with an enmeshed family it is useful for the therapist to specifically require each member to speak *only* for himself or herself, saying what (s)he wants from the other person(s), speak only in the first person, not answer for another. This approach is designed to strengthen individual boundaries and block the diffusion. When the therapist doubts the genuiness of a family member's remark, the therapist may step in and express his or her own doubts, trying to urge greater reflection and candor. When angry body language and a screaming voice surrounding a remark assure that the informational content of the communication will neither be heard nor addressed, the therapist may act as a signal extractor: "Setting aside the violent temper, what I just heard A. say was. . . . Would you prefer to discuss the temper, or what A. was trying to say?"

5. Deal with structural and systems process issues: Minuchin et al (1978) describe a number of tactics for challenging the family's rigidity, conflict avoidance, and maladaptive processes. Each member is asked to assume responsibility for his or her own views and desires: Overdirective patterns are pointed out and interrupted; triangulations, detouring maneuvers, and coalitions are pointed out; individual autonomy and competence is supported; children are kept out of parental arguments and are removed physically or temporally when parents need to deal with conflicts that they are avoiding; the therapist points out discordance between words and body language messages so that mixed messages are picked up and explored, and connotations identified and made explicit. These procedures are repeated over and over again until they seem to be actually received and integrated by the family members. When indicated by the course of therapy, the parents are offered separate couples therapy to deal with conflicts that have otherwise been avoided.

Family members are often given prescriptions to perform specific homework assignments. These may be designed to strengthen the parental tie, modify the parent-child interaction or even, paradoxically, prescribe the symptomatic behavior to provoke change. All these behaviors are designed to inject what in cybernetic terms are called new "constraints" into the family system in an effort to destabilize the ongoing maladaptive patterns (Hoffman, 1981). For example, a couple may be asked to do something as "simple" as hold hands for 15 minutes a night as a prelude to restoring communication. Sometimes these techniques work, and sometimes they don't, but in each instance the therapist acquires new information about underlying resistances.

Selvini-Palazzoli and her Milan associates (1978) have operated in a team of four psychiatrists using a one-way screen (two in front and two in back) to create an intensive systems oriented family therapy. Although the method contains "high theater," it is designed to allow a great deal of cross-checking and consultation in assessing and prescribing for the family. The prescriptions they produce often appear paradoxical. They frequently reframe the symptom with a positive connotation, pointing out essentially all the comfort and secondary gain accruing to the family system (often the extended one) as a result of the symptom *and* the ongoing pathological patterns. They may, for example, compliment a child with anorexia nervosa on having provided the family something substantial to worry about so that the mother can be spared having to reflect about the emptiness in her life; the grandmother can have a good excuse to intrude into the family and instruct the mother on caring for the anorexic child; and the parents feel obliged to stay together rather than divorce because of their mutual concern for the child. In a similar fashion, White may ask that the symptoms be continued "for everyone's best interest." He uses the term "conservative approach" in prescribing symptoms in this manner, his way of distancing himself from underlying perjorative connotations that often accompany the concept of paradoxical prescription (White, 1983).

ASSESSMENT OF FAMILY THERAPY

In Chapter 23 of this volume, Kennedy and Garfinkel review the literature on prognosis. Few systematic studies of family therapy for anorexia nervosa and none for family therapy of bulimia are available. Minuchin et al (1978) have presented the largest series so far available. Minuchin's claim of success in over 80 percent of his patients should be regarded with interest, but also with caution. Selection bias exists in his patient sample; they are mostly younger in age and have intact families who are willing to come to therapy. These important factors may themselves account in part for their better than average prognosis. Although not specifically studied, these families may have what Wertheim (1973) has called *open external boundaries*, meaning that they are relatively accessible for therapy in contrast to walled off families with closed external boundaries. She speculates that this would be a good prognostic sign for many conditions. And, to put Minuchin and his associates' results into further perspective, in another follow-up study of 30 children whose age at onset ranged from 9½ to 16 years, Goetz et al (1977) reported that five to 20 years after initial treatment, outcome was poor in only 17 percent; treatment for that group was generally short term, averaging six months, and included only supportive therapy for parents and some individual therapy for patients.

It is also not clear that family interventions change family patterns in directions consistent with their formulations. Family interviews and structured tests following recovery would have to be made to ascertain whether treated families are indeed less enmeshed, overprotective, rigid, and conflict-avoiding than they were at the start. And since changes in these dimensions may partly reflect the spontaneous resolution of a family stress response rather than an effect of therapy, control families should be observed as well. Serious evaluation of family therapy for anorexia nervosa is needed, and remains to be explored. Nevertheless, even with these limitations, the consensus of contemporary clinicians strongly endorses including family assessment and therapy as a treatment component for virtually all adolescent patients with anorexia nervosa. Family therapy for the older anorexia nervosa patient is often of great value but may not be as critical as for younger patients.

BULIMIA

From the preceding discussion, and from the discussions in other chapters in this section, it should be evident that a continuum of psychopathology is thought to be present among patients with bulimic anorexia nervosa, normal weight bulimia, and bulimic obesity. Although we may assume that family characteristics of normal weight bulimics may resemble those already described for bulimic anorexia nervosa patients (and our clinical experience validates this speculation to some extent) available data are inadequate to make this assertion conclusively.

This area is further complicated by the growing awareness of the heterogeneity of clinical syndromes that are subsumed within normal weight bulimia. This group includes a large number of context-related, "trendy" experimental binge eaters and vomiters who are found in large numbers on college campuses, as well as the smaller number of "hard core" bulimics, those who would meet only the stricter definitions. Among the entrenched bulimics are several subgroups, including those in whom an affective component is highly apparent, those whose bulimia represents one manifestation of an impulse-ridden personality disorder (often not the most troubling manifestation), those who have been severely obese and for whom bulimia with purging is a preferable alternative to being superfat, those who have previously had frank anorexia nervosa, and possibly an "epileptoid" subgroup as well. Clearly, one or even a handful of family patterns may not be expected in every case.

With these limitations in mind, we can examine family aspects of normal weight bulimia. The prevalence of eating disorders among family members of normal weight bulimics has received little attention. In one survey 746 respondents reported, for their mothers and fathers respectively, anorexia nervosa in three percent and one percent, binge eating in 22 percent and nine percent, obesity in 41 percent and 28 percent, and "other weight problems" in 20 percent and 13 percent. No differences in family prevalences were reported by bulimics who never had anorexia nervosa, bulimic anorexia nervosa respondents, or nonbulimic anorexia nervosa respondents (Yager et al, 1983).

Relatively more attention has been given to the prevalence of other psychiatric disorders in families of normal weight bulimics. In the families of normal weight bulimics, higher than expected prevalences of depression, particularly in mothers, and of alcoholism, especially in fathers, have been reported (Pyle et al, 1981; Hudson et al; 1983, Yager et al, 1983).

The literature on family therapy of bulimia, aside from anorexia nervosa, is sparse and consists primarily of case examples (for example, Madanes, 1981; Schwartz, 1982). For families of normal weight bulimics, patterns of enmeshment, parental discord, triangulation, and the like resemble pathological family systems described for anorexia nervosa families. Family system interventions have been of benefit. In our clinic, short-term multiple family groups for bulimic patients and their families, using an educational and dynamic format, have been well received. Many of our bulimic young adults, in their mid twenties, are still quite involved with their parents even though they no longer live in the parental home. For them, family assessment and sometimes therapy is indicated. Couples assessment and therapy is often useful for the older patient who is married or involved in a long-term relationship.

OBESITY

It is well known that obese families raise obese children. Children with one or two obese parents are much more likely to become obese than children with two thin parents (Garn and Clark, 1976; Mayer, 1968), and more than 60 percent of obese patients have one or more obese parents (Bray, 1976). Various lines of evidence suggest that "nature" and "nurture" each contribute roughly 50 percent to this occurrence.

In general, no typical psychopathological pictures have been established for obese families. Individual cases, including some described for morbidly obese persons, have resembled the enmeshed families described by Minuchin et al (1978), but clearly these patterns are neither necessary nor sufficient to account for the obesity.

Several studies have examined the potential contribution of family members to the treatment of obesity, but the results thus far are inconclusive. Stuart and Davis (1972) studied marital interactions based on tape recorded mealtime conversations involving a group of overweight women and their husbands; they found many of the husband's comments and behaviors to be both critical of their wife's eating while also undermining their efforts to lose weight.

Based on these and other observations, Wilson and Brownell (1978) conducted the first study to systematically manipulate and evaluate family interactions in the treatment of obesity using a standard behavior program. Those obese persons treated alone received behavior therapy. For the group treated with their family, family members attended all of the treatment sessions in the eight-week program. During this time they were all instructed in the basic principles of behavioral weight reduction programs, were told to stop being critical of the obese relative's eating habits and weight, and were urged to help their relatives in attempts to restructure their environments to improve their self-control. Relatives included not only spouses but some siblings and children as well. Disappointingly, at both the end of the eight-week treatment and six-month follow-up periods, no differences were found between the two groups.

In a subsequent study, Brownell and co-workers (1978) compared three groups using a ten-week treatment program: subjects treated with their cooperative spouses in couples training, subjects with cooperative spouses who were treated alone without spouse involvement, and subjects whose noncooperative spouses refused to participate. At the end of the treatment phase, the differences in weight loss among the groups were not significant, but the couples-treated group had lost more weight. However, it should be noted that after the six months maintenance phase (during which time monthly booster sessions were held) the couples-treated group had lost considerably more than initially, a mean weight loss of thirty pounds, significantly more than the other treatment groups.

This study was followed by a series of others, reviewed by Brownell (1983), which showed mixed results. Most studies did show a beneficial effect for family or couples interventions, particularly when the partner played an active role in treatment. But several studies do not support this. Furthermore, in a study by Brownell and Stunkard (1981) which compared the interactions of drug treatment with couples training, patients with untreated cooperative spouses, and patients with uncooperative spouses, results differed markedly from those of the earlier Brownell et al (1978) study. In the latter study no effect could be found due to couples training.

The treatment of obesity in young patients also invites interest in the potential involvement of family members. Stunkard reviews the most pertinent studies in Chapter 22 of this volume. Suffice it to say that this area merits further investigation; preliminary data suggest that family involvement may be important in affecting the outcome of weight loss programs.

While waiting for the research data to come forth, the clinician faced with an obese patient seeking treatment should inquire about the weight histories and eating habits of other family members, and about their overt and covert attitudes toward obesity and weight loss in the identified patient. Among patients successfully treated for morbid obesity, a number of cases have been described in which the nonobese spouse becomes depressed and/or the marriage breaks up (Neill et al, 1978). The assumption here is that, according to the initial marital "contract," the obese spouse was supposed to *remain* obese, and the subsequent weight loss was experienced as a threat by the partner. Conversely, following treatment for morbid obesity, the newly treated and slimmer patient may choose to leave a spouse he or she viewed as inadequate all along, or may need to "try out" the new body and self-image with other partners. But these are in the minority. Most marriages are unchanged or improved (Kuldau and Rand, 1980).

Furthermore, just as the treatment of an alcoholic may be extremely difficult if not impossible in the presence of an uncooperative alcoholic spouse, the same may be true of foodaholics. And since obesity in both members of a couple is a common occurrence (Garn and Clark, 1976) this issue may frequently contribute to the difficulties that some obese patients experience in adhering to weight reduction programs.

At the very least, such issues suggest that an evaluation of family patterns and dynamics around eating and obesity may help the clinician to plan more effective treatments.

CONCLUSION

Eating disorders remain perplexing, serious, and challenging problems for clinicians and researchers. Major questions remain regarding the role of the family in their etiology and pathogenesis, the specificity or nonspecificity of characteristic family systems for the appearance of these syndromes, the role of the family in maintaining or alleviating the patient's symptoms, and the value of family therapy in comprehensive treatment. Although an overenthusiastic endorsement of a family approach as the only major meaningful intervention is unwarranted, accumulated evidence supports the value of family therapy as an important component of treatment in anorexia nervosa and in many cases of bulimia as well. Attention to family issues also seems warranted in assessment and treatment planning for the obese patient.

REFERENCES

Anderson AE, Hedblom JE, Hubbard FA: A multidisciplinary team treatment for patients with anorexia nervosa and their families. International Journal of Eating Disorders 2:181-192, 1983

Beavers WR, Voeller MN: Family models: comparing and contrasting the Olson Circumplex Model with the Beavers System Model. Fam Process 22:85-97, 1983

Beumont PJV, Abraham SF, Argall WJ, et al: The onset of anorexia nervosa. Aust NZ J Psychiatry 12:145-149, 1978

Bray GA: The Obese Patient. Philadelphia, W.B. Saunders, 1976

Brownell KD: Obesity: treatment effectiveness and adherence to behavioral programs, in Eating and Weight Disorders. Edited by Goodstein RK. New York, Springer, 1983

Brownell KD, Stunkard AJ: Couples training, pharmacotherapy and behavior therapy in the treatment of obesity. Arch Gen Psychiatry 38:1224-1229, 1981

Brownell KD, Heckerman CL, Westlake RJ: The effect of couples training and partner cooperativeness in the behavioral treatment of obesity. Behav Res Ther 16:323-333, 1978

Bruch H: Eating Disorders: Obesity, Anorexia Nervosa and the Person Within. New York, Basic Books, 1973.

Bruch H: The Golden Cage: The Enigma of Anorexia Nervosa. Cambridge, Harvard University Press, 1978

Cantwell D, Sturnzenberger S, Burroughs J, et al: Anorexia nervosa: an affective disorder? Arch Gen Psychiatry 34:1087-1093, 1977

Cobb S: Borderlands of Psychiatry. London, Oxford University Press, 1943

Crisp AH: Anorexia Nervosa: Let Me Be. New York, Grune and Stratton, 1980

Crisp AH, Kalucy RS: Aspects of the perceptual disorder in anorexia nervosa. Br J Med Psychol 47:349-361, 1974

Crisp AH, Harding B, McGuinness B: Anorexia nervosa: psychoneurotic characteristics of parents: relationship to prognosis. J Psychosom Res 18:167-173, 1974

Crisp AH, Hsu LKG, Harding B, et al: Clinical features of anorexia nervosa. J Psychosom Res 24:179-191, 1980

Dally P: Anorexia Nervosa. London, Heinemann Medical Books, 1969

Dally P, Gomez J: Anorexia Nervosa. London, Wm. Heinemann, Ltd., 1979

Dare C: Family therapy for families containing an anorectic youngster, in Understanding Anorexia Nervosa and Bulimia. Columbus, Ohio, Ross Laboratories, 1983

Garfinkel PE, Garner DM: The role of the family, in Anorexia Nervosa: A Multidimenional Perspective. Edited by Garfinkel PE, Garner DM. New York, Brunner/Mazel, 1982

Garfinkel PE, Moldofsky H, Garner DM: The heterogenity of anorexia nervosa. Arch Gen Psychiatry 37:1036-1040, 1980

Garfinkel PE, Garner DM, Rose J, et al: A comparison of characteristics in families of patients with anorexia nervosa and normal controls. Psychol Med 13:821-828, 1983

Garn SM, Clark DC: Trends in fatness and the origins of obesity. Pediatrics 57:443-456, 1976

Garner DM, Garfinkel PE, O'Shaughnessy M: Clinical and psychometric comparison between bulimia in anorexia nervosa and bulimia in normal weight women, in Understanding Anorexia Nervosa and Bulimia. Columbus, Ohio, Ross Laboratories, 1983

Gershon ES, Hamorit JR, Schreiber JL, et al: Anorexia nervosa and major affective disorders associated in families: a preliminary report, in Childhood Psychopathology and Development. Edited by Guze SB, Earls FJ, Barrett JE. New York, Raven Press, 1983

Goetz PL, Succop RA, Reinhart JB, et al: Anorexia nervosa in children: a followup study. Am J Orthopsychiatry 47:597-603, 1977

Goldstein M: Family factors associated with schizophrenia and anorexia nervosa. Journal of Youth and Adolescence 10:385-405, 1981

Hall A, Brown, LB: A comparison of the attitudes of young anorexia nervosa patients and nonpatients with those of their mothers. Br J Med Psychol 56:39-48, 1983

Halmi KA, Goldberg SC, Eckert E, et al: Pretreatment evaluation in anorexia nervosa, in Anorexia Nervosa. Edited by Vigersky RA. New York, Raven Press, 1977

Halmi KA, Struss A, Goldberg SC: An investigation of weights in the parents of anorexia nervosa patients. J Nerv Ment Dis 166:358-361, 1978

Harper G: Varieties of parenting failure in anorexia nervosa: protection and parentectomy revisited. J Am Acad Child Psychiatry 22:134-139, 1983

Hoffman L: Foundation of Family Therapy: A Conceptual Framework for Systems Change. New York, Basic Books, 1981

Hudson JL, Pope HG Jr, Jonas JM, et al: Family history study of anorexia nervosa and bulimia. Br J Psychiatry 142:133-138, 1983

Kalucy RS, Crisp AH, Harding B: A study of 56 families with anorexia nervosa. Br J Med Psychol 50:381-395, 1977

Kantor D, Lehr W: Inside the Family. San Francisco, Jossey-Bass, 1975

Kaplan DM, Smith A, Grobstein R, et al: Family mediation of stress. Social Work 18:60-69, 1973

Kay DWK, Leigh D: The natural history, treatment and prognosis of anorexia nervosa based on a study of 38 patients. Journal of Mental Science 100:411-431, 1954

Kob E, Pierloot R, Vandereycken W: Methodologic considerations of family research in anorexia nervosa. International Journal of Eating Disorders 2:79-84, 1983

Kuldau JM, Rand CSW: Jejunoileal bypass: general and psychiatric outcome after one year. Psychosomatics 21:534-539, 1980

Lazarus RS, Averill JR, Opton EM Jr: The psychology of coping: issues of research and assessment, in Coping and Adaptation. Edited by Coehlo GV, Hamburg DA, Adams JE. New York, Basic Books, 1974

Liebman R, Sargent J, Silver M: A family systems orientation to the treatment of anorexia nervosa. J Am Acad Child Psychiatry 22:128-133, 1983

Madanes C: Strategic Family Therapy. San Francisco, Jossey-Bass, 1981

Mayer J: Overweight: Causes, Costs and Controls. Englewood Cliffs, NJ, Prentice-Hall, 1968

Miller BC, Rollins BC, Thomas DL: On methods of studying marriages and families. Journal of Marriage and the Family 44:851-873, 1982

Miller JG, Miller JL: General living systems theory and small groups, in Comprehensive Group Psychotherapy, 2nd edition. Edited by Kaplan HI, Sadock BJ. Baltimore, Williams and Wilkins, 1983

Minuchin S, Rosman BL, Baker L: Psychosomatic Families: Anorexia Nervosa in Context. Cambridge, Harvard University Press, 1978

Morgan HG, Russell GFM: Value of family background and clinical features as predictors of long term outcome in anorexia nervosa: four year followup study of 41 patients. Psychol Med 5:355-371, 1975

Morgan HG, Purolog J, Welbourne J: Management and outcome in anorexia nervosa: a standardized prognostic study. Br J Psychiatry 143:282-287, 1983

Neill JR, Marshall AR, Yale CE: Marital changes after intestinal bypass surgery. JAMA 240:447-450, 1978

Nichols M: Family Therapy: Concepts and Methods. New York, Gardner Press, 1984

Nowlin NS: Anorexia nervosa in twins: case report and review. J Clin Psychiatry 44:101-105, 1983

Olson DH, Russell CS, Sprenkel DH: Circumplex model of marital and family systems: VI. Theoretical update. Fam Process 22:69-83, 1983

Pierloot R, Wellens W, Houben M: Elements of resistance to a combined medical and psychotherapeutic program in anorexia nervosa. Psychother Psychosom 26:101-117, 1975

Pyle R, Mitchell JE, Eckert ED: Bulimia: a report of 34 cases. J Clin Psychiatry 42:60-64, 1981

Reiss D: The Family's Construction of Reality. Cambridge, Harvard University Press, 1981

Sargent J: The family and childhood psychosomatic disorders. Gen Hosp Psychiatry 5:41-48, 1983

Schwartz RC: Bulimia and family therapy: a case study. International Journal of Disorders 2:75-82, 1982

Selvini-Palazzoli M: Self-Starvation. New York, Jason Aronson, 1978

Sours JA: Starving to Death in a Sea of Objects: The Anorexia Nervosa Syndrome. New York, Jason Aronson, 1980

Stern S, Whitaker CA, Hagemann NJ, et al: Anorexia nervosa: the hospital's role in family treatment. Fam Process 20:395-408, 1981

Strober M: The significance of bulimia in juvenile anorexia nervosa: an exploration of possible etiologial factors. International Journal of Eating Disorders 1:28-32, 1981

Strober M: Familial Depression in Anorexia Nervosa. Paper presented at American Psychiatric Association Annual Meeting, New York, 1983

Strober M, Salkin B, Burroughs J, et al: Validity of the bulimia-restrictor distinction in anorexia nervosa: parental personality characteristics and family psychiatric morbidity. J Nerv Ment Dis 170:345-351, 1982

Stuart RD, Davis B: Slim Chance in a Fat World: Behavioral Control of Obesity. Champaign, Ill., Research Press, 1972

Szmuckler GI: A study of family therapy in anorexia nervosa: some methodological issues, in Anorexia Nervosa: Recent Developments in Research. Edited by Darby PL, Garfinkel PE, Garner DM, et al. New York, Alan R. Liss, 1983

Theander S: Anorexia nervosa: a psychiatric investigation of 94 female patients. Acta Psychiatr Scand (Suppl) 214:38-51, 1970

Vandereycken W, Meerman R: Has the family to be treated? in Anorexia Nervosa: A Clinician's Guide to Treatment. Edited by Vandereycken W, Meerman R. Berlin-New York, Walter de Gruyter-Aldine, 1984

Vandereycken W, Pierloot R: Anorexia nervosa in twins. Psychother Psychosom 35:55-63, 1981

Wertheim E: Family unit therapy and the science and typology of family systems. Fam Process 12:343-376, 1973

White M: Anorexia nervosa: a transgenerational system perspective. Fam Process 22:255-273, 1983

Will D: Some techniques for working with resistant families of adolescents. J Adolesc 6:13-26, 1983

Wilson GT, Brownell KD: Behavior therapy for obesity: including family members in the treatment process. Behavior Therapy 9:943-945, 1978

Winokur A, March V, Mendels J: Primary affective disorder in relatives of patients with anorexia nervosa. Am J Psychiatry 137:695-698, 1980

Wold P: Family structure in three cases of anorexia nervosa: the role of the father. Am J Psychiatry 130:1394-1397, 1973

Yager J: Family issues in the pathogenesis of anorexia nervosa. Psychosom Med 44:43-60, 1982

Yager J, Landsverk J, Lee-Benner K, et al: Bulimia spectrum disorder: The Glamour Survey. Paper presented at American Psychiatric Association Meeting, New York, 1983

Chapter 26

Psychological Issues in the Diagnosis and Treatment of Anorexia Nervosa and Bulimia

by David M. Garner, Ph.D. and Paul Isaacs, Ph.D.

THEORETICAL ACCOUNTS

A complete psychology of anorexia nervosa should take into account the patient characteristics that predispose to anorexia nervosa, the variety of developmental experiences that interact with these factors to initiate anorexia nervosa, the psychology surrounding the symptom picture (including the phenomenology), the maintaining variables, and the key variations in the symptom picture. The various treatment options would then grow out of an analysis of a particular patient's history.

While clinical experience and research have converged regarding the personality structure and phenomenology of the typical anorexic patient, there is much less agreement concerning etiology. The nature of the disorder is such that plausible, if not provable theories have been constructed to account for its development from a wide variety of conceptual vantage points. Accordingly, there are theories emphasizing Freudian drive constructs, object relations, ego functions, self phenomena, family interactional patterns, developmental arrest and underlying cognitive assumptions. Most theories generalize to anorexia nervosa from a set of constructs which were originally developed in another context. These diverse models are not necessarily mutually exclusive and can be selectively integrated in the understanding of the varied etiological pathways which may lead to both anorexia nervosa and bulimia (Garner et al, 1982; Guidano and Liotti, 1983; Swift and Stern, 1982).

The theories which have been proposed to account for the central symptom pattern in classical anorexia nervosa differ in their relative emphasis on patients' phenomenology at the time of their illness, vs. the remote developmental history. Thus, for some, the formulations emphasize events which are remote in time from the expression of symptoms, while others concentrate on events that are closer in time to the development of the disorder. While all theories acknowledge the role of earlier experiences in helping to set the background for the development of anorexia nervosa, those which especially emphasize early events (distal theories) postulate specific developmental sequences. Formulations based on issues that appear later in psychological development (proximal theories) emphasize the role of current attitudes, beliefs, and relationships in bringing about and maintaining the disorder. These latter accounts view anorexia nervosa as a common solution to a more varied set of problems. The implications of regarding the theories along the earlier vs. later psychological issues dimension are central to the development of a multifaceted psychotherapy which may be systematically applied to the different problem areas associated with these disorders.

At the extreme of those theories that focus on later issues are formulations based on analyses of the immediate causal factors, maintaining variables and self-perpetuating symptom patterns.

Cognitive and Behavioral Concepts

The assumption that reinforcement contingencies maintain anorexia nervosa is the cornerstone of the numerous reports on behavioral treatment (Garfinkel and Garner, 1982). Recently, several authors have systematically examined the functional relationships between antecedent events, positive reinforcers, and negative reinforcers in the development of anorexia nervosa (Garner and Bemis, 1982, 1984; Slade, 1982) as well as bulimia (Loro and Orleans, 1981; Rosen and Leitenberg, 1984). According to Slade (1982) there are both positive and negative reinforcing consequences of dieting behavior. The positive reinforcement derives from the feelings of success, of being in control, and of self-satisfaction, feelings which are magnified in a person who perceives the rest of her existence as failure. The negative reinforcement derives from the successful avoidance of the feared weight gain.

Slade (1982) attempts to explain why anorexia nervosa is the disorder of choice for some persons with low self-esteem. Noting the perfectionist tendencies that have been strongly associated with anorexia nervosa (Bruch, 1978; Garner et al, 1983c; Halmi et al, 1977; Kalucy et al, 1977; Strober, 1980), he postulates that the combination of perfectionism and low self-esteem leads to a need for absolute control over some aspect of the patient's life situation. In most aspects of life, being dependent on the behavior of others does not afford such an opportunity. Self-control in general, and control over the body, in particular, are two of the few areas offering this kind of certainty. Anorexic patients generally opt for control over both.

The cognitive approach to the analysis of anorexia nervosa emphasizes the way in which the symptom pattern derives logically from the faulty assumptive world of the patient. An analysis of these assumptions (Garner and Bemis, 1984; Garner et al, 1982) reveals the ways in which deficits in self-esteem as well as deficits in awareness of affect and bodily sensations combine with idiosyncratic beliefs concerning food and weight, to maintain anorexia nervosa. The approach involves untangling the skein of beliefs that has at its center the belief that "it is absolutely essential that I be thin" (Garner and Bemis, 1982). The surplus meaning that has come to be attached to this belief accounts for the current behavior and provides a window into the anorexic patient's broader system of self-evaluation. The formal errors in the patient's thinking—such as the use of dichotomous thinking when dealing with topics having emotional impact, or the bizarre correlating of unrelated events with body size—help to establish and maintain the disorder. For example, it is very hard to establish moderation in eating if one thinks in extremes and does not allow for the "in betweens" (Garner and Bemis, 1982). The proximal formulations of the cognitive approach do not depend upon any particular early developmental sequence for symptom development and thus they are not necessarily incompatible with other theoretical accounts.

Fears of Psychosexual Maturity

Crisp (1980) has emphasized a slightly earlier developmental explanation for anorexia nervosa. According to this model, the body image which is feared represents a state of psychosexual maturity. He postulates that this particular meaning is central for all anorexic patients and is essential to the understanding of the syndrome. The age distribution of anorexic patients and the frequently expressed fears associated with becoming a teenager offer some support for the theory. According to this view, anorexia nervosa is an attempt to cope with intense fears of psychobiological maturity. The dieting and "weight phobia" have the physical effect of a regression to a prepubertal state (Crisp, 1965). This is often accompanied by an active rejection of the adult sexual role. Dieting and resulting starvation become the mechanisms by which the patient regresses to a prepubertal appearance, hormonal status, and experience (Crisp, 1980). This regression is reinforced by the relief it provides from adolescent turmoil and related conflicts within the family. Crisp (1981) views the causes of bulimia as similar to those precipitating anorexia nervosa, the major difference being that the nonemaciated bulimic patient has failed to achieve the much coveted prepubescent shape.

Family Conflicts

A number of theorists have ascribed a causative role to family factors in the genesis of anorexia nervosa (Minuchin et al, 1978; Yager, 1982) and bulimia (Schwartz et al, 1984). A tendency for families of anorexics to emphasize appearance and performance has been noted. These families have also been described as denying feelings and events that do not confirm their idealized image of themselves. Minuchin et al (1978) view the entire syndrome as a family interactional problem. Schwartz et al (1984), on the other hand, have integrated principles from structural and strategic family therapy with those of psychodynamic models to account for the development of bulimia. Apart from noting that emphasis on family factors may be thought of as somewhat remote in time from the onset of the condition than the formulations described earlier, we will not cover this topic, as it is dealt with in Chapter 25 by Drs. Yager and Strober, in this volume.

Developmental Theories

The following theories look for the causes of anorexia nervosa in the developmental history and are, therefore, closer to the earlier end of the explanatory continuum.

Hilde Bruch (1962, 1973) feels that the low self-esteem, sense of personal ineffectiveness, and confusion in concepts about the body are rooted in early disturbances in parenting. Bruch postulates that for healthy development to occur the child must learn the connections between internal physiological signals and appropriate social and behavioral responses. This learning is fostered by the mother's responsiveness to the child's needs. For example, according to Bruch (1962, 1973), "hunger awareness" is normally achieved when the mother's reaction to the child's state of food deprivation confirms the meaning of the child's own internal physiological experiences. When the mother does not respond to the child's own bodily needs but superimposes her own inaccurate perceptions of those needs, then the child is unable to validate her own internal experiences. For Bruch this confusion about needs is quite general in anorexia nervosa and applies not only to visceral sensations related to satiety, sexual feelings, and fatigue, but also to affective awareness. Being "deprived of inner guideposts," the anorexic is unable to define and take responsibility for satisfying her own inner needs. This leaves her dependent on others and leads to feelings of helplessness and loss of self-control. Linking her views to Piaget's theory of cognitive stages, Bruch feels that the deficiencies in self-initiated behaviors result in a blockage of normal cognitive development. Not having fully acquired the capacity for abstract thinking, the anorexic is "stuck" at the preconceptual stage of concrete operations. This may be manifest as literal-mindedness, a characteristic which has been noted in anorexia nervosa by various clinicians (Goodsitt, 1984). Much of the anorexic's behavior is captured by what Bruch (1978) calls "narrow-minded good behavior [which] reflects the moral judgment of a very young child" (p. 55). The anorexic's childhood is often one of extreme compliance with the demands of others, to such an extent that the normal degree of childhood self-assertiveness is missing. While parents and teachers may regard the preanorexic girl as a model child, her inner experience is adrift in the never-ending attempt at second guessing others in order to be accepted. Upon reaching adolescence she is poorly prepared for meeting the newly salient demands for autonomy and self-mastery. The assertion of total control over her own body represents a maladaptive effort to meet those demands and to define her self.

A more specific interpretation of the anorexic's fear of her body's growth is offered by Selvini-Palazzoli (1978). She feels that as physical maturation occurs, the breast development and beginning feminine curves enhance the anorexic's perception of her body as "the maternal object." Her experience of her body as powerful and threatening, yet self-sufficient, is due to her equating her body with the incorporated mother. The development which leads to this is similar to that described by Bruch, namely, experiences of being overwhelmed by the mother in the early feeding followed by later development of a compliant stance.

Masterson (1977) has applied object relations theory to the phenomena of anorexia nervosa, stressing that different psychodynamic explanations are appropriate depending upon the level of development of the underlying personality structure. According to object relations theory, psychotic, borderline and neurotic personality structures result from arrest at the symbiotic, separation-individuation and "approaching object constancy" stages of development, respectively. Masterson acknowledges that anorexia nervosa can occur within any of these personality structures, but thinks that the borderline personality is predominant. He feels that most anorexics show the concerns which characterize arrest at the symbiotic or separation-individuation phases. Their problems derive from fears of loss of self or loss of the good object and are associated with feelings of emptiness and struggles over autonomy (Masterson, 1977). Masterson's formulation of the anorexic's underlying intrapsychic constellation does not differ from the more general descriptions of borderline psychopathology. The early parent-child interactions which are thought to promote the borderline character structure involve the rewarding of clinging, dependent behavior and parental withdrawal in response to exploratory growth behavior. This pattern sets up expectations that growth and initiative will lead to abandonment. Masterson (1977) links various specific anorexic features to this general description. The pursuit of thinness is seen as relieving the anxiety that would be created by the loss of the object which would inevitably follow physical, sexual, or emotional growth by literally blocking such growth. The obsessive controls surrounding eating are viewed as substitutes for feelings and thoughts of individuation. The emaciation is seen as expressing the patient's hostility towards her mother. Helplessness and lack of initiative are consequences of the fears of loss associated with mastery behavior. Precipitating events, described by Bruch in general terms as having to do with demands for increased autonomy, are seen by Masterson to have their power by virtue of "threatening the relationship with the person to whom the patient is clinging" (p. 492) or by requiring individual coping. Either of these features threatens the patient's defensive system. Masterson does not account for the specific development of anorexia nervosa instead of more typical borderline presentations.

Goodsitt (1984) has applied the concepts of Kohut's self psychology to anorexia nervosa. Goodsitt views anorexia nervosa as a maladaptive attempt to solve several specific problems. First, the strict controls on eating and the frequently seen pattern of bulimia and vomiting are interpreted as attempts at tension regulation, suggesting a serious defect in the anorexic's abilities to regulate tension internally. Secondly, the adoption of anorectic symptomatology provides a framework of pseudo-meaningfulness for the patient's very existence, thus suggesting a basic defect in the capacity for self-organization. These defects in self are related to a failure to acquire the capacity for using transitional objects for self regulation, the consequences of which are that the anorexic is dependent on other people to act as self-objects (that is, as extensions of herself). According to Goodsitt (1984), the anorexic's pseudo self-sufficient stance is a defense against symbiotic needs. This symbiotic attachment is associated with feelings of guilt over the very act of being different from or conflicting with the parents in any way. The whole symptom pattern is initiated when the realities of adolescence begin to convey the message that symbiotic attachments must be given up. The anorexic does not feel that she has a right to a life of her own and engages in many actions which tend to deny her very selfhood. Existing is seen as selfish, eating as "an unjustifiable self indulgence" (Goodsitt, 1984). Extolling the virtues of self-denial, discipline, and asceticism provides the intellectual rationale for the negation of the self's independence. In therapy, the anorexic often expresses the concern that if the eating disorder is cured, there will be nothing of significance left in her life.

A MULTIDIMENSIONAL PERSPECTIVE

It is our view that anorexia nervosa and bulimia represent a final common pathway that may be arrived at from a number of distinctly different developmental routes (Garfinkel and Garner, 1982; Garner and Bemis, 1984) some of which have been captured by the specific etiologies described above. Having embarked on an anorexic or bulimic course, the patient becomes caught up in a self-perpetuating pattern of disordered thinking, feeling, and behaving, in which the residue of the developmental path is of variable significance (Garner and Bemis, 1982, 1984; Garner et al, 1982).

The concept of multiple pathways and multiple determinants can be illustrated with reference to how self-esteem becomes linked to the body image in those who go on to develop anorexia nervosa or bulimia. We can construct a list of hypothesized contributing factors. Included might be disturbances in early feeding (Bruch, 1962), family emphasis on eating and physical attractiveness (Kalucy et al, 1977), socio-cultural pressures (Garner et al, 1983a) and peer group expectations. More interactive hypotheses would include the notion that the body becomes the only arena in which perfectionism can have full reign, a hypothesis that presumes a separate set of factors that create the perfectionistic traits (Garner and Bemis, 1982; Slade, 1982). Another hypothesis is that the concrete thinking style, which is said to be typical of anorexics, interacts with an other-directed personality to amplify an emphasis on external appearances. These hypothesized mechanisms are not mutually exclusive nor is there any a priori reason why different patients could not have become preoccupied with their body shape for different reasons. It is certainly possible to study the relative frequency of each of these factors in the histories of anorexic or bulimic patients, but there is no need to assume a uniformity where none exists.

We believe that there is no single basis for the crystallization of self-esteem onto body shape or weight that applies to all patients. Neither is there one family constellation which describes all families of anorexic or bulimic patients (Schwartz et al, 1984). From the review of theories presented above, it is apparent that some of them are describing the same kinds of patients using a different language or perspective. Other theories seem to be describing different patients, or at least patients for whom different issues are salient. We believe that there are different subgroups of patients which are best described by individual theories. A patient for whom fears of becoming a teenager are paramount is different from the more disturbed borderline patient. For the borderline patient, such fears, if present, are secondary to a more fundamental disorganization. Although no single factor theory will encompass all cases of anorexia nervosa, this does not imply that there are an infinite number of factors at work, either. From a research point of view, the multidimensionality may be reduced to typologies based on frequently observed groupings.

SUBTYPES AND TYPOLOGIES

The underlying heterogeneity among patients diagnosed as having anorexia nervosa has recently become more prominent in the literature (Beumont, George and Smart, 1976; Casper et al, 1980; Garfinkel and Garner, 1982; Sours, 1980; Strober, 1980, 1981, 1983; Yager, 1982). This has rekindled interest in the definition of subtypes of patients who are more homogenous. Two major methods have been used to define subgroupings of anorexic patients: The first is based on patterns of symptoms; the second is based on personality characteristics.

Symptom-Based Typologies

The most salient symptoms of anorexia nervosa are those pertaining to the variations in food intake and elimination. Bulimia (gorging) is the major variant in the first category and the bulimia–restricter distinction has generated the most typological research. Bulimia has received much recent attention as a symptom in its own right. There is now ample evidence that bulimia occurs not only in anorexic patients but also in obese (see, for example, Loro and Orleans, 1981) and in normal weight women (Fairburn and Cooper, 1982; Halmi, Falk, and Schwartz, 1981)*. Typically it is associated with vomiting, but this is not always the case (Russell, 1979). A number of studies have examined the behavioral, personality, and familial differences between bulimic anorexics and restricting anorexics, as described by Kennedy and Garfinkel in Chapter 23 of this volume. In brief, bulimics seem to engage in more behaviors that have an addictive or impulsive quality than do restricters (Casper et al, 1980; Garfinkel et al, 1980; Strober, 1981; Strober et al, 1982). Thus, bulimics tend to show a greater frequency of usage of alcohol and street drugs. They are more likely to engage in compulsive stealing, to have had prior suicide attempts, and to have engaged in self-mutilation, particularly genital self-mutilation. They are also more likely to be outgoing, to express a greater interest in sex, and to be heterosexually experienced. They show more lability of mood in a psychiatric interview and are also more depressed than restricters. They weigh more than restricters, are more likely to have been obese and to have had an obese mother. Their prognosis is also poorer than that of restricters (Garfinkel and Garner, 1982).

It has been suggested that bulimics often have a borderline personality organization (Sours, 1980). This could possibly account for the association between bulimia and the litany of symptoms just cited.

One study has shown that bulimic anorexics may be closer in symptomatology, personality, and demography to a group of normal weight bulimics than to the restricting anorexics (Garner et al, 1983b). In general, the descriptions of restricting anorexics come much closer to the high striving, perfectionistic, and rigid personality style that has been associated with the classical description of anorexia nervosa. Their families are also more likely to conform to the prototypical anorexic family, in which there is more of a surface calm and control than appears in the chaotic families of the bulimic.

Despite the utility of the bulimia–restricter distinction, the dichotomy between these two subtypes of anorexia nervosa may be somewhat specious. Vandereycken and Pierloot (1983) divided their sample of anorexia patients into dieters, bulimics, and vomiters/purgers on the basis of the most prominent and most frequently occurring symptom. They found evidence that bulimia could emerge as a symptom quite some time after the onset and initial treatment of the anorexia nervosa; moreover, it was not uncommon for patients to meet different criteria depending on when they were assessed. These authors call into question the whole notion of the stability of symptom-based typologies.

Personality-Based Typologies

The research on the personality characteristics of anorexics has tended to confirm clinical descriptions. For example, Strober (1980) summarizes his research findings: "the prototype of the young female anorexic is one who is markedly obsessional in character makeup; introverted and socially insecure; self-denying, deferential and given to overcompliant adaptation; prone to self-abasement with limited spontaneity and self-directed autonomy; and overly formalistic and stereotyped in thinking despite being industrious, planful and intellectually efficient" (p. 358).

Despite this confirmation of classical descriptions, it is reasonable to ask if there are definable subgroups whose personality style differs significantly from this prototype. Strober (1983) was able to empirically define three personality subtypes on the basis of a cluster analysis of MMPI scores from a group of 130 anorexia nervosa patients. There were highly significant differences in background, symptom pattern, and short-term prognosis among the three groups. Cross validation of this research is clearly needed, as is a longer period of follow-up.

Garner et al (1984a) found cluster analytic procedures useful in distinguishing subgroups of weight-preoccupied college women who superficially resemble subclinical anorexia nervosa from those who display more serious psychopathology. These results underscore the importance of a multidimensional evaluation of the psychopathology of anorexia nervosa and bulimia.

Having a reliable personality-based typology with good predictive power would be a decided advantage for planning treatment. The personality structure of the patient is, presumably, more stable than the symptom picture which often fluctuates over the course of time. Strober's (1983) choice of the MMPI represents a reasonable starting point for research, in which the testing approach could be tailored to capture the specific issues important in anorexia nervosa or bulimia.

IMPLICATIONS FOR THERAPY

Many types of psychotherapy have been advocated for treating anorexia nervosa. Often the approach is tied to a conventional model of psychotherapy, with no emphasis on the anorexic patient's special problems, such as her unwilling participation in therapy or the need to deal with food and weight issues. It is our impression that the orthodox practice of many traditional methods without attention to these special areas may alienate the patient, frustrate the therapist, and result in treatment failure (Garner et al, 1982). By way of contrast, traditional methods may be adapted usefully to accommodate these special needs (Goodsitt, 1984; Rosen and Leitenberg, 1984; Schwartz et al, 1984). Indeed, the descriptions of therapy with anorexics by those who have specialized in this area, regardless of theoretical orientation, point to certain common strategies that have evolved independently on the basis of experience. Our view of these disorders as multidetermined has led to the development of a multifaceted treatment strategy which incorporates principles from differing therapies (Garfinkel and Garner, 1982; Garner and Bemis, 1982, 1984; Garner et al, 1984b).

Throughout the course of therapy we recommend a conscious "two track" strategy on the part of the therapist. The first track pertains to the patient's current eating behavior and physical condition. The therapist must be aware of these at all times and must carefully plan specific interventions aimed at normalizing them. The second track pertains to the overall context for the disorder, namely the features of the patient's personality which may tend to maintain the disorder or promote relapse, and the more general issues of psychological adjustment that may be unrelated to the eating disorder. We feel that these two tracks demand different therapeutic strategies which, nevertheless, must be

•

coordinated. At no time is this more critical than during the initial contact with the patient.

The Initial Phase of Therapy

The circumstances surrounding the initiation of treatment and the way in which the therapist deals with these circumstances are particularly important in anorexia nervosa and bulimia. Unlike more typical psychiatric patients who readily admit to psychological discomfort, it is often not the anorexic patient, but her relatives who perceive a problem. If the patient arrives under some duress with a view of the therapist as executor of the family's wishes, she may respond by remaining unconcerned, negativistic or defiant. In this event, care must be taken to enlist the cooperation of the patient and her family, and to avoid blaming any one family member for the presence of the disorder. Other patients arrive on their own initiative, sometimes with a longstanding eating disorder for which they have received either no treatment at all or inappropriate treatment. Usually, there is less denial with the bulimia patient; however, some minimize the dangers associated with bingeing, vomiting, or laxative abuse and will only consent to treatment if it does not result in weight gain. With the increasing media coverage of anorexia nervosa and bulimia, we are seeing more patients who seek treatment soon after symptom development. These patients are more motivated and are somewhat older.

For both anorexic and bulimic patients it is useful to begin by taking a complete weight history to determine the patient's current position in her "weight range" (Garner et al, 1982, 1984). This informs the patient that the therapist has a reality orientation in regard to this dimension. If the patient is quite emaciated, but relatively cooperative, it may be useful to describe in detail the effects of starvation derived from studies with normal volunteers (Keys et al, 1950) and identified in anorexia nervosa (Dally, 1969; Russell, 1970, Lucas et al, 1976; Casper and Davis, 1977; Garner and Garfinkel, 1980). Many of these symptoms, including dry skin, hair loss, lanugo, paresthesia, sensitivity to noise, and hypothermia, may have become quite distressing to the patient. Psychological disturbances such as anxiety, depression, labile moods, feelings of inadequacy, fatigue, food preoccupations, poor concentration, episodes of bulimia, and social withdrawal are also heightened by starvation and are felt to be unpleasant by the patient. We have suggested that these same principles may apply to individuals who present with bulimia but are at a normal weight. Many of these formerly obese patients have starved themselves to reach a weight which is unrealistic given their higher "set point" for body weight (Garner et al, 1984b). The description of the "starvation state" helps patients to integrate a confusing set of symptoms. Moreover, describing these symptoms as in part "physiologically derived" serves to allay some of the guilt which many patients have around the development of "psychiatric symptoms." This approach may contrast sharply with previous experiences with therapists who are unfamiliar with eating disorders, thus establishing a degree of trust in the therapist's expertise. This will be very important, as one of the goals of the initial sessions is to help the patient accept the need for weight restoration.

We believe that it is essential that the patient accept the need to attain physiological normalcy through direct work on her eating behavior. One of the real dangers of a traditional, insight-oriented approach is that it suggests to the patient that her highly valued, but self-destructive eating patterns are not expected to change until a certain degree of insight is attained. This approach unwittingly encourages these patients to strive endlessly for "perfect insight" while making no progress in normalizing their eating.

A Two-Track Therapeutic Strategy

The two-track approach demands that discussion be extended to issues other than eating and weight. While this is helpful for all patients, it is most important for establishing a working alliance with those patients, described above, who have come for treatment under some external pressure. Emphasizing the uniqueness of the patient's concerns and personality in noneating-related areas helps shape the subsequent patient-therapist interactions, which will emphasize that self-esteem is to be derived, not from control over eating, but from expression of a developing individuality. For some patients, a natural introduction to these broader issues may follow from their answer to a hypothetical question posed during the discussion of weight. Patients are asked: "Although I understand that you would prefer not to gain weight, if you were to gain, at what point would you begin to experience panic?" (Garner et al, 1982). Most patients have not considered the question in this way, but are able to identify that they would begin to panic at a particular weight (Crisp, 1980). This weight may often represent the threshold for return of menses. In responding to the question, some patients seize the opportunity to elaborate upon fears of "growing up." The relevance of this issue must be judged for each patient.

In introducing a recommendation for therapy, it is useful to explicitly acknowledge that a two-track approach will be used. By not entirely subsuming the patient's eating disorder under a broader category of "deep-seated psychological disturbance," an opportunity is left open to tackle the disordered eating by means of behavioral and cognitive behavioral methods. On the other hand, by not ignoring the underlying psychological problems, the patient is given the message that therapy is not contingent on her having a manifest eating disorder and that the therapist is committed to deal with whatever difficulties are encountered over a longer period of time. As therapy progresses, certain themes are likely to emerge. We feel that the most helpful stance for the clinician is to be familiar with the base rate probabilities for these various themes. By systematically exploring for the presence of each, the therapist can tailor the therapy to the requirements of each patient.

Emergent Themes

Dramatically different results will be obtained with different patients as behavioral change in abnormal eating patterns is attempted. For some bulimic patients, a structured plan for altering the behavior, combined with the decoupling of the disturbed eating from psychological issues that we have advocated, is sufficient to normalize well-entrenched patterns in a matter of a week or two (Garner et al, 1984). For most patients, particularly those who are starved or who have long histories of bulimic eating patterns, normalization of eating is a more difficult process during which many issues begin to surface with much intensity.

For most patients the initial increased food consumption or introduction of new foods into their diet leads to fears that they will lose total control of their eating. At a later stage, as their weight begins to approach the critical weight for the resumption of menses, fears associated with attaining a mature shape may emerge. At any weight the linkage of self-esteem to an idealized appearance may wax and wane in importance. Specific approaches to each of these and other themes from the cognitive behavioral viewpoint is provided elsewhere (Garner et al 1982; Garner and Bemis, 1984).

Many themes which are commonly found to pervade the psychology of eating disorder patients are not tied directly to food or weight issues. These themes vary in prominence from patient to patient. Poor self-esteem, feelings of incompetence, and lack of personal trust are often reported. Many times these occur in the context of an individual who is having difficulty with issues of separation and autonomy. Impoverished affective experience or expression is also common, especially among restricting anorexics. Therapeutic strategies for dealing with these themes in eating disordered patients need not be that different from those applied to other psychiatric populations. We agree with Bruch's (1973) position that it is harmful to adopt an attitude in which interpretations of the patient's feelings or thoughts seem to imply that the therapist is more knowledgeable about the patient's inner life than is the patient herself.

SUMMARY

There is not one psychology of either anorexia nervosa or bulimia. Both disorders are final common pathways that derive from individual, familial, and cultural predisposing factors that vary across a heterogenous patient population. This chapter has described some of the most common psychological themes encountered, and has proposed a multifaceted treatment aimed at cognitive, behavioral, affective, and interpersonal deficits.

REFERENCES

Beumont PJV, George GC, Smart DE: "Dieters" and "vomiters and purgers" in anorexia nervosa. Psychol Med 6:617–622, 1976

Bruch H: Perceptual and conceptual disturbances in anorexia nervosa. Psychosom Med 24:187–194, 1962

Bruch H: Eating Disorders. New York, Basic Books, 1973

Bruch H: The Golden Cage. New York, Basic Books, 1978

Casper RC, Davis JM: On the course of anorexia nervosa. Am J Psychiatry 134:974–978, 1977

Casper RC, Eckert ED, Halmi KA, et al: Bulimia. Arch Gen Psychiatry 37:1030–1035, 1980

Crisp AH: Some aspects of the evolution, presentation and follow-up of anorexia nervosa. Proceedings of the Royal Society of Medicine 58:814–820, 1965

Crisp AH: Anorexia Nervosa: Let Me Be. New York, Grune and Stratton, 1980

Crisp AH: Anorexia nervosa at a normal weight! The abnormal-normal weight control syndrome. Int J Psychiatry in Medicine 11:203–233, 1981

Dally PJ: Anorexia Nervosa. New York, Grune and Stratton, 1969

Fairburn CG, Cooper PJ: Self-induced vomiting and bulimia nervosa: an undetected problem. Br Med J 284:1153–1155, 1982

Garfinkel PE, Garner DM: Anorexia Nervosa: a Multidimensional Perspective. New York, Brunner/Mazel, 1982

Garfinkel PE, Moldofsky H, Garner DM: The heterogeneity of anorexia nervosa. Arch Gen Psychiatry 37:1036–1040, 1980

Garner DM, Bemis KM: A cognitive-behavioral approach to anorexia nervosa. Cognitive Therapy and Research 6:123–150, 1982

Garner DM, Bemis KM: Cognitive therapy for anorexia nervosa, in A Handbook of Psychotherapy for Anorexia Nervosa and Bulimia. Edited by Garner DM, Garfinkel PE. New York, Guilford Press, 1984

Garner DM, Garfinkel PE: Sociocultural factors in the development of anorexia nervosa. Psychol Med 10:649–656, 1980

Garner DM, Garfinkel PE, Bemis KM: A multidimensional psychotherapy for anorexia nervosa. International Journal of Eating Disorders 1:3–46, 1982

Garner DM, Garfinkel PE, Olmsted MP: An overview of the sociocultural factors in the development of anorexia nervosa, in Anorexia Nervosa: Recent Developments. Edited by Darby PL, Garfinkel PE, Garner DM, et al. New York, Alan R. Liss, 1983a

Garner DM, Garfinkel PE, O'Shaughnessy M: Clinical and psychometric comparison between bulimia in anorexia nervosa and bulimia in normal-weight women, in Understanding Anorexia Nervosa and Bulimia. Report of the Fourth Ross Conference on Medical Research. Columbus, Ohio, Ross Laboratories, 1983b

Garner DM, Olmstead MP, Polivy J: Development and validation of a multidimensional eating disorder inventory for anorexia nervosa and bulimia. International Journal of Eating Disorders 2:15–34, 1983c

Garner DM, Olmsted MP, Polivy J, et al: A comparison between weight-preoccupied women and anorexia nervosa. Psychosom Med 46:255–266, 1984a

Garner DM, Rockert W, Olmsted MP, et al: Psychoeducational principles in the treatment of bulimia and anorexia nervosa, in a Handbook of Psychotherapy for Anorexia Nervosa and Bulimia. Edited by Garner DM, Garfinkel PE. New York, Guilford Press, 1984b

Goodsitt A: Self-psychology and the treatment of anorexia nervosa, in A Handbook of Psychotherapy for Anorexia Nervosa and Bulimia. Edited by Garner DM, Garfinkel PE. New York, Guilford Press, 1984

Guidano VF, Liotti G: Cognitive Processes and Emotional Disorders: A Structural Approach to Psychotherapy. New York, Guilford Press, 1983

Halmi KA, Goldberg SC, Cunningham S: Perceptual distortion of body image in adolescent girls: distortion of body image in adolescence. Psychol Med 7:253–257, 1977

Halmi KA, Falk JR, Schwartz E: Binge-eating and vomiting: a survey of a college population. Psychol Med 11:697–706, 1981

Kalucy RS, Crisp AH, Harding B: A study of 56 families with anorexia nervosa. Br J Med Psychol 50:381–395, 1977

Keys A, Brozek J, Henschel A, et al: The Biology of Human Starvation. Minneapolis, University of Minnesota Press, 1950

Loro AD, Orleans CS: Binge-eating in obesity: preliminary findings and guidelines for behavioral analysis and treatment. Addict Behav 6:155–166, 1981

Lucas AR, Duncan JW, Piens V: The treatment of anorexia nervosa. Am J Psychiatry 133:1034–1038, 1976

Masterson JF: Primary anorexia nervosa in the borderline adolescent—an object-relations view, in Borderline Personality Disorders. Edited by Hartocollis P. New York, International Universities Press, 1977

Minuchin S, Rosman BL, Baker J: Psychosomatic Families: Anorexia Nervosa in Context. Cambridge, Harvard University Press, 1978

Rosen JC, Leitenberg H: Exposure plus response prevention treatment of bulimia nervosa, in A Handbook of Psychotherapy for Anorexia Nervosa and Bulimia. Edited by Garner DM, Garfinkel PE. New York, Guilford Press, 1984

Russell GFM: Anorexia nervosa: its identity as an illness and its treatment, in Modern Trends in Psychological Medicine. Edited by Price JH. New York, Appleton-Century-Crofts, 1970

Russell GFM: Bulimia nervosa: an ominous variant of anorexia nervosa? Psychol Med 9:429–448, 1979

Schwartz RC, Barrett MJ, Saba G: Family therapy for bulimia, in A Handbook of Psychotherapy for Anorexia Nervosa and Bulimia. Edited by Garner DM, Garfinkel PE. New York, Guilford Press, 1984

Selvini-Palazzoli M: Self-starvation: From Individual to Family Therapy in the Treatment of Anorexia Nervosa. New York, Jason Aronson, 1978

Slade PD: Towards a functional analysis of anorexia nervosa and bulimia nervosa. Br J Clin Psychol 21:167–179, 1982

Sours JA: Starving to Death in A Sea of Objects: The Anorexia Nervosa Syndrome. New York, Jason Aronson, 1980

Strober M: Personality and symptomatological features in young, non-chronic anorexia nervosa patients. J Psychosom Res 24:353–359, 1980

Strober M: The significance of bulimia in anorexia nervosa: an exploration of possible etiological factors. International Journal of Eating Disorders 1:28–43, 1981

Strober M: An empirically derived typology of anorexia nervosa, in Anorexia Nervosa: Recent Developments. Edited by Darby PL, Garfinkel PE, Garner DM, et al. New York, Alan R. Liss, 1983

Strober M, Salkin B, Burroughs J, et al: Validity of the bulimia-restricter distinction in anorexia nervosa. J Nerv Ment Dis 170:345–351, 1982

Swift WJ, Stern S: The psychodynamic diversity of anorexia nervosa. International Journal of Eating Disorders 2:17–36, 1982

Vandereycken W, Pierloot R: The significance of subclassification in anorexia nervosa: A comparative study of clinical features in 141 patients. Psychol Med, 1983

Yager J: Family in the pathogenesis of anorexia nervosa. Psychosom Med 44:43–60, 1982

Afterword

by Joel Yager, M.D.

The broad perspective on the eating disorders presented in the preceding chapters may reflect our wish not to overlook anything important (because of the large lacunae in our current state of knowledge) more than it may reflect any one truth about these disorders. The fact that research, theory, and clinical approaches extend to every level of biopsychosocial organization may simply mean that as yet we lack the Rosetta stones—if any in fact exist—that will one day help us to unravel primary from secondary aspects of these disorders. But, while we await such illuminating discoveries, the comprehensive perspective emphasized in this section represents the most prudent one, one that leaves the clinician in the position of being least likely to neglect those aspects which may be most relevant in any given case, and one which invites researchers to pursue a myriad of currently supportable hypotheses.

Each chapter raises more questions than it answers. We are far from understanding causes and far from delineating effective prevention or treatment programs. We are, historically, in a position resembling that of nineteenth century clinicians faced with "dropsy" or Bright's Disease, essentially final common pathway syndromes which, as we now know, actually encompassed an incredibly large group of diseases. To some extent we are like clinicians who witnessed the ravages of tuberculosis before antibiotics, who could prescribe primarily nonspecific supportive treatment programs rather than scientifically based specific interventions. An honest admission of our ignorance and limitations may help us contend with the frustrating feelings of impotence that even the most experienced clinicians feel in relation to some patients. And, nondefensive humility is in order to assure that we don't too quickly claim credit for clinical improvements which may occur *at least* in part due to "nonspecific" therapeutic factors.

ADDITIONAL CONSIDERATIONS

Let us consider some of the questions raised.

Diagnosis

The need for better definition and delineation of these disorders is pressing, especially regarding subtypes and the dimensions that will more accurately predict outcome. The variability of each of the disorders is great: For anorexia nervosa, the restricter versus bulimic subtype is a start, but even regarding this dichotomy there is dispute as to how valid these subtypes are. A large number of other psychological, biological and clinical dimensions suggest themselves as well. For bulimia, some of the dimensions that currently seem relevant have been enumerated, and now must be empirically tested. For obesity, the classification scheme according to severity alone is at best primitive.

Better definitions of where the syndromes begin and where "normal" weight preoccupation and dieting end are required. No doubt, as with alcoholism, the disorders begin where health and social function are adversely affected. For the more severe cases, it would appear that health and functioning are affected not only as the disturbed eating patterns themselves increase, but also as other psychological and family disturbances are loaded in. Some aspects of severe cases may differ from those of milder cases only in degree; others may be categorically distinct. As these issues are being worked out it would be worthwhile for workers in the field of eating disorders to develop some conventions for complete case reporting analogous to those already suggested by Kupfer and Rush (1983) for depressive disorders.

Pathogenesis

Current knowledge, and fashion as well, draw our attention to a variety of neurohormones, brain-gut peptides and hypothalamic releasing factors. Each month's journals pour forth the results of the work of dedicated scientists who meticulously measure alterations in various brain secretions and their peripheral consequences in patients with eating disorders. But, which of these alterations is central to the appearance of these syndromes is unknown. The sensitivity of the hypothalamic-ovarian axis, with the onset of amenorrhea even prior to major weight loss in a substantial minority of patients with anorexia nervosa, is noteworthy and suggests hypothalamic sensitivity. The occasional patient whose eating disorder is precipitated by starting or stopping birth control pills, or whose condition is improved or worsened by pregnancy, suggests that, in addition to the psychological factors associated with these major events, physiological factors, too, may be at work—perhaps in the regulation of gonadotropin releasing hormones, or in their neurophysiological and neurohumoral antecedents.

Do the parallels between eating disorders and addictive states imply common pathophysiologic elements, perhaps associated with the regulation of endorphins? To what extent do the hyperactivity and obsessional ritualized behaviors of the restricter anorexia nervosa patient resemble those of the amphetaminized animal? What are the implications?

Can we develop animal models of eating disorders that are superior to those currently available, perhaps produced by combinations of behavioral and biological means?

Prospective studies of "at risk" populations are needed. Such populations might include girls who intend to train in fields where a high prevalence of eating disorders appear, such as ballet dancers and fashion models, and in the younger siblings and offspring of patients who have already developed eating disorders. Twin studies and adoption studies would be particularly revealing. Such studies might reveal biological and/or psychological markers for subsequent vulnerability. That biological changes can be the consequence of behavioral events is obvious to students of starvation. The trick is identifying those that may be present before the onset of the disorder. Similarly, studies of persistent abnormalities not only following weight recovery but in those with complete clinical remission are essential.

We need better means for determining ideal body weight for each individual based on a variety of biological measures such as fat cell numbers, amount of brown fat, metabolic patterns, distribution patterns of fat, and so forth. We need to know what determines the "set point," just how set this point is, and the influences that may alter its regulation. This would help us to know more precisely for any given patient what she or he is up against in desiring to lose weight.

The above discussion is relevant not only for obesity, but for so-called normal weight bulimia as well: The question is "normal for whom?" To the extent that we can better delineate the weight tendency of each person, we may find that some so-called normal weight bulimics are, relatively speaking, still starving.

Psychopathology

Numerous questions exist regarding psychological causation and psychopathology. To what extent are the disturbances of thinking—such as concrete thinking, obsessionality and rigidity, feelings of ineffectiveness, body image distortions, and the cognitive distortions described by Drs. Garner and Isaacs in Chapter 26—epiphenomena of starvation? How can we test the validity of the psychological theories? Only through prospective studies will we be able to assess the extent to which difficulties in achieving autonomy, psychosexual maturity, in judging enteroceptive sensations including affect, and difficulties in moving beyond the stage of concrete operations precede and contribute to the development of eating disorders. And, we still need to know why such difficulties lead to eating disorders in these patients rather than to other disorders which might also serve as vehicles for the expression of such difficulties.

What is the relationship of personality to anorexia nervosa and bulimia? It's simply not true that all eating disorder patients have borderline personality disorganization. What drives the distortions and reinforces their persistence? Do the tension reduction mechanisms provided by anorexia nervosa and bulimia bear similarity to those of the addictive states? To displacement behaviors?

It might be worthwhile to delineate the prevalence of each proposed type of personality difficulty among patients with eating disorders. In this manner individual patient profiles with prognostic value might emerge.

The study of family interactions is likely to be informative. It is striking that poorer prognosis in both anorexia nervosa and schizophrenia is associated with families characterized by high negative expressed emotion; if confirmed, such a finding would suggest that this family pattern might constitute an important "nonspecific toxicity" factor possibly predictive of poor prognosis in a wide variety of disorders, not only those in which it has thus far been specifically examined.

Treatment

With regard to the treatment of the eating disorders, we are still in an early stage of development. There are as yet no controlled treatment studies for anorexia nervosa, for example, to demonstrate convincingly that *any* form of intervention is ultimately more successful in affecting long-term prognosis than any other. Can we expect more specific biological or psychological treatments in the future? While some studies have shown the ability of certain therapies to produce behavioral and weight improvement over the short term, good long-term follow-up studies following these treatment trials are not yet available.

At least for now we must acknowledge that many anorexia nervosa patients are extremely difficult to treat. They can leave the clinician feeling therapeutically impotent, and extremely exasperated. Willfully resistant anorexia nervosa patients may evoke highly negative countertherapeutic countertransference feelings in the otherwise well-integrated clinician. These patients are often maligned by staff as manipulative, sociopathic and obstinate when in fact they are defending a psychobiological position that may be the best they can do. With this in mind, the clinician should be on guard against acting out against the frustrating patient. A therapeutic stance of benign interest, firmness, and limit setting, where appropriate, is usually indicated. And since the clinician who stumbles in treatment of these cases is in good company, he or she should have the good sense to seek consultation without feeling too defensive or defeated.

Accumulated wisdom requires that therapy be directed both to behavior (that is, assuring nutritional rehabilitation) and to the psychological experience of the patient. The patient's self-esteem must be respected, but the patient cannot be permitted to have total control, if that control will lead to further starvation. As patronizing as it sounds, the starving anorexia nervosa patient is a regressed person who requires an affectively benign but nevertheless authoritative and firm intervention. Further research is needed on the way behavioral and psychodynamic elements can best be combined.

An important unresolved treatment question concerns how to determine the optimum length of hospital stay. Given economic realities and diagnosis-related groups (DRG) considerations, pressure may be exerted to keep anorexia nervosa patients in hospitals for much shorter stays than has customarily been the case. Might ultrashort stays be totally ineffective or actually detrimental? Are day programs feasible? Multicenter studies that compare long versus short stay treatment programs utilizing inpatient, day hospital, and outpatient modalities are necessary.

At this time, unresolved legal and ethical issues also lurk just beneath the surface. The clinician who treats anorexia nervosa will occasionally come up against a patient who absolutely refuses treatment in spite of the obvious need. Is the adult patient with anorexia nervosa capable of making judgments about treatment? Since few patients are so psychotic as to merit conservatorship over other areas of their lives, requests for conservatorship to treat such patients on an involuntary basis may be refused by some judges and juries. I have seen a 56-pound woman set free by a jury, in spite of her obvious lack of desire to stop her anorexic behavior. The jury felt that she had the right to make her own decisions about self care. Fortunately, most patients, even the more severe cases, can usually be persuaded by the combined influences of family and staff to remain in the hospital for treatment. But, when the rare, determined, intransigent patient refuses care, what should be the opinion of the law? A study group to consider this question for anorexia nervosa patients would be of help.

For bulimia, several controlled treatment trials, none perfect in design, show that several different psychological and/or biological interventions are superior to placebo treatment or no treatment. Important questions to be answered are those regarding the design of the right treatment menu for the individual case: What therapies in what combinations are best suited for what clinical profiles?

The same questions apply for the treatment of obesity. Whereas short-term results can be gratifying, the real demonstration of lasting long-term improvement for substantial numbers of those patients who actually *need* to be treated for obesity has been elusive.

Social and Cultural Issues

Still lacking are good epidemiologic studies on the prevalence of eating disorders in the United States. Most "guesstimates" are based on extrapolations from limited surveys, many of which were not based on random sampling methods. What endemic areas exist? Do certain health clubs breed eating disorders? What is the prevalence of bulimia in males? What are the child-rearing practices of women with eating disorders? What about the cultural pressures that seem to shape the expression of these disorders? From one point of view, anorexia nervosa is a perversion of the optimum—the golden girl dream pushed to the absurd. Will our society ever stop glamorizing women who are too thin? My own belief is that this can certainly take place. Although current pressures in the media for thinness remain great, and a virtual reorientation of beauty standards would be required, fad and fashions are capable of relatively rapid change in our society. The "thin is in" tendency spread like an epidemic over just a few decades, so conceivably a rapid reversal is possible, too. But it will take the right women to model a healthier, more realistic weight trend, and the right men to reinforce this value. Can we get away from equating thin shape with self-worth? This would not be easy, but it is possible.

However, should eating disorders become less prevalent I suspect that other new disorders will replace them as a means for expressing underlying maturational conflicts, personality disturbances, and tensions. Phenotypes might change, but the genotype is likely to remain, even if the "genotype" is partly biological and partly the result of early experience.

Finally, attention should be drawn to national organizations concerned with eating disorders. Stunkard mentions several lay-led groups for the obese. Many eating disorders groups publish newsletters which contain articles, book reviews, and notices of interest to patients and their families. Those involved in the treatment of eating disorder patients are advised to become acquainted with local and national groups. Among those worth writing to are:

- American Anorexia Nervosa Association, Inc. (AANA)
  133 Cedar Lane, Teaneck, New Jersey 07666
- Anorexia Nervosa and Related Eating Disorders, Inc. (ANRED)
  Box 5102, Eugene, Oregon 97405
- National Anorexia Aid Society, Inc. (NAAS)
  P.O. Box 29461, Columbus, Ohio 43229
- National Association of Anorexia Nervosa and Associated Disorders (ANAD)
  Box 271, Highland Park, Illinois

Since many patients are likely to be interested in the potential value of such self-help groups, clinicians are urged to become acquainted with them in order to assist patients to obtain whatever help they may currently provide.

Patients with eating disorders should be offered the full array of professional and self-help treatment opportunities. At present, for many patients, there seem to be multiple roads to improvement.

REFERENCES

Kupfer DJ, Rush J: Recommendations for Depression Publications. Arch Gen Psychiatry 40:1031, 1983

V

The Therapeutic Alliance and Treatment Outcome

Section

V

Contents

The Therapeutic
Alliance and
Treatment
Outcome

Section V

The Therapeutic Alliance and Treatment Outcome

Introduction

by John P. Docherty, M.D., Section Editor

The field of psychotherapy research is currently experiencing unparalleled vitality and vigor. The findings presented in the chapters of this section represents only a portion of the work taking place in this active, developing field. The basis for this resurgence in psychotherapy research lies in the fact that we have, over the last several years, addressed ourselves to some hard issues. We are no longer in the position of the man who lost his key on the dark side of the street, and then spent hours looking for it on the other side, "because that's where the street light is." Rather, through dedicated effort, we have devised methods to illuminate the relevant dark side.

As Donald Klein noted in Volume III of Psychiatry Update: the APA Annual Review, "Science is the art of the soluble." More formally stated, science is the systematic organization and accumulation of empirically verified knowledge. It is an enterprise highly dependent on adequate conceptualization and effective technology. At the heart of the experiment, as indeed of every other pragmatic endeavor, is the issue of feasibility: It is feasibility that translates the wish into the work. I will briefly review just a few of the important recent innovations in psychotherapy research that have enhanced the feasibility of this field in productive scientific work.

The most essential recent development is the standardization of psychotherapeutic treatment. For many years, psychotherapy research has been plagued by the fact that there has been no assurance that the treatment studied in one setting under a given rubric (for example, "client centered," "psychodynamic," "gestalt") was the same as that being studied in another setting; or, indeed, that there was consistency of treatment from one session to the next. If we compare this to drug therapy, this is the equivalent of not being certain that a drug called by a common name is the same drug from dose to dose or from setting to setting. Two steps have been taken to effectively address this issue. The first is the development of procedures for standardizing "treatment packages." In the area of depression, examples of such treatment packages are "interpersonal psychotherapy" (Klerman et al, 1984) and "cognitive behavior therapy" (Beck et al, 1979). These treatment packages have been standardized by addressing three questions. The first is, "What is the therapy?" This has been answered through the use of detailed manuals describing the rationale, strategies, tech-

---

This Introduction was written by Dr. Docherty in his private capacity. No official support or endorsement by NIMH is intended or should be inferred.

---

niques and boundaries of the therapy and, through the use of audiovisual tape libraries, illustrating the application of the therapy. The second question is, "Are the therapists in a given situation competent to conduct the therapy?" This has been addressed through the development of standardized training procedures and quantitative rating scales applied to videotaped examples of the therapists' work, as well as through reviews given by outside experts. The third question is, "Do the therapists carry out the indicated treatment during the course of the study?" This issue has been addressed through the use of multicomponent procedures for assessing the "adherence" of the therapist to the study therapy, and for interventions to keep therapists "on track" should they demonstrate "drift." The second forward step has been a development of useful taxonomies of therapeutic interventions that are not restricted to particular "treatment packages," but are more broadly applicable (for example, Hill, 1978).

These developments have highlighted another group of research issues. One is the need to assess psychotherapy as "an emergent phenomenon": that is, the recognition that psychotherapy is an interactive process and that the specification of therapists' behavior is not, in itself, sufficient to determine its success. A second issue is the assessment of the "absorption of the psychotherapy." The fact that the treatment is being delivered as prescribed does not reveal what has been "taken in" by the patient. A third issue is the standardization of the therapeutic relationship. One of the hoary debates in the field of psychotherapy has been the relative importance of the relationship, versus the specific techniques, of the therapy. To a large extent this has been framed within the infamous "specificity/nonspecificity" debate: That is, does successful outcome depend upon the power of specific techniques, or upon a felicitous set of circumstances and procedures that produces a feeling of optimism, trust, security and "a way out?" Since the history of the development of psychotherapy has been characterized by the emergence of competing technique-based "schools of treatment," this has been a passionately debated topic. It is thus of great interest that systematic procedures for controlling and standardizing the technique variables in psychotherapy have intensified the focus on the relationship variable. In this context, other questions for further understanding the nature and impact of the therapeutic relationship have assumed greater salience: What are the requisite capacities of the therapist to permit a therapeutic relationship to be readily formed? What degree of basic competence is necessary for adequate standardization of a therapeutic relationship? Are standardization requirements for the therapeutic relationship the same in different types of treatment?

In understanding the historical importance of the construct "therapeutic alliance" that is dealt with in this section, it is also important to understand that the current focus on this particular construct is a convergent one. Broadly speaking, psychotherapy research can be divided into two major domains: outcome research and process research. As has just been noted, the remarkable developments in the standardization of the technique variable in outcome research have reciprocally required the development of efforts to standardize the therapeutic relationship variable. Developments in the process research field have also come to focus on the therapeutic relationship: in particular, on the aspect of the therapeutic relationship known as therapeutic alliance. With the important conceptual and methodological contributions in the late 1970s by Bordin and

Luborsky, research in this area began to flourish. Bordin's organization of workshops on this topic at meetings of the Society for Psychotherapy Research helped to stimulate this research by bringing together interested researchers who, for the most part, shared a psychoanalytic orientation. The field of process research is currently undergoing a healthy resurgence. Investigators in this area have clearly identified major conceptual and methodological problems that have limited previous investigations on the therapeutic alliance and other important dimensions of the psychotherapeutic change processes. A fundamental appreciation is that change process constructs must be conceived in a more complex and more highly differentiated way in order to reflect important clinical realities. To quote Bill Pinsoff (1980), "Interventions come in different sizes." Analysis of psychotherapeutic change mechanisms must take into account the type of intervention, the context in which the intervention occurs, the skillfulness and manner with which it is delivered and the phase of treatment during which it occurs.

Two major methodological developments reflect the successful effort to construct more refined measures of important, clinically based structures in psychotherapy. One of these is the concept of "critical events." This refers to a set of procedures used to describe change-relevant recurrent moments in therapy that have an identifiable regularity of characteristics (see, for example, Rice and Greenberg, 1984). The identification of such moments permits the more accurate examination of the effect of different interventions on such "moments" (for example, insight events, misperception events). Greenberg's (1980) work, which examined the effect of interventions during therapy on a particular pattern of patient behavior (marked by a "split"), is nicely illustrative of this research approach.

The second major area of development has been in the progressive articulation and quantification of the therapeutic alliance. Essentially, current research has demonstrated the importance of a positive therapeutic alliance for a good outcome of psychotherapeutic treatment. Research has also begun to demonstrate that the notion of a therapeutic alliance is, in fact, a complex construct and, further, has begun to suggest that the development and maintenance of a good therapeutic alliance is inextricably bound with the skillful selection and application of psychotherapeutic techniques. The interventions through which a therapist handles critical events in psychotherapy may have major impact on the strength and durability of the therapeutic alliance. An exciting exploration and delineation of the ways in which these two may interact was begun at a recent workshop on Psychotherapy Process Research sponsored by the Psychosocial Treatments Research Branch of the National Institute of Mental Health. This concept has caught the imagination and generated great excitement in the field, not only because of the therapeutic potential clearly inherent in the phenomenon of therapeutic alliance itself, but also because empirical investigation offers a road toward the resolution of the longstanding and debilitating conflict over relationship versus technique. Technical competence in the conduct of a psychotherapy requires a positive therapeutic alliance; a positive therapeutic alliance requires technical competence.

Finally, it has been noted before that the strength of a field of science can be assessed by the number of salient testable hypotheses it generates. Such hypotheses regarding the relationship of the therapeutic alliance to the outcome of psychotherapy are now too numerous to fully list. Some of the questions, which can now be approached through the scientific method, include the following: What is the relationship between diagnosis and the therapeutic alliance? Are different techniques more or less useful for the development of a therapeutic alliance with different diagnostic groups? What are the particular problems or obstacles toward the development of a therapeutic alliance presented by different diagnostic groups? For example, Bordin (1983) has hypothesized that borderline patients tend to use the relationship as an end in itself, rather than to use it for purposes of change; and that schizophrenic patients are beset by a longstanding mistrust of the self and others that must be overcome. Thus, for both of these diagnostic groups, the most arduous and most modifying part of the treatment is represented in its initial phase. In addition, the methodological, conceptual development of the therapeutic alliance construct now allows us to ask more basic and very interesting questions regarding the interaction of pharmacological and psychotherapeutic treatments. We can now begin the development of a new field, which David Janowsky (personal communication) has referred to as "the pharmacotherapy of interpersonal processes." For example, we can now ask, "Can certain drugs be used to modify a negative therapeutic alliance?" More specifically, "Can hostility be significantly modulated in some depressed patients to permit a positive therapeutic alliance to form where it was otherwise not possible?"

In the chapters that follow, some of the major issues relating to therapeutic alliance are covered. Selection of these chapters was made with the intention of addressing not only the basic scientific work attempting to understand this phenomenon, but also with the intention of addressing some of the key clinical issues related to this central aspect of psychotherapeutic endeavor. Chapter 27, by Dr. Dianna Hartley, is an overview of the state of the art of research on the therapeutic alliance. In Chapter 28, Drs. Lester Luborsky and Arthur Auerbach review the research evidence for the role of the therapeutic relationship and therapeutic alliance in psychotherapy, particularly psychodynamic and exploratory forms of psychotherapy, and draw some major clinical implications of this work. Chapter 29, by Dr. A. John Rush, focuses on the role of the therapeutic alliance in brief focused forms of psychotherapy. In Chapter 30, Drs. Mardi Horowitz and Charles Marmar discuss some of the major barriers in the development of a therapeutic alliance and suggest methods for overcoming such impediments. In Chapter 31, Dr. Susan Blumenthal, Dr. Enrico Jones and Janice Krupnick examine the critical issue of the influence of gender and race on the therapeutic alliance and the outcome of psychotherapy. Chapter 32, by Drs. John Docherty and Susan Fiester, examines the importance and central role of the therapeutic alliance and other psychosocial variables in the effective conduct of psychopharmacological treatments. Finally, in my Afterword, I discuss each of the chapters, raising some of the important questions that current and future research must address.

REFERENCES

Beck AT, Rush AJ, Shaw BF, Emery G: Cognitive Therapy of Depression. New York, Guilford Press, 1979

Bordin E: Myths, realities, and alternatives to clinical trials. Paper presented at International Conference on Psychotherapy, Bogota, Colombia, 1983

Greenberg L: The intensive analysis of recurring events from the practice of Gestalt Therapy. Psychotherapy, Theory, Research & Practice 17:143-152, 1980

Hill LE: The development of a system for classifying counselor responses. J Consult Clin Psychol 47:453-458, 1978

Janowsky D: Personal communication.

Klein D: Introduction to part five: the anxiety disorders, in Psychiatry Update: Vol. III. Edited by Grinspoon L. Washington, D.C., American Psychiatric Press, Inc., 1984

Klerman G, Weissman M, Rounsaville B, Chevron E: Interpersonal Psychotherapy of Depression. New York, Basic Books, 1984

Pinsoff WM: Family therapy process research, in Handbook of Family Therapy. Edited by Gurman AE, Kniskern D. New York, Bruner/Mazel, 1980

Rice LN, Greenberg LS: Patterns of Change. New York, Guilford Press, 1984

Waskow IE: Specification of the technique variable in the NIMH Treatment of Depression Collaborative Research Program, in Psychotherapy Research: Where Are We and Where Should We Go? Edited by Williams J, Spitzer R. New York, Guilford Press, 1984

Chapter 27

Research on the Therapeutic Alliance in Psychotherapy

by Dianna E. Hartley, Ph.D.

THE CONCEPT OF THE THERAPEUTIC ALLIANCE

All forms of individual psychotherapy have, as their basis, a relationship between two persons. One person, the patient, feels unable to change a situation that is causing distress, and seeks the assistance of a therapist who is assumed to be competent to help with such problems. These two persons undertake a series of interactions that both believe will bring about desired changes in the patient's feelings, attitudes and behavior. Since most psychotherapists practicing in this country identify themselves either as psychodynamic or as "eclectic," using psychodynamic principles along with other techniques (Garfield, 1980), we can assume that the concept of therapeutic alliance is relevant across a broad range of therapies currently practiced. My goals here are to present current clinical practices and theories about therapeutic alliance and its role in the effectiveness of psychotherapy, and to relate empirical findings to those ideas. I will focus on research involving individual outpatient psychotherapy and measures taken during the therapy process.

In the earliest writings of modern psychotherapy, Breuer and Freud (1895/1955) spoke of the patient as an active collaborator in treatment. In most of his subsequent work on the psychoanalytic relationship, Freud focused on transference and resistance. He did, however, also recognize the role of friendliness and affection as "the vehicle of success in psychoanalysis" (Freud, 1912/1958, p. 105). Sterba (1934) was the first to explicate the role of positive identification with the therapist in leading the patient to work toward the accomplishment of common therapeutic tasks. Later, Freud (1940) described the analyst and patient as banding together against the patient's symptoms in a "pact" based on free exploration by the patient, and discretion and competent understanding by the therapist. Beginning with Zetzel (1956), psychoanalytically oriented therapists have been increasingly attentive to the notion that the therapeutic alliance, which depends to a large degree on basic trust and relatively high levels of ego functioning of the patient (as well as on the therapist's active participation and partnership), is essential to the effectiveness of any therapeutic intervention. Greenson (1967) carefully spelled out the theoretical and clinical implications of considering these aspects of therapeutic interaction separately from those aspects that are regarded as more irrational or transferential, while recognizing that the boundary is somewhat artificial.

While it is hard to find a clear, jargon-free definition, a consensus seems to be evolving that the therapeutic alliance has two components: the real relationship and the working alliance (Greenson, 1967; Bordin, 1975; Dickes, 1975; Marziali, et al, 1981; Hartley and Strupp, 1983). The real relationship refers to the mutual human response of the patient and therapist to each other, including undistorted perceptions and authentic liking, trust and respect for each other, which exist along with the inequalities inherent in the therapy situation. The working alliance depends upon and reflects the ability of the dyadic partners to work purposefully together in the treatment they have undertaken. It begins with the decision of two people to work toward the alleviation of the problems experienced by the patient. The aura of mystery and authority with which the therapist is often initially endowed is ideally replaced by a sense that the two are collaborating adults, each with certain roles and responsibilities. During the process of mutual agreement about the definition of the problems, the goals of therapy and the methods to be employed, the patient develops a more accurate perception of the treatment and an allegiance to the contract. When a patient understands what is expected and why certain tasks can be helpful, he or she can more fully participate in personal exploration, communicate more openly and try out new, potentially more productive modes of behavior.

Although the concept of therapeutic alliance is psychoanalytic in origin, the importance of the real relationship between patient and therapist and of the working "contract" are acknowledged by theorists of other schools of therapy as well. Carl Rogers (1957) probably took the most radical relationship-oriented stance when he advocated the idea that warmth, genuineness and empathic understanding are the necessary and sufficient conditions for therapeutic benefit. At the other end of the continuum, behavior therapists have traditionally claimed that their techniques alone carried therapeutic impact. More recently, a few behavioral theorists (Wilson and Evans, 1976; Goldfried, 1980) are beginning to examine seriously the effects of interpersonal dynamics between therapists and patients. The basic model of behavior therapy, however, remains one of an expert directing the therapy and making decisions to be carried out by the patient. A more integrative approach is emerging from proponents of interpersonal psychotherapy based on the teachings of Harry Stack Sullivan, in which the focus is on transactions in a two-person system with both therapist and patient seen as active participants (Cashdan, 1973; Anchin and Kiesler, 1982).

One of the most widely accepted findings of psychotherapy research is that all forms of therapy that have been examined have some positive effect, but that none is consistently superior to the others (Smith and Glass, 1977; Bergin and Lambert, 1978). Despite recent progress toward specifying the techniques of various psychotherapies in treatment manuals from several research projects, we still have scant evidence that techniques per se differentiate successful from unsuccessful therapies. The current emphasis on the technology of therapy seems to represent another swing of the pendulum from an earlier relationship-centered focus, and also to stem from an aspiration to develop clinical methods that demonstrate effects above and beyond those of the interpersonal context in which they are applied. Debating the relative importance of relationship and technique has a long history, and will undoubtedly continue. However, it may be unproductive to conceptualize the two as separate dimensions—relationship versus technique, or specific versus nonspecific factors. Rather, it may be more useful to view the two as interacting processes, with the concept of therapeutic alliance capturing this interaction. Research using this conceptualization of the therapeutic alliance has the potential to integrate research among therapist, patient, relationship and technique variables, since all are taken into account.

Bordin (1976) has suggested that the capacity and willingness of both therapist and patient to undertake particular tasks with each other determines the outcome of any therapy. He delineated three components of the therapeutic alliance: *bonds*, referring to the optimal social relationship between patient and therapist and factors that either facilitate or hinder its formation; *tasks*, including the techniques used by the therapist, and role expectations and behaviors of the patient; and *goals*, denoting movement toward the desirable outcome of treatment. The alliance, then, can be viewed as a goal-directed system, with the cognitive and interpersonal styles of the patient and therapist interacting with each other and with the chosen techniques of the therapy.

RECENT RESEARCH FINDINGS

Several researchers have developed methods to examine the role of the alliance in psychotherapy (Luborsky, 1976; Marziali et al, 1981; Hartley and Strupp, 1983; Horvath and Greenberg, in press; Allen et al, in press). Most past psychotherapy process research involved variables that overlap, to some extent, with the alliance concept as defined here. A reexamination of these studies yields support for the hypothesis that the strength of the alliance is positively correlated with therapeutic outcome (Orlinsky and Howard, 1978).

Modern psychotherapy research began with Carl Rogers looking for associations between personal growth in psychotherapy and what came to be known as the "facilitating conditions" provided by the therapist—warmth, empathy, respect and genuineness. His research group started taping therapy sessions, so that the perspective of outside observers could be incorporated into research designs. In the intervening 25 years, numerous studies of psychotherapy process and outcome were undertaken; but few linked process with outcome variables, or included measures of both patient and therapist variables in ways that permitted statements about their interactions. As recently as 1978, Parloff and colleagues found that "the category of studies dealing with experimental research on therapist and patient interactions within the treatment setting remains essentially null" (p. 234). Since their review was written, however, the number of such studies has increased and the quality of process research has improved. The concept of therapeutic alliance has become a focus of research in several settings. While each research group defines the alliance in slightly different ways, the emerging consensus is that the alliance is a multifaceted dyadic interaction to which both the patient and the therapist contribute.

The Therapist's Contribution

The therapist contributes to the alliance in terms of both personal attitudes and professional therapeutic behavior. Bordin's (1976) formulation involves the willingness and the ability of the therapist, as well as the patient, to establish a relationship and to carry out the tasks of the therapy that is undertaken. Consequently, both personal qualities and professional expertise are essential aspects to be considered, in clinical practice and in research.

Practitioners across most major schools of therapy agree that there are certain ideal personal qualities of a good therapist. Such a person is sensitive, tolerant, warm, logical, straightforward and committed to the integrity and dignity of all persons. He or she restrains personal reactions in the service of therapeutic commitment and focuses on the tasks and goals of therapy, but is also flexible. Although the idea that the personality of the therapist is an important element of therapeutic effectiveness has gained wide acceptance, surprisingly little research evidence supports it. Particularly when studies have been formulated in terms of a positive statement (such as, more mature, well-adjusted therapists produce better outcomes), results are generally null. Slightly more evidence has accumulated for the notion that psychological disturbance in the therapist makes poor outcomes more likely. Research in this area is hampered by several problems. To begin with, chances of finding statistically significant associations are greatly reduced by the fact that therapists who participate in most research projects do not vary greatly in the kinds of personal qualities being considered. This lack of variance, combined with vague general operationalizing of concepts and adherence to traditional research designs that may be ill-suited to the relevant questions is no surprise. Very promising research was done by Vandenbos and Karon (1971), who investigated the quality of good and poor therapists for schizophrenics. They specifically defined and operationalized the concept of "pathogenic" therapists—those who, on projective measures, showed tendencies to use dependent persons to satisfy their own personal needs. They found that such therapists were not effective treating schizophrenics and could cause deterioration.

A good psychotherapist has personal characteristics similar to those of any other mature, responsible person. Little is likely to be gained by investigating such global qualities. Personality traits of therapists become relevant variables in therapy research to the extent that they are linked to what he or she actually does in therapy and to his or her ultimate impact on patients. A more productive pursuit may be to delineate the specific characteristics necessary for therapists to form optimal therapeutic relationships, and to carry out specific procedures with specific kinds of patients; and, conversely, to delineate the characteristics that are significant impediments to effective practice. The role of therapist requires one to regulate transactions across the spatial and temporal boundaries that differentiate the therapy relationship from other social encounters. The therapist promises confidentiality, keeps external interruptions and distractions to a minimum, and limits contact with the patient outside the therapy environment. The therapist is an expert who takes the responsibility for defining the tasks of the therapy. Thus, the success of therapy may depend upon the therapists' ease in assuming the role of a legitimate, benign authority figure, teacher, or manager (Newton, 1973).

The most thoroughly researched hypotheses in psychotherapy research have been Rogers' (1957) assertions that the therapist's warmth, empathic understanding and genuineness in themselves produced personality change in patients. Numerous studies of these variables, each one with serious methodological flaws, indicate a small but consistent correlation with outcome. Such qualities play some role in the establishment of a therapeutic alliance, but are not in themselves the most important ingredients of therapy. Rogers actually specified that the patient's *perception* of the therapist's facilitating qualities was the essential ingredient of therapy. As he might have expected, research using the Barrett-Lennard Relationship Inventory (1962) assessing relationship qualities from the patient's perspective does show a stronger, more consistent association with outcomes, but still leaves unanswered the question of how therapists bring about or enhance patients' perceptions of them as understanding and helpful.

Defining the therapists' contribution purely in terms of providing a positive interpersonal climate led researchers, until very recently, to ignore the more technical or professional aspects of the working alliance. A psychotherapy relationship is formed because the therapist offers expert help with certain kinds of problems. Attempts to operationalize and investigate therapist expertise have been, by and large, unsuccessful. The most common strategy has been to use years of experience as an index of greater competence. This operational definition has led to mixed findings. Usually, we have seen differences in process variables, but not differences in outcome (Parloff et al, 1978). Neither amount of training nor professional discipline has shown a consistent relationship to process or outcome.

Another approach to studying therapist competence has been proposed by Schaffer (1982, 1983a, 1983b). He argues persuasively for directly measuring the "skillfulness" with which therapists use their techniques. Interventions of all types, from the most molecular to the most molar, can potentially be assessed for the competence with which they are delivered. Three dimensions are essential for such measures: type of therapist behavior; skillfulness; and interpersonal manner. Since these variables are relatively independent, all three should be considered for each intervention, yielding a profile of the therapist's behavior. His scheme is compatible with the conceptualization of therapeutic alliance proposed here, in that it allows investigation of both "specific" and "nonspecific" factors and of their interaction. For example, Greenberg and Rice (1981) statistically controlled for the level of the therapists' skill in carrying out either a client-centered or a Gestalt therapy interaction. They demonstrated specific differences in patient behavior in response to these two different techniques as measured by the Experiencing Scale (Klein et al, 1970).

Another approach to the study of therapist competence is illustrated by the Vanderbilt Negative Indicators Scale, developed from a survey of psychotherapy experts (Strupp et al, 1977). Using this scale, Sachs (1983) found that, contrary to her expectations, patient and therapist personal qualities were only slightly predictive of therapy outcome and that the therapist category "Errors in Technique" accounted for most of the variance in her sample.

Several recent studies of therapeutic alliance have indicated that therapist-offered relationship variables are weak predictors compared to patient variables (Marziali et al, 1981; Hartley and Strupp, 1983; Luborsky et al, 1983; O'Malley et al, 1983). It is likely that with more careful attention to measurement of the interpersonal as well as the technical realms, we can get a sharper picture both of how therapists relate to patients and how they do the work of psychotherapy.

The Patient's Contribution

The most important determinants of a patient's readiness to form a sound therapeutic alliance lie in his or her previous experiences with important persons.

The demands made of patients entering a therapy relationship vary along several dimensions: the type and degree of self-observation and self-disclosure, the range and complexity of cognitive processing, the extent of dependence on or compliance with the therapist, and the degree of ambiguity inherent in the relationship (Bordin, 1975). To engage in productive therapeutic work, the patient must feel some degree of confidence in and attraction to the therapist, both as a healer and as a person. In addition to being open to help from another person, a patient has to be willing to cooperate with the ground rules of the particular form of therapy offered by the therapist. Thus, the patient's behavior in therapy may also be considered in terms of two dimensions: interpersonal behavior and task behavior. Even though patient process variables usually show more variance than therapist variables, and are thought to be more important in determining outcome, far fewer studies of patient behavior have been conducted.

Research growing out of the client-centered framework has included several measures of the patient's role in therapy, as well as the therapist-offered conditions discussed earlier. Several measures of patient behavior were developed by the Rogers group, including the Experiencing Scale (Klein et al, 1970). At the low end of the scale, discourse is impersonal and superficial; and at the high end, feelings are explored and self experience is the reference for understanding and problem solving. Research utilizing this scale indicates that in many varieties of psychodynamic and experiential therapies, self exploration is positively correlated with outcome. However, it has not been shown that a *change* in level of experiencing or self-exploration occurs over the course of treatment in successful cases. A similar pattern of results exists for other patient measures, such as the Depth of Exploration Scale (Truax and Carkhuff, 1967) and Voice Quality Index (Rice and Wagstaff, 1967). These measures of the patient's emotional expressiveness, internal focus, or free association show positive correlations with outcome, but it is not clear that patients change along this dimension during treatment. Two possibilities exist. It may be that by using some intervention strategy, patients can be helped to develop these attributes. Another approach is to use such variables as selection criteria for predicting which patients might do well in exploratory, expressive therapies.

Several of the therapeutic alliance scales mentioned earlier have been used to assess various aspects of the alliance from the patient's, the therapist's, or the observer's perspective. In several multivariate studies using these scales, two consistent findings have emerged: One is that patient variables are more highly correlated with outcome measures than therapist variables, and the second is that ratings of these variables made early in therapy (approximately the third to sixth sessions) are highly correlated with outcome (Luborsky, 1976; Gomes-Schwartz, 1978; Marziali et al, 1981; Hartley and Strupp, 1983; Marmar et al, in press). In a pioneering study, Luborsky (1976) inferred the presence of a simple helping alliance from counting, in transcripts of therapy sessions, the number of times patients stated that they felt better, that therapy was helping, or that they felt understood by the therapist. This was called a Type I alliance. A second type of alliance, Type II, was defined by a sense of the patient and therapist working together with shared responsibility for achieving treatment goals. Comparing the ten most improved and ten least improved patients in the Penn Psychotherapy Research Project, he found that improvers demonstrated positive attitudes early in therapy while nonimprovers showed negative attitudes. Very few of the dyads in his sample achieved mutual, responsibility-sharing relationships. One problem with this method of measuring alliance is that it depends upon the patients' saying in the session that he or she experiences help or improvement—or the opposite—so that the measure may actually be predicting long-term outcome from immediate gains.

A research group at the Menninger Foundation (Allen et al, in press) has developed a method for closely examining the patient's contribution to the alliance, which they define as the patient's *collaboration* in work appropriate to the therapy. The degree of collaboration is judged by looking at six different components: to what extent does the patient bring in significant issues and material?; how openly does the patient share information and express feelings?; how well does the patient use the efforts of the therapist to clarify or change problems?; how actively does the patient work on the therapy tasks?; how extensively does the patient apply therapeutic learning to his or her life outside therapy?; and how does the patient identify with the therapist in adopting "therapist-like" behaviors toward himself or herself?

Several other rating systems measure various aspects of the patient's positive and negative contributions to the alliance. These scales usually contain between 40 and 80 items, about half relevant to the therapist's behavior and half to the patient's behavior. In several studies, all the patient items of these scales have been collapsed into a global Patient Contribution or Patient Involvement score by summing the ratings or computing factor scores. This composite Patient Involvement measure has correlated highly with outcome (Gomes-Schwartz, 1978; Marmar et al, in press). In a study using the Vanderbilt Therapeutic Alliance Scale (Hartley and Strupp, 1983), factor analysis showed four different patient subscales. Two were positive: motivation and responsibility; and two were negative: active resistance and anxiety. In the initial phase of therapy, patients with poorer outcomes were noted to be more hostile, defensive and anxious; those who had better outcomes were seen as more willing to take an active, responsible role in the therapy. The two groups were rated as equally distressed and motivated for therapy. One implication of this finding is that patients contribute to the alliance in two ways: One is to acknowledge personal difficulty and the need for help; the second is to actively engage in the tasks of therapy and to apply what is learned there to one's life outside the therapy relationship. Most patients can do the first, but both the Penn and the Vanderbilt projects indicate that establishing a sense of mutual responsibility for the treatment is a harder-won achievement.

Patients' positive attitudes toward and attachment to the therapist have consistently been linked with positive outcome, while the expression of negative attitudes has predicted poorer outcome. These findings stand in contrast to the results of four studies in which the expression of hostility was found to predict better outcomes (Mintz et al, 1971; Crowder, 1972). The relationship between the alliance and the expression of negative feelings toward the therapist or about the treatment process is not clear. Certainly some therapists—for example, Kernberg and Sifneos—encourage the active expression and exploration of these negative feelings whenever they occur, and especially in the early phases of treatment. They see such exploration as vital to the alliance, since it is likely that such feelings, unaddressed, will build to disruptive proportions or go underground, silently eroding the therapeutic relationship and limiting the amount of progress the patient can make.

Patients' in-therapy behavior from early sessions has consistently been found to predict therapy outcome. To examine this phenomenon further, Moras and Strupp (1982) tried to determine the extent to which these relationship patterns are due to a predisposition of the patient. Using the Patient Involvement Scale from the Vanderbilt Psychotherapy Process Scale (Gomes-Schwartz, 1978), they found that the quality of the patients' pretherapy interpersonal adjustment was significantly correlated with positive engagement in treatment. Closer examination, however, showed that the correlation was determined mostly by those patients with the highest ratings on both dimensions; that is, those who had good relationships with others established a good relationship with the therapist. For patients with low or moderate pretherapy interpersonal relationship scores, the kind of relationship established with the therapist was not predictable. While these studies represent first crude steps toward operationalizing and empirically examining the formation of a therapeutic alliance, we have much to learn before we will understand the process of a patient's engagement with a therapist in carrying out the tasks of therapy.

Patient-Therapist Interactions

In addition to viewing the patient and therapist as separate persons, researchers have looked at their interactions in sessions. This research has been conducted either directly, by rating interactions, or indirectly, by rating separate variables and examining their interactions in complex research designs. A few such studies exist, which shed light on both interpersonal and task aspects of interactions. The results of Saltzman and his colleagues (1976) studying the formation of a therapeutic relationship at a university counseling service indicate that it is of fundamental importance that the therapist and patient experience a caring attachment to each other. A relationship characterized by mutual feelings of warmth, respect, caring, openness and understanding was associated with fewer premature terminations, better patient satisfaction, and greater improvement. At the same time, important dissatisfactions and disruptions in the relationship were noted by both patient and therapist by the third session in cases which went on to either premature termination or poor outcome.

Another method of addressing the therapist-patient interaction is to collect ratings of characteristics of a good or a poor session from patients', therapists', and observers' perspectives. An observer is typically another clinician who listens to a tape or reads a transcript of a session. Such studies indicate that therapy sessions are evaluated along two dimensions. Stiles (1980) calls the first Depth/Value and the second Smoothness/Ease. These two factors replicate those found by Orlinsky and Howard (1975). Therapists tend to value depth of exploration more highly, even if it is difficult, while patients rate warm, easy sessions more highly, at least immediately afterwards. There is also evidence that independent observers (who are also clinicians) view the goodness of an hour along different dimensions from either participant (Hoyt et al, 1983). Unfortunately, none of the research on good hours has been linked to outcome variables, so we do not know how these variables "add up" in producing therapeutic change.

An extremely promising model for measuring interactional concepts is based on the circumplex concept (Leary, 1957; Wiggins et al, 1981). This method involves arranging behaviors or attitudes on a surface defined by two axes. The horizontal axis reflects the affiliative domain and has as endpoints words such as *love–hate* or *attack–shared ecstasy*. The vertical axis is concerned with autonomy and control and has endpoint labels like *freedom–control* or *dominate–submit*. The regions between the axes may be subdivided in various ways, but the most psychometrically desirable is usually eight regions (Benjamin, 1982). While this approach is still in early stages of development as a measure of both process and outcome in psychotherapy research, the work of Benjamin (1974, 1979, 1982) on the Structural Analysis of Social Behavior (SASB) shows its enormous potential. SASB is based on a general model of interpersonal behavior that can be used across a wide variety of situations and theoretical approaches to therapy. Psychometric and validation studies have established it as a viable measure. Further, it can be used to assess interpersonal behavior at both the overt level and at the level of intrapsychic representation. A study by Ben-Torvim and Greenup (1983) showed that a similar model could be used to trace changes in a patient's perception of the therapist and to relate these changes to the therapist's interventions.

FUTURE DIRECTIONS AND NEW RESEARCH STRATEGIES

Current Status of Therapeutic Alliance Scales

Developing a measure of any aspect of the psychotherapy process requires a large program of methodological research, which often takes years (Kiesler, 1973; Bordin, 1974). Attention must be paid to such issues as the selection of key variables; the operational definition of abstract concepts; sampling relevant patients, therapists and portions of the therapy process; and the selection of who should make the ratings. Once these decisions are made, scales such as those recently developed to measure therapeutic alliance need to be carefully assessed for reliability, dimensionality and validity. Table 1 shows a brief synopsis of the measurement systems that have recently been developed to assess the therapeutic alliance. For each of these systems, the goal of the research team has been to devise a method that is applicable across a broad range of therapies, although all explicitly acknowledge that their conceptual framework derives from the work of Greenson (1967) and other psychoanalytic theorists. The therapies to which the scales have been applied have been generally brief and exploratory in nature (psychoanalytic, client-centered and Gestalt). Therefore, the question of their applicability to other approaches, such as cognitive or behavioral therapies, remains unanswered.

All these scales have shown moderate to very good levels of internal consistency and reliability when used by judges who are clinically trained. Since none of them have been used outside the groups in which they were developed, there is no information about reliability when they are used by others. However, each group has written a manual, making application to other data bases possible. While lack of cross-validation makes empirical comparison of the systems in terms of either reliability or validity impossible at this time, all have shown adequate levels to be considered viable research tools.

One problem that has not been adequately addressed in the process of developing these scales is that of identifying signs of alliance in the sessions. The choice of units for measurement has not been empirically examined for any system. Therefore, we do not know, for example, if more stable measurements result from rating a whole session than from rating 15 minutes. Even more important is the underlying assumptions that the alliance is relatively homogeneous across time. Kiesler (1966) pointed out the pitfalls involved in psychotherapy researchers assuming that all patients, all therapists, or all treatments are the same and that random sampling is a valid procedure. The rationale for selecting units has often been indicated (for example, early sessions versus late sessions; or the beginning, middle and end of a session). A sharper conceptual focus on this issue and empirical investigation is called for.

A more critical problem is that of data reduction. Each of the scales or rating systems has multiple items, ranging from ten for the Penn Helping Alliance Rating Method to 80 for the Vanderbilt Psychotherapy Process Scale, because their developers believed the concept was of sufficient complexity to warrant a multidimensional approach. Usually, however, scales have been used additively and collapsed, resulting in much lost information. For example, ratings of patients' expression of negative attitudes may be reverse-scored and added to the ratings of positive attitudes. The result is used as a measure of positive engagement with the therapist and is found to be correlated with outcome. Unfortunately, no one has yet gone back to untangle this dimension and look more closely at the complex relationship between the expression of negative feelings and therapeutic alliance and eventual outcome.

The Importance of a Tripartite Model of the Therapeutic Alliance

Just as each participant and observer had a different story to tell in the Japanese film *Rashomon* (Mintz et al, 1973), each participant and nonparticipant observer of a psychotherapy session will see and attribute meaning to it in a different way. For example, in one study there was only a .18 correlation between the ratings of psychodynamic therapists who conducted the sessions and those of psychodynamically oriented clinician/observers who listened to tapes on a measure of the "goodness" of a session (Hoyt et al, 1983). Orlinsky (1983) emphasized this point: "Anyone who would study therapy process may legitimately study it from any one of these perspectives: what the patient experienced; what the therapist experienced; what the nonparticipant observer experienced. On the other hand, anyone who wants to study psychotherapy process as a whole must study it from all three perspectives and must include the congruences and divergences of these perspectives as part of the data" (p. 5).

The formation and maintenance of a therapeutic alliance is a complex process; to capture it for research requires multiple variables. The question is, then, how to make a meaningful whole of these measures. As patients, clinicians and supervisors, we do it all the time. The ideal goal of research should be to reproduce as fully as possible a comprehensive picture of how a therapy relationship system does its work.

Table 1. A Synopsis of Research with Therapeutic Alliance Measuring Instruments

Scale	Conceptual Definition	Unit of Process	Population	Factor Structure	Empirical Findings
Penn Helping Alliance Methods (Luborsky, 1976; Morgan et al, 1982; Luborsky et al, 1983)	Observers' perspective. Patient and therapist items. Two levels of alliance are accepting help (Type 1) and mutual collaboration on problems (Type 2). Either counting literal references or judges' inference.	First 20 minutes of 2 early and 2 late sessions from transcripts; sometimes collapsed into a single rating.	Nonpsychotic general clinic outpatients, treated by residents and staff, psychiatrists in psychoanalytic psychotherapy.	A priori division into Type 1 and Type 2. Correlation of .91 between Type 1 and Type 2 suggests one dimension.	No change in alliance ratings from early to late sessions. Patient-related alliance scores positively correlated with outcome in 10 most and 10 least improved cases. Correlated with patient-therapist demographic similarity.
Vanderbilt Psychotherapy Process Scale (Gomes-Schwartz, 1978; Moras and Strupp, 1982; O'Malley et al, 1983)	Observers' perspective. Patient, Therapist, Interactional Items. Eclectic orientation to examine therapist-offered relationship, patient involvement, and exploration.	10-minute random segments; First + middle + last 5-minutes from Audiotapes of sessions over course of therapy.	Neurotic college students in broad range of brief ($\leq$25 sessions) dynamic therapies with professional and nonprofessional therapists.	Patient: Participation, Hostility, Exploration, Psychic Distress. Therapist: Warmth, Negative Attitude, Exploration.	Positive patient involvement (by Session 3) predicts outcome. Pretherapy goal relationships predict patient involvement.
Vanderbilt Therapeutic Alliance Scale (Hartley and Strupp, 1983)	Observers' perspective (Patient and therapist versions also exist). Patient, Therapist, Interaction items. Eclectic but primarily psychodynamic orientation. Items measure interpersonal bonds and task-related dimensions.	First + middle + last 5-minutes of session across course of therapy.	Same as VPPS above.	Patient: Motivation, Responsibility, Resistance, Anxiety. Therapist: Positive Climate, Intrusiveness.	Alliance did not predict dropouts, only initial phase scores discriminated between good and poor outcome groups. Patient variables were more predictive of outcome, especially negative attitudes with poorer outcome.

Table 1. A Synopsis of Research with Therapeutic Alliance Measuring Instruments—Continued

Scale	Conceptual Definition	Unit of Process	Population	Factor Structure	Empirical Findings
Therapeutic Alliance Rating System (Marziali et al, 1981; Horowitz et al, 1984; Marmar et al, in press)	Observers' perspective (Patient and therapist scales also exist). Focus on affective and attitudinal aspects. Assesses patient positive and negative and therapist positive and negative contributions.	20-25 minute segments from sessions across course of therapy from audio- or videotapes.	Neurotic-level stress response reactions in brief (12 session) psychodynamic therapy by faculty-level psychiatrists, psychologists, social workers.	A priori scales supported by item analysis and factor analysis: Patient: Positive Contribution, Negative Contribution. Therapist: Positive Contribution, Negative Contribution Sometimes Collapsed to Patient and Therapist Total Contribution.	Patient contribution predicts outcome. Patient contribution correlated with maturity of self concept, but not level of disturbance. Alliance variables predict outcome differently at different levels of motivation.
Working Alliance Inventory (Horvath and Greenberg, in press)	Patients' and therapists' self report inventories. Explicitly developed items based on concepts of bonds, tasks, goals (Bordin, 1976). Eclectic orientation to apply to wide variety of approaches.	Rated at end of third session for relationship up to that time.	Volunteers in individual psychotherapy in a variety of outpatient settings with wide variety of approaches and therapists.	A priori scales: Goals, Bonds, Tasks. High correlations found between Goals and Tasks suggests overlap.	Overall alliance predicts patient self report of outcome well; Task dimension is most highly correlated with outcome.
Menninger Therapeutic Alliance Scales (Allen et al, in press)	Observers' perspective (can be used by therapist). Alliance defined primarily as patient's active collaboration with therapist, mediated by certain patient attitudinal variables. Acknowledgement of primary orientation toward psychoanalytic therapy and psychoanalysis.	Transcripts of whole sessions.	15 Tapes from Vanderbilt Psychotherapy Research Project (see above) and one from Dr. Merton Gill.	Collaboration as major variable with Mediating variables (Trust, Acceptance, Optimism, Affect Expression) and component scales (Significant material, active work, Use of therapist, Reflection, Application outside therapy, Motivation to Change, Resistance, Work with resistance). High intercorrelations, but no formal factor analysis.	Research has focused thus far on definition, reliability, and dimensionality. No available information for relationship with other variables.

Choosing Units to Study

Most research on therapeutic alliance and variables related to it has been conducted in ways that are not consistent with clinical practice and clinical knowledge, making the task of communication between practitioner and researcher even more difficult than it needs to be. Typically, as researchers, we have used a fixed segment of time (say, five minutes) on a speech unit; rated it; summed the ratings; and then averaged across raters, segments, hours and cases to get a data-point for statistical analyses. The yield of such research is statements of probabilities that hold for groups in the long run, but are subject to varying interpretations and do little to inform the treatment of individual cases.

Recently, several approaches to more intensive analysis of the therapy process have been suggested (Elliott, 1983; Rice and Greenberg, 1984). These proposed methodologies share certain features: They focus at a clinically meaningful point in the therapy; they attend to the context of the behavior being studied; they seek patterns of behavior, not just frequency counts; and they use intensive designs for single cases or carefully defined groups. Rather than using random sampling, researchers study "key events" chosen by reference to some formal or informal theory about the nature of the change process in psychotherapy, or through some empirical process such as a session report questionnaire, Interpersonal Process Recall, or therapist notes. Some researchers have focused on patient markers (for example, Greenberg and Rice, 1981), while others propose to begin with therapist strategies (Goldfried, 1980) or intentions (Hill, 1983). Since each variable has its own logical unit of analysis, different amounts of time are sampled for rating different variables. Greenberg (1980), for example, used two-minute segments to examine changes in level of experiencing after Gestalt therapy intervention using the two-chair technique. Ben-Tovim and Greenup (1983), who were looking for changes in transference dispositions toward the therapist, found the most change in their measure in a session two weeks after a significant interpretation by the therapist.

Another promising strategy was used by Strupp (1980a,b). He picked cases for analysis based on knowledge of outcomes. He compared a more and a less successful case from the same therapist on a number of relationship and task dimensions, using a range of quantitative measures, and also listening to tapes of all the sessions to integrate information and form a clinical impression.

With regard to therapeutic alliance, most research so far has focused primarily on the initial phase of therapy. The clinical literature, however, suggests that while the initial phase is important for establishing the bond, other aspects of the alliance might be more salient at other stages. Even the bonding process may be different for different kinds of patients. A neurotic patient with an adjustment disorder might form an adequate bond for brief psychotherapy in one hour, while a meaningful working alliance with a schizophrenic patient can take years to build. Bordin (1976) has suggested the intensive study of the middle phase of therapy, when the process of repairing the alliance when it is weakened or disrupted actually becomes the work of the treatment.

Large–N and/or Small–N Studies

Most psychotherapy researchers, like other clinical researchers and social scientists, have used standard methodological approaches while lamenting their inappropriateness. A few investigators have moved in the direction of the single-case study, usually done in a more systematic way than a simple report of the treater's impressions (for example, Horowitz, 1979). For good reasons, calls to abandon large–N, classical-design studies are increasing. It is important to remember that both group designs and N–of–one studies have advantages and disadvantages. Group designs allow us to argue for both the robustness and the generalizability of our findings. Large studies also offer the chance to look at the interactions of multiple variables, and thus to develop and test complex hypotheses. Particularly if the inclusion/exclusion criteria are well-defined and the contrast groups are well-chosen, large studies can contribute substantially to progress in clinical research. While many criticisms are valid, coping strategies do exist; for example, emphasizing nonparametric statistics when assumptions of normal distribution are not met (Kraemer, 1981).

The use of N–of–one or time-series designs can be one solution. These designs are most helpful in behavioral and biological research when baseline and interventions can be clearly marked off from each other. However, they may not be applicable to most variables of interest in the area of therapeutic alliance. We are not usually looking for the impact of a single intervention, but for logical orderly sequences that can be "discovered" much in the way Piaget and Kohlberg described unfolding developmental phases. The best research strategy seems to be one of alternating between large–N and small–N studies, either building up a number of single cases to test and eliminating various hypotheses, or closely examining the data available in group studies. Too often we stop when we know the significance level of the t– or F–test, when we could learn much more from doing comparisons, partial correlations, and further tests of differences in variance. Individual cases can be studied within the context of large–N designs. For example, one might pick a case that prototypically exemplifies the phenomenon of interest or that is the "exception that proves the rule." The goal of this research strategy is to build understanding of what happens from the level of molecular interaction, to whole sessions, to the course of therapy and to lasting benefits at long-term followup.

The Question of Prediction and the Quest for Understanding

The goal of scientific understanding is often described as the ability to predict and control the behavior under investigation. In psychotherapy research, as well as in practice, the more appropriate and realistic goals are to understand and to exert some degree of influence, while accepting that any impact will not be great because of the vast number of other influencing persons and events. The number of events and variables that influence the kind of therapeutic alliance established by any dyad is much too large to incorporate in a comprehensible way in any research design. Fortunately the mind of the clinician is capable of weighing and processing this information in ways beyond the capacity of the most sophisticated computer. Even the best sequential designs are reductionistic, allow analysis of only a small number of variables and a few points in time and, thus, do not convey the clinical realities of the therapy.

For progress in the area of therapeutic alliance, we need to define as specifically as possible for each tradition of therapy what kind of personal attachment between therapist and patient is optimal, what tasks are essential for the patient and for the therapist, what are the critical incidents upon which effective therapy hinges, and how a therapist best responds to these incidents. To know what it takes to be "willing and able" to undertake a certain therapy will inform us also about who might be unwilling or unable to succeed in certain therapies; this, in turn, will lead to reductions in negative effects and in wasted effort where change is highly unlikely.

In our search for predictors, we seldom attend to the fact that of all the pretherapy and process variables that correlate reasonably well with outcome at termination, almost none are consistently associated with long-term gain as measured in followup studies one to five years after treatment. We know little about what is necessary or sufficient to maintain the benefits of therapy. This question moves from the realm of psychotherapy process into that of the mechanisms of change which, I think, are largely determined by the emotional, cognitive and interpersonal predispositions of the patient; they influence the ways in which the therapist and the therapeutic relationship are internalized. The therapeutic alliance, from this perspective, begins when the patient first decides to seek help; it takes place not just for 50-minute sessions, but continuously in the patient's mind as he or she experiences the presence of the therapist; and it fades gradually from active memory rather than abruptly terminating. To understand such a complex interpersonal and intrapersonal sequence, we need to use all our clinical and research resources as creatively as possible; to employ multidimensional, multiperspective designs, as well as intensively tracing single variables; to quantify what we can, while recognizing that much of the action of psychotherapy transcends quantification; and, therefore, to complement research findings with qualitative understanding based on broader knowledge of the humanities, arts and sciences.

REFERENCES

Allen JG, Newson GE, Gabbard GO, et al: Assessment of the therapeutic alliance from a psychoanalytic perspective. Bull Menninger Clin 48:5:383-400, 1984

Anchin JC, Kiesler DJ: Handbook of Interpersonal Psychotherapy. New York, Pergamon Press, 1982

Barrett-Lennard GT: Dimensions of therapist response as causal factors in therapeutic change. Psychol Monogr, 76, No 43, Whole No. 562, 1962

Benjamin LS: Structural analysis of social behavior. Psychol Rev 81:392-425, 1974

Benjamin LS: Use of markov chains to study dyadic interactions. J Abnorm Psychol 88:303-319, 1979

Benjamin LS: Use of structural analysis of social behavior (SASB) to guide interventions in psychotherapy, in New Perspectives in Interpersonal Psychotherapy. Edited by Anchin JC, Kiesler DJ. New York, Pergamon Press, 1982

Ben-Tovim DI, Greenup J: The representation of transference through serial guides: A methodological study. Br J Med Psychol 56:255-261, 1983

Bergin AE, Lambert M: The evaluation of therapeutic outcomes, in Handbook of Psychotherapy and Behavior Change. Edited by Garfield SL, Bergin AE. New York, Wiley, 1978

Bordin, ES: Strategies of Psychotherapy Research. New York, Wiley, 1974

Bordin ES: The generalizability of the concept of working alliance. Presented at the annual meeting of the Society for Psychotherapy Research, Boston, June, 1975

Bordin ES: The working alliance: basis for a general theory of psychotherapy. Presented at the annual meeting of the American Psychological Association, Washington DC, September, 1976

Breuer J, Freud S: Studies on hysteria, in The Standard Edition of the Complete Psychological Works of Sigmund Freud, vol 2, Edited and translated by Strachey J. London, Hogarth, 1895/1955

Cashdan S: Interactional Psychotherapy: Stages and Strategies in Behavioral Change. New York, Grune and Stratton, 1973

Crowder JE: Relationship between therapist and client interpersonal behaviors and psychotherapy outcome. Journal of Counseling Psychology 19:68-75, 1972

Dicks R: Technical considerations of the therapeutic and working alliances. Int J Psychoanal Psychother 4:1-24, 1975

Elliott R: Fitting process research to the practicing psychotherapist. Psychotherapy Theory, Research and Practice 20:47-55, 1983

Freud S: The dynamics of the transference, in Standard Edition of the Complete Works of Sigmund Freud, vol 12. Edited and translated by Strachey J. London, Hogarth, 1912/1958

Freud S: The technique of psychoanalysis, in Standard Edition of the Complete Works of Sigmund Freud, vol 23. Edited and translated by Strachey J. London, Hogarth, 1940/1964

Garfield SL: Psychotherapy: An Eclectic Approach. New York, Wiley, 1980

Goldfried MR: Toward the delineation of therapeutic change principles. Am Psychol 35:991-999, 1980

Gomes-Schwartz BA: Effective ingredients in psychotherapy: prediction of outcomes from process variables. J Consult Clin Psychol 46:1023-1035, 1978

Greenberg L, Rice LN: The specific effects of a gestalt intervention. Psychotherapy Theory, Research and Practice 18:31-37, 1981

Greenson RR: The Technique and Practice of Psychoanalysis. New York, International Universities Press, 1967

Hartley DE, Strupp HH: The therapeutic alliance: its relationship to outcome in brief psychotherapy, in Empirical Studies of Psychoanalytical Theories, vol 1. Edited by Masling J. Hillsdale, NJ, Erlbaum, 1983

Hill C: Therapist intentions in selecting intervention within psychotherapy sessions. Paper presented at Society for Psychotherapy Research, Sheffield, England, July 1983

Horowitz MJ: States of Mind: Analysis of Change in Psychotherapy. New York, Plenum, 1979

Horowitz MJ, Marmor C, Weiss DS, et al: Brief psychotherapy of bereavement reactions: the relationship of process to outcome. Arch Gen Psychiatry 41:438-448, 1984

Horvath AO, Greenberg L: The development of the working alliance inventory, in Psychotherapeutic Process: A Research Handbook. Edited by Greenberg L, Pinsoff W. New York, Guilford Press, in press

Hoyt, MF, Xenakis SN, Marmor CR, et al: Therapist's actions that influence their perceptions of "good" psychotherapy sessions. J Consult Clin Psychol 171: 400-404, 1983

Kiesler DJ: Some myths of psychotherapy research and the search for a paradigm. Psychol Bull 65:110-136, 1966

Kiesler DJ: The Process of Psychotherapy: Empirical Foundations and Systems of Analysis. Chicago, Aldine, 1973

Klein MH, Mathieu PL, Gendlin ER, et al: The Experiencing Scale: A Research and Training Manual. Madison, Wisconsin Psychiatric Institute, 1970

Kraemer HC: Coping strategies in psychiatric clinical research. J Consult Clin Psychol 49:309-319, 1981

Leary T: Interpersonal Diagnosis of Personality. New York, Ronald Press, 1957

Luborsky LL: Helping alliances in psychotherapy, in Successful Psychotherapy. Edited by Claghorn J. New York, Brunner/Mazel, 1976

Luborsky LL, Crits-Christoph P, Alexander L, et al: Two helping alliance methods for predicting outcomes of psychotherapy. J Nerv Ment Dis 171:480-491, 1983

Marmor CR, Marziali E, Horowitz MH, et al: The development of the therapeutic alliance rating system, in The Psychotherapeutic Process: A Research Handbook. Edited by Greenberg L, Pinsoff W. New York, Guilford Press, in press

Marziali E, Marmor C, Krupnuick J: Therapeutic alliance scales: development and relationship to psychotherapy outcome. Am J Psychiatry 138:361-364, 1981

Mintz J, Auerbach A, Luborsky L, et al: Patient's, therapist's and observer's views of psychotherapy: a "Rashomon" experience, or a reasonable consensus: Br J Med Psychol 46:83-89, 1973

Mintz J, Luborsky L, Auerbach AH: Dimensions of psychotherapy: a factor analytic study of ratings of psychotherapy sessions. J Consult Clin Psychol 36:106-120, 1971

Moras R, Strupp HH: Pretherapy interpersonal relations, patients' alliance, and outcome in brief therapy. Arch Gen Psychiatry 39:405-409, 1982

Morgan R, Luborsky L, Crits-Christoph P, et al: Predicting the outcomes of psychotherapy by the Penn helping alliance rating method. Arch Gen Psychiatry 39:397-402, 1982

Newton P: Social structure and process in psychotherapy: a sociopsychological analysis of transference, resistance and change. Int J Psychiatry 11:480-526, 1973

O'Malley SS, Suh CS, Strupp HH: The Vanderbilt psychotherapy process scale: a report on the scale development and process-outcome study. J Consult Clin Psychol 51:581-586, 1983

Orlinsky DE: Who's on first, what's on second, I don't know is on third: Reflections on the significance of observational perspective for the study of psychotherapeutic processes. Presented at NIMH Workshop on Psychotherapy Process Research, Bethesda, MD, September 22-23, 1983

Orlinsky D, Howard K: Varieties of Psychotherapy Experience. New York, Teachers College Press, 1975

Orlinsky D, Howard K: The relation of process to outcome in psychotherapy, in Handbook of Psychotherapy and Behavior Change. Edited by Garfield SL, Bergin AE. New York, Wiley, 1978

Parloff MB, Waskow IE, Wolfe BE: Research on therapist variables in relationship to process and outcome, in Handbook of Psychotherapy and Behavior Change. Edited by Garfield SL, Bergin AE. New York, Wiley, 1978

Rice LN: Therapists' style of participation and case outcome. J Consult Clin Psychol 29:155-160, 1965

Rice LN, Greenberg LS: Patterns of Change: Intensive Analysis of Psychotherapy Process. New York, Guilford Press, 1984

Rice LN, Wagstaff AK: Client voice quality and expressive style as indexes of productive psychotherapy. J Consult Clin Psychol 31:557-563, 1967

Rogers CR: The necessary and sufficient conditions of therapeutic personality change. J Consult Clin Psychol 21:95-103, 1957

Sachs JS: Negative factors in brief psychotherapy: an empirical assessment. J Consult Clin Psychol 51:557-564, 1983

Saltzman C, Luegart MS, Roth CH, et al: Formation of a therapeutic relationship: experiences during the initial phase of psychotherapy as predictors of treatment duration and outcome. J Consult Clin Psychol 44:546-555, 1976

Schaffer ND: Multidimensional measures of therapist behavior as predictors of outcome. Psychol Bull 92:670-681, 1982

Schaffer ND: Methodological issues of measuring the skillfullness of therapeutic techniques. Psychotherapy Theory, Research and Practice 20:486-493, 1983a

Schaffer ND: The utility of measuring the skillfullness of therapeutic techniques. Psychotherapy Theory, Research and Practice 20:330-336, 1983b

Smith ML, Glass GV: Meta-analysis of psychotherapy outcome studies. Am Psychol 132:752-760, 1977

Sterba R: The fate of the ego in analytic therapy. Int J Psychoanal 15:117-126, 1934

Stiles WB: Measurement of the impact of psychotherapy sessions. J Consult Clin Psychol 48:176-185, 1980

Strupp HH: Success and failure in time limited psychotherapy: a systematic comparison of two cases. Arch Gen Psychiatry 37:595-603, 1980a

Strupp HH: Success and failure in time limited psychotherapy: a systematic comparison of two cases (comparison 2). Arch Gen Psychiatry 37:708-716, 1980b

Strupp HH, Hadley SW, Gomes-Schwartz B: Psychotherapy for Better or Worse: The Problem of Negative Effects. New York, Jason Aronson, 1977

Truax CB, Carkhuff RR: Toward Effective Counseling and Psychotherapy. Chicago, Aldine, 1967

Vandenbos GR, Karon BP: Pathogenesis: a new therapist personality dimension related to therapeutic effectiveness. J Pers Assess 35:252-260, 1971

Wiggins JS, Steiger JH, Gaelick L: Evaluating circumplexity in personality data. Multivaried Behavior Research 16:263-289, 1981

Wilson GT, Evans IM: Adult behavior therapy and the therapist-client relationship, in Annual Review of Behavior Therapy, vol 2. Edited by Franks CM, Wilson GT, New York, Brunner/Mazel, 1976

Zetzel E: Current concepts of transference. Int J Psychoanal 37:369-376, 1956

Chapter 28

The Therapeutic Relationship in Psychodynamic Psychotherapy: The Research Evidence and Its Meaning for Practice

by Lester Luborsky, Ph.D. and Arthur H. Auerbach, M.D.

Two classes of factors are often considered when exploring the gains from psychodynamic psychotherapy (Luborsky, 1984). These are the relationship of the patient with the therapist, and the understanding achieved by the patient. The first is thought to be essential in order for the second to be meaningful. Clinical and research evidence has been assembled to support the influence of each on the outcome of psychotherapy (Luborsky et al, in press (b)). The clinical evidence is massive for each of these factors; however, there is more quantitative evidence to support the influence of the relationship factor than there is to support the influence of the understanding factor.

In the first half of this chapter, we will summarize the research evidence on the role of the therapeutic relationship as a predictor of outcome. The research based on psychodynamically oriented psychotherapy has been more completely summarized than it has been for other therapies. In the second half of the chapter, we will discuss the implications for clinical practice and further research.

What researchers have done is to extract certain elements from the totality of the therapeutic relationship, measured them and judged their importance by correlating them with outcome. When we say that a certain factor (such as the patient's problem-solving attitude) predicts outcome, we mean that this patient factor tends to be associated with a good outcome. However, a correlation may be greater than chance and still play only a small part in determining the outcome of therapy. Degree of improvement is the product of many factors. Naturally, we are interested in the magnitude of the correlation between any particular factor and outcome; that is, in how large a part that factor may play in producing outcome.

THE RESEARCH EVIDENCE ON THE ROLE OF THE RELATIONSHIP

Three categories of research studies will be reviewed: research focusing on patient factors, therapist factors and relationship factors. In these studies, judgments are based on the patient-therapist interaction in psychotherapy sessions. There are 20 to 30 studies representing each of the three categories.

Patient Factors as Judged From the Sessions

Three types of patient factors were examined in these studies: likeability, problem solving attitude and capacity for experiencing.

A clinician's judgment that a patient is likeable tends to be associated with a favorable psychotherapeutic outcome. Likeability was examined in four studies, and two of the four showed a significant prediction of outcome: Stoler (1963, 1966) and Strupp et al (1963) were significant, and Bowden et al (1972) and Gottschalk et al (1967) were not. The pretreatment judgment that a patient is likeable tends to be associated with the expectation that the patient is suitable for psychotherapy. In the course of psychotherapy, this expectation may actually provide favorable conditions for the patient's development, similar to those Rosenthal and Jacobson (1968) found for the performance of school children whose teachers had positive expectations of them.

A problem solving attitude implies that the patient shows during the sessions that he is trying to find ways of coping with his problems. Such an attitude appears to demonstrate that the patient is doing what a patient should do in psychodynamically oriented psychotherapy. It proved significantly predictive of a favorable outcome in all three studies of this quality (Fiske et al, 1964; Kirtner and Cartwright, 1958; and Gomes-Schwartz, 1978).

Patients who show more of the capacity for "experiencing" tend to have better outcomes of their psychotherapy than patients who show less of such capacity. This concept requires that the patient be capable of two behaviors in sequence: to be able to experience deeply and immediately; and to be able to be reflective about this experience (Rogers, 1959; Gendlin et al, 1968). Six out of seven studies using client-centered psychotherapy showed significant correlation between the patient's capacity for experiencing and his improvement (Gendlin et al, 1960; Gendlin et al, 1968; Kirtner et al, 1961; Tomlinson, 1967; Tomlinson and Hart, 1962; Walker et al, 1960). The one study using psychoanalytically oriented psychotherapy (Luborsky et al, 1980) was nonsignificant.

Therapist Factors as Judged From Treatment Sessions

Two main categories of therapist factors as judged from treatment sessions have been subjects of research studies: empathy and other "therapist facilitative conditions" (such as warmth and genuineness); and factors mostly related to therapist's technical competence.

Measures of empathy as judged from the sessions have been studied for many years, beginning with Rogerian client-centered research. Empathy was significant in five of the ten studies when rated from brief tape samples (Rogers et al, 1967; Truax, 1963; Truax et al, 1966, Kurtz and Grummon, 1972; Melnick and Pierce, 1971). These empathy measures were nonsignificant in studies by Bergin and Jasper (1969), Rogers et al (1967), Mintz et al (1971), and Mullen and Abeles (1971). Mitchell et al (1977) concluded that the evidence is still inadequate for observed ratings of empathy.

Empathy as rated by the patient and by the therapist tends to predict positive outcome somewhat better than ratings by an observer listening to sessions. Four out of six such studies were significant (Barrett-Lennard, 1962; Feitel, 1968; Lesser, 1961; and Kurtz and Grummon, 1972) and two were nonsignificant (Cartwright and Lerner, 1963; Lesser, 1961).

Until the last decade there had been relatively little evidence in support of the predictive value of any components of technique as judged from psychotherapy sessions, but now several studies confirm its importance. These technique variables achieved significant predictive success: avoidance of errors in therapist technique, using the Vanderbilt negative indicator scale (Sachs, 1983); the therapist's freshness of language (Rice, 1965); the therapist's rating of understanding the patient (Saltzman et al, 1976); the therapist using ways of facilitating the patient's helping alliance (Morgan et al, 1982); the therapist's "purity" of technique, in the sense of following the recommended techniques of the intended treatment and not using techniques from other forms of treatment (Luborsky et al, in press (a)); the therapist's use of transference interpretations (Marziali, 1984); the therapist's encouragement of the patient's independence (Lorr, 1965); and the therapist's behaving in a nonauthoritarian fashion (Lorr, 1965). The predictions in two studies were nonsignificant: the patient's ratings of the therapist's strength (Melnick and Pierce, 1971) and the therapist's use of reflective techniques and topical focus (Rounsaville et al, 1981). In summary, eight of the ten studies of aspects of therapist performance showed significant relationships to outcome.

It is noteworthy that two of the variables we have mentioned showed more recently a reduced predictive power more recently than they had when they were first tested. These were experiencing (under the patient factors) and empathy (under the therapist factors) (Mitchell et al, 1977). An obvious basis for the reduction is that these variables had predicted well within the client centered framework but not as well outside of it. There are also some other likely reasons. One is that the level of the facilitative conditions in the group as a whole should not be deficient. Another is that variation among therapists needs to be considerable in order to achieve a significant correlation. Third, these conditions may be necessary but not sufficient conditions; they may interact with other therapeutic conditions.

Relationship Qualities

Relationship qualities are even more strongly related to the benefits patients achieve than therapist factors and patient factors. Twelve qualities from almost as many studies were significantly related to the achievement of the patient's benefits in psychotherapy. These are listed here in order of the date of their appearance: positive evaluation of others (Rosenman, 1955); a positive relationship on the Barrett-Lennard Relationship Inventory (Barrett-Lennard, 1962); feeling understood by the therapist (Feitel, 1968); the therapist's positive regard and understanding as rated by the patient (Feitel, 1968); mutual understanding rated by the patient (Saltzman et al, 1976); favorable feelings toward the therapist (Saltzman et al, 1976); involvement in the therapy rated by a clinical observer (Gomes-Schwartz, 1978); and the patient's experience of the helping alliance with the therapist (Morgan et al, 1982; Luborsky et al, 1983; Luborsky et al, in press(a); Marziali et al, 1981; Hartley and Strupp, in press). This is an amazingly consistent predictive record and it extends Gurman's earlier one (1977). As we will discuss below, this must imply that positive relationship qualities, such as the patient's experience of the helping alliance, are crucially involved in the curative process in psychotherapy.

Nineteen studies have dealt with some form of similarity between the therapist and patient. Thirteen of these showed a positive correlation with the outcomes of the patient's treatments—greater similarity was associated with better outcomes.

The significant studies were: Graham, 1960; Hollingshead and Redlich, 1958; Landfield and Nawas, 1964; Lesser, 1961; Sapolsky, 1965; Schonfield et al, 1969; Sheehan, 1953; Tuma and Gustad, 1957; Welkowitz et al, 1967; Carr, 1970; Melnick, 1972; Dougherty, 1976; and Luborsky et al, 1980. These studies were based on a variety of similarities, including social class, interests, values, and compatibility of orientation to interpersonal relations. Of these, similarity of interests had especially strong evidence supporting it; it was significant in four out of four studies.

Our research has produced evidence of a substantial mediating link between certain basic similarities between patient and therapist and the development of a helping alliance. The term "helping alliance" refers to the degree to which the patient experiences the relationship with the therapist as helpful or potentially helpful in achieving the patient's goals in psychotherapy. We found (Luborsky et al, 1983) that basic background similarities between patient and therapist, such as age and religious activity, were highly correlated with the helping alliance measure (for example, the sum of ten similarities correlated .60 ($p<.01$) with early positive helping alliance counting signs): for example, "Our work together has made me feel less depressed than when I started." The helping alliance measure is one in which a judge goes through the samples of the transcripts and counts literal or almost literal helping alliance signs. The correlation of patient–therapist similarities with the helping alliance implies that these similarities create an environment in which the helping alliance can develop. The presence of these similarities probably heightens the sense, in both participants, that they have something in common in terms of shared membership in groups and shared interests and values. This creates an alliance that helps the patient to achieve therapeutic goals. Evidence in support of these causal inferences is provided by the fact that the similarities were known to be present before the treatment from results of a questionnaire (Luborsky et al, in press (a)).

IMPLICATIONS FOR PRACTICE AND NEW RESEARCH DIRECTIONS

We have reviewed three types of psychotherapy research dealing primarily with judgments of psychotherapy sessions. These have focused on the patient, the therapist and the relationship, respectively. We are now ready to consider what these observations imply about practice and new research directions.

The Development and Management of the Therapeutic Relationship

IMPORTANCE OF THE RELATIONSHIP. The development and management of the therapeutic relationship is of primary importance. This view derives from new, consistent evidence of the predictive power of the therapeutic relationship on the outcome of psychotherapy. Certainly this idea will not surprise clinicians. However, the research provides a verified account of the *specific* ways in which the treatment relationship is predictive.

To illustrate the implications of this research we will draw from the findings of the 12 studies of the therapeutic relationship and especially from the largest subcategory of them, the helping alliance.

The research has distinguished two types of patients' expressions of the experience of the helping alliance, (Luborsky et al, 1983). In type one, the therapist is seen as providing help to the patient and the patient as receiving it. In type two, the patient and therapist are seen as working together, in a team effort, to help the patient. These two types of helping alliance tend to be highly correlated. Type one tends to occur earlier in the treatment than does type two. Evidences of both types are commonly found in the early sessions, even as early as the first session. One patient, for example, decided at the end of the first session that things would go well in the treatment.

Therapist: "How did you decide?"

Patient: "You remind me of my boyfriend, and I see from the fact that your shoes aren't shined that you're not vain, so I will get on with you well."

In this way, this patient (who ultimately improved) revealed one basis for the rapid development of a positive relationship.

It has also been found that the positive versus negative signs of the helping alliance have different predictive capacities. The early positive signs have considerable consistency from early to late in psychotherapy and are substantial predictors of the outcomes of psychotherapy (Luborsky et al, 1983). On the other hand, the early negative signs of the helping alliance are not negative predictors of outcome; they are unrelated to outcome. The clinical lore that these positive signs are "honeymoon phenomena" and should be discounted as unreliable predictors is not supported by this evidence. Our findings suggest that the positive and negative are much more consistent with the observation about love relationships, that "yes" means "yes" and "no" means "maybe." Furthermore, it could be valuable to examine those patients who, early in therapy, were negative; then to trace the conditions that became influential in either changing or not changing the helping alliance. Changes will often stem from the employment of the usual techniques of psychodynamic psychotherapy: for example, the therapist's degree of focus on the signs of a negative relationship. Presumably, in those instances in which the relationship begins negatively but a positive outcome results, the therapist has resolved the negative relationship.

There is some evidence to support the inference that therapist activity is partly responsible for establishing the helping alliance; we have found a high correlation between therapist facilitating conditions and the helping alliance (Luborsky et al, 1983).

Another powerful basis for the patient's experience of the helping alliance must come from the patient's experience of a good match between patient and therapist. As we have already noted, we base this inference on the high correlations between similarities in age, occupation, marital status and other characteristics with the helping alliance. Not only are these similarities highly correlated with the helping alliance measures, but they are significantly correlated with psychotherapy outcomes (Luborsky et al, 1980; Luborsky et al, in press (b)). Such similarities, even though they are probably not completely known to the patient and therapist, apparently make a sizeable contribution to the development of a positive relationship. According to social psychological studies (French and Raven, 1959; Tedeschi and Lindskold, 1976) similarities in values induce a trusting, favorable feeling in the patient.

The findings about good matches should have clinical applications, particularly in assigning patients to therapists on the basis of such similarities. However, some cautions are necessary about the carrying out of this recommendation. There is no evidence that all similarities are predictive—only those for which research evidence is available. Second, the application of these similarities in matching patients and therapists should have considerable effect on facilitating the development of a helping alliance; however, the effects on the outcomes of treatment would not be expected to be large, since the correlation of similarities with the outcome measures are not large (in the Penn Psychotherapy study they are around .2 to .3, which is approximately the level in other studies).

In further research, other similarities should be explored. In addition, with only one exception (McLellan et al, 1983), the existing studies did not involve samples in which similarities were used as a basis for matching. Instead, similarities that happened to be already present between patient and therapist were examined. Therefore, studies should be done to use similarities as a basis for matching. The one exceptional study in which matching was deliberate (McLellan et al, 1983) found significant advantages when compared with the results that nonmatching might have produced.

IMPORTANCE OF PATIENT AND THERAPIST. Assessments of psychotherapy show two other classes of factors to be predictive of success in psychotherapy: patient factors and therapist factors; although these are less predictive than are relationship factors. The most predictive patient factors were likeableness, problem-solving attitude and capacity for experiencing. The last of these, however, has not continued to be predictive outside of the client-centered approach. Among therapist factors, the two most predictive were empathy and technical performance and competence. The second of these shows even more promise than the first in both clinical and research implications.

TRAINING FOR RELATING. Training therapists to establish therapeutic relationships may significantly improve the therapist's effectiveness. The clinical and research evidence points to the therapeutic relationship as the main facilitator of the benefits of psychotherapy. The evidence also indicates that the therapist's facilitative behaviors are highly correlated with the development of the helping alliance. These two findings suggest that it would be valuable to know the extent to which therapists can be trained to establish, to formulate and to respond to the therapeutic relationship, and then to discover how much difference such training makes for therapists' success with their patients.

Clinicians differ in their views about the difficulty of establishing a therapeutic relationship. According to some clinicians, if one follows certain undemanding principles, the therapeutic relationship may be relatively easy to establish—it may be merely a matter of letting the relationship develop. Freud (1913) had this view when he recommended that the therapist should do nothing to interfere with the natural inclination of the patient to become attached: "It remains the first aim of the treatment to attach (the patient) to it and to the person of the doctor . . . if one exhibits a serious interest in him . . . and avoids making certain mistakes, he will of himself form such an attachment . . . it is certainly possible to forfeit this first success if from the start one takes any standpoint other than that of sympathetic understanding" (page 139-140).

There are no studies of this training principle; nor are there studies of the effectiveness of any training methods in establishing therapeutic relationships, although every training program assumes that training is beneficial. The fact that experienced therapists establish better relationships with their patients than inexperienced therapists (Auerbach and Johnson, 1977) is consistent. Research on the benefits of training would probably confirm that training is better than no training; it would probably reveal the specific ways the training is helpful; and it might well point to ways to increase that helpfulness.

Several types of studies are needed. Studies to evaluate the capacities of the therapist for establishing therapeutic relationships at the beginning of the therapist's training are needed. The capacity to form good therapeutic relationships may be a talent that is present before specific training is provided. Supervisors of psychotherapists in training often notice that therapists differ widely in their capacities at the very beginning of training.

Studies of variations in therapist's effectiveness with patients are needed. There are more than 600 studies of the comparative effectiveness of different forms of psychotherapy; however, in comparison with control groups (Smith et al, 1980; Luborsky et al, 1975), there are hardly any studies showing differences in effectiveness among different therapists. The first systematic study of this (Luborsky et al, in press (a)) revealed tremendous differences among therapists in effectiveness as measured by their patient's benefits. The most prominent basis for these differences appeared to be the capacity of the therapist to form a helping relationship (as measured by the Helping Alliance Questionnaire, Alexander and Luborsky, in press).

Much more research needs to be done on the basis for the difference in therapists' success and the source of their power to influence. Such studies should take up the leads provided by the social psychological research (French and Ravin, 1959; Tedeschi and Lindskold, 1976). These studies suggest that the patient estimates the therapist's trustworthiness, confidence and attractiveness to the degree that he or she shares similar values with the patient. A source of the therapist's influence has been found to be transmitted through the impact of the therapist's behavior on the patient's self-esteem (Janis, 1982, 1983).

More studies of the benefits of different methods of training are needed: such studies as those by Rogers (1957), Ekstein and Wallerstein (1958), and Luborsky (1984). Some research from the client-centered school has indicated that client-centered training produces an increase from low to moderate levels of empathy, warmth and genuineness. Training has a greater effect on the therapist's level of empathy than on warmth and genuineness. This may be because the client-centered school has an easily specified definition of empathy.

The use of psychotherapy manuals should be investigated for their contribution to training. For comparative studies of psychotherapies, reliance on manuals has become virtually mandatory in the past decade, constituting a small revolution in research practice (Luborsky and DeRubeis, 1984). Several advantages derive from the use of manuals in the training of psychotherapists (Luborsky 1976, 1984). First, the rate of learning is improved because of the manual's organized presentation of principles and techniques accompanied by examples;

and, second, the degree to which the therapist conforms to the chosen form of psychotherapy can be determined by independent judgments by other clinicians. The last advantage matters because there is evidence that therapists who conform most closely to their intended techniques achieve more benefits for their patients than do therapists who deviate from these techniques. This is the implication of the correlation between the "purity" of technique and benefits achieved for patients (Luborsky et al, in press (a)).

RELATING VS. UNDERSTANDING.   The achievement of a good therapeutic relationship appears to be more basic than the achievement of increased understanding. The relative weighting of these two curative factors should not be a surprise. It has been known for centuries that a helping relationship can be therapeutic, and that its loss can have unhealthy consequences both psychically and somatically (Schmale, 1958).

Of course, a good therapeutic relationship and the achievement of increased understanding ordinarily work together as curative factors; they have been isolated here only for purposes of comparison. The most common agenda of both the patient and the therapist in psychodynamic psychotherapies is the achievement of such understanding, because it is considered to be the main vehicle to resolution of symptoms once a therapeutic relationship has been established. In fact, when the patient and therapist achieve increased understanding of the symptoms and the related relationship problems, the therapeutic relationship is also strengthened (as discussed in Luborsky, 1984).

While the importance of the therapeutic relationship in helping the patient achieve the goals of the treatment is supported by much research evidence, the importance of increased understanding is not so supported. An example taken from the Penn Psychotherapy Project (Luborsky et al, 1980) illustrates that there are some treatments in which the patient achieves significant benefits without much change in understanding. For example, an intelligent woman formed a strong helping alliance with an experienced analyst. Despite the fact that the patient did achieve her goals for the relief of severe symptoms, she did not achieve much by way of understanding of her basic relationship problems. This example is extreme because, for most patients, the two factors work together in accordance with the principles of the theory of the therapy.

Psychotherapy research has so far slighted the assessment of the benefits of greater understanding. Practitioners, researchers and, ultimately, patients might all benefit from studies providing increased insight into the relevance of reality-based and transference-based core relationship problems as a predictor of the outcomes of psychotherapy (Luborsky, 1984). Such research is now within the capacity of the available technology.

SUMMARY

Eighty-five studies of psychotherapy sessions have been summarized in terms of three factors: the patient, the therapist and the relationship between them.
1. About 70 percent of these studies show significant prediction of treatment outcomes.
2. Relationship factors are more highly predictive than patient or therapist factors.

3. Within the relationship factors, most often predictive are measures of the helping alliance and the match of the patient with the therapist.

4. The results apply both to psychodynamically oriented psychotherapy and to closely related forms of psychotherapy.

5. When the entire group of 85 studies is divided into short-term and longer-term psychotherapies, two major differences appear: Patient factors are likely to be more often significantly predictive in studies of short-term therapy, while the therapist and relationship factors are more often predictive in studies of longer therapies.

6. Research is needed on the benefits of various methods of training (such as through treatment manuals) in establishing and dealing with the relationship of patient and therapist.

7. Of the two main curative factors—the relationship established between patient and therapist and the understanding gained—this brief review has focused on the results of the relationship because most of the research has concentrated on this factor. Future research should remedy the imbalance.

REFERENCES

Alexander L, Luborsky L: Research on the helping alliance, in Psychotherapeutic Process: A Research Handbook. Edited by Greenberg L, Pinsoff W. New York, Guilford Press, in press

Auerbach A, Johnson M: Research on the therapist's level of experience, in Effective Psychotherapy. Edited by Gurman A, Razin A. Oxford, Pergamon Press, 1977

Barrett-Lennard GT: Dimensions of therapist response as causal factors in therapeutic change. Psychological Monographs 76:43 (Whole No. 562), 1962

Bergin AE, Jasper LG: Correlates of empathy in psychotherapy: a replication. J Abnorm Psychol 74:477-481, 1969

Bowden C, Endicott J, Spitzer R: A–B therapist variables and psychotherapeutic outcome. J Nerv Ment Dis 154:276-286, 1972

Carr J: Differentiation similarity of patient and therapist and the outcome of psychotherapy. J Abnorm Psychol 76:361-369, 1970

Dougherty F: Patient-therapist matching for prediction of optimal and minimal therapeutic outcome. J Consult Clin Psychol 44:889-897, 1976

Ekstein R, Wallerstein R: The Teaching and Learning of Psychotherapy. New York, Basic Books, 1958

Feitel B: Feeling understood as a function of a variety of therapist activity. Unpublished doctoral dissertation, Teachers' College, Columbia University, 1968

Fiske DW, Cartwright DS, Kirtner WL: Are psychotherapeutic changes predictable? Journal of Abnormal and Social Psychology 69:418-426, 1964

French JRP, Raven B: The bases of social power, in Studies in Social Power. Edited by Cartwright D. Ann Arbor, University of Michigan, 1959

Freud S (1913): On beginning the treatment, in Standard Edition. Edited by Strachey J. London: Hogarth Press, 1958, pp. 123-144

Gendlin ET, Jenney R, Shlien J: Counselor ratings of process and outcome in client-centered therapy. J Clin Psychol 16:210-213, 1960

Gendlin ET, Beebe J, Cassens J, et al: Focusing ability in psychotherapy, personality, and creativity, in Research in Psychotherapy, vol. 3. Edited by Shlien JM, Hunt HF, Matarazzo JD, et al. Washington DC, American Psychological Association, 1968

Gomes-Schwartz B: Effective ingredients in psychotherapy: predictions of outcome from process variables. J Consult Clin Psychol 46:123-135, 1978

Gottschalk LA, Mayerson P, Gottlieb AA: Prediction and evaluation of outcome in an emergency brief psychotherapy clinic. J Nerv Ment Dis 144:77-96, 1967

Graham SR: The influence of therapist character structure upon Rorschach changes in the course of psychotherapy. Am Psychologist 15:415, 1960

Gurman AS: The patient's perception of the therapeutic relationship, in Effective Psychotherapy. Edited by Gurman A, Razin A. Oxford, Pergamon Press, 1977

Hartley D, Strupp H: The therapeutic alliance: its relationship to outcome in brief psychotherapy, in Empirical Studies of Psychoanalytic Theories, vol. 2. Edited by Masling J. Hillsdale, NJ, Laurence Erlbaum Associates Inc., in press

Hollingshead AB, Redlich FC: Social Class and Mental Illness. New York, Wiley, 1958

Janis IL: Counseling on Personal Decisions: Theory and Research on Short Term Helping Relationships. New Haven CT, Yale University Press, 1982

Janis IL: The role of social support in adherence to stressful decisions. Am Psychologist 38:143-160, 1983

Kirtner WL, Cartwright DS: Success and failure in client-centered therapy as a function of initial in-therapy behavior. Journal of Consulting Psychology 22:329-333, 1958

Kirtner WL, Cartwright DS, Robertson RJ, et al: Length of therapy in relation to outcome and change in personal integration. Journal of Consulting Psychology 25:84-88, 1961

Kurtz R, Grummon D: Different approaches to the measurement of therapist empathy and their relationship to therapy outcomes. J Consult Clin Psychol 39:106-115, 1972

Landfield AW, Nawas MM: Psychotherapeutic improvement as a function of communication and adoption of therapist's values. Journal of Counseling and Psychology 11:336-341, 1964

Lesser WM: The relationship between counseling progress and empathic understanding. Journal of Counseling and Psychology 8:330-336, 1961

Lorr M: Client perceptions of therapists: a study of therapeutic relations. Journal of Consulting Psychology 29:146-149, 1965

Luborsky L: A Treatment Manual for Supportive-Expressive (SE) Psychoanalytically Oriented Psychotherapy. Lester Luborsky, 1976

Luborsky L: Principles of Psychoanalytic Psychotherapy—A Manual for Supportive-Expressive (SE) Methods. New York, Basic Books, 1984

Luborsky L, DeRubeis R. The use of psychotherapy treatment manuals: a small revolution in psychotherapy research style. Clinical Psychology Review, 4:1984

Luborsky L, Singer B, Luborsky Lise: Comparative studies of psychotherapies: is it true that "everybody has won and all must have prizes"? Arch Gen Psychiatry 32:995-1008, 1975

Luborsky L, Mintz J, Auerbach A, et al: Predicting the outcomes of psychotherapy—findings of the Penn psychotherapy project. Arch Gen Psychiatry 37:471-481, 1980

Luborsky L, Crits-Christoph P, Alexander L, et al: Two helping alliance methods for predicting outcomes of psychotherapy: a counting signs vs. a global rating method. J Nerv Ment Dis 171:480-492, 1983

Luborsky L, McLellan AT, Woody G, et al: Therapists' success and its determinants. Arch Gen Psychiatry, in press(a)

Luborsky L, Mintz J, Auerbach A, et al: Psychotherapy: Who Will Benefit and How? Factors Influencing the Outcomes of Psychotherapy. McGraw-Hill Book Co, in press (b)

Marziali E: Prediction of outcome of brief psychotherapy from therapist interpretative interventions. Arch Gen Psychiatry 41:301-304, 1984

Marziali E, Marmar C, Krupnick J: Therapeutic alliance scales: development and relationship to psychotherapy outcome. Am J Psychiatry 138:361-364, 1981

McLellan AT, Woody G, Luborsky L, et al: Increased effectiveness of substance abuse treatment: a prospective study of patient treatment "matching." J Nerv Ment Disease, 171:397-603, 1983

Melnick B: Patient-therapist identification in relation to both patient and therapist variables and therapy outcome. J Consult Clin Psychol 38:97-104, 1972

Melnick B, Pierce R: Client evaluation of therapist's strength and positive-negative evaluation as related to client dynamics, objective ratings of competence and outcome. J Clin Psychol 27:408-410, 1971

Mintz J, Luborsky L, Auerbach AH: Dimensions of psychotherapy: a factor-analytic study of ratings of psychotherapy sessions. J Consult Clin Psychol 36:106-120, 1971

Mitchell KM, Bogarth JD, Krauft CC: A re-appraisal of the therapeutic effectiveness of accurate empathy, nonpossessive warmth and genuineness, in Effective Psychotherapy. Edited by Gurman A, Razin A. Oxford, Pergamon Press, 1977

Morgan R, Luborsky L, Crits-Christoph P, et al: Predicting the outcomes of psychotherapy by the Penn Helping Alliance Rating Method. Arch Gen Psychiatry 39:397-402, 1982

Mullen J, Abeles N: Relationship of liking, empathy and therapist's experience to outcomes of psychotherapy. Journal of Consulting Psychology 38:97-104, 1971

Rice LN: Therapist's style of participation and case outcome. Journal of Consulting Psychology 29:155-160, 1965

Rogers C: Training individuals to engage in the therapeutic process, in Psychology and Mental Health. Edited by Strother CR. Washington DC, American Psychological Association, 1957

Rogers CR: A tentative scale for measurement of process in psychotherapy, in Research in Psychotherapy, vol. 1. Edited by Rubinstein EA, Parloff MB. Washington DC, American Psychological Association, 1959

Rogers CR, Gendlin E, Kiesler D, et al: The Therapeutic Relationship and Its Impact: A Study of Psychotherapy with Schizophrenics. Madison, University of Wisconsin Press, 1967

Rosenman S: Changes in the representation of self, other and interrelationship in client-centered therapy. Journal of Counseling and Psychology 2:271-278, 1955

Rosenthal RI, Jacobson L: Pygmalion in the Classroom. New York, Holt, Rinehart & Winston, 1968

Rounsaville B, Weissman M, Prusoff B: Psychotherapy with depressed outpatients: patient and process variables as predictors of outcome. Br J Psychiatry 138:67-74, 1981

Sachs J: Negative factors in brief psychotherapy: an empirical assessment. J Consult Clin Psychol 51:557-564, 1983

Saltzman C, Luetgert M, Roth C, et al: Formation of a therapeutic relationship: experiences during the initial phase of psychotherapy as predictors of treatment duration and outcome. J Consult Clin Psychol 44:546-555, 1976

Sapolsky A: Relationship between patient-doctor compatibility, mutual perception, and outcome of treatment. J Abnorm Psychol 70:70-76, 1965

Schmale A: Relationship of separation and depression to disease. Psychosom Med 20:259-277, 1958

Schonfield J, Stone A, Hoehn-Saric R, et al: Patient-therapist convergence and measures of improvement in short-term psychotherapy. Psychotherapy: Theory, Research, and Practice 6:267-271, 1969

Sheehan JG: Rorschach changes during psychotherapy in relation to the personality of the therapist. Am Psychologist 8:434, 1953 (Abstract)

Smith M, Glass G, Miller T: The Benefits of Psychotherapy. Baltimore, Johns Hopkins Press, 1980

Stoler N: Client likeability: a variable in the study of psychotherapy. Journal of Consulting Psychology 27:175-178, 1963

Stoler N: The relationship of patient-likeability and the A–B psychiatric resident types. (Doctoral dissertation, University of Michigan) Ann Arbor, Michigan, University Microfilms, 1966

Strupp HH, Wallach MS, Jenkins JW, et al: Psychotherapists' assessments of former patients. J Nerv Ment Dis 137:222-230, 1963

Tedeschi JT, Lindskold S: Social Psychology. New York, Wiley, 1976

Tomlinson TM: The therapeutic process as related to outcome, in The Therapeutic Relationship and Its Impact. Edited by Rogers CR. Madison, University of Wisconsin Press, 1967

Tomlinson TM, Hart JT: A validation of the process scale. Journal of Consulting Psychology 26:74-78, 1962

Truax CB: Effective ingredients in psychotherapy: an approach to unraveling the patient-therapist interaction. Journal of Consulting Psychology 10:256-263, 1963

Truax C, Wargo D, Frank J, et al: Therapist empathy, genuineness and warmth and patient outcome. Journal of Consulting Psychology 30:395-401, 1966

Tuma AH, Gustad, JW: The effects of client and counselor personality characteristics on client learning in counseling. Journal of Counseling Psychology 4:136-141, 1957

Walker A, Rablen RA, Rogers CR: Development of a scale to measure process change in psychotherapy. J Clin Psychol 16:79-85, 1960

Welkowitz J, Cohen J, Ortmeyer D: Value system similarity: investigation of patient-therapist dyads. Journal of Consulting Psychology 31:48-55, 1967

Chapter 29

The Therapeutic Alliance in Short-Term Directive Therapies

by A. John Rush, M.D.

The therapeutic alliance refers to the working relationship between therapist and patient that facilitates the application of therapeutic techniques and constructive changes in behavioral, emotional and cognitive patterns. This alliance is based on the nonneurotic, rational rapport that the patient has with the therapist and includes an identification with the sympathetic, empathic understanding part of the therapist. Various psychodynamic thinkers such as Melanie Klein and Otto Kernberg have identified a number of defenses against trust and the formation of this alliance. These defenses include denial, derogation, control, triumph, reading negatives into what the therapist does, and bursts into activity. Denial refers to the patient's recognition of a fact while he maintains the position that the fact has "no meaning." Derogation refers to the patient's tendency to belittle the therapist and/or the therapy process. Triumph refers to the patient's belief that he/she does not need or want the therapist. The tendency of depressed patients to view neutral statements by the therapist or interactions with the therapist as attacks or accusations is referred to as reading negatives into the situation (Rush, 1980).

Short-term therapies, in particular, demand careful and skillful management of this alliance because these therapies create a demand for therapeutic change that is far more pressured than time-unlimited or nondirective approaches. That is, both the predefined time limit (usually ten to 20 weeks) and the therapist's role as a guide and prescriber of techniques creates a focus on immediate issues and on change to be accomplished in short order. Many patients may be uncomfortable with such pressure and may respond by dropping out or failing to comply with therapist directives or suggestions. Others may even experience symptom exacerbation.

On the other hand, depending upon the therapist, a time-limited, more concrete directive approach may actually increase optimism and compliance, and facilitate more rapid change than nondirective, time-unlimited approaches. It would appear that certain patients will quickly form meaningful stable therapeutic alliances in short-term directive therapies, while others will balk at this essential first step. In the former cases, the particular techniques can be easily applied and therapy will proceed apace. In the latter cases, however, the therapist is required to focus on the development of the alliance itself, employing available techniques to develop, shape and establish the alliance. Only later can the therapist employ those techniques aimed at guiding the patient into behavioral, emotional and cognitive changes in interpersonal relationships other than that of the therapist-patient dyad. Alternatively, the time limit itself may have to be modified or renegotiated on a prescheduled basis. Several short-term therapists have suggested that sharp time limits with directive techniques are not indicated (unless modified) for particular patients (for example, those with borderline or schizotypal personality disorders) who have notable difficulty in forming therapeutic alliances or other collaborative interpersonal relationships (Rush, 1983; Beck et al, 1979).

The first section of this chapter provides guidelines for identifying those patients who will have difficulty forming a therapeutic alliance. Next, patient and therapist variables that may obstruct the formation of such alliances are discussed. Particular disorders or symptom patterns may require modification of the usual short-term directive approaches. Case examples are provided to illustrate some of these points in greater detail.

The ideas and guidelines contained in this chapter are developed largely from clinical experience. That is, little research data are available to test these notions at present. Further, they are derived from clinical work with behavioral, cognitive and structured family therapy approaches. While these notions may apply to other short-term directive therapies, data are lacking to support the generalizability of these observations to other forms of short-term treatment. It is hoped that the notions contained in this chapter will provide some guidelines for the practitioner as well as hypotheses that can be empirically tested by psychotherapy researchers.

THE CAPACITY TO FORM A THERAPEUTIC ALLIANCE

Most practitioners of short-term therapies provide specific guidelines for patient selection, among which is the ability to rapidly form a therapeutic alliance. Psychodynamic (Zaiden, 1982) as well as cognitive (Beck et al, 1979), interpersonal (Rounsaville and Chevron, 1982) and behavioral (Lewinsohn et al, 1982) approaches all provide some specification as to inclusion or exclusion criteria for patients to be treated.

How might the clinician rapidly assess a particular patient's capacity to form a therapeutic alliance? For the purposes of discussion, evidence that bears on this question can be divided into that obtained from the clinical interview, as well as that derived from the patient's past history. When the therapy involves the use of homework assignments, the therapist will often begin by suggesting a relatively simple homework task. The patient's response to this task is often a useful clue as to whether meaningful collaboration will shortly ensue.

To illustrate: In cognitive therapy, the first task asked of the patient is to read a five-page pamphlet, *Coping with Depression* (Beck and Greenberg, 1976) following the initial descriptive and medical diagnostic interviews. The first therapy session begins with a review of this task. Patients' responses to it vary from a meaningful, "Yes, I can see how my negative thinking can make my situations worse," to a hostile, "I don't think this approach has anything to do with me. Furthermore, I lost the pamphlet." Other responses might include, "I read the pamphlet, and I got more depressed," or, "I was too depressed to do it." The first response calls for a further probing of just what the patient learned from the pamphlet; was it as helpful as initially stated, or is the patient simply acting in a compliant manner? The second hostile comment suggests that the patient was somehow personally affronted at being asked to read the pamphlet and that he or she is angry at something or someone (probably the therapist). Here, a gentle exploration of the anger and cognitions associated with it is indicated. If the patient responds by escalating the denigration of the therapist or therapy, one might have encountered a defense against trust and forming an alliance. If so, then the patient may not be as suitable for a time-limited approach. In this case, the fears, fantasies and cognitions about the therapist and therapy must become the initial targets for treatment (see Case 1, p. 568).

The patient who felt more depressed while doing the task appears willing to participate in the therapy but is expressing, perhaps, a fear of symptom exacerbation. This patient would be further questioned about the particulars in the pamphlet that led to greater sadness. What cognitions occurred as he read the material? Was the description too confusing, leading to the notion that, "I can't even do this simple task. Therefore, I'll never get better," or was it that the patient realized that negative thinking had been present for years and had interfered with job and family to a much greater degree than initially thought? Again, this would appear to be a patient who tries to perform the task and is able to directly express the pain and frustration that ensues. A therapeutic alliance is likely to develop.

The patient who was too depressed to read the pamphlet is thinking globally and perhaps too pessimistically to initiate new behaviors. This patient may respond to the therapist's further exploration of this cognition and attempts to specify the details of how the depression stopped the patient. On the other hand, the patient may be attempting to establish a passive role, thereby placing all of the responsibility on the therapist to magically cure the problem without the patient's participation. Is this an attempt to avoid establishing a therapeutic alliance, so that if therapy fails, the patient can blame the therapist or therapy, while avoiding further injury to his already negative view of himself? Again, further discussion about the details of this apparent noncompliance will determine whether it can be easily dispelled, or whether it is the tip of the iceberg that points toward diffculties in forming a collaborative relationship with the therapist.

This brings us to the second interview-based observation, which portends the degree of ease or difficulty in forming a therapeutic alliance—that is, how easy is it to discuss and detail the reasons for noncompliance and convert the patient into a more willing collaborator? Can the patient report the negative expectations and fears associated with compliance? Does the patient take personally and respond negatively to such a discussion, or is he able to view the dialogue with some objectivity, to hear it as the therapist's attempt to help him review, observe and respond to his initial negative cognitions? Patients who are severely ill or psychotic do not easily establish the alliance and are more likely to respond negatively to such probing discussions. That is, such patients have more difficulty in objectively evaluating the therapist-patient dialogue. The patient who is more likely to negatively personalize such discussions is even less able to form an alliance. As one patient recently commented, "I came here with an emotional problem, and now you're telling me I have a thinking disorder too!" This patient felt personally attacked even by a very gentle discussion of her moment-to-moment thinking pattern in the first interview; she thought that the therapist was attacking her personally by such discussions. This behavior should alert the potential short-term therapist that particular attention must be paid to the alliance.

Finally, as short-term therapies adhere to a time limit, the willingness of the patient to participate in agenda setting and the allocation of available time is often another clue to whether a therapeutic alliance can be easily formed. If the patient insists repeatedly over several interviews that there is not enough time for all of his problems, or if he repeatedly strays from the agenda and is offended at being drawn back to it by the therapist—perhaps commenting, "You don't care about me. You're preoccupied with time"—then the formation of the alliance should take precedence over methods aimed more directly at the ultimate objectives of therapy (for example, cognitive change, interpersonal problem solving, and so forth).

In addition to interview behaviors, patients' past histories often provide clues to the potential difficulty or ease in forming an alliance. Does the patient have a history of relatively constant parenting figure(s)? Did he have a "best friend" with whom mutual intimate exchanges occurred and that lasted for several years during latency or adolescence? Is there a history of relative consistency in employment, heterosexual relationships, or in child rearing? All of these data give clues to the patient's capacity to form longer lasting relationships and indirectly have implications for the formation of a therapeutic alliance.

A second relevant historical variable is the lack of history of impulsiveness. Does the patient, when confronted with interpersonal difficulties, leave the relationship? Does he make efforts to solve such difficulties, or are the feelings of rejection, anger, loneliness and the like immediately converted into impulsive behaviors?

Third, patients who suffer from severe personality disorders that are likely to interfere with the rapid formation of the therapeutic relationship are poor candidates for time-limited, directive approaches. These disorders would include borderline, antisocial, schizotypal and, perhaps, others. In such cases, a revision of the time limit may be needed to allow sufficient time for the formation of the alliance, before the particular symptoms or behavioral patterns are addressed. Alternatively, the main objective of treatment might shift to the treatment of the personality difficulties while treating the Axis I disorder with medication, depending upon the diagnosis.

DIFFICULTIES IN FORMING THE THERAPEUTIC ALLIANCE

There are three major groups of contributors to the formation of the alliance: those due to the patient, those due to the therapist and those due to the disorder. As such contributors are manifold, I will briefly illustrate each of these three groups by examples, rather than attempt an encyclopedic enumeration. For the practitioner of short-term directive therapies, it is important to keep in mind that any one of these groups (the patient, the therapist, or the disorder) can, at any particular moment, present obstacles. When such obstacles are encountered, they must be identified and differentially dealt with.

Let us first turn to patient contributants. Consider the depressed patient who is in cognitive therapy. One important variable is the patient's cognitive set. It is well known that such patients see themselves, their immediate future and those with whom they interact (including the therapist) in negative ways. One patient, who was particularly sensitive to the therapist's behavior, appeared upset when I arrived ten minutes late to our session. When queried, the patient reported to be thinking, "He isn't interested in me. I must be the worst patient he has." For the next session I purposely arrived and began early. This time the patient reported her thinking as, "I must be sicker than all the other patients; that's why he's spending extra time." At the following session I was punctual to the moment. This time she reportedly thought, "He's just running a factory here. He's not taking a personal interest in me." While these negative interpretations may be exacerbated by the presence of major depression, many patients will have a lifelong tendency to closely scrutinize and erroneously disparage the therapeutic relationship. In such instances, greater focus on these tendencies is required before and during the assignment of directive homework tasks. For such a patient, homework is likely to be viewed as a harsh demand without purpose and is likely to contribute to disruption of the alliance.

This brings us to a second patient variable—the response to homework assignments or directives in the interview. In order to ameliorate the potentially disruptive effects of such tasks, it is imperative that these tasks follow logically from the therapist-patient dialogue and that the rationale or basis for such requests be clearly stated at the onset. Furthermore, the patient's participation in the creation of such tasks is essential, not only to improve the likelihood of compliance, but also to ensure that the alliance is either strengthened or at least not weakened when such a request is made. Finally, once the patient attempts such tasks, the therapist should ask the patient, not simply about what he did or did not do, but about his feelings, thoughts and attitudes about the undertaking. This review should be conducted at the beginning of each session, in order to decipher the patient's feelings about the previous session, and at the end of each session in order to review the transactions between patient and therapist in that particular session. Patients shold be encouraged to share especially those feelings of frustration, annoyance, hopelessness and other negative emotions about the therapist and therapy. In this way, the therapist can gauge whether his behavior is viewed as or is actually contributing to a weakening of the alliance.

A third patient variable consists of the style by which information is organized and processed. This style may or may not be associated with a particular personality disorder. While some disorders are notorious for suggesting severe problems in interpersonal relationships (for example, borderline, schizotypal), other personality styles (for example, hysterical or obsessive-compulsive) can interfere with communication in a short-term approach and secondarily disrupt the alliance. For example, a patient with obsessive-compulsive personality may fail to be cognizant of the therapist's affective tone or try to comply in too great detail, thereby sidetracking the dialogue into a web of thoughts that have little or no emotional relevance. On the other hand, those with a more hysterical style will think in global terms and will balk, at least initially, at what appears to be picky details of homework tasks. Those with such personality styles will be more consumed with wanting to please, entertain or win the approval of the therapist. Again, a greater focus is needed on the relationship itself and on how the patient's style of processing information affects the alliance.

The therapist can contribute in manifold ways to the disruption or weakening of the alliance. The short-term directive therapist must constantly judge whether he is too active and directive (for example, talking over the patient while failing to listen). On the other hand, the therapist may be too passive, hesitating to initiate action for fear he has not fully understood the problem or patient. Perhaps the most useful guideline to reduce the probability of either error is to ask the patient his view when conceptualizing a problem or designing a task—to ask the patient whether the conceptualization seems realistic or whether the task appears feasible and reasonable.

In general, the degree of therapist activity/direction should be titrated against the patient's need for such direction. Early on in these therapies a greater degree of directiveness is typical. Later, however, the patient will have acquired more understanding and familiarity with the techniques and approaches. Therefore, more patient and less therapist initiative are to be expected during the latter phases of therapy.

Many short-term directive therapies espouse particular techniques (such as thought stopping, cognitive reattribution, keeping schedules, and so on). The way these techniques are applied has implications for the alliance. Techniques may be misapplied in an impersonal, mechanical fashion, leaving the patient feeling uncared for. Alternatively, some therapists will prematurely switch from one technique to the next when the first appears ineffective. This leads the patient to feel confused and frustrated, and confidence in the therapist may drop. On the other hand, the dogged persistence with one technique that is not helping can lead to similar feelings. Careful attention to these dangers, as well as continual dialogue with the patient about the therapist's reasons for persistence with or change of technique (and the patient's feelings about these events), is required.

Let us turn to contributants derived from the disorder itself that can impair the alliance. The contribution of personality difficulties that impair the formation of the alliance has already been mentioned. Where reality testing is impaired (for example, with hallucinations or delusions) or where there is marked suspiciousness, the therapist's directives may be confusing or misunderstood. In one study we attempted to modify schizophrenic delusions with direct cognitive techniques. These techniques exacerbated the delusions in some patients, and lead to marked hostility toward and suspiciousness of the therapist (Hole, Rush and Beck, 1979).

Where memory, concentration or abstraction abilities are impaired, written instructions, telephone reminders and a greater focus on specific, concrete, simple tasks and concepts is required. Within the session, a dialogue to summarize each step is often needed. Sometimes the therapist and patient need to create a written summary of the session. Alternatively, an important other person might be asked to assist the patient in carrying out certain tasks.

Finally, not all disorders respond to short-term directive or even long-term nondirective approaches. Some depressions, perhaps those with endogenous or melancholic symptom features, may not respond at all or may respond only in part. The therapist must keep this fact in mind. When failure is encountered, the therapist should consider a revision in the treatment plan and even a new diagnostic evaluation. For example, one woman with migraine headaches and a nonendogenous unipolar major depression had little symptom relief after 20 sessions of cognitive therapy. Upon reevaluation, it was found that she had been taking alphamethyldopa for hypertension—a fact not reported in her initial assessment. Once the medication was stopped, she became asymptomatic.

CASE EXAMPLES

These case vignettes illustrate some potential obstacles to formation of the therapeutic alliance, and ways that these obstacles might be managed.

Case 1:

This 22-year-old schoolteacher became depressed after her 26-year-old husband died from cancer of the kidney. Immediately after his death, she began to fly about the country trying to "run away." Within a month, she ingested all the medication she had on hand and was accidentally found comatose by her mother, who had returned home unexpectedly. She had recurrent visions of her dead husband calling her to join him and had put her name on his tombstone, expecting to join him shortly. (The latter fact was not disclosed until she had been in treatment for several months.) The first therapy session was conducted in the Medical Intensive Care Unit. She was extremely angry and ordered the therapist to leave; she refused to talk for most of the session.

The patient offered several clues that the therapeutic alliance would be critical and not easily established: hostility to the therapist's presence as well as questions, impulsiveness and visual hallucinations. Further, she had previously not had a "best friend" except for her deceased husband. Therefore, a revision in the time limit and early focus on the alliance was necessary. Her descriptive diagnosis was unipolar major depression, nonrecurrent, with melancholic and psychotic features.

After three weeks of doxepin (400 mg per day) and chlorpromazine (250 mg per day), she began outpatient treatment. Initially, she offered little more than one- or two-sentence responses; she would become irritated or angry with no apparent provocation. The therapist inquired about how she thought and felt about the therapist and therapy. Did she feel accused or hurt when the therapist asked her questions? Did she view the therapy as hopelessly doomed to failure? Did she fear trying to participate in treatment because she couldn't stand another failure? In essence, the beliefs that precluded the alliance became the initial targets in therapy. The patient appeared relieved to see that someone could apparently put some of her thoughts into words and, therefore, might understand how she felt.

The maintenance of the alliance continued to be critical for the first several months of treatment. Even rather superficial intellectual discussions of specific notions, such as "Life isn't worth it," irritated her. She frequently derogated the therapy and the therapist, or she refused to speak. Ten- to 20-second silences were often followed by her angry query, "What are you thinking?" Gradually, these angry responses became cues for exploring her own thinking at that moment. She expressed ideas such as "You can't depend on anybody else." She believed that the therapist was thinking "I'm bored. I can't stand to see you. You are the worse patient I have. I can't listen to all this," during the silences. This repeated focus on her thoughts and feelings about the therapist (that is, the alliance) in the session allowed her to gradually see that she was assuming the most negative possibilities within the therapy session, and later in her interpersonal interactions. Initially, her tendency to read negatives into the therapeutic alliance and to burst into activity were the focus of discussion. Later in the treatment, the patient was able to evaluate more objectively her stream of negative cognitions and to identify the specific silent assumptions supporting these thoughts (such as, "getting close to another person only leads to rejection"). At this point, techniques that focused on changing symptoms and interpersonal patterns could be employed. Had the techniques been used early, when the therapeutic alliance was not established, she probably would have dropped out of treatment. Given the fact that the alliance was the main target of treatment for the first several months, the time limit was initially set at six months. A second contract (agreement) was established for another six-month period. Therapy ended after one year.

Case 2:

This 27-year-old divorced white woman was referred by the Neurology department, complaining of severe, incapacitating right retrobulbar headaches of four years' duration and two episodes of major depression. Although the headaches were present without depression, they became more severe when she was dysphoric. The headaches were associated with pain, nausea, vomiting and photophobia. She had failed to respond to anxiolytic, antidepressant, antimigraine and analgesic medications as well as a right occipital neurectomy. She had been unable to work for nine months. Her Hamilton Rating Scale (HRS–D) (Hamilton, 1960) and Beck Depression Inventory (BDI) (Beck et al, 1961) were both 30. Treatment consisted of cognitive therapy only. Below is her response to treatment:

Week	1	3	5	7	9
BDI	30	22	7	5	4

In session one, the patient expressed great skepticism about psychiatric treatment because of previous therapy failures. She reported the following automatic thoughts associated with her headaches: "No one cares about my headaches. There's something wrong with my brain; I can't cope. I am afraid I will lose my mind." She was willing to consider the possibility that these thoughts might be related to worsening of the headaches. As homework, she was asked to record the events, automatic thoughts and moods associated with exacerbations in her headaches.

In session two, the patient complained of excruciating headaches, was distraught and had a patch over one eye. She had not done any homework and reported that she awoke with a headache and had distressing thoughts and feelings of hopelessness and helplessness. A pre–post session headache severity rating (on a scale of 0–10) revealed a decrease from nine to five in her headaches during the session. The therapist used these data to demonstrate the degree to which thoughts and feelings expressed in treatment were related to her somatic complaints. Shortly after the session, she presented to the Emergency Room with a headache and, failing to respond to several injections of narcotics, was admitted to the Psychiatric Inpatient Service.

Sessions three and four were conducted while she was hospitalized. She was still not recording her automatic thoughts. She described herself as the "black sheep" in her very religious family. She was irritated at being unemployed and having to be at home with her constantly critical parents (her view). She was fearful of taking a job, as she expected to fail because of her headaches and depression. From this and other history, the therapist inferred that she would endorse the belief, "I must be perfect in order for people to like me," to which she partially agreed. Her anticipations about the positive and negative benefits of working were explored; she agreed to test out her negative predictions by applying for part-time work.

These first four sessions focused largely on establishing the therapeutic alliance. Her reasons for noncompliance were the focus of treatment. Repeated failures with previous interventions led her to be untrusting of this therapist and therapy. Symptom exacerbation was encountered early. A past history of being isolated as well as poor interpersonal relationships was noted. Her tendency to somatize rather than communicate and emote also pointed toward the need to focus on the alliance first. In this case, her fear of trust was converted into curiosity about whether she could work or not. By making this a neutral question that could be answered by action on her part, a tenuous alliance with the therapist was established. Subsequently, techniques that focused on symptom reduction were employed.

In sessions five to nine, the mastery and pleasure technique was used to determine whether she devalued her own efforts. She recorded each activity every hour while awake and noted the degree of achievement (mastery) and enjoyment (pleasure) that accompanied each undertaking. She also recorded the severity of head pain that accompanied each activity. Furthermore, she was to record her thoughts before going to bed each evening, because her headaches were more intense on awakening.

She was unable to record her thinking. However, the activity record indicated that she consistently undervalued her efforts. The therapist tried to elicit the cognitions associated with her attempts to record her thoughts. The theme in this thinking was that she believed that she needed to resolve her problems before presenting them, and that she needed to write only relevant or important thoughts in order to please the therapist. The therapist indicated that thought recording was only an experiment to see whether writing down her thoughts would result in reduced symptoms. She visited the neurologist again to see if he would give her more medication, which he refused to do.

She had begun working. She was dissatisfied with her job because "I am not accomplishing anything." She endorsed the theme, "I must accomplish great things in order to be happy" and reported her secret desire to become a missionary in Africa.

By session eight, she had begun to record some thoughts. Her activity record showed her headaches were reduced after activities in which she felt mastery and/or pleasure. A list of enjoyable activities was created. She used the headaches as cues to participate in one of these undertakings for 30 minutes. She continued to have difficulty in recording cognitions. However, her capacity to carry out much of the homework suggested the therapeutic alliance was developing further.

At session nine, her symptom record showed that she had experienced a severe headache while watching a television show in which a couple was making love. The therapist suggested that a number of beliefs surrounding sexuality might be critical to her head pain, particularly in light of her divorce and her reported rape at age 12.

In sessions ten to 11, she began to record self-critical thoughts and negative interpretations of others' feelings toward her (such as, my parents think I am crazy, a dope addict, and so forth). She practiced answering these thoughts; that is, she and the therapist considered evidence for and against each conceptualization, and she gradually developed alternative, more realistic ideas that better fit the data.

She attended an "R" rated film to determine if her headaches were related to silent assumptions about sexuality. The film precipitated a severe headache and feelings of intense anger. She recalled having fantasies of wanting to kill her husband, and having to get drunk to have sex with him. During the session, she vividly and emotionally recalled being raped at age 12, her family's blaming her, and her father saying, "You are ruined for life." The cognitions that surrounded the event included: "I'm bad, good girls don't get raped; I'm ruined for life; if I had listened to my parents, it wouldn't have happened; I must do good work to make up for being bad." Such attitudes probably contributed to her initial difficulties in establishing the therapeutic alliance. She was asked to continue recording thoughts that surrounded the rape and her marriage.

In sessions 12 to 13, the thoughts and beliefs that surrounded the rape and her current headaches were examined and corrected as she and the therapist considered the evidence she presented in support of each belief (such as, "I am ruined for life because I'm not a virgin; good girls don't get raped"). Furthermore, the therapist explored how she dealt with feelings of anger. She believed, "People won't like you if you show anger." To gain objectivity about these feelings, she decided to write (but not mail) letters to people with whom she was angry. These letters allowed her to see how she blamed herself even while expressing anger (for example, "I am angry with you but it is my fault").

She also wrote a letter to the therapist expressing anger at the upcoming termination. The associated cognitions included, "Now I will have no one. I can't make it alone." With discussion, she was able to see how these ideas were related to her underlying theme, "I am defective and incapable." The negative bias in these ideas was reduced as she considered the progress in therapy and her new-found ability to control her headaches for several weeks. Note that the impending disruption in the alliance (termination) had to be dealt with earlier than it would for other patients who might form the alliance with greater ease.

In sessions 14 to 15, several behavioral experiments were used to assess the evidence for or against various beliefs. She moved into her own apartment to see if she could get along "without anyone." She discussed the rape with her father and mother to see if they would endorse the attitudes she attributed to them. Her father denied blaming her and recalled how he had previously tried to get her to discuss the incident with him. Her mother had felt responsible and blamed herself.

In sessions 16 to 17, discussion focused on beliefs about termination. She believed that she would fail and only have the Emergency Room for relief. These and other negative anticipations were related to her basic belief of being defective and incompetent. She reviewed her accomplishments in treatment and rehearsed responses to anticipated stressful events, which allowed her to better gauge her capacity to cope and see alternative solutions.

This case illustrates several points. First, patients with severe depressions, particularly those with somatic complaints, may find it difficult to carry out particular assignments—especially to verbalize or record their thoughts. This "resistance" was reconceptualized in terms of cognitions and beliefs about expressing thoughts and about the therapeutic alliance. These ideas were then subjected to empirical testing. Second, somatic complaints may serve as cues for attending to distorted thinking and problematic silent assumptions or schemas derived from past experiences. The schemas can often be inferred from stereotyped recurrent conceptualizations of specific events. Further, these beliefs are also operative both during and between therapy sessions. Third, repeated experiences are usually needed to correct such long standing beliefs and each may strengthen the alliance. Thus, several behavioral experiments were used to help the patient assess and test those notions that she held with such certainty.

Several techniques were described which should be applied with great care (such as writing letters to clarify specific notions and feelings). The therapist must weigh the potential risks (such as acting out angry impulses) against the potential gains (clarifying the cognitions underlying these feelings) when considering one of these methods. Finally, particular attention to the termination is needed for patients who initially have difficulty developing the alliance to begin with.

CONCLUSIONS

A variety of time-limited, directive therapies have been recently developed. However, careful patient selection for these approaches is required. The patient's behavior in the initial sessions and his response to task assignments, as well as past history, provide clues about suitability of these approaches. Personality disorders and certain personality styles may require modification of the techniques or time limits. Because the therapist is rather active, great care in the application of techniques, as well as frequent assessments of the impact of therapist behavior on the patient, are needed. Patients with psychotic disorders, defenses against trust and memory problems are likely to require greater focus early in treatment on establishment of the therapeutic alliance before symptom relieving techniques can be applied. Should the patient fail to respond to a short-term, directive approach, a reevaluation and modification in the treatment plan is called for.

REFERENCES

Beck AT, Greenberg R: Coping with Depression. Philadelphia, Center for Cognitive Therapy, 1976

Beck AT, Ward CJ, Mendelson, M, et al: An inventory for measuring depression. Arch Gen Psychiatry 4:561-565, 1961

Beck AT, Rush, AJ, Shaw, BF et al: Cognitive Therapy of Depression. New York, Guilford Press, 1979

Hamilton M: A rating scale for depression. J Neurol, Neurosurg Psychiatry, 23:56-62, 1960

Hole R, Rush AJ, Beck AT: Cognitive change methods with delusional patients. Psychiatry 42:312-319, 1979

Lewinsohn PM, Sullivan JM, Grosscup SJ: Behavioral therapy: clinical applications, in Short-Term Psychotherapies for Depression. Edited by Rush AJ. New York, Guilford Press, 1982

Rounsaville BJ, Chevron E: Interpersonal psychotherapy: clinical applications, in Short-Term Psychotherapies for Depression. Edited by Rush AJ. New York, Guilford Press, 1982

Rush AJ: Psychotherapy of the affective psychoses. Am J Psychoanal 40:99-123, 1980

Rush AJ: Cognitive therapy for depression, in Affective and Schizophrenic Disorders: New Approaches to Diagnosis. Edited by Zales MR. New York, Brunner/Mazel, 1983

Zaiden J: Psychodynamic therapy: clinical applications, in Short-Term Psychotherapies for Depression. Edited by Rush AJ. New York, Guilford Press, 1982

Chapter 30

The Therapeutic Alliance With Difficult Patients

by Mardi Horowitz, M.D. and Charles Marmar, M.D.

THE PSYCHOTHERAPIST'S EXPERIENCE OF "DIFFICULTY"

There is at the present time very little empirical information that would allow one to describe the characteristics of a difficult patient. Instead, it is helpful to regard difficulty as a feeling that emerges either in the therapist or in some other clinician who reviews the psychotherapeutic process. The experience that one is dealing with a difficult patient may reach conscious recognition as a sense of foreboding when approaching or anticipating an interview with a certain patient or a sense of frustration during a session, and will often manifest itself in a communication to colleagues such as "I just had a session with a difficult patient." While colleagues know what is meant, the details of that difficulty and how to handle it are considerably less clear.

For certain therapists, a specific type of patient may be the most difficult. Some therapists feel especially stymied or frustrated when dealing with patients who are highly suspicious, very angry, demanding, dependent, or who have conflicts that are active and unresolved in the therapist himself. For most therapists, it is not the sickest patients who are necessarily the most difficult. Rather, difficulty seems to result from a composite of traits affecting the relationship that can be established between the patient and therapist. With a difficult patient, establishing a therapeutic alliance is a formidable and perhaps an impossible task.

Preceding chapters in this section have dealt with definitions and quantitative studies of the therapeutic alliance. The pertinent empirical literature will not be reviewed again here. Myerson (1977, 1979) has reviewed the clinical descriptive literature and has provided an important summary formulation. He follows Balint (1968) and others in describing the therapist's subjective experience of difficulty. It is as if, when dealing with a difficult patient, there is a shell surrounding that patient. Because of this insulation the therapist feels screened

The authors gratefully acknowledge Nancy Wilner, Reed Brockbank, Barry Levine, and Robert Sokol who viewed videotapes and conducted dilemma analyses, as well as Robert Rosenbaum, Karen Cliffe, and Stephen Shane who viewed videotapes and conducted difficulty analyses, thus clarifying both concepts. This paper was prepared while Dr. Horowitz was a Fellow at the Center for Advanced Studies in the Behavior Sciences, Stanford University, and supported by a fellowship grant from the John D. and Catherine T. MacArthur Foundation. Additional research support was derived from an NIMH Clinical Research Center Award to the Center for the Study of Neuroses at the Langley Porter Psychiatric Institute of the University of California, San Francisco.

off, left out, unable to connect. The metaphor uses a "hard," interposed, protective shield because the "shell" is not simply due to unfamiliarity with the opportunities for honest expressiveness provided by the usual psychotherapeutic situation. It is not modified by the patient's chance to learn that the therapist is a safe person with whom to discuss ideas and feelings. Similarly, the shell is not due to a justifiable early alertness to seeing whether this therapist is a good one or not. Instead, the shell is carried about, from one relationship to the next, from this therapist to that one, and constitutes not only a part of the patient's difficulty, but an obstacle in the path of work upon that difficulty.

The role-relationship model that is manifested by the shell is formed, as Myerson describes it, in early development. The important figures, such as parents, in that development may have been either overstimulating and intrusive, or more likely they have been ungratifying, as well as unwilling or unable to mitigate the distress of the child who grows up into the patient. The shell is a character defense based on the expectation that the other person cannot or will not help, and/or that the other person will be invasive in a dangerous manner.

The particular type of shell discussed by Myerson and others is especially frustrating because it does not fulfill the hopes of the patient. The patient, when alone, can imagine a close relationship in which there is a helpful, mutual, give-and-take of honestly disclosed ideas and feelings. When with someone, as when with the therapist, this imagined closeness cannot be established. There is a frustrating difference between the relationship expected when the patient is alone, and the relationship that the patient can actually offer when not alone. This frustrating difference between the two models of relationship is transmitted to the therapist in the process of either blaming the therapist, or signaling to the therapist that the patient does wish to establish a closer contact, but cannot do so.

The presence of these difficulties has been felt to be especially high in persons with narcissistic or borderline personality organizations, as described by Winnicott (1965), Modell (1976), Hartocollis (1977), Kohut (1977), Kernberg (1975) and Horowitz et al (1984).

Patients at this level of personality organization tend to have high state mobility (as, for example, with rapid and unstable shifts from rage to hopelessness, to paralyzing guilt or terrifying emptiness), uncontrolled surges of emotion, distortions in the perception of intentions of other persons, a tendency to regressive shifts in self and object representations, and to present in polysymptomatic syndromes that shift over time. Most authors, however, in recognizing this composite of attributes, do focus on the difficulty as the therapist's sense of frustration in establishing the kind of relationship that the therapist would like to establish, and usually does establish. This relationship has been described as the therapeutic alliance, reviewed in preceding chapters. In order to further discuss the difficulty in the path of establishing a therapeutic alliance, it is helpful to contrast this model of a relationship with two others: the social alliance and transference relationships.

ROLE RELATIONSHIP MODELS IN PSYCHODYNAMIC PSYCHOTHERAPY

Any individual patient can be described in terms of varied role-relationship models that he or she may use to organize expectations and intentions as they take place during psychotherapy. Generalizing across patients, three types of relationship models may characterize the transactive patterns as conceptualized by either party. The therapeutic alliance is a term used to designate that relationship pattern in which both the patient and therapist have the shared goal of progressive understanding and resolution of the patient's problems. The therapist is characterized as an expert, the patient as a person seeking and motivated to obtain help from that expert. The aim of each party is a mutual give-and-take that will lead to gradual, full disclosure of problems, and discussion of possible modes of their solution in relationship to "if/then/but" blocks to their solution.

Transference relationship phenomena have been well described and lie at the very core of the psychodynamic approach to psychotherapy (Freud, 1912, 1914; Gill, 1982). The transference relationship models may be composed of varied negative and positive intentions or expectations. They are derived from wishes and fears based on earlier experiences, and unconsciously transposed into the psychotherapy opportunity. This is not necessarily antitherapeutic; instead, comparison of the role-relationship models of a therapeutic alliance with the role-relationship models of the manifested transference relationship allows for insight and modification.

A third type of relationship model in psychotherapy is the social alliance (Horowitz, 1979). The social alliance may serve as a resistance to establishing a therapeutic alliance, for it is based on a role-relationship model that might take place were the two parties to meet in ordinary life, but not for the purposes of psychotherapy. The social alliance might have aims between the parties of friendly conversation about matters of mutual but superficial interest, banter, sexuality or a coalition to criticize some third party.

These three models of relationship, the therapeutic alliance, social alliance, and transference relationship, all involve some kind of "transference" in terms of their formation. That is, any role-relationship model used to organize expectations, appraisals and intentions in an interpersonal transaction will derive elements from the repertoire of schematic forms carried into the situation by the patient and the therapist. The therapeutic alliance is formed on the basis of a choice of elements within an available repertoire, the elements that most closely resemble the realistic possibilities within the ground rules of what constitutes dynamic psychotherapy. The social alliance deflects from these aims of therapy as therapy, substituting instead the aims and scripts of courtship, friendship or games.

In patients who are not perceived by therapists as being especially difficult, dynamic psychotherapy proceeds by interpretations of the social alliance when it serves as a resistance to the therapeutic alliance, and of transference as an inappropriate set of ideas and emotions based on past but not necessarily current realities or fantasies. The therapy proceeds with a gradual deepening of the therapeutic alliance; in that deepening it loses some of the properties transferred from preexisting role-relationship models imposed upon the situation, and schematizes the new transactional properties found in the growing mutuality and intimacy of the actual therapeutic give-and-take. Deepening and development of the role-relationship model of the therapeutic alliance is, in and of itself, one of the advances made in the course of the psychotherapy, for it involves development of both the patient's self-concept and capacities for relating with others. In difficult patients there is some type of impasse interfering with this type of development and deepening.

One of the major early findings in clinical observation of dynamic interchanges was that transference manifestations did not necessarily obstruct the aims of symptom resolution and improved adaptation in relation to personal problems. Instead, the manifestation of transference-relationship models, the allowance of regression, and expression of usually warded-off wishes and fears, often created an opportunity for deepened insight and working through of conflicts to points of new decision. Interpretation of transference became one of the key ingredients in psychoanalytically oriented psychotherapy.

Nonetheless, the facilitating effect of transference interpretation was not found in all cases. In a difficult case, as noted by Myerson (1977), the usual efforts at transference interpretation often have little positive effect and may possibly have a negative effect. Horowitz et al (1984) have reported some empirical evidence supporting the clinical impressions reported by Myerson (1977) and have summarized impressions by other clinicians and psychotherapy researchers. Especially in cases where at treatment onset there is low motivation and reality relationship capacity in the patient, transference interpretations may not lead to a deepening of the therapeutic alliance.

In summary, then, it may be stated that the utilization by the patient of either a social alliance or transference-relationship model for organizing the expected or intended relationship between patient and therapist is not necessarily a source of difficulty. Either of these impositions can be interpreted and contrasted with the potentials for a therapeutic alliance, leading to gains. Impasses occur when social alliances or regressive transferences are imposed and there is interference with this route to change. In such instances the therapist recognizes the presence of an impasse.

IMPASSES

In an empirical analysis of elements in the psychotherapeutic process, Orlinsky and Howard (1975) distinguished five kinds of impasse. These included: unproductive contact, which is similar to Myerson's (1977) concept of the "shell" as a prevention to relatedness; defensiveness; ambivalent nurturance-dependence aims leading to excessive and frustrating dependency; uncomfortable types of involvement; and conflictual erotization. Themes such as ambivalence, dependency and erotization do not necessarily complicate therapy. But they do lead to impasses when they are caught up in the kind of conflicts suggested by Orlinsky and Howard. That is, there might be some kind of double-binding situation tying up both the patient and the therapist.

The double bind, in this formulation, is present not only in the patient, but as Kiesler (1979) has pointed out, is evoked in the therapist by means of "command messages" sent by the patient and reacted to unconsciously by the therapist. Strupp has indicated such factors, as well, in the difference between success and failure in dynamic psychotherapy (Strupp, 1980). Lang has written extensively about this type of impasse (1975, for example). Ryle (1979) has offered an especially illuminating formulation, writing at just about the same time as Myerson.

Ryle defined what he called "dilemmas, snags, and traps" as various types of impasse in psychotherapy, and offered these as potentially key focal concerns that might center attention in brief psychotherapy. Stimulated in part by the work of Kelly (1955) on personal constructs, and based on his own empirical research using the repertory grid technique (1975), Ryle defined dilemmas as false dichotomizations into "either/or" expectations or excessively limited, or rigid "if/then" kinds of beliefs. Ryle gave examples of two common dilemmas. In one of these, the patient feels that "in relationships I am either close to someone and feel smothered, or I am cut off and feel lonely." The second example would be stated by a patient like this: "I feel that if I am feminine, then I feel that I have to be insensitive" (pp. 47-48).

Ryle is aware that such dilemmas have long been described in the psychoanalytic psychotherapy literature, and that sometimes they are even used to describe particular kinds of personality disorder (as in *DSM-III*). The progressive aspect of the work, as found in other cognitive approaches such as those reported by Beck (1967, 1976) is that the actual propositions in these patterns are clearly stated in a way that is not only pertinent to an individual, but may also represent a typology or set of patients.

As already mentioned, Ryle divided impasses into dilemmas, snags, and traps. He defined traps as the result of relating to others in terms of such "either/or" or "if/then" dilemmas. One of the examples that he gave features the alternatives between being accommodating or unreasonably angry. As a patient might word this, were it conscious and clear as a pattern: "I am unduly accommodating to others; the result of this is that I often feel abused or invaded by them: this leads to my being irritable or unreasonably angry; as a result of this I feel guilty and that makes me unduly accommodating to others." The trap is that the person cannot escape from this cycle but is ensnared within it. This leads Ryle to define a snag as an obstacle to change that results from the combination of dilemmas and traps. It is like the third feature in a double bind that keeps the person from leaving the field. It says in effect, "I want to change, but if I do then the snag will be. . . ."

Following these definitions, Ryle identifies six main groups of dilemmas, snags and traps. They can be summarized in this way:

1. A distance/closeness dilemma: either the patient feels excessively isolated or at risk from being too close.
2. A controlled/controlling dilemma: the patient feels either helplessly submissive to another, or excessively powerful over another.
3. A must/won't dilemma: the patient feels that he either has to have feelings or to communicate ideas at the expense of being chaotic, or that he has to be in tight control, in which he cannot or will not reveal ideas and feelings that ought to be revealed according to the roles of therapy.

4. A forced choice dilemma: the patient feels that only two roles are being offered; that he or she must choose one or the other, with the loss of some opportunity in giving up one, when in reality there is an opportunity to select components of both roles and combine them in some way.

5. A trap in which a problematic role relationship can only be reversed, so either the self or the other is in a given role, such as being either aggressor or victim, with unacceptable consequences of being in either position.

6. A snag that usually involves a wish to enact some transaction with either a parent or sexual partner, coupled with a belief that such aims always lead to a bad consequence such as punishment, guilt, shame or anxiety.

CONFIGURATIONAL ANALYSIS OF IMPASSES

A dilemma, in the sense provided by Ryle, would be exemplified by a patient who cannot remain in a social alliance, because then therapy would not proceed; but the patient cannot leave the social alliance, because then the more emotional give-and-take would lead into a feared transference-relationship model rather than a therapeutic alliance. A difficult patient would be one who could not imagine or project a therapeutic alliance, and would thus be trapped in this dilemma. Another aspect of a trap would be a situation in which the patient and therapist would endlessly blame each other, shifting roles as to who was guilty of failing to make the therapy "work."

A method for systematically formulating the different components of such forms of impasse has been called "configurational analysis" (Horowitz, 1979; Horowitz et al, 1984). This method provides a series of steps and formats for description and explanatory clinical inferences about the states of mind, self-concepts, role-relationship models and modes of processing information that take place within the therapy situation. It focuses on the integrative function of the mind, resulting from the interaction and conflict of multiple component functions.

Utilizing this method of explanatory description, Horowitz and colleagues have identified compromise states of mind and role-relationship models that are used to prevent *both* establishment of the therapeutic alliance and the emergence of dreaded emotions in more regressive or projective relationship phenomena. We have located two types of difficulties that are pertinent to this discussion. One is a kind of impediment to the development of the therapeutic alliance generated by the active presence of regressive or projective role-relationship models. The other type of difficulty has to do with the absence of a superordinate self-concept and role conceptualizing system; in such a case, the patient cannot allow the kind of parallel processing that permits recognition of inappropriate but active relationship views to be simultaneously compared with reality, or with the actual possibility of a therapeutic alliance (Horowitz and Zilberg, 1983).

In our detailed analyses of change processes in psychotherapy, using the configurational analyses method, we have found that many such instances of impasse have three characteristics. These are:

1. The patient indicates to the therapist that he or she should be more than

usually active in order to facilitate a halting or disabled level of therapeutic work (as follows the finding of Kiesler, 1979).

2. The patient then indicates to the therapist, often in a barely conscious way, that there is some pitfall standing in the path of the very activity that is being solicited.

3. Unfortunately, in such patients that are found by the therapist to be difficult, there is hardly any zone of safety between either ignoring the provocation (1) or responding to it (2).

The therapist is thus on the horns of a dilemma.

Dilemmas are best described with clinical detail such as analyzed transcripts from the individual psychotherapy. Such detail is provided elsewhere (Horowitz, 1979; Horowitz et al, 1984) and so here a simple, general model will be provided. The first horn of such a dilemma can be illustrated by a patient who displays chaotic thoughts and intense fear and confusion, suggesting an inability to structure inner experiences, with difficulty in communication.

Such fear and confusion, signaled to the therapist, is not uncommon and does not lead to the sense of difficulty described here in the therapist. Instead it usually tends to call forth very positive responses in which the therapist helps the patient to focus on a line of thought, and organize it into a coherent sequence of memories, responses and plans. With an especially difficult patient, when the therapist answers the call for help in this usual way, something untoward happens. The therapist then encounters the second horn of the dilemma.

As described by Myerson and Ryle, the second horn occurs when the patient feels that the therapist is invading his or her autonomy and privacy, fears merger with the therapist, and so responds oppositionally. The therapist finds himself in a "damned if you do and damned if you don't" position in response to these horns of a dilemma. When the therapist tries interpreting both horns simultaneously, the patient becomes confused. Both parties experience the session as difficult (and so does the supervisor or consultant).

A dozen sample dilemmas, following this form of two horns, are listed in Table 1. These dilemmas have been developed from configurational analyses and scrutiny of videotapes by a team of colleagues, seeking to specify such dilemmas. It is not an exhaustive list but it does illustrate this approach. At the present time we seek to determine if clinicians can reach consensual agreement as to whether a given dilemma is present on a given segment of recorded psychotherapy and, if so, to analyze the process of its solution. The example just given is listed as the first of these dilemmas.

An expanded view of the first dilemma listed in Table 1 is provided by the following example. A nonworking state of mind indicates the need for some change in the therapy situation. We will refer to this state as that of *social chit-chat*. In this state, the patient's self-concept is presented as that of a peer aiming at friendly interchange, to pass the time amiably with the therapist. The therapist is viewed as if a casual companion by the patient. During this social chit-chat state of mind there is leakage of emotions, anguish and rage over a recent loss. The slight, momentary shimmers of these warded-off emotions activate the therapist to act against the resistence of the social chit-chat state. This is the role-relationship model of horn *a* of the first dilemma listed in Table 1.

Table 1. A Dozen Sample Dilemmas

1. **a.** The patient is constantly frightened of inability to structure inner experiences and control chaotic thoughts and emotions.

   b. *But if* the therapist attempts to structure the communication of these ideas and feelings, the patient will see this as an invasion of autonomy and privacy, will fear domination or merger and will oppose it.

2. **a.** The patient manifests helplessness and dependency upon the therapist for caretaking.

   b. *But if* the therapist addresses this attitude or indicates the necessity for assuming personal responsibility, the patient will feel so neglected or overwhelmed by demands that regression or withdrawal will follow.

3. **a.** The patient is so deflated and demoralized that very little impetus to engage in work is present.

   b. *But if* the therapist addresses this attitude or encourages the patient to a more positive view, then the patient will feel the therapist is too unempathic and unrealistically optimistic and will feel increasingly hopeless.

4. **a.** The patient feels entitled to more than the therapist can give within the usual boundaries of psychodynamic psychotherapy and so feels neglected and abandoned.

   b. *But if* the therapist allows boundaries to become flexible the patient will feel too special to have to work in therapy.

5. **a.** The patient exhibits a tendency or likelihood to act out.

   b. *But if* the therapist interprets this as maladaptive and needing increased control, the patient will see this as criticism and become increasingly rebellious.

6. **a.** The patient does little besides repetitively express personal suffering.

   b. *But if* the therapist addresses this pattern and encourages other work, the patient will feel so misunderstood that only increased expressions of suffering or withdrawal will take place.

A tentative series of efforts by the therapist does not alter the social chit-chat situation and he then intervenes vigorously. Responses at such times indicate another role-relationship model, one underlying Horn *b* of the dilemma. In this role-relationship model the patient is like a dangerously vulnerable, empty and damaged person frightened by a ruthless invader and manipulator. This concept of the situation leads to a fearful, chaotic state of mind in which thoughts are experienced as confusing jumbles. The patient cannot process what the therapist means. As the therapist backs off, the patient gradually resumes the social chit-chat state of mind.

Between these two role-relationship models there was little zone of safety

Table 1. A Dozen Sample Dilemmas—Continued

---

7.   **a.** The patient is so passive that all initiative is placed with the therapist.

    b. *But if* the therapist becomes active in fostering communication, the patient will comply dependently without processing meanings personally.

8.   **a.** The patient maintains such a distance in regard to key issues that the therapist is not trusted with intimate communications.

    b. *But if* the therapist interprets the avoidance or encourages the patient toward increased intimacy, the patient will become fearful and back off further.

9.   **a.** The patient is preoccupied with challenging the therapist to show competency and strength.

    b. *But if* the therapist addresses this challenge by reassuring the patient about an ability to tolerate whatever the patient expresses, the patient will either obstinately increase the level of the challenge or submit obsequiously and inauthentically.

10.   **a.** The patient does not express some ideas and feelings central to core aspects of important topics.

    b. *But if* the therapist addresses this avoidance or mentions these warded-off ideas, the patient would experience this as corrosively scornful criticism.

11.   **a.** The patient presents in a contrived manner in which substitute emotions are used to hide more primary and authentic ones.

    b. *But if* the therapist confronts the defense and the warded-off affects, the patient will become confused.

12.   **a.** The patient presents in an overcontrolled manner that avoids emotional expression.

    b. *But if* the therapist discusses this avoidance and the warded-off emotions, the patient will either be overwhelmed by experiencing them, or distraught with fear of being unable to tolerate the experience.

---

because there was no role-relationship model of cooperative mutuality in this patient's repertoire of mental schemata. Conflictual and infantile patterns of interpersonal behavior with both parents persisted into adulthood, and there were no restorative figures such as siblings or peers in her surrounding social network. The absence of an intimate, equal relationship was compounded by never having had even a good teacher-to-student relationship during school years. There were few elements in the patient's repertoire upon which to build a therapeutic alliance. The therapist felt left out: his real attributes and the real opportunities in the situation were unrecognized, contributing frustration to his sense of difficulty.

Two impediments to development of a therapeutic alliance have been mentioned. One is generated by the type of linked and threatening expectations just explicated as the two horns of a dilemma. The second is the relative absence of supraordinate concepts of self and relationship. The patient in the present example has not fully developed a supraordinate self-concept, and an equivalent schematic form for synthesizing varied role-relationship models. As a consequence of this difficulty in psychic schematizations of meaning, it was hard for the patient to modulate one relationship view (one horn of the dilemma) with another (the relationship model characterizing the other horn of the dilemma). Thus the patient was entirely "in" one state or the other, with abrupt shifts between states. This also meant that the therapist could not engage the patient in parallel processing, a simultaneous examination of both threatening relationship models involved in the dilemma.

EMPIRICAL STUDIES

Previous chapters by Hartley and Luborsky have summarized psychotherapy research studies, indicating that aspects of the therapeutic alliance can be reliably measured. Our own work has followed such leads and found an empirical support for the clinical postulate that the alliance could be divided into patient and therapist relationship contributions, each with an enhancing (positive) or impairing (negative) component (Marmar et al, 1984). In a study involving 52 cases of pathological grief treated with brief dynamic psychotherapy, high levels of negating patient contributions were found to be associated with poorer outcome, controlling for the effects of pretherapy symptomatic severity (Horowitz et al, 1984). The dilemmas discussed may be an aspect of these alliance-impairing factors, as suggested by our intensive analysis of some cases in this sample using configurational analysis for descriptive explanation (Horowitz et al, 1984), and Strupp's (1980) intensive studies of paired cases, ones having good and poor outcomes, as treated by the same therapist.

The techniques that in clinical observations may help resolve dilemmas will be discussed below. Foreman and Marmar, in work still in preparation, have studied in an empirical manner the techniques that might help reduce patient alliance-impairing relationship contributions. Their pilot study examined six cases from the sample of 52 mentioned above. Each of these six cases manifested high patient-negative contributions towards a therapeutic alliance early in the brief psychotherapy for neurotic-level mental disorders precipitated by a bereavement. Half of the cases assessed to have initially negative patient contributions to the therapeutic alliance went on to improve the alliance, and to have a favorable outcome. Half of the cases maintained patient-negative contributions to the alliance over the course of the brief therapy and had a poor outcome. The most salient and consistent finding that differentiated the two groups of three cases was that, in the patients who improved, the therapist had addressed the defenses of the patient against expressing feelings about relationships both in and outside of the therapy. It appeared that the alliance scores did not improve until the therapist did address the patient's defenses within the patient-therapist relationship pattern. Of eight therapist actions assessed, in each therapy session this was the only one that seemed to correspond closely to the time frame of the decline of scores for the patient's negative contributions to the relationship as assessed by independent judges. This empirical finding, in a pilot study of a small number of well-selected cases, accords with general clinical suggestions, such as those of Kernberg in discussing issues of technique for psychotherapy of the borderline patient (1975).

In order to study dilemmas of the relationship as contributors to poor outcome in psychotherapy, and to arrive at a method for early identification, Rosenbaum, Wilner, Horowitz and Marmar have embarked on studies assessing the components and reliability of clinicians' assessments of patient difficulty; they used independent operations, assessments of such dilemmas as described in Table 1. The results of such quantitative studies of validity, reliability, and predictive utility should help refine the concept of dilemmas.

HOW TO HANDLE DILEMMAS

Understanding the components of an impasse in forming a therapeutic alliance is essential if the therapist is to resolve the situation. In many instances, a minor difficulty is handled intuitively by the therapist without conscious recognition of the obstacle in the path of deepening or developing a therapeutic alliance. Analytic review and understanding is indicated when the operation of intuition alone is not sufficient to resolve the difficulty.

A relationship dilemma can be analyzed in terms of the horns that lead to a "damned if you do and damned if you don't" response. Once both horns are identified, the therapist may then attempt to puzzle out a way to clarify, for the patient, a middle zone that does not enter fully into either of the threatening positions. As that middle zone of safety is developed, the therapeutic alliance is deepened; and the threat of either of the horns can be examined within that zone, utilizing the usual methods of helping the patient to re-examine events and to discriminate reality from fantasy projections.

This remedy is relatively straightforward with some difficult patients, but with the "difficult" difficult patients there is no middle ground; the horns of the dilemma overlap. When the therapist attempts to clarify the threat embodied within each horn of the dilemma, hoping to indicate the possibility for a therapeutic alliance between them, the patient instead feels impaled by both problems simultaneously. To avoid flooding the patient and risking a drop-out, the therapist may avoid excessive interpretation while at the same time avoiding being provoked into any action that could be interpreted by the patient as a version of the threatening relationship expectations. This leads to the type of empathic holding treatment described by Kohut (1977) and Modell (1976), and the principles of therapeutic change with persons of lower organizational levels of self-concept development, as described by Gedo and Goldberg (1975).

The goal of building a therapeutic alliance may be explicitly stated and discussed as a shared focus for attention during sessions. A hierarchy of technical approaches may build on this understanding. The first general tactic is to interpret horn a, the manifest surface of the dilemma, and to observe how the patient processes this information. The therapist may then add clear description of the potential alliance by repeatedly defining his own attributes, expectations and intentions.

An important aspect of such an approach is to ask the patient what he or she has heard the therapist say. This inquiry aims to find out the patient's several appraisals after the session as well as during it.

The next technique in this hierarchy of therapist actions to counteract a dilemma is to interpret the *b* horn, the more hidden aspect of the dilemma. In so doing the therapist may, with the most difficult patients, say explicitly and repeatedly what safeguards are incorporated into the real situation to reduce this threatening expectation. The usual techniques of showing the activity, meaning and developmental origin of the patient's negative expectations and transferences are used in this approach. The added emphasis is on helping the patient learn the real potentials and attributes of the relationship of the therapeutic alliance.

REFERENCES

Balint M: The Basic Fault: Therapeutic Aspects of Regression. London, Tavistock, 1968

Beck A: Depression. New York, Harper & Row, 1967

Beck A: Cognitive Therapy and Emotional Disorders. New York, International Universities Press, 1976

Freud S (1912): The dynamics of transference. Standard edition 12:99-108. London, Hogarth, 1958

Freud S (1914): Remembering, repeating, and working through. Standard edition 12:147-156. London, Hogarth, 1958

Gedo J, Goldberg S: Models of the Mind. New York, International Universities Press, 1975

Gill M: Analysis of Transference: Theory and Technique. New York, International Universities Press (Psychol Issues #53), 1982

Hartocollis P: Borderline Personality Disorders. New York, International Universities Press, 1977

Horowitz MJ: States of Mind. New York, Plenum, 1979

Horowitz M, Zilberg N: Regressive alterations in the self-concept. Am J Psychiatry 140:284-289, 1983

Horowitz M, Marmar C, Krupnick J, et al: Personality Styles and Brief Psychotherapy. New York, Basic Books, 1984

Horowitz M, Marmar C, Weiss D, et al: Brief psychotherapy of bereavement reactions: the relationship of process to outcome. Arch Gen Psychiatry, in press

Kelly GA: The Psychology of Personal Constructs. New York, Norton, 1955

Kernberg O: The Borderline Conditions and Pathological Narcissism. New York, Aronson, 1975

Kiesler DJ: An interpersonal communication analysis of relationship in psychotherapy. Psychiatry 42:299-311, 1979

Kohut H: The Restoration of the Self. New York, International Universities Press, 1977

Langs R: Therapeutic misalliances. Int J Psychoanal Psychother 4:77-105, 1975

Marmar C, Marziali E, Horowitz M, et al: The development of the therapeutic alliance rating system, in The Psychotherapeutic Process: A Research Handbook. Edited by Greenberg L, Pinsoff W. Philadelphia, Guilford Press, in press

Modell AH: The holding environment and the therapeutic action of psychoanalysis. J Am Psychoanal Assoc. 24:285-308, 1976

Myerson P: Therapeutic dilemmas relevant to the lifting of repression. Int J Psycho-Anal 58:458-463, 1977

Myerson P: Issues of technique where patients relate with difficulty. Int Rev Psycho-Anal, 6:363-375, 1979

Orlinsky DE, Howard K: Varieties of Psychotherapeutic Experience. New York, Teachers College Press, 1975

Ryle A: Frames and cages. New York, International Universities Press, 1975

Ryle A: The focus in brief interpretive psychotherapy: dilemmas, traps, and snags as target problems. Br J Psychiatry 134:46-54, 1979

Strupp HH: Success and failure in time-limited psychotherapy, a systematic comparison of two cases: comparison one. Arch Gen Psychiatry 37:595-603, 1980a

Strupp HH: Success and failure in time-limited psychotherapy, a systematic comparison of two cases: other comparisons. Arch Gen Psychiatry 37:831-841; 947-954, 1980b

Winnicott DW: Ego distortion in terms of the true and false self, in Natural Process and the Facilitating Environment. New York, International Universities Press, 1965

Chapter 31

The Influence of Gender and Race on the Therapeutic Alliance

by Susan J. Blumenthal, M.D., Enrico E. Jones, Ph.D. and Janice L. Krupnick, M.S.W.

Previous papers in this Section have discussed the influence of the "match" between therapist and patient in the formation of a successful therapeutic alliance. Although there are many variables that may influence this match (such as cognitive style, ethnic background, personality type) there are two of current social and political importance: gender and race. Questions have frequently been raised over the past decade concerning the role of gender and race in psychotherapy. The emergence of gender and race as themes in both the clinical and research literatures is a reflection of contemporary social issues. As women and minorities have increasingly begun to reexamine their roles in society, concern has mounted over the means by which traditional values are instilled and maintained. One expression of this social movement has been a challenge to the institution of psychotherapy. Yet, little direct research data regarding the influence of gender and race on the therapeutic alliance is currently available. In order to convey what is known about the impact of gender and race on the process and outcome of psychotherapy, we will review a somewhat broader base of research data. In the area of gender, we will review issues of sex role bias and stereotyping in psychotherapy, and the influence of gender on the process and the outcome of psychotherapy. In the area of race, clinical research literature bearing upon the effects of race on psychotherapy will be reviewed, concluding with some practical implications for the treatment of the black patient. Parloff et al (1978) articulate two major questions that have been generated from recent social criticism questioning the adequacy of treatment provided by psychotherapists for minorities and women. The first is, do stereotypes and biases held by therapists about such patients result in inadequate treatment of these patients? And, second, does an absence of shared experience and values interfere with the therapist's ability to establish rapport and, thus, to treat these patients effectively? This paper will summarize the relevant research findings in these areas and discuss implications for clinical practice and training.

GENDER

The rise of the Women's Movement in the late 1960s has led to a reexamination of the impact of various social institutions on the functioning and wellbeing of American women. One of the "institutions" scrutinized has been psychother-

This chapter was coauthored by Dr. Blumenthal in her private capacity. No official support or endorsement by NIMH is intended or should be inferred.

apy, particularly as it has been traditionally practiced (Chesler, 1971; Howard and Howard, 1974; Siassi, 1974; Hare-Mustin, 1980). The fact that the majority of recipients of mental health treatment are women, while the providers are most often men (Brodsky and Hare-Mustin, 1980; Marecek and Johnson, 1980) has given rise to some uncertainty and concern about the effectiveness of this particular gender match in promoting change and psychological wellbeing in women patients.

This concern over the pairing of male therapists with female patients centers on several potentially negative areas of impact. For example, Chesler (1971) doubts the ability of men raised in this society to be helpful to women, while Rice and Rice (1973) express the concern that men may be unable to truly empathize with a woman's innermost feelings. Studies of client preference for counselors of one or the other gender appear to support this concern. College samples of both men and women were found to prefer counselors of the same sex, if personal problems were the expected focus of counseling (Fuller, 1964; Boulware, 1970). Similarly, Simons and Helms (1976) found that noncollege women subjects viewed female counselors as more genuinely interested in helping them and better able to understand their problems than males, and reported expectations of greater comfort and ease of expression with female than with male counselors. It is possible that some clinicians intuitively agree with this expectation. Shullman and Betz (1979) report that in a university counseling center, clients were predominantly referred to same-sex counselors regardless of presenting problem, or the sex of the intake evaluator. Some writers suggest that the basis for this preference may lie, in part, in the ability of female therapists to serve as role models for female patients and to facilitate open expression of feelings (Brodsky, 1973; Kronsky, 1971). Other writers suggest that male and female therapists are appropriate at different life stages, or may function better for some patients as cotherapists (Fodor, 1974a, 1974b). Still others are very cautious about such arrangements, fearing that such a cotherapy situation might simply reinforce sex role stereotypes (Barrett et al, 1974).

Feminist assertions about gender-matching in psychotherapy have led some researchers to investigate the actual effects of therapist and patient gender on psychotherapy process and outcome. Even so, much of what is believed about this subject continues to rest more on theoretical and ideological biases and assumptions than on empirical data. As in much of psychotherapy research, where determining the effects of a single variable on outcome is difficult, ascertaining how a therapist's gender affects a patient's progress has been fraught with considerable difficulty. Some research evidence is available, but the validity of the data remains questionable.

Most reviews of the research data in this area (for example, Meltzoff and Kornreich, 1970; Garfield, 1978; Parloff et al, 1978; Orlinsky and Howard, 1980) have been highly critical of both the limited quantity and quality of the studies that have been conducted. Among the methodological problems they have identified as possibly contributing to the lack of research clarity include: the failure of most investigators to use control groups; use of small samples drawn from varied populations; and lack of random assignment (Maffeo, 1979; Parloff et al, 1978). As Parloff and colleagues (1978) note, most of the studies on gender-matching and psychotherapy outcome were not originally designed to investigate this particular problem and so the designs and methods which have been used are far from ideal.

Another major problem in this area of research is the fact that analogue studies comprise a good deal of the research that has been conducted. As Jones and Zoppel (1982) note, "frequently these studies involve single interview situations employing subjects drawn from college populations, or, they are investigations of therapists' attitudes and expectations that rely, for example, on ratings of hypothetical case descriptions." These authors question how effectively studies of this sort capture meaningful dimensions of psychotherapy. Naturalistic designs that reflect the process and effectiveness of psychotherapy as it is actually conducted are clearly superior (Maffeo, 1979). However, most studies of treatment situations have been limited to relatively small samples.

Research on gender-matching and psychotherapy has generally tended to focus on three main topics: the presence or the absence of sex-role bias and stereotyping in psychotherapists' attitudes; the effect of therapist gender on psychotherapy process; and the relationship between therapist and patient gender and psychotherapy outcome. Findings from each of these areas will be summarized and implications of these findings for the therapeutic alliance will be discussed.

Sex-Role Bias and Stereotyping

The majority of studies on gender-matching in psychotherapy have focused on the problem of sex-role bias and stereotyping in psychotherapists' attitudes. Some attention has been paid to problems of sex bias influencing diagnosis as well as method and duration of treatment, but the primary focus has been on the attempt to document whether psychotherapists do, in fact, harbor stereotyped attitudes regarding so-called "appropriate" sex-role behaviors which might negatively affect their clinical practice with women. There has also been interest in determining whether male therapists hold more biased attitudes toward their female patients than do female therapists. The assumption is that if male therapists do hold more prejudicial attitudes regarding women than do female therapists, they may be less helpful than their female counterparts and might even bring psychological harm to the female patients they treat. Different standards of "ideal" behavior for men and women may result in psychotherapist's discouraging certain types of actions in women, such as those which might be labeled "aggressive" or "assertive" (Ticho, 1972; Friedman, 1977).

Broverman and colleagues' (1970) early and highly influential study in this area showed that mental health professinals of both genders indeed did hold different concepts of mental health for male and female clients. Seventy-nine psychiatrists, psychologists and social workers were asked to describe "a mature, healthy, socially competent" female, male, and adult (gender unspecified). Based on responses to a Sex-Role Stereotype Questionnaire, therapists were found to believe that emotionally healthy women were less independent, less adventurous, less aggressive, less competitive, more emotional and more submissive than the emotionally healthy male. In addition, these researchers found that both male and female therapists were less likely to ascribe traits of a healthy adult (gender unspecified) to a healthy woman than to a healthy man. Subsequent studies (Miller, 1974; Bowman, 1976; Neulinger et al, 1976; and Tanney and Birk, 1976) have supported this finding of sex-role stereotyping among both male and female clinicians.

Other studies, however, have shown that sex-role stereotyping is more pronounced among male therapists than among their female counterparts. For example, Persons (1973) found that male counselors-in-training predicted higher prestige occupations for the same clinical protocol when the subject was said to be male, than when the subject was said to be female. Also, in a series of studies (Maslin and Davis, 1975; Delk and Ryan, 1975, 1977; Kahn, 1977; Aslin, 1977) aimed at extending Broverman and colleagues' (1970) findings, it was determined that male therapists were more likely than female therapists to hold stereotypically feminine standards for emotionally healthy females. In a study conducted by Fabrikant (1974) in which mental health clinicians were asked to respond to questions about various sex-role traits and behaviors, it emerged that the majority of male therapists—in contrast to the majority of women therapists and patients in the study—believed that most women could be satisfied and fulfilled by the wife/mother role alone. Observing the behavior of male trainees in psychotherapy supervision, Alonso and Rutan (1978) similarly noted a "subtle but persistent absence of data regarding ambition, creativity, financial planning and long-term career goals in the material male therapists presented on their female patients," leading these authors to conclude that the male therapists in their sample held traditional female sex-role stereotypes.

It should be noted that there are serious limitations on the conclusions that can be drawn from the data on sex-role bias and stereotyping. Most of the studies are analogue studies that may not generalize to the clinical situation. In addition, many of the studies discussed above were conducted at least a decade ago, which probably limits their utility at the present time. Since the past decade has been a period of considerable change in terms of attitudes regarding "appropriate" roles and behaviors for women, studies conducted as little as five years ago may already be outdated.

Psychotherapy Process

A number of authors have theorized that gender-matching in psychotherapy will facilitate processes that will positively influence outcome. Process studies on therapist and patient gender have provided interesting empirical data regarding variables that may be involved in these processes; but they are few in number and have generally been derived from studies of counseling rather than psychotherapy. Findings from these studies (for example, Brooks, 1974; Grantham, 1973; Hill, 1975; Fuller, 1963) suggest that therapist gender may influence the expression of affect, with women therapists on the average demonstrating a superior capacity to facilitate such expression. Studies show that in therapeutic dyads including a woman, there is more self-disclosure and more display of emotion than in male dyads. Furthermore, expression of feelings seems to increase in pairs containing at least one woman (Fuller, 1963). Hill (1975) and Aries (1976) both found women therapists to be more active and empathic, with a tendency to elicit more feelings from their clients than male therapists.

This handful of process studies provides some insight into variables that may influence treatment outcomes, suggesting that therapist gender may influence patient expression of feelings, self-disclosure and self-explanation. Generalizations are difficult, however, since higher scores on one or another of these variables have been reported for some same-sex dyads (Hill, 1975), for opposite-sex dyads (Brooks, 1974) and for dyads that include a woman as either a patient or therapist (Fuller, 1963). For example, Persons et al (1974) found that women clients were especially responsive to women therapists and males to male therapists in terms of patients' post-therapy descriptions of therapy process. In addition, results of this research are confounded, since there is no control for other therapist variables, including experience and status of the therapist.

Psychotherapy Outcome

Studies of the outcome of psychotherapeutic treatment present a more equivocal picture of the influence of gender match on psychotherapy. The most direct way to assess the influence of gender-matching on therapeutic outcome is to review the results of outcome studies that focus on the predictive value of this variable. Data on the influence of gender-matching on therapeutic outcome are sparse, with reviews of the literature providing varying conclusions. For example, Luborsky et al (1971) assert that superior results occur in psychotherapy when the therapist and patient are matched in terms of gender. In contrast, other reviewers of the outcome literature (for example, Meltzoff and Kornreich, 1970; Garfield, 1978; Parloff et al, 1978; Orlinsky and Howard 1980) feel that because the data are inconsistent, a clear relationship between the gender composition of a therapeutic dyad and outcome cannot be established at this time.

Some investigators assert that gender-matching may be important for only specific subgroups of patients. Based on responses to questionnaires sent to all women members of the American Psychiatric Association and an equal number of randomly selected male members on the significance of therapist gender in the treatment of special groups of patients, Ivey (1960) suggested that gender-matching in psychotherapy may be particularly important for adolescents, patients with identification problems, marital and/or sexual problems and homosexual patients, although he notes that the majority of women respondents, unlike their male colleagues, thought a homosexual patient should be treated by a therapist of the opposite sex. Scher (1975) also concluded that for some types of problems, such as sex role identity difficulties, it might be advisable to match clients and therapists on the basis of gender.

Empirical studies of psychotherapy outcome in actual psychotherapy situations are not only somewhat inconsistent in their findings but are also limited in number. Studies generally favor pairing women patients with female therapists, although this finding is not universal. Investigating the relationship between therapist and patient gender on ratings of patients' symptom relief and satisfaction with therapy, Scher (1975) found no gender differences. Strassberg and Anchor (1977) similarly found no significant differences in male versus female trainee therapist's ratings of improvement for clients of both genders. In contrast, Hill (1975) found that clients of both genders treated at a university counseling center reported greater satisfaction with therapy when they had been seen by female rather than male clinicians. In a retrospective outcome study using university patient ratings of their therapies, Kirshner et al (1978) also found that both male and female patients reported greater levels of satisfaction and improvement from therapy when their therapists had been women rather than men.

In a similar vein, Cartwright and Lerner (1963) reported that, when the therapist is experienced, same-sex pairs have better therapist-rated outcomes than do gender-mixed dyads. In a study of the relationship between gender-matching and patient satisfaction, Howard et al (1970) found that female patients seen by female therapists have more helpful experiences and express greater satisfaction with treatment than those seen by male therapists. In studies of women patients, Orlinsky and Howard (1976, 1980) found no primary effects due to gender-matching, but did find significant interactions when certain antecedent patient characteristics such as age, marital status and diagnosis were considered. They found that young, single, depressed women had significantly better outcomes when they were treated by female rather than male therapists.

In a major study aimed at assessing the impact of client and therapist gender on psychotherapy process and outcome using relatively large samples of therapists and patients, Jones and Zoppel (1982) found a number of significant effects associated with the gender composition of the therapy dyad. Based on retrospective reports using both interview and rating scale data derived from actual patients treated in clinical settings, these investigators reported the following findings: Therapists in same-gender pairings were able to achieve neutrality more readily than therapists in mixed-sex dyads; female clients in same-sex pairings experienced greater emotional intensity than those in mixed-sex dyads; female therapists in general were able to achieve more effective therapeutic alliances than their male counterparts; female therapists were rated as more effective than male therapist in terms of their actual therapy behavior by former patients; both male and female therapists rated their patients, regardless of gender, as having improved as a consequence of therapy; and women therapists rated themselves as achieving more successful outcomes, particularly with women patients.

Summary and Discussion of Research Findings

As many of the reviewers of the research literature caution, it may be unwise to put too much stock in the findings that have been obtained thus far. A major difficulty with these studies is that the conclusions about the effects of therapist gender on therapy process and outcome have been made from studies not originally designed for this purpose and are therefore complicated by problems such as lack of random assignment, little attention to outcome measures, confounding by other variables (Parloff et al, 1978) and poor generalizability to clinical settings.

Research on sex-role bias and stereotyping has come under particularly heavy fire. According to Smith (1980), it is the psychological literature itself that demonstrates problematic bias, rather than clinicians. Based on a meta-analysis of both published and unpublished studies of sex bias in counseling and psychotherapy, she found little evidence of sex-role bias toward women. According to her findings, published studies reveal only a small sex-bias effect against women; unpublished studies show "the same magnitude of bias toward men and a degree of rigor in research designs at least as good as that evident in published studies." Smith asserts that the motivation to conduct this type of research has frequently been ideological, and notes that small but significant effects became sweeping, categorical conclusions that were then widely disseminated. She concludes that journals have shown a tendency to publish studies that have shown a sex-bias effect, regardless of the study's quality.

Furthermore, even if psychotherapists, and especially male clinicians, do hold stereotypic views of women, it is not clear that such attitudes have significant effects in the process and outcome of psychotherapy. Chesler (1971) and Maffeo (1979), for example, insist that stereotypes do invade and negatively influence treatment; but Whitley (1979) cautions against such conclusions. Emphasizing social psychological observations that people's attitudes toward an object bear little relationship to their behavior, he asserts that there is little evidence to suggest that mental health care providers' sex-role stereotypes affect their professional judgments or treatment goals. He suggests that clinicians may adhere more to therapeutic norms that stress autonomy and the development of the patient's personal values and talents than to personal cultural biases and stereotypes. Thus, in terms of the literature on sex-role bias and stereotyping, it is not only unclear whether substantive therapist prejudice against female patients actually exists, but if it does exist, whether it translates into detrimental therapeutic behavior in the actual clinical setting.

It is similarly difficult to draw conclusions from studies of gender-matching and psychotherapy process. As already noted, process studies in this area have generally been investigations of counseling rather than psychotherapy, and therefore little is known about the effect of therapist and patient gender on actual psychotherapy process. Furthermore, it is not clear how the findings regarding psychotherapy process relate to outcome. Most of the studies in this area suggest that dyads including a woman are more emotionally expressive than all-male pairs, but they do not necessarily demonstrate that all-female dyads are the most emotionally expressive therapist-patient combination. Even if they did, one could not necessarily conclude that this would result in superior outcomes. One might speculate that greater expression of patient affect might imply greater patient involvement, a variable which has been positively correlated with outcome (Gomes-Schwartz 1978). This hypothesis was empirically tested by Jones and Zoppel (1982), who found that female patients in same-gender pairings tended to experience greater emotional intensity in psychotherapy and that this intensity was significantly correlated with outcome.

Data on gender-matching suggest that women patients who are treated by female rather than male psychotherapists are likely to be more satisfied with their therapy experience than women who are seen by male therapists. There are no studies that demonstrate such trends with male therapists (Kirschner et al, 1978). In addition, findings from outcome studies do suggest that for certain subgroups of women (that is, single, younger women), having a female therapist may result in greater satisfaction with and benefit from psychotherapy, although the data here are sparse and sometimes inconsistent. According to Orlinsky and Howard (1980), who seem to represent the majority viewpoint of reviewers of these data, there is "not much directly relevant research in this area, not much consistent quality, and not much by way of results."

Only one of the studies reviewed here (Jones and Zoppel, 1982) was done since the Orlinsky and Howard article was published. This study attempted to improve upon earlier work by investigating actual psychotherapy as it is practiced in the field with relatively large samples of therapists and patients. However, this study has several limitations, including varied length of treatment (from eight to more than 100 sessions), sampling problems (the use of patients from different clinic settings), the retrospective nature of the study, and the preponderence in the sample of young, single women (that is, those most likely to benefit from seeing a woman therapist. This study suggests that sex bias is not sufficient to explain the complexity of the impact of gender on psychotherapy. Female patients did not directly identify any sort of sex bias in this study. They judged women therapists as forming better therapeutic alliances, which the authors felt might be related to differences in women therapist's emotional capacities, abilities and skills. It should be kept in mind that although it did have some impact, gender was not an "overriding" influence in psychotherapy outcome.

Based on the inconsistency of findings, there seems to be a clear need for further investigation of the relationship between therapist/patient gender and therapy outcome. Studies of both short- and long-term psychotherapy, which use opposite and same-sex pairings and which employ proper control groups, would contribute significantly to our knowledge in this area. Prospective designs with adequate sample sizes and improved measures of social functioning that reflect new roles for both sexes are needed. Good studies should focus on multidimensional measures of outcome, such as social functioning, work functioning and self-esteem, as well as symptoms. Controlling for other variables such as therapist discipline, therapeutic skill and experience, age, type and length of therapy are also necessary to improve the quality of studies.

Therapeutic Alliance

It has been well established that important sex differences exist in many psychological variables, ranging from cognitive functioning to personality characteristics (Maccoby and Jacklin, 1974). It might be reasonable to expect that the implication of such extensive differences as these would extend into the realm of psychological intervention processes, notwithstanding the failure of past methodologically flawed studies to produce consistent findings (Maracek and Johnson, 1980). The most recent evidence (Jones and Zoppel, 1982), however, suggests that the gender variable may have sufficient impact on the treatment process to serve as a vehicle for further investigation of elements of critical importance for psychotherapy in general. For example, one of the most important findings of the Jones and Zoppel study (1982) is that a factor analysis of the patient interview items yielded an item "therapeutic alliance," which accounted for 67.6 percent of the variance in outcome, and that women therapists, in the perception of both male and female patients, tend to create more effective therapeutic alliances.

Clinical and theoretical speculation in the psychoanalytic literature may help shed light on the ways in which the gender of the patient and therapist may influence the therapeutic relationship. Gender effects in psychotherapy may be most profound in the intrapsychic and interpersonal experience of the therapeutic alliance. Mogul (1982) skillfully reviewed psychoanalytic positions regarding gender of the analyst and found that there is no consensus among psychoanalysts about the effects of gender on the psychoanalytic therapeutic relationship. There is some agreement that gender may influence the content and sequence of the transference in analyzable neurotic patients, but it may not significantly influence the outcome of the analysis (Mogul, 1982).

Different problems may arise at different stages of therapy with same-sex and opposite-sex therapist-patient pairs. For example, there is some evidence that gender effects on the therapeutic alliance may be different in less intensive and/or shorter-term psychotherapies, where more partial transference reactions are present and where symptom alleviation may be of foremost concern. Some research studies suggest that female patient-therapist dyads may be more helpful and satisfying in shorter-term work. Zetzel (1970) examined therapist gender in distinguishing between outcomes in psychotherapy and psychoanalysis. She postulates that for a woman, psychotherapy with a woman therapist may lead to increased self-esteem, positive identification and positive transference. Goz (1973) also reports that women may experience greater advantages with women therapists in short-term psychotherapy.

Some researchers suggest that women are more likely to possess certain traits, such as greater sensitivity, nurturance and patience (Blain, 1968; Notman, 1965; Roeske, 1973) that might make them better psychotherapists than men, or more helpful to certain patients. For cultural reasons, women may more easily assume "masculine" traits, while men may find acquisition of "feminine" qualities as difficult or threatening (Kaplan, 1979). This may explain why men have been reported to have more difficult countertransference problems with women patients. (Kaplan, 1984; Orlinsky and Howard, 1976). Of course, the effects of gender must also be understood in the context of the time course of psychotherapy. In longer-term therapy and analysis in which preoedipal issues may become more salient, women seeing female therapists or analysts may experience more difficulties than their counterparts who are treated by men. Thus, patient-therapist gender match may have differentiating effects on the therapy process, depending upon the phase of the psychotherapy.

Some contemporary theorists have suggested that there are significant differences between male and female world views (Kaplan, 1984; Miller, 1976; Gilligan, 1982), which may affect the conduct of psychotherapy. Men and women have different courses of psychological development, different modes of communication, different experiences at home and in the work force, and have "different values by which moral reasoning is constructed" (Kaplan, 1984). Miller (1976) asserts that these differences stem from different concepts of the self in which women's reactions are more often relational, while men's responses may be more influenced by an autonomous and separate sense of self. Kaplan (1984) believes that this theory translates into different therapeutic behaviors for male and female therapists, but cautions that careful research is necessary to assess the validity of this theory. She suggests that a woman therapist "might be especially cognizant of present, interactional considerations in her clinical work and more receptive to the client's ongoing affective experience." Furthermore, she suggests that the female therapist may be more empathic and sensitive to the "danger of overstepping boundaries . . . and likely to check out the meaning of her decisions for her client—or wonder if a decision was the best one." A male therapist "might build less on affective connectedness and more on questioning or interpreting the client's remarks. Affect might be handled more in terms of its transferential implications and less as a process of mutual exploration within the ongoing therapy relationship." She also speculates that male therapists may have to pay special attention to relational issues in the therapeutic relationship with women patients, a formulation that is supported by Orlinsky and Howard's (1978) study of 118 female clients. In this sample, more eroticized affection, anger, depression and inhibition was reported by patients seeing male therapists than by those seeing female therapists. Following the therapy, women who had been in treatment with male therapists viewed themselves as less open, less self-possessed, and more self-critical than did women who had been in treatment with female therapists.

Kaplan (1984) further hypothesizes that a key component of female psychotherapist's success in establishing a relational bond may be their capacity for empathy; that is, "the capacity to internalize and appreciate the affective life of another while maintaining a sense of self to permit cognitive restructuring of the experience." This capacity is critical to the formation of a therapeutic alliance. Orlinsky and Howard (1976) have written that "the positive quality of the relational bond, as exemplified in the reciprocal interpersonal behavior of the participants, is more clearly related to patient improvement than are any of the particular treatment techniques used by therapists."

Finally, men and women have different experiences over the course of the life cycle. There are certain areas of experience that people of the same sex share that may not be well understood by people of the opposite sex: for example, gender linked, reproduction related life events. It is possible that if such issues are the focus of treatment, the therapeutic alliance may be enhanced by same-sex therapist-patient dyads. This may be especially true if the treatment is short term.

It may be specifically hypothesized that most patients will experience a similar outcome with a therapist of either sex. However, there may be differences for some groups of patients where a therapist of a paticular gender would be more beneficial to the outcome of the psychotherapy. The influence of gender on psychotherapy outcome will not be clarified until appropriate subtypes of patients have been identified who will benefit from a particular gender match with a therapist. Operational criteria need to be developed to clearly identify subgroups of women and men who will respond selectively to psychotherapy with the same-sex or opposite-sex therapist.

In the research literature, the male-male therapist-patient match has been relatively underaddressed. A number of issues that have been discussed for female-female therapist-patient pairing, such as role modeling, similarity of certain life experiences and empathy, are not well described for men. It is recommended that researchers investigate the impact of all male dyads in future research.

Finally, gender match alone will not override technique in producing good therapeutic outcome. There are multiple interactions that occur in the therapeutic process. It must be kept in mind that gender match alone accounts for only a part of the variance in outcome. Many other factors, such as therapist characteristics (including experience, skill and personality style) and patient characteristics (including personality style and developmental level), are important variables that must be considered to influence the therapeutic alliance. For example, gender effects have been shown to be less apparent with experienced therapists than with inexperienced therapists (Howard and Orlinsky, 1979; Kirschner et al, 1978). In addition, Horowitz et al (1984) note that there is an interaction between the therapeutic approach and a patient's pretherapy developmental level and degree of motivation to determine outcome.

Clinical Implications and Training Issues

This review provides strong if somewhat inconsistent evidence for the impact of gender on the process (particularly on the therapeutic alliance) and on the outcome of psychotherapy. The demonstrated effect of gender in psychotherapeutic treatment has important implications for clinical and research training in psychotherapy. Training programs should make necessary changes to adequately incorporate and integrate current knowledge about the effects of gender on psychotherapy. Didactic training and supervision should emphasize sex and gender-related psychological, biological and sociocultural differences over the life cycle. Particular emphasis should be given to understanding commonalities and differences between men's and women's psychological realities, and their biological life courses. In addition, there should be encouragement of open and active discussion of such information, and of the attendant social and political issues.

Changes in the practical aspects of psychotherapy training are also necessary. Standard approaches to teaching psychotherapy tend to emphasize cognitive elements such as psychodynamic formulations and intervention techniques. Greater emphasis needs to be placed on relational bonds and the development of a capacity for empathic understanding. In addition, residents should treat patients of both genders and should be supervised by both men and women. Such supervision helps to deal with cultural blind spots, countertransference problems and other gender issues (Nadelson and Notman, 1977; Alonso and Rutman, 1978). This emphasis on the importance of sex and gender-related issues in didactic training and supervision should commence at the beginning of residency training and continue throughout the training program, in order to provide a foundation for continued work in understanding similarities and differences in women's and men's experiences. Only through the encouragement of such explicit awareness of gender, gender roles and gender stereotypes is it possible for psychotherapists engaged in training and treatment to move toward a more genuine understanding and acceptance of such issues, and to have this understanding reflected in clinical practice and research.

RACE

The role played by the therapist's race and the impact of racial matching of the therapist/patient dyad on the process and outcome of psychotherapy is an area of particular social concern. This topic has been examined in a number of articles (Parloff et al, 1978; Sattler, 1977; Harrison, 1975; Griffith, 1977), to which the reader is referred for comprehensive reviews of this subject. The influence of race is a controversial issue that is highly vulnerable to biases and misperceptions. As with gender and psychotherapy, many conceptions about race and psychotherapy are influenced by ideology and must await systematic investigation. Although there are special concerns affecting psychotherapy for different racial and ethnic groups, the psychotherapy research literature in this area is very limited. The research that has been done on race and psychotherapy is relatively recent and has focused primarily on the black patient and/or therapist (Parloff et al, 1978). Therefore, this review will examine selected psychotherapy process and outcome research relevant to the treatment of black patients.

Research on racial factors in psychotherapy has generally been of three types: epidemiological studies that examine numbers of patients, clinical diagnosis, method and length of treatment; analogue studies that examine same and differing race interviewer-interviewee interactions in a laboratory setting; and outcome studies of actual psychotherapy.

Epidemiological studies reveal that blacks: use psychiatric services at a lower rate than expected based on their proportion in the population in the community; they tend to receive more severe diagnoses; and they are given different treatments than are white patients (Jackson et al, 1974; Mayo, 1974). Some researchers (Sue, 1977; Sue et al, 1974) challenge these findings, reporting that blacks are only slightly more likely to receive less intensive forms of treatment. Nonetheless, Jones and Zoppel (1982) point out that one finding is consistent across studies: Black patients remain in treatment for shorter periods of time than do white patients. Socioeconomic factors have been the focus of much of the research on premature termination. It is important to distinguish the effects of social class and other cultural factors from the influence of race in evaluating the research literature (Varghese, 1983). For example, Jones (1974) documented that members of lower socioeconomic groups are less likely to be accepted for treatment and to remain in treatment than are members of higher socioeconomic groups. Black patients may be particularly affected in these situations (Jackson et al, 1974; Raynes and Warren, 1971) because a greater proportion may be in lower socioeconomic groups. However, some research exists suggesting that social class is not the most critical factor determining continuation in therapy by black patients. Sue (1977) demonstrated that even when education and income were controlled, over 50 percent of a sample of approximately 1,000 black clients did not continue in psychotherapy after the first session.

Patient-therapist matching on the race variable is the second major focus of research. The most broadly investigated question has been the effect of a white therapist-black patient match. Another important issue is whether black therapist-black patient match has a more beneficial effect on the development of the therapeutic alliance and on the outcome of psychotherapy.

The role of social bias has been raised as a factor influencing psychotherapy for black patients. Parloff et al (1978) review the role of social biases in therapist's attitudes on the therapeutic relationship. White therapist's racial biases and stereotypes about blacks have been investigated as a variable affecting a successful therapeutic relationship. One study (Bloombaum et al, 1968) found that 75 percent of therapists responding to structured interviews had beliefs and attitudes reflecting racial biases and stereotypes. Such therapists' attitudes may also be responsible in part for the higher dropout rates and less frequent meetings that have been reported for black patients. For example, a study by Yamamoto et al (1967) demonstrated that therapists who scored high on ethnocentricity were not as likely to see their black patients six or more times in treatment, while they were likely to see their white patients at least this number of times.

As with studies of gender and psychotherapy, most studies that have examined the effects of race in psychotherapy have been analogue studies. Many of these studies have used nonpatient (usually college student) "clients" (Banks, 1972; Banks, Berenson and Carkhuff, 1967; Cimbolic, 1972; Bryson and Cody, 1973; Grantham, 1973; Ewing, 1974; Gardner, 1972; Carkhuff and Pierce, 1967), and most have focused on the process of the interview, although some included measures of outcome, patient satisfaction and willingness to return to psychotherapy (Cimbolic, 1972; Grantham, 1973; Ewing, 1974). The majority of these studies suggest that blacks respond better (Grantham, 1973), feel better understood (Bryson and Cody, 1973), engage in more self-exploration and experience a better rapport with black counselors than white counselors (Banks, 1972; Bryson and Cody, 1973). In one study that used an actual patient population in a single interview situation (Carkhuff and Pierce, 1967), significant effects of patient and therapist race and social class matching were reported. This study was flawed, however, by major methodological weaknesses.

Again, as with the gender and psychotherapy research literature, uncertainty exists about the extent to which these analogue studies should be generalized to the actual psychotherapy situation. In addition, reviewers reach different conclusions based on the same research. Griffith (1977), while acknowledging the limitations of these studies, states that they provide major support for the negative impact of racial differences on therapy outcome. Sattler (1977) notes, however, that there is some evidence to suggest that race has little effect on nonclinical interviews. Jones (1978) seriously questions the generalizability of findings based on these analogue studies, given his own findings of changes on process measures from initial to subsequent sessions of psychotherapy.

The few studies of actual psychotherapy with black patients, most of which involved small samples, have shown similar but somewhat weaker effects than the analogue studies (Jones, 1982; Jones, 1978; Krebs, 1971). The results of these studies are inconclusive. Parloff et al (1978), in their review of these studies, present evidence on both sides. For example, Lerner (1972), reporting on the treatment of black and white patients including many disturbed patients and patients from lower socioeconomic classes, concludes that white therapists can be helpful to black patients. In a review of the literature, Sattler (1977) describes a number of studies that generally report benefits from black patient-white therapist matches. The lack of a comparison group of black patients treated by black therapists seriously flaws these studies. Also, Winston et al (1972) found that a sample of black patients treated in individual psychotherapy by white psychiatrists in an inpatient milieu showed more improvement than a control group of white patients during hospitalization. However, these effects could not be separated from the effects of the milieu where many of the nursing staff were black. Two additional studies (Goldberg, 1973; Winston et al, 1972) report greater improvement in black than in white patients seen by white therapists.

On the other side, Warren et al (1973) administered structured interviews to black and white families treated by white therapists in a child guidance clinic. While this study has been cited as demonstrating that black families found therapy to be less beneficial than whites, it is unclear that this conclusion can be drawn from the data. Only one measure (40 percent of the patients felt that therapy had been impeded by the therapists' inability to understand the patient) among many assessments demonstrated significant differences. In a large-scale study of black outpatients seen by white therapists, Krebs (1971) found that blacks attended therapy sessions at a significantly lower rate and tended to terminate earlier than white patients.

Jones (1978) investigated psychotherapy process and outcome in a naturalistic study examining a small number of racially similar and dissimilar patient-therapist dyads. While this study is limited by the homogeneity of the sample (well-educated women) and the fact that assessments were made after the first ten sessions of open-ended therapy, it is nonetheless of importance. Contrary to expectations, the outcome of therapy was not affected by racial similarities or differences in patient/therapist match; however, the quality of the interaction was affected by the race of the therapist and patient. A factor analysis of therapy process ratings yielded a number of factors that varied significantly across racial pairings. The significant factors were related to the quality and depth of therapeutic experience and the presence of race as an important issue in treatment. This finding has social significance, as well as intriguing theoretical and clinical implications. It suggests that different qualities of patient-therapist interaction may still lead to the same outcome.

In a recent study of the impact of race on psychotherapy, and the only one where longer-term therapy is systematically examined, Jones (1982) studied 169 black and white patients, half in racially similar therapist-patient dyads and half in racially dissimilar pairings. Employing a retrospective design, the therapists of these patients furnished an evaluation and a description of their perceptions of their clients. Patients were seen for a mean of 31 treatment hours. Results showed that white therapists generally rated their patients as psychologically more impaired in areas of symptomatology and in quality and nature of family relationships than did black therapists. This was especially true for black patients. Crawford (1969) showed that black and white therapists have different conceptions of mental illness, and that certain types of behavior that may be seen as "disturbance" by white psychotherapists may be viewed as adaptive among blacks (Grier and Cobb, 1968). Jones (1982) concluded that it appears likely that cultural and value differences are reflected in the ratings of adjustment by black and white therapists. The most important finding of this study (Jones, 1982), that therapist-patient match has little influence on outcome in longer-term psychotherapy, is consistent with research on actual treatment situations that have not shown racial differences.

In interpreting the results of this study (Jones, 1982), it is important to note that patients who did not continue in treatment for more than eight therapy sessions were not included. Yet, it may be precisely in this early phase of treatment that racial matching is most likely to have its greatest impact. Jones (1982) suggests that if a white therapist can establish an effective therapeutic alliance relatively rapidly, successful outcomes can be achieved.

In summary, more systematic investigation is needed of the effects of various therapist/patient pairings across different racial and ethnic groups on the process and outcome of psychotherapy. Such studies should control for additional variables such as social class and gender. There are still too few studies available comparing cross-racial or cross-cultural therapist-patient matches over time to draw definitive conclusions.

Clinical Implications and Training Issues

The data reflecting the influence of the racial variable on the outcome of psychotherapy is limited; and the question, like that of gender and psychotherapy, needs more systematic investigation. What is evident and important from this literature is that it seems to bear out a finding of the more general therapeutic alliance literature. The early phase (in this case the first eight sessions in psychotherapy) is critical to the formation of a therapeutic alliance, and it is here that the influence of the racial variable seems most profound. If patients do not drop out of treatment during this initial phase, the effect of race on outcome appears to be much less significant.

It may be that certain cultural forms of expression and characteristic patterns of thought are essential to establishing the early sense of positive regard and trust in the therapeutic relationship, which is an important factor in keeping a patient in treatment. Psychotherapists working with patients of different ethnic backgrounds need to be aware of their patient's feelings about racial and cultural differences in order to facilitate effective treatment and to understand potential transference reactions. In addition, the critical role of countertransference and empathy (Jones, 1984) must be considered. Failures in empathy may lead to an increased likelihood of negative countertransference reactions, which may involve antitherapeutic cultural stereotypes (for example, the patient being "unmotivated for treatment"). A therapist's self-knowledge and continual self-awareness are important factors in preventing these personal reactions from interfering in the therapy. This self-understanding, as well as cultural understanding on the part of the therapist, is of basic importance in cross-racial therapist-patient matches.

In summary, just as with the issue of gender, training in psychotherapy should attend to cultural, ethnic and racial issues. Didactic and supervisory teaching should include: emphasis on understanding the patient's racial and ethnic background; exposure to minority faculty and clinical supervisors; and seminars on racial and cultural issues. In addition, there is a pressing need to train more minority clinicians and researchers who can bring their backgrounds and experiences to the training of psychotherapists and to the treatment of minority patients. Jones et al (1970) point out that race is often "glossed over or avoided" during residency training. Supervisory and didactic sessions where racial and ethnic issues are openly discussed are critical to the training of psychotherapists. Varghese (1983) notes that the trainee's failure to bring up these issues in supervision is matched by the supervisor's unwillingness to discuss them. Open discussion of racial and cultural similarities and differences in training will encourage awareness in trainees of their own attitudes and countertransference reactions, as well as increase their sensitivity to racial or culturally related transference reactions in their patients.

As a final note, while a review of the research literature on the effects of gender and race on psychotherapy demonstrate effects of these two variables on the process and outcome of psychotherapy, it should be emphasized that these studies are based on group comparisons of therapists and patients and do not tell us a great deal about what might be most effective or helpful with a particular patient. Psychotherapy is a highly individualized endeavor. Generalizations made from the research literature about gender and race on the process and outcome of psychotherapy may not apply to every patient. The effects of gender and race on psychotherapy are embedded in a continually evolving sociocultural context. In part, the individual therapist's and patient's experience of this context will govern his or her response to gender, ethnic similarities, or differences in psychotherapy. Clearly, in psychotherapy practice, research and training, the effects of gender and race deserve careful attention as significant factors affecting therapeutic interaction.

REFERENCES

Abramowitz SI, Roback HB, Schwartz JM, et al: Sex bias in psychotherapy: a failure to confirm. Am J Psychiatry 133:706-709, 1976

Alonso A, Rutan J: Cross-sex supervision for cross-sex therapy. Am J Psychiatry 135:928-931, 1978

Aries E: Interaction patterns and themes of male, female, and mixed groups. Small Group Behavior 7:7-18, 1976

Aslin A: Feminist and community mental health center psychotherapists' expectations of mental health for women. Sex Roles 3:537-545, 1977

Banks G, Berenson BG, Carkhuff RR: The effects of counselor race and training upon counseling process with Negro clients in initial interviews. J Clin Psychol 23:70-72, 1967

Banks WM: The differential effects of race and social class in helping. J Clin Psychol 28:90-92, 1972

Barrett CJ, Berg PI, Eaton EM, et al: Implications of women's liberation and the future of psychotherapy. Psychotherapy: Theory, Research and Practice 11:11-15, 1974

Bart PB: Sexism and social silence: from the gilded cage to the iron cage, or the perils of Pauline. Journal of Marriage and the Family 33:734-745, 1971

Bergin AE, Lambert MJ: The evaluation of therapeutic outcomes, in Handbook of Psychotherapy and Behavior Change: An Empirical Analysis, 2nd ed. Edited by Garfield SL and Bergin AE. New York, Wiley, 1978

Blain D: Women in psychiatry, in Careers in Psychiatry. Edited by Burch C. New York, Macmillan Publishing Co, 1968

Block C: Diagnostic and treatment issues for black patients. The Clinical Psychologist 37:51-54, 1984

Bloombaum M, Yamamoto J, James Q: Cultural stereotyping among psychotherapists. J Consult Clin Psychol 32:99, 1968

Boulware DW, Holmes DS: Preference for therapists and related expectancies. J Consult Clin Psychol 35:269-277, 1970

Bowman P: The relationship between attitudes toward women and the treatment of activity and passivity. Dissertation Abstracts International, 1976, 36, 5779B

Brodsky A: The consciousness-raising group as a model for therapy with women. Psychotherapy: Theory, Research and Practice. 10:24-29, 1973

Brodsky A, Hare-Mustin R: Psychotherapy and women: priorities for research, in Women and Psychotherapy: An Assessment of Research and Practice. Edited by Brodsky A, Hare-Mustin R. New York, The Guilford Press, 1980

Brooks L: Interactive effects of sex and status of self-disclosure. Journal of Counseling Psychology 21:469-474, 1974

Broverman I, Broverman D, Clarkson F, et al: Sex-role stereotypes and clinical judgments of mental health. J Consult Clin Psychol 34:1-7, 1970

Bryson S, Cody J: Relationship of race and level of understanding between counselor and client. Journal of Counseling Psychology 20:495-498, 1973

Carkhuff RR, Pierce R: Differential effects of therapist race and social class upon patient depth of self-exploration in the initial clinical interview. Journal of Consulting Psychology 31:632-634, 1967

Cartwright R, Lerner B: Empathy, need to change, and improvement with psychotherapy. Journal of Consulting Psychology 27:138-144, 1963

Chesler P: Marriage and psychotherapy, in The Radical Therapist. Edited by Agel J. New York, Collective Ballantine Books, 1971

Chester P: Women and Madness. New York, Doubleday, 1972

Cimbolic P: Counselor race and experience effects on black clients. J Consult Clin Psychol 39:328-332, 1972

Crawford F: Variations between Negroes and whites in concepts of mental illness, its treatment and prevalence, in Changing Perspectives in Mental Illness. Edited by Plog S and Edgerton R. New York, Holt, Rinehart and Winston, 1969

Delk J, Ryan T: Sex-role stereotyping and A-B Therapist status: who is more chauvinistic? J Consult Clin Psychol 43:589, 1975

Delk J, Ryan T: A-B status and sex stereotyping among psychotherapists and patients. J Nerv Ment Dis 164:253-262, 1977

Dent JK: Exploring the psycho-social therapies as revealed by the personalities of effective therapists. DHEW Publication No. (ADM) 77-527, Rockville, MD, National Institute of Mental Health, 1978

Ewing TN: Racial similarity of client and counselor and client satisfaction with counseling. Journal of Counseling Psychology 21:446-449, 1974

Fabrikant B: The psychotherapist and the female patient: perceptions, misconceptions, and chance, in Women in Therapy. Edited by Franks U, Burtle M. New York, Brunner/Mazel, 1974

Fodor IE: Sex role conflict and symptom foundation in women: can behavior therapy help? Psychotherapy: Theory, Research and Practice 11:22-29, 1974a

Fodor IE: The phobic syndrome in women: implications for treatment, in Women in Therapy: New Psychotherapies for a Changing Society. Edited by Franks V and Burle V. New York, Brunner/Mazel 1974b

Friedman HJ: Special problems of women in psychotherapy. Am J Psychother 31:405-416, 1977

Freud S: Female sexuality (1931), in Standard Edition of the Complete Psychological Works of Sigmund Freud, vol. 21. Edited by Strachey J. London, Hogarth, 1961

Fuller F: Influence of sex of counselor and of client on client expressions of feeling. Journal of Counseling Psychology 10:34-40, 1963

Fuller FF: Preferences for male and female counselors. Personnel and Guidance Journal 42:463-467, 1964

Gardner LM: The therapeutic relationship under varying conditions of race. Psychotherapy: Theory, Research and Practice 8:78-87, 1971

Gardner WE: The differential effects of race, education and experience in helping. J Clin Psychol 28:87-89, 1972

Garfield S: Research on client variables in psychotherapy, in Handbook of Psychotherapy and Behavior Change: An Empirical Analysis, 2nd ed. Edited by Garfield S, Bergin A. New York, John Wiley and Sons, 1978

Gilligan C: In a different voice. Cambridge, Harvard University Press, 1982

Glaser K: Women's self-help groups as an alternative to therapy. Psychotherapy: Theory, Research and Practice 13:77-81, 1976

Goldberg M: The black female client, the white psychotherapist: an evaluation of therapy through clients' retrospective reports. Dissertation Abstracts International 33:3302B, 1973

Goldenholz N: The effect of the sex of therapist-client dyad upon outcome of psychotherapy. Dissertation Abstracts International, 36:4687B-4688B, 1976

Goldstein A: Structural Learning Therapy: Toward a Psychotherapy for the Poor. New York, Academic Press, 1973

Gomes-Schwartz B: Effective ingredients in psychotherapy: prediction of outcomes from process variables. J Consult Clin Psychol 46:1023-1035, 1978

Gove WR: The relationship between sex roles, marital status and mental illness. Social Forces 51:34-44, 1972

Goz R: Women patients and women therapists: some issues that come up in psychotherapy. Int J Psychoanal Psychother 2:298-319, 1973

Grantham R: Effects of counselor sex, race, and language style on black students in initial interviews. Journal of Counseling Psychology 20:553-559, 1973

Greenson RR: The technique and practice of psychoanalysis. New York, International Universities Press, 1967

Grier WH, Cobb PM: Black Rage. New York, Basic Books, 1968

Griffith MS: The influence of race on the psychotherapeutic relationship. Psychiatry 40:27-40, 1977

Griffith MS, Jones EE: Race and psychotherapy: changing perspectives, in Current Psychiatric Therapies. Edited by Masserman JH. New York, Grune and Stratton, 1979

Hare-Mustin, R. An appraisal of the relationship between women and psychotherapy: 80 years after the case of Dora. American Psychologist 38:593-601, 1983

Harrison IK: Race as a counselor-client variable in counseling and psychotherapy: a review of the research. The Counseling Psychologist 5:124-133, 1975

Heine, R, Trossman H: Initial expectations of the doctor-patient interaction as a factor in continuance in psychotherapy. Psychiatry 23:275-278, 1960

Hill C: Sex of client and sex and experience level of counselor. Journal of Counseling Psychology 22:6-11, 1975

Horner MS: Toward an understanding of achievement-related conflicts in women. Journal of Social Issues 28:157-175, 1972

Horowitz M, Marmar C, Weiss D, et al: Brief psychotherapy of bereavement reaction: the relationship of process to outcome. Arch Gen Psychiatry 41:438-448, 1984

Howard E, Howard J: Women in institutions: treatment in prisons and mental hospitals, in Women in Therapy. Edited by Franks V, Burtle V. New York, Brunner/Mazel, 1974

Howard K, Orlinsky D: What effect does therapist gender have on outcome for women in psychotherapy? Presentation at the Conference of the American Psychological Association, New York, 1979

Howard K, Orlinsky D, Hill J: The therapist's feeling in the therapeutic process. J Clin Psychol 25:83-93, 1969

Howard K, Orlinsky D, Hill J: Patient's satisfaction in psychotherapy as a function of patient-therapist pairing. Psychotherapy: Theory, Research and Practice 7:130-134. 1970

Ivey E: Significance of the sex of the psychiatrist. Arch Gen Psychiatry 2:622-631, 1960

Jackson AM: Problems experienced by female therapists in establishing an alliance. Psychiatric Annals 3:6-9, 1973a

Jackson AM: Psychotherapy: factors associated with the race of the therapist. Psychotherapy: Theory, Research and Practice 10:273-277, 1973b

Jackson A, Berkowitz H, Farley G: Race as a variable affecting the treatment involvement of children. J Am Acad Child Psychiatry 13:20-31, 1974

Jones BE, Lightfoot OB, Palmer D, et al: Problems of black psychiatric residents in white training institutions. Am J Psychiatry 127:798-803, 1970

Jones EE: Social class and psychotherapy: a critical review of research. Psychiatry 37:307-329, 1974

Jones EE: The effects of race on psychotherapy process and outcome: an exploratory investigation. Psychotherapy: Theory, Research and Practice 15:226-236, 1978

Jones EE: Psychotherapists' impressions of treatment as a function of race. J Clin Psychol 38:722-731, 1982

Jones EE: Some reflections on the black patient and psychotherapy. The Clinical Psychologist 37:62-65, 1984

Jones EE, Korchin SJ: Minority mental health perspectives, in Minority Mental Health. Edited by Jones EE and Korchin SJ. New York, Praeger, 1982

Jones EE, Zoppel C: Impact of client and therapist gender on psychotherapy process and outcome. J Consult Clin Psychol 50:259-272, 1982

Kahn L: Effects of sex and feminist orientation of therapists on clinical judgments. Dissertation Abstracts International 37:3613B, 1977

Kaplan A: Toward an analysis of sex-role related issues in the therapeutic relationship. Psychotherapy 42:112-120, 1979

Kaplan AG: Female or male psychotherapists for women: new formulations. Wellesly College Work in Progress No. 83-02, 1984

Kirsh B: Consciousness-raising groups as therapy, in Women in Therapy. Edited by Franks V and Burtle V. New York, Brunner/Mazel, 1974

Kirshner L, Genack A, Hauser S: Effects of gender on short-term psychotherapy. Psychotherapy: Theory, Research and Practice 15:158-167, 1978

Klauber S: The psychoanalyst as a person. Br J Med Psychol 41:315-322, 1968

Kravitz DF: Consciousness-raising groups and group psychotherapy: alternative mental health resources for women. Psychotherapy: Theory, Research and Practice 13:66-71, 1976

Krebs RL: Some effects of a white institution on black psychiatric outpatients. Am J Orthopsychiatry 41:589-596, 1971

Kronsky BJ: Feminism and psychotherapy. Journal of Contemporary Psychotherapy 3:89-98, 1971

Lazarus AA: Women in behavior therapy, in Women in Therapy: New Psychotherapies for a Changing Society. Edited by Franks V and Burtle V. New York, Brunner/Mazel, 1974

Lerner B: Therapy in the Ghetto: Political Impotence and Personal Disintegration. Baltimore, Johns Hopkins University Press, 1972

Linehan ML, Goldfried MR, Goldfried AP: Assertion therapy: skill training or cognitive restructuring? Behavioral Therapy 10:372-388, 1979

Lorion RP: Research on psychotherapy and behavior change with the disadvantaged: past, present, and future directions, in Handbook of Psychotherapy and Behavior Change. Edited by Garfield SL and Bergin AE. New York, John Wiley, 1978

Luborsky L, Auerbach A, Chandler M, et al: Factors influencing the outcome of psychotherapy: a review of quantitative research. Psychology Bulletin 75:145-184, 1971

Maccoby EE and Jacklin CN: The psychology of sex differences. Stanford, California, Stanford University Press, 1974

Maffeo P: Thoughts on Stricker's "Implications of research for psychotherapeutic treatment of women." American Psychologist 34:690-695, 1979

Marecek J, Johnson M: Gender and the process of therapy, in Women and Psychotherapy: An Assessment of Research and Practice. Edited by Brodsky A, Hare-Mustin R. New York, The Guilford Press, 1980

Marecek J, Kravetz D: Women and mental health: a review of feminist change efforts. Psychiatry 40:323-329, 1977

Maslin A, Davis J: Sex-role stereotyping as a factor in mental health standards among counselors-in-training. Journal of Counseling Psychology 22:87-91, 1975

Mayo J: The significance of sociocultural variables in the psychiatric treatment of black patients. Comprehensive Psychiatry 15:471-482, 1974

Meltzoff J, Kornreich M: Research in Psychotherapy. New York, Atherton Press, 1970

Menaker E: The therapy of women in the light of psychoanalytic theory and the emergence of a new view, in Women in Therapy. Edited by Franks V and Burtle V. New York, Brunner/Mazel, 1974

Mendelsohn G, Geller M: Structure of client attitudes toward counseling and their relation to client-counselor similarity. Journal of Consulting Psychology 29:63-72, 1963

Miller D: The influence of the patient's sex on clinical judgment. Smith College Studies in Social Work, 44:89-100, 1974

Miller JB: Toward a New Psychology of Women. Boston, Beacon Press, 1976

Mogul KM: Overview: the sex of the therapist. Am J Psychiatry 139:1-11, 1982

Morgan R, Lubovsky L, Crits-Christoph P, et al: Predicting the outcomes of psychotherapy by the Penn Helping Alliance Rating Method. Arch Gen Psychiatry 39:397-402, 1982

Nadelson CC, Notman MT: Psychotherapy supervision: the problem of conflicting values. Am J Psychother 31:275-283, 1977

Neulinger J, Stein MI, Schillinger M, et al: Perceptions of the optimally integrated person as a function of therapists' characteristics. Perception and Motor Skills 30:375-384, 1970

Notman M: Twelve years later: a woman psychiatrist. Psychiatric Opinion 2:27-32, 1965

Orlinsky D, Howard K: The effects of sex of therapist on the therapeutic experiences of women. Psychotherapy: Theory, Research and Practice 13:82-88, 1976

Orlinsky D, Howard K: The relation of process to outcome in psychotherapy, in Handbook of Psychotherapy and Behavior Change: An Empirical Analysis. Edited by Garfield SL and Bergin AE. 2nd edition. New York, John Wiley & Sons, 1978

Orlinsky D, Howard K: Gender and psychotherapeutic outcome, in Women and Psychotherapy. Edited by Brodsky A, Hare-Mustin R. New York, Guilford Press, 1980

Parloff M, Waskow I, Wolfe B: Research on therapist variables in relation to process and outcome, in Handbook of Psychotherapy and Behavior Change. Edited by Garfield S, Bergin A. New York, Wiley, 2nd ed., 1978

Persons R, Persons M, Newmark I: Perceived helpful therapist's characteristics, client improvements, and sex of therapist and client. Psychotherapy: Theory, Research and Practice 11:63-65, 1974

Persons W: Occupational prediction as a function of the counselor's racial and sexual bias, Dissertations Abstracts International 34:139A-140A, 1973

Rawlings EI, Carter DK: Feminist and nonsexist psychotherapy, in Psychotherapy for Women. Edited by Rawlings EI and Carter DK. Springfield, Illinois, Charles C Thomas, 1977

Raynes A, Warren G: Some distinguishing features of patients failing to attend a psychiatric clinic after referral. Am J Orthopsychiatry 41:581-588, 1971

Rice JK, Rice DG: Implications of the women's liberation movement for psychotherapy. Am J Psychiatry 130:191-199, 1973

Roeske NA: Women in psychiatry: past and present areas of concern. Am J Psychiatry 130:1127-1131, 1973

Sattler JM: The effects of therapist-client racial similarity, in Effective Psychotherapy: A Handbook for Research. Edited by Gurman AS and Razin AM. New York, Pergamon, 1977

Scher M: Verbal activity, sex, counselor experience and success in counseling. Journal of Counseling Psychology 22:97-101, 1975

Schullman SL and Betz NE: An investigation of the effects of client sex and presenting problem in referral from intake. Journal of Counseling Psychology 25:140-145, 1979

Siassi I: Psychotherapy with women and men of lower classes, in Women in Therapy. Edited by Franks V, Burtle V. New York, Brunner/Mazel, 1974

Simons JA and Helms JE: Influence of counselor's marital status, sex, and age on college and noncollege women's counselor preferences. Journal of Counseling Psychology 23:380-386, 1976

Smith M: Sex bias in counseling and psychotherapy. Psychological Bulletin, 87:392-407, 1980

Strassberg D, Anchor K: Ratings of client self-disclosure and improvement as a function of sex of client and therapist. J Clin Psychol 33:239-241, 1977

Sue S: Community mental health services to minority groups. American Psychologist 32:616-624, 1977

Sue S, McKinney H, Allen D, et al: Delivery of community mental health services to black and white clients. J Consult Clin Psychol 42:794-801, 1974

Tanney M, Birk J: Women counselors for women clients? A review of the research. The Counseling Psychologist 6:28-32, 1976

Tennov D: Feminism, psychotherapy and professionalism. Journal of Contemporary Psychotherapy 5:107-111, 1973

Ticho EA: The effects of the analyst's personality on psychoanalytic treatment. Psychoanalytic Forum 4:137-151, 1972

Varghese F: The racially different psychiatrist—implications for psychotherapy. Aust NZ J Psychiatry 17:329-333, 1983

Warren RC, Jackson AM, Nugaris J, et al: Differential attitudes of black and white patients toward treatment in a child guidance clinic. Am J Orthopsychiatry 43:384-393, 1973

Waskow IE: Summary of discussion following workshop (workshop on research on psychotherapy in women). Psychotherapy: Theory, Research and Practice 13:96-98, 1976

Weems L: Awareness: the key to black mental health. Journal of Black Psychology 1:30-37, 1974

Whitehorn J, Betz B: A study of psychotherapeutic relationships between physicians and schizophrenic patients. Am J Psychiatry 111:321-332, 1954

Whitley, B: Sex roles and psychotherapy: a current appraisal. Psychol Bull 86:1309-1321, 1979

Winston A, Pardes H, Papernick DS: Inpatient treatment of blacks and whites. Arch Gen Psychiatry 26:405-409, 1972

Yamamoto J, James QC, Bloombaum M, et al: Social factors in patient selection. Am J Psychiatry 124:84-90, 1967

Zeldow PB: Sex differences in psychiatric evaluation and treatment. Arch Gen Psychiatry 35:89-93, 1978

Zetzel ER: The doctor-patient relationship in psychiatry, in The Capacity for Emotional Growth. New York, International Universities Press, 1970

Chapter 32

The Therapeutic Alliance and Compliance With Psychopharmacology

by John P. Docherty, M.D. and Susan J. Fiester, M.D.

Haynes suggests that the first recorded incident of human noncompliance occurred with Eve in the Garden of Eden (Haynes 1979b). Concern over the more specific issue of medication noncompliance was later noted by Hippocrates, who admonished the physician to "keep aware of the fact that patients often lie when they state that they have taken certain medicines" (Haynes, 1979). Since that time, a massive amount of research has been carried out in an attempt to answer the perplexing question of why patients do not follow physicians' treatment recommendations, particularly those having to do with the taking of medication.

Noncompliance is a widespread problem that faces every physician in practice, and it is one with potentially serious consequences. It has been estimated that between 25 and 50 percent of medical patients are noncompliant with their prescribed medication regimen (Becker, 1979; Blackwell, 1972; Christensen, 1978; Davis, 1966; DiNicola and DiMatteo, 1982; Fox, 1962; Ley, 1982; Marston, 1970; Mazzula and Lasagna, 1972; Mitchell, 1974; Sackett, 1976; Sackett and Snow, 1979; Stimson, 1974). Estimates of drug noncompliance in psychiatric populations have been similar, with noncompliance rates of approximately 40 to 50 percent (Blackwell, 1973, 1976; Ley, 1982; Stimson, 1974). These high rates of drug noncompliance can have a significant impact on patient health, on physician management and on society in general. Asburn estimates that 20 to 25 percent of all hospitalizations may be the result of noncompliance with the medication regimen (Asburn, 1981). Furthermore, approximately 30 percent of patients misuse their medications in a manner that poses a serious threat to their health (Boyd, 1974). Thus, noncompliance can result in personal and societal costs by increasing morbidity and mortality, and necessitating hospitalization, resulting in enormous economic costs to society as well as personal economic and social costs to the individual. This is all the more regrettable given the availability of current pharmacological treatments that have increased specificity and efficacy for treating acute illness, as well as for prophylaxis.

DEFINITION AND ASSESSMENT OF COMPLIANCE

Traditionally, compliance (or the alternative term, adherence) has been regarded as the extent to which patients follow the prescribed preventive or therapeutic

---

This chapter was written by Drs. Docherty and Fiester in their private capacities. No official support or endorsement by NIMH is intended or should be inferred.

regimens of health care providers. Two primary approaches have been used to characterize compliance (Gordis, 1979). In the categorical approach, a rationale is chosen for dichotomizing patients into either compliers or noncompliers. The rationale can be based on statistical criteria (above or below the mean or median for a population), on arbitrarily selected criteria or on clinical criteria (drug taking behavior which is felt to be at sufficient variation from the prescribed regimen to compromise the therapeutic outcome). In contrast, compliance has been regarded in much of the research literature as a continuous variable, with "zones of compliance" in which a patient is compliant a certain proportion of the time or compliant within given ranges of medication dosages. Although it would be ideal to have a biological definition of compliance (a point below which the desired preventive or therapeutic result is unlikely to be achieved), such biological criteria unfortunately does not exist in most treatment situations (Gordis, 1979).

Physicians wishing to assess compliance can use either direct or indirect methods (Christensen, 1978; Gordis, 1979). Indirect methods include the determination of the degree to which the expected outcome has been attained; the degree to which side effects or other metabolic consequences of drug activity are present; the degree to which prescriptions have been filled; and the degree to which the number of pills remaining coincides with the number of pills expected according to the prescription. The physician may also determine compliance by interviewing the patient, family members or third parties, such as nursing staff, about the patient's drug taking behavior, or by developing a general impression about the degree to which the patient is complying. Direct measures involve sampling blood or urine for the presence and/or levels of medication, metabolites or tracers. The choice of measurement may differ, depending upon whether compliance is being assessed for research or clinical purposes, with each of these methods having advantages and disadvantages. With direct measures, the clinician must be aware of the possibility that significant individual variations may exist in absorption, metabolism and excretion. Indirect measures involve other inherent problems. Use of outcome as a criterion requires that the treatment be effective, with a good correlation between compliance with the regimen and outcome, and denies the influence of environmental or other factors on outcome. Interviews that are of questionable reliability and validity tend to grossly overestimate compliance, and pill counts also tend to somewhat overestimate compliance. Physician impression of the degree of noncompliance is notoriously poor.

Besides assessing noncompliance in a quantitative fashion, the physician should also determine the type of noncompliance, the pattern of noncompliance and the conscious or unconscious reasons underlying noncompliance. Several types of noncompliance can occur (Malahy, 1966). Failure to take the medication is probably the most common type, but patients can also take the medication for the wrong reason, take the wrong dosage, or take the medication at the wrong time or in the wrong sequence. Some patients may also take more medication than is prescribed or take additional medications of which the physician is not aware. In addition to assessing the type of noncompliance, determining patients' individual patterns of compliance and noncompliance can also be important. For example, two individuals may ingest the same total weekly dosage of medication, although one takes the medication daily and the other erratically, making up for missed doses by increasing subsequent doses.

Finally, a patient's reasons for noncompliance can be extremely variable, ranging from the presence of practical obstacles (lack of money or transportation), to capriciousness, deliberate refusal or confusion about the details of the treatment regimen. Determining the meaning of the noncompliance to the individual patient can be critical. For example, capricious noncompliance as a result of carelessness or forgetfulness is quite different from a patient's consciously deciding to regulate his own dosage as a way of asserting control. Likewise, deliberate drug refusal as a result of paranoid delusions is quite different from a decision to refuse the drug based on information about a relative's negative experience with the drug. In summary, specific diagnosis and assessment of noncompliance, including the degree, type, pattern and reasons underlying noncompliance, is essential. Understanding the nature and context of noncompliant behavior is crucial if the physician is to develop effective strategic interventions to alter compliance behavior.

DETERMINANTS OF COMPLIANCE

For a physician to think of compliance or noncompliance as a characteristic behavior pattern for a given individual can be extremely misleading. Research has shown that compliance may vary over time in a given individual and can depend on many intervening factors. It is perhaps more useful to think of compliance as an outcome in an individual treatment situation that is determined by multiple and complexly interacting variables. For purposes of highlighting the most important factors in compliance, we have grouped these determinants into several major categories: the patient; the physician; the treatment regimen; the clinical setting; and the doctor-patient relationship. In addition, we will also discuss particular characteristics of psychiatric patients and psychiatric illness that can affect compliance. Since there have been several comprehensive reviews of the determinants of compliance (Baekeland and Lundwall, 1975; Becker, 1976, 1979; Becker and Maiman, 1980; Blackwell, 1972, 1973, 1976, 1979; Christensen, 1978; Evans and Spelman, 1983; Haynes, 1976, 1979a; Ley, 1982; Stimson, 1974), we will only briefly mention the primary variables in each category and then focus in detail on the final category, the doctor-patient relationship.

The Patient

Although some controversy exists, it is generally felt that demographic variables such as age, sex, race, marital status, social class and educational and occupational levels have little effect on compliance to medical regimens (Becker, 1979; Christensen, 1979; Haynes 1976, 1979a; Stimson, 1974). Studies do suggest that at the extremes of age (children and the elderly) there is generally decreased compliance (Blackwell, 1973; Christensen, 1979). Type and severity of illness also appear to bear little relationship to compliance (Becker, 1976; Christensen, 1978; Evans and Spelman, 1983; Haynes, 1976, 1979a); however, particular aspects of the illness, such as the nature and type of symptomatology, may be relevant. For example, compliance is greater in diseases where the consequences of decreased medication are immediate, serious and unpleasant, and in situations where medication is prescribed for the actual treatment of symptoms rather than for prophylactic purposes (Blackwell, 1973, 1976; Christensen, 1979). In schizophrenic patients, different constellations of symptoms on relapse have also been found to be related to differential compliance with prophylactic neuroleptic regimens. Schizophrenics who display symptoms such as grandiosity and paranoia during psychotic relapse tend to have poor compliance with prophylactic neuroleptic treatment, while those with symptoms such as anxiety and depression who lack grandiosity show better compliance (Evans and Spelman, 1983; Van Putten, 1978).

Patients' level of understanding and education about the illness and about the therapy in general has very little effect on compliance; however, a patient's attitudes and beliefs about his illness can have a very potent effect on compliance (Becker, 1974, 1979; Becker et al, 1979), as has been shown with the development of the Health Belief Model. This model, developed by Becker, Rosenstock and others, states that the patient's perception of personal susceptibility to an illness, the severity and consequences of the condition, the potential benefits of therapy and the financial, social and psychological costs of the therapy, will determine the patient's compliance with a particular treatment regimen. Studies testing the utility of this predictive model have shown each factor to be clearly related to compliance (Becker, 1976; Becker et al, 1979).

Although personality characteristics per se do not appear to be related to compliance (Becker, 1979; DiNicola and DiMatteo, 1982), patient hostility (especially covert hostility) and unfavorable attitudes toward authority or parental figures are negatively related to compliance (Raskin 1961; Richards 1964). Other psychological factors such as motivation may also be important determinants of compliance (Evans and Spelman, 1983). When illness serves a positive function, compliance may be decreased, as in patients who prefer remaining in hospital to being discharged to noxious home environments. Likewise, when illness serves a negative function, such as producing a threat of job loss, compliance may be improved.

In addition to the personal characteristics mentioned above, specific characteristics of psychiatric patients and psychiatric illness may contribute to poor compliance. Pervasive denial of illness is particularly common in psychiatric patients and can result in severe compromise of compliance with treatment. In contrast, insight into illness has been shown to be associated with increased compliance (Evans and Spelman, 1983; Van Putten, 1978). When psychiatric illness involves an element of cognitive disorganization and confusion, as in the psychosis accompanying schizophrenia and unipolar or bipolar affective illness or in organic brain syndromes, this disorganization can seriously compromise the patient's capacity to understand and carry out the treatment regimen. To the extent that anxiety is a major element of psychiatric disorder, it can generate avoidance behavior that may result in impaired ability to comply. Patients' irrational beliefs, as well as negative symbolic meanings that are attributed to the illness or medication, are also particularly important as contributors to noncompliance in psychiatrically ill patients. This can involve factors such as paranoid delusions, fears of addiction, or externalization of the patient's feelings of deficiency or worthlessness onto the medication.

The patient's family and general sociocultural milieu can have a profound impact on the patient's compliance behavior. General family health beliefs and attitudes, family attitudes toward the patient's particular illness and treatment, normal family roles and the way in which they interact with the patient's sick role and therapeutic regimens, and irrational beliefs within the family system can all affect compliance behavior (Becker, 1979; Blackwell, 1976; Evans and Spelman, 1983). The extent of the family's support and external monitoring is also important; it has been shown that the absence of a stable support network or person to function in a supervisory role (as is the case with many socially isolated psychiatric patients or the elderly) is associated with low levels of compliance (Blackwell, 1973, 1976; Stimson, 1976). Finally, cultural, ethnic or religious factors within the family or in the broader sociocultural context can have a significant impact on compliance (Becker, 1979; Blackwell, 1973; Christensen, 1978; Evans and Spelman, 1983; Stimson, 1974).

The Physician

Several attributes of the physician, including his or her attitudes toward medication and general competence and skills, can have a significant impact on compliance. Patients are more likely to comply with medication regimens if their physicians believe in the efficacy and importance of the medication (Baekeland and Lundwall, 1975; Blackwell, 1976; Davis and VonderLippe, 1968; Evans and Spelman, 1983). Appropriateness of the prescribed medication is also important. Physicians who prescribe inappropriate medications for patients as a result of incorrect diagnosis or inadequate treatment (for example, prescribing major tranquilizers for depressed patients) are likely to contribute to noncompliance (Baekeland and Lundwall, 1975; Wilcox et al, 1965). Competence in the ongoing supervision of patients' treatment regimens is also important. One study showed that physicians who had more treatment dropouts and medication deviators were less conscientious and skillful in supervising their patients' drug taking (Rickels and Cattell, 1969).

Treatment Regimen

Patient attitudes regarding particular drugs and the drugs' effects can be powerful factors in noncompliance. Patients will adhere to a regimen to the degree that they find the effects of a specific agent acceptable. The greater the degree to which the drug effects are synchronous with the patient's idiosyncratic likes and dislikes, the more likely the compliance; the greater the quantity and severity of treatment emergent side effects, the less likely the compliance (Baekeland and Lundwall, 1975; Blackwell, 1973, 1976; Christensen, 1978; Evans and Spelman, 1983). It is important to note that mild or subclinical side effects (such as akathisia) that go unrecognized by the physician may also interfere with compliance (Van Putten, 1978).

Several other factors involving the drug itself or the treatment regimen can affect compliance. The greater the number of drugs prescribed, the greater the frequency of dosing; the longer the duration of the therapy and the greater the cost of treatment, the lower the compliance (Becker and Maiman, 1980; Blackwell, 1973, 1979; Christensen, 1978; Evans and Spelman, 1983; Haynes, 1976, 1979a; Ley, 1982; Stimson, 1974). The agent who administers the drug, the route of administration and the drug packaging can also affect compliance, with the following factors decreasing compliance: self-administration, the oral versus the parenteral route of administration, and the presence of safety caps on medication bottles (Blackwell, 1976; Evans and Spelman, 1983; Haynes, 1976, 1979a; Stimson, 1974). One study found that offering the liquid form of chlorpromazine rather than the pill form for schizophrenics increased compliance significantly. Placing pills in special containers that visually indicate the dosage schedule and obviate the need to read and interpret a prescription label will also increase compliance (Haynes, 1976, 1979; Stimson, 1974). Finally, to the extent that the therapeutic regimen requires change in the patient's behavior or habits, compliance will be diminished (Becker and Maiman, 1980; Haynes, 1979a; Marston, 1970).

Clinical Setting

A number of factors associated with the clinical setting can have a significant impact on patients' compliance. Continuity of care (repeated contact with a particular provider), which fosters feelings of familiarity and comfort, is associated with increased patient medication compliance (Becker, 1979; Blackwell, 1973, 1976, 1979; Ettlinger and Freedman, 1981; Evans and Spelman, 1983; Haynes, 1979a; Ley, 1982). Decreasing degrees of supervision and support in the treatment setting—for example, inpatient treatment versus day hospital treatment versus outpatient treatment—is associated with decreases in compliance. Finally, factors such as decreased waiting time, which increases convenience and decreases frustration for the patient, can lead to improved compliance.

INFLUENCE OF THE DOCTOR-PATIENT RELATIONSHIP ON COMPLIANCE

All doctors and patients bring to the therapeutic situation preexisting ideas, beliefs, attitudes and expectations about the nature of the therapeutic encounter. During the therapeutic encounter, doctor and patient are involved in verbal and behavioral interaction in which roles are established, problems are defined, goals are set and a method of achieving these goals is determined. This all takes place within an interpersonal context that is colored by an affective element. Kasl notes that in the doctor-patient relationship, "the crucial element . . . is probably not the exchange of information and facts but the nature of the expectation each one has about his own role and the role of the other person in the dyad, the congruence and mutuality of such expectations and the potential for exploring and revising these expectations" (Kasl, 1975).

Despite views such as Kasl's, the doctor-patient relationship has been a relatively neglected area of compliance research (Eisenthal et al, 1979). However, results of recent studies have begun to demonstrate the importance of this element in patient compliance. As we review the research literature in order to elucidate the ways in which the doctor-patient relationship is related to compliance, we will individually consider several of the most important components of the relationship. Garrity (1981), in a review of the clinician-patient relationship and medical compliance, organized the literature into four headings, which we have slightly altered into the following four components: role relationships; expectations; communication; and affective tone. For each of these components we will first review the literature on medical compliance and the doctor-patient relationship, and then relate findings from the psychotherapeutic literature on therapeutic alliance to findings from the medical compliance literature. It is important to keep in mind that although we are examining these components separately, they are not necessarily independent and that considerable overlap exists among these components.

ROLE RELATIONSHIPS

The traditional view of the doctor-patient relationship in medicine has been one in which the patient is seen as a relatively passive agent who is bound to accept the doctor's advice and unquestioningly carry out the recommended therapeutic regime. However, in recent years there has been an increased emphasis on the consumer perspective in medical care, which has brought pressures for change in the traditional attitudes, roles and behaviors of physician and patient. These pressures have resulted in a trend toward the more equitable distribution of power, information, responsibility and decision-making in the doctor-patient relationship. Evidence has begun to accumulate which suggests that this trend toward more cooperation, collaboration and reciprocity in the doctor-patient relationship can lead to improved patient compliance and therapeutic outcome.

A number of studies have examined the patient role in the doctor-patient relationship in terms of the dimension of "patient activity" or "patient participation." Caplan (1979) describes a model of the doctor-patient relationship based on this dimension. This "patient participation model" provides fairly explicit views about the respective roles of doctor and patient, and their rights and responsibilities toward one another. This model is based on a number of assumptions, such as: The provider gives expert information and advice to the patient and functions as a sounding board. However, the patient is also assumed to be an "expert," in that he is more informed than the doctor about his own values and life goals. Thus, the patient has the right to choose whether to follow the doctor's advice and the right to determine which aspects of the advice to follow.

Studies have generally found that the establishment of doctor-patient roles in which the patient has increased participation (activity) and assumes increased responsibility results in increased compliance. Schulman (1979) found that patients who received care aimed at involving them as active participants in treatment ("active patient orientation") had better control of blood pressure and greater adherence to the treatment regimen. Eisenthal et al (1979) investigated the relationship of the degree of negotiation in an initial interview to adherence to treatment disposition, and found that degree of perceived negotiation was significantly related to patient adherence. The negotiation factor that correlated best with adherence was participation in treatment planning. Roter (1977) found that an intervention which encouraged patients to ask more questions of the physicians resulted in greater attendance at clinic appointments over four months at followup. In a study by Glanz (1979), dieticians who more actively influenced their patients and involved patients more in sessions had better compliance with dietary regimens. Tracy (1977), in a study comparing a traditional intake procedure versus an intake procedure involving treatment goals negotiated with the patient, found attrition to be significantly less in the negotiated group.

Studies of the behavioral technique of contingency contracting corroborate the above findings regarding increased patient participation and its effect on compliance. Contingency contracting involves agreement by both parties on a treatment goal, clarification of the responsibilities of both parties in achieving the goal and the establishment of a time frame for the contract. The development of such contracts in the medical setting necessitates the clarification of doctor and patient expectations and requires increased responsibility and involvement of the patient in the therapeutic process. Contingency contracting has been found in numerous studies to increase compliance and has been effectively used in the treatment of a wide range of medical and psychiatric disorders in children and adults (Becker and Maiman, 1980).

One of the ways in which increased patient involvement and reciprocity may influence compliance is by increasing the patient's sense of control in the therapeutic situation. A wide variety of studies suggest that greater feelings of control have a positive relationship to psychological well-being and physical health, and enhance satisfaction and performance, while decreased feelings of control impact negatively on both psychological and physical health (Schorr and Rodin, 1982). The crucial variable appears to be the perception of control regardless of the actual degree of control. Greater feelings of control in aversive health and/or treatment situations also produce an increased ability to cope.

It should be noted that the respective doctor and patient roles are components of a dynamic interactive system and that changes in the role of one party may have interactive effects with the role of the other party. With regard to the doctor's role, Davis (1971) showed that the doctor's passive acceptance of the patient's active participation is likely to induce patient noncompliance. Increased compliance is associated with the doctor's actively providing suggestions and orientation. Thus, feedback is critical if a more participatory patient role is to produce a positive result in terms of compliance and outcome.

Although research suggests that increased activity and control on the part of the patient is generally beneficial, an extreme degree of reciprocity in the doctor-patient relationship may not be totally desirable. Caplan (1979) points out that too much reciprocity in the doctor-patient relationship can undermine trust and the legitimate expert role of the doctor, whereas too little reciprocity may not provide enough of a sense of control for the patient. As a result, it is necessary for doctor and patient to come to a clear understanding about the areas in which reciprocity and choice are legitimate and the areas in which they are not.

Likewise, the relationship between perceived control and compliance does not appear to be a simple one. Other conditions can affect the potential benefits of perceived control. An increased perception of control can be stress-inducing if it increases a patient's feelings of responsibility for the outcome (Schorr and Rodin, 1982). If a patient experiences increased control in the context of inadequate information on which to base decisions, increased stress can also result. Individual psychological factors, such as locus of control and feelings of self-efficacy, can also interact with control to produce positive or negative outcomes. Patients who have greater feelings of self-efficacy and those with an internal locus of control appear to respond more positively to the opportunity for control

(Schorr and Rodin, 1982). In contrast, patients with high needs for independence have low health-seeking and low adherence behaviors (Becker, 1979).

In summary, it has been shown that doctor and patient roles that are more reciprocal as evidenced by active patient participation and involvement, increased patient control and responsibility, and negotiation between doctor and patient involving clarification of mutual goals and respective responsibilities, can all result in increased compliance. However, factors such as individual patient's needs and capacities can interact in a complex way to mitigate or enhance the more general effects of increased patient activity and control on compliance.

EXPECTATIONS

A number of researchers have examined the expectations that doctors and patients have about the therapeutic encounter and have investigated the impact these expectations have on compliance. Two related areas of inquiry have received the most attention: the degree of similarity and/or difference between doctors' and patients' expectations about the therapeutic encounter; and the effect of mutuality or nonmutuality of expectations on compliance. With regard to the first area, research suggests that doctors and patients may have very different expectations. For example, one study of the provision of information surveyed the percentage of physicians and patients who believed that the patient should be given various types of information about medications, such as the name of the medication and risks involved in taking the medication. This study found that a greater percentage of patients than physicians felt that they should be given information on each of the different aspects of the drug (Fedder, 1982). This discrepancy is undoubtedly responsible for the widespread patient dissatisfaction with information provided in the treatment setting and for the actual lack of knowledge that patients often demonstrate (Garfield and Wolpin, 1963). These discrepancies are particularly important in light of the fact that in one study, 65 percent of the expectations held by patients were not even communicated to the physician (Korsch et al, 1968).

Regarding the degree of mutuality of expectation and its effect on compliance and outcome, research findings consistently show that congruence of doctor-patient expectations and, in particular, patients' perceptions that their doctors have met their expectations, has a positive effect on compliance (Kasl, 1975, Garrity, 1981, Downing et al, 1975). For example, a series of studies of various acute medical illnesses found compliance to be associated with fulfillment of patient expectations. These studies found that compliance was poorer when expected tests and treatments were not done, and when explanations about the cause of the illness were not provided (Korsch et al, 1968; Francis et al 1969). Hulka et al (1975) and Hulka (1979) also found that agreement about the specifics of the therapeutic regimen resulted in increased compliance.

Studies from the psychotherapy literature are also relevant and support the general findings from the medical compliance literature. For example, one study of the relationship of the client's expectations to length of stay in psychotherapy found that certain expectancies differentiate short stay versus long stay in treatment (Heine and Trosman, 1960). Early terminators stressed passive cooperation (versus active collaboration), expected specific advice and had the least accurate expectations about the doctor's role (medical orientation) and activity level. Overall and Aronson (1963), in a study of psychiatric patients, found that to the extent that patient expectations about therapists' activity, medical orientation and supportiveness were not fulfilled, patients were less likely to comply with attendance at their next appointment. It should be pointed out that unfulfilled expectations at the crucial time of the initial contact or visit may have an especially noxious effect in that they may disrupt the therapeutic relationship and produce dropout from treatment (Kasl, 1975).

COMMUNICATION

A recent review of the research literature on patient satisfaction concluded that 35 to 53 percent of patients were dissatisfied with communication in the doctor-patient encounter (Ley, 1982). Since satisfaction with communication is strongly related to satisfaction with the medical encounter in general and is also related to the recall of information, the pervasiveness of this dissatisfaction is especially worrisome (Ley, 1982). Looking at the roots of this dissatisfaction it has been found that, as previously noted, patients are often provided with less information than they wish or expect to receive from their doctors. In addition, patients frequently either fail to understand or tend to forget the information that has been presented to them by their physicians (Ley, 1982).

Despite this dismal picture, it is encouraging to note that the most frequently investigated component of the doctor-patient relationship is the communication process (Kasl, 1975). Research on doctor-patient communication falls into two primary areas of investigation: the quality of the communication and the content or type of information communicated. Studies have consistently found a relationship between various aspects of doctor-patient communication and compliance. Regarding the quality of the communication, a series of studies by Ley et al (1976a, 1976b) showed a consistent relationship between the understandability and comprehensibility of instructions and medication compliance. Svarstad (1974) found that the clarity, explicitness and consistency of doctors' instructions and the provision of written information correlated with medication compliance, and that greater explicitness of communication produced greater agreement between doctor and patient about the patient's task. Research by Hulka (1975, 1979) showed that the adequacy of the doctor-patient communication as measured by agreement on issues discussed was related to compliance. Finally, Davis (1968) studied communication patterns in the doctor-patient relationship and found that deviant communication patterns, especially negative interactions (where there was no tension release; where the doctor was formal, rejecting and controlling; and where the doctor disagreed completely with the patient or interviewed the patient at length without subsequent feedback) were associated with poor compliance.

Other authors have noted the following factors in the quality of communication that appear to increase compliance: brevity of the communication; presentation of the most important information first; the combined presentation of oral and written information; and the avoidance or adequate explanation of medical terms (Becker and Maiman, 1980; Ley, 1982). In the psychotherapy literature, Duehn and Proctor (1977) found that the presence of therapist responses acknowledging the content of the patient's preceding communication, and therapist responses in which the content was relevant to the expectations of the patient, correlated with continuation versus termination from treatment.

Regarding the type of information, it has been found that general knowledge and information about a disease does not necessarily increase compliance, although specific knowledge about the purpose of the treatment and about particular aspects of the medical regimen may improve compliance. For example, Hulka (1975, 1979) found that patients who were provided with more information about their drugs had better compliance. She also found that misconceptions about dosage scheduling were significantly related to noncompliance. However, it should be noted that knowledge about how to take medications does not guarantee compliance. Wartman et al (1983) found that although 75 percent of patients understood how to take the medication, noncompliance occurred in 50 percent of patients.

It should be noted that, just as an inordinate amount of patient involvement and responsibility can be detrimental, the provision of too much information may also be harmful. Although the provision of more information per se does not necessarily lead to adverse effects (Becker, 1979), the presentation of too much information to certain patients can result in decreased compliance. Patients' needs for information and their abilities to process and assimilate information vary and depend on many factors. In addition, other patient variables may affect the degree to which the provision of increased information to the patient can potentially affect compliance. For example, one study found a significant association between knowledge and compliance only in patients with little prior disease experience (Tagliacozzo and Ima, 1970). Thus, the physician should take into account each patient's individual needs and abilities in determining the optimal amount of information he or she will provide, and in determining the optimal manner in which this information will be presented.

AFFECTIVE TONE

A positive "affective tone" is defined by Garrity (1981) as "emotional support in the therapeutic relationship." Achieving such support may involve the doctor's providing the ingredients of positive support such as sympathy, understanding, encouragement, warmth and friendliness. There has been a paucity of research on this important element of the doctor-patient relationship. However, the little existing research has consistently found that a positive affective tone in the doctor-patient relationship—as manifest by qualities such as friendliness, warmth and understanding—is correlated with compliance. Svarstad (1974) found physician approachability (based on characteristics of the physician's behavior, such as friendliness, interest and respect) to be related to compliance. Freemon et al, (1971) found that the affective tone of the doctor-patient interaction (friendliness and solidarity versus disagreement, tension and antagonism) was related to compliance. Francis et al (1969) found that in a pediatric population, compliance was better if the mothers felt the physician was friendly. They also found that friendliness, concern, and a pleasant personality on the part of the physician increased compliance less than an actively unpleasant manner on the part of the physician decreased it. Charney et al (1967) found that a warm relationship of a longstanding nature between doctor and patient produced better compliance.

Turning to the psychotherapy literature, Downing et al (1975), in a study of neurotic outpatients, found that "deviators" from a medication regimen were less well liked by their doctors. Shapiro (1974) found that therapists' affective responses were more positive and prognosis more optimistic for patients who continued in treatment. Reynolds (1965) also found that patients who were more compliant were offered more hope of benefit by their therapists. Only one study provided findings which were contradictory. Davis and Eichorn (1963) found that a formal relationship between doctor and patient produced better compliance than a friendly one.

As is true for the other components of the doctor-patient relationship, patient and illness variables can interact with the affective tone of the relationship to alter the expected effects of affective tone on compliance. For example, a few researchers have found that warmth may have a negative impact on psychotherapy outcome in patients with particular diagnoses, such as schizophrenia and certain neuroses (Parloff, 1978). Also, a study by Freedman et al (1958) rating warmth of the therapist in a drug treatment situation found no relationship between warmth and dropout. However, warmth interacted with patient expectations, so that patients high on denial of illness who received warmth tended to drop out, while patients accepting of their illnesses who received warmth tended to continue in treatment.

MECHANISMS

A small body of research has shed light on possible mechanisms by which the previously examined components of the doctor-patient relationship might exert their effects on compliance (Kasl, 1975). The effects may be direct or may involve mediating factors. Satisfaction is one of the most frequently investigated potential mediating variables. A number of studies have found that patient level of satisfaction with the visit, therapist or clinic is correlated with compliance (Ley, 1982). Thus, patient satisfaction may be a final common pathway that facilitates increased compliance with mutuality of expectations, adequate communication or acceptable role relationships leading to patient satisfaction and patient satisfaction then leading to increased compliance. Other sequences have been postulated. Svarstad (1974) has suggested that when a patient perceives the physician as friendly (positive affective tone), there is an increase in the patient's activity (role relationships), which leads to increased communication and ultimately to increased compliance. In addition, a study of a special pharmacist intervention program that provided ongoing "educational" visits resulted in increased compliance while the visits continued, but after termination, compliance returned to its original levels (Becker and Maiman, 1980). This suggests that the visits may have really functioned to increase motivation, and that motivation and not increased information may have been the critical mechanism affecting compliance behavior.

SUMMARY

Although the doctor-patient relationship has been the least well studied of the three elements of the therapeutic encounter (the doctor, the patient and the relationship), evidence consistently supports the importance of its effect on compliance. The following components of the relationship appear to be factors that contribute to increased compliance: increased reciprocity in the respective doctor-patient roles, which of necessity involves increased patient control, activity, participation and responsibility; mutuality of expectations, which may involve negotiation between doctor and patient; improved quality of communication, with optimal provision of information in an optimal manner; and the existence of an ambience with a positive affective tone in the doctor-patient interaction.

RESEARCH ON THE THERAPEUTIC ALLIANCE

The basic nature of the therapeutic relationship or, for that matter, any helping relationship, is defined by the presence of a help seeker, a help provider and the interpersonal interaction that occurs between them in the process of pursuing shared goals. It may be useful to first place this concept in a historical framework. The therapeutic relationship was first conceptualized in the psychoanalytic writing of Freud, who acknowledged the existence of the relationship, but saw it as relatively unimportant compared to technical factors in producing therapeutic change (Freud 1940, 1964). Later psychoanalytic theorists gave increased attention to the importance of the therapist-patient relationship; however, it still did not gain primacy within the psychoanalytic framework (Gomes-Schwartz 1978). With the surge of interest in client-centered therapy during the 1950s and 1960s and its focus on accurate empathy, nonpossessive warmth and genuineness, the therapeutic relationship finally moved to the forefront. This triad of "facilitative conditions" was accorded primacy over technique in the therapeutic encounter and was seen as both a necessary and sufficient condition for change (Rogers, 1957). Frank (1971) also emphasized the importance of the doctor-patient relationship as one of the following six nonspecific factors in psychotherapy: an emotionally charged confiding relationship; a therapeutic rationale; the provision of new information; the strengthening of the patient's expectations for help; the provision of success experiences; and the facilitation of emotional arousal. Frank took a more middle ground in viewing the therapeutic relationship as a necessary but not sufficient condition for therapeutic change. Finally, with the advent of the behavioral therapies, the focus has again shifted to an increased emphasis on the technical aspects of treatment and a relative deemphasis of the importance of the therapeutic relationship.

We will now present four major findings from the therapeutic alliance literature and then examine the relationship of these findings to the compliance literature already reviewed. We will attempt to show how research on the therapeutic alliance can provide additional support for findings from the medical compliance literature, and how this research can further illuminate our understanding of the way in which the doctor-patient relationship can effect compliance with psychopharmacology.

1). The overall quality of the therapeutic alliance correlates highly with outcome, and certain aspects of the relationship are more powerful than others in predicting outcome.

Several researchers have developed instruments for assessing the therapeutic alliance and have then used these instruments to investigate the relationship of the quality of the therapeutic alliance to outcome in psychotherapy. Barrett-Lennard (1962) was the first to develop an instrument for rating the therapeutic alliance. This instrument assessed five aspects of therapist attitude: level of regard (negative versus positive affective response), unconditionality of regard, degree of empathic understanding, congruence in the relationship (sincerity, honesty, directness) and willingness to be known. He found that the first four factors were positively related to therapeutic change. Strupp et al (1963) found a high correlation between emotional/attitudinal variables relating to the quality of the therapeutic relationship and ratings of therapy outcome. Specifically, they found that the therapist's liking the patient, enjoying working with the particular type of patient, therapist warmth toward patient, patient warmth toward therapist, therapist emotional investment, patient motivation and quality of the working relationship correlated with outcome. Lorr (1965), in a factor analysis of five dimensions of perceived therapist behavior, found that therapist understanding and acceptance were significantly positively correlated with both client- and therapist-rated improvement and were also correlated with patient satisfaction. In addition, he found that authoritarianism and critical/hostile behavior on the part of the therapist was significantly negatively correlated with improvement.

Saltzman et al (1976) looked at various therapist and client dimensions and found that a number of dimensions predicted either client- or therapist-rated outcome. In this study, client feeling that the therapist understands and allows the patient to take responsibility predicted client-rated outcome. Client feeling that the therapist understands, respects the client, is open, offers security, continuity and movement (progress), and therapist feeling of respect for the patient and a positive prognosis, predicted therapist-rated improvement. They also found that certain dimensions could predict the viability of the therapeutic relationship early on, by the third session. Factors predicting dropout included low ratings on therapist's respect, confidence in the therapist, and patient and therapist involvement in the therapy. Gomes-Schwartz (1978), using the Vanderbilt Psychotherapy Process Scale, looked at the relationship of three process factors to outcome: exploratory process, participatory involvement and therapist-offered relationship, and found that patient participation involvement (defined as patient willingness and ability to become actively involved in the therapeutic interaction) most consistently predicted outcome. Marziale et al (1981) developed a therapeutic alliance scale that looked separately at patient and therapist contributions to the therapeutic attitudinal/affective climate and found that only the patient's contribution was predictive of outcome.

Luborsky et al (1983) and Morgan et al (1982) recently developed a helping alliance measure consisting of two types of patient statements. Type 1 consists of four subtypes—feels therapist is helping; feels changed; feels rapport; feels optimism and confidence in the therapist and the treatment—and reflects the patient experience of the therapist as providing help which is needed. Type 2 consists of three subtypes—experiences self as working with the therapist in a joint effort; shares similar conceptions about the source of problems; and demonstrates qualities similar to those of the therapist—and reflects the patient's experience of treatment as a process of working together with the therapist toward the goals of treatment. Both aspects of this helping alliance scale have significant power in predicting outcome. Furthermore, early signs of a positive helping alliance correlated significantly with rated benefits, and these early positive signs were better predictors of outcome than negative signs were predictors of negative outcome. Finally, one study of the therapeutic relationship in psychopharmacology found that pharmacotherapies in which therapists were actively involved with their patients and provided more interview structure had fewer dropouts with a lower class population than therapists who were less involved and provided less structure (Howard et al, 1970).

Two previous reviews have also concluded that the nature of the therapist-patient relationship has an effect on outcome. A recent review of psychotherapy research on the Rogerian triad of accurate empathy, nonpossessive warmth and genuineness (Mitchell et al, 1977) concluded that the evidence for the relationship between high levels of these facilitative conditions and positive outcome is equivocal, but does suggest there may be a weak relationship to outcome. The evidence is strongest for the empathy factor (Mitchell et al, 1977). Orlinsky and Howard (1977), in their review of the therapeutic alliance literature, conclude that therapist activity and positive instrumental task behavior, and warmth and respect for the patient, produced better psychotherapy outcome. They state, "the quality of the relational bond . . . is more clearly related to patient improvement than are any of the particular treatment techniques . . ." (Orlinsky and Howard, 1977).

In summary, besides the overall quality of the relationship, the following factors in the therapeutic relationship have been most frequently and consistently found to be related to outcome: *Therapist factors:* level and unconditionality of regard and respect; empathy, understanding and acceptance; congruence; warmth, liking and a feeling of emotional investment; optimism about the outcome; security and continuity; providing help and structure. *Patient factors:* participatory involvement, motivation, warmth toward the therapist, and experience of therapist as providing help which is needed. *Interactive factors:* progress in the therapy; experience of treatment as a process of working together towards goals.

2). There is evidence for a strong positive relationship between the patient's perception of the therapeutic conditions and outcome; this relationship is even more powerful when therapeutic conditions are rated by the patient as compared to an independent judge. Furthermore, there is very little agreement between therapist and patient perception of the quality of the therapeutic relationship.

Since there are many studies of patient perception of the therapeutic relationship, we will primarily refer to previous reviews which have summarized this extensive literature. Gurman's (1977) excellent review of the patient's perceptions of the therapeutic relationship, as well as a previous review by Howard and Orlinsky (1972), both conclude that the patient's perceptions are strongly related to outcome. Looking more closely at therapist factors that are correlated with patient perceptions, studies have found that the actual behavior of the therapist has a greater impact on the patient's perception of the therapeutic conditions than therapist attributes such as "expertness" or "prestige"

(Gurman, 1977). There is also some evidence that a patient perception of the therapist as being authoritarian, dominant, or dogmatic is predictive of a poor therapeutic relationship (Gurman, 1977). In addition, therapist "experiencing level" and therapist self-confidence are correlated with patient perception of the therapeutic conditions. Patient factors have also been found to be related to the patient's perception of the therapeutic relationship. Psychological-mindedness is correlated with higher levels of perceived therapeutic conditions, as is external locus of control. Surprisingly, "sicker" clients' perceptions appear to be better predictors of outcome than perceptions of less "sick" clients.

3). Experienced therapists establish better therapeutic relationships with patients; however, this does not necessarily lead to better outcome. Thus, outcome is not solely dependent upon the goodness of the therapeutic relationship.

It may be most enlightening to first look at the specific aspects of the therapeutic relationship that differentiate experienced from inexperienced therapists. Fiedler (1950a,b) studied therapists of different orientations and different experience levels and developed a description of the ideal therapeutic relationship. He then rated therapists' sessions in three areas: communication, emotional distance and status role, and found that experienced therapists more closely approximated the ideal than inexperienced therapists. Experienced therapists were most different from inexperienced therapists on communication items (ability to understand and communicate the understanding). Barrett-Lennard (1962) also studied differences between experienced versus inexperienced therapists using the Relationship Inventory, and found that experienced therapists scored higher on level of regard, unconditionality of regard, empathic understanding, and congruence in the relationship than inexperienced therapists. Others have found that experienced therapists kept less defensive distance between themselves and patients than inexperienced therapists (Cartwright and Lerner, 1963), were more empathic (Muellen and Abeles, 1971) and provided more unconditional positive regard (Beery, 1970). One additional study found that clients had more positive attitudes toward experienced therapists (Ivey et al, 1968).

Looking at the association between the goodness of the therapeutic relationship and outcome, reviews by Auerbach and Johnson (1977), Luborsky et al (1971), Parloff et al (1978) and Baekeland and Lundwall (1975) have generally concluded that there is no significant relationship between therapist experience and outcome. Baekeland and Lundwall (1975) did, however, find a significant relationship between therapist experience and length of study in treatment.

4). Mutuality of expectations, particularly congruence of expectations about roles, has a positive effect on continuance of the therapeutic relationship.

An excellent review by Berzins (1977) on expectancies and preferences notes that there are few studies which simultaneously assess both patient and therapist expectancies on the same measures. There is some evidence that mutuality of expectations facilitates the continuation of the relationship, even if it is not positively related to outcome (Parloff, 1978). It should be noted that much of the research in this area is based on the assumption that therapists prefer certain behaviors, such as active participation, and that in most cases mutuality has been rated on the degree the patient role agrees with that expected by the therapist. The evidence for mutuality of expectations is best for role expectancies (kinds of personal attributes or behaviors participants expect are appropriate during therapy sessions) as compared to prognostic expectancies.

Several authors have suggested the use of a "role induction" interview to channel expectancies in the psychotherapeutic situation. Interviews directed toward inducing certain expectancies in the patient have been most commonly used, although some research has investigated the use of therapist induction interviews, particularly in the treatment of lower-class patients. Garfield (1978) and Orlinsky and Howard (1978) have reviewed these studies and conclude that this approach is effective in producing increased continuation in therapy. Parloff et al (1978) also concluded that induction procedures in psychotherapy produce increased patient involvement, increased continuation in therapy and improved outcome. Finally, Bordin (1983) postulates that in the psychotherapy situation, the strength of the therapeutic alliance is related to outcome, and that the strength of the alliance is dependent on the degree of agreement between therapist and client about change goals and methods or tasks involved in achieving these goals.

RECOMMENDATIONS

In concluding, we will outline an ideal doctor-patient relationship conducive to compliance, and we will then discuss ways of achieving such a relationship through the presentation of a clinical case vignette. Based on review of the medical compliance and psychotherapeutic alliance literature, the following type of overall doctor-patient relationship should result in an optimal degree of compliance: a relationship in which there is reciprocity of roles, with the patient feeling a sense of control and being involved as an active participant, and with the doctor actively sharing information, encouraging discussion of issues and providing feedback; a relationship in which mutuality of expectations is achieved through a process of sharing both parties' expectations about treatment goals and the mechanisms of achieving these goals, and in which negotiation and collaborative decision-making take place; a relationship in which there is clarification of the rights and responsibilities of both parties; in which there is the provision of an optimal quantity of information in a comprehensible form on which decisions can be based (especially information about the treatment regimen); a relationship in which a therapeutic "environment" is created where the patient experiences the doctor as warm, friendly, sympathetic, interested, respectful, concerned and generally positive and supportive, not authoritarian, dominant, dogmatic, critical or distant; a relationship in which the patient is motivated and has a positive attitude; in which the patient's individual needs, abilities and life circumstances are actively considered in the general therapeutic process; in which there is active inquiry about and adequate attention given to the patient's perception of all these factors, particularly the patient's perception of the therapeutic relationship; and, finally, in which special attention is given to these factors in the critical early visits when the relationship is first being established.

Given this view of the ideal therapeutic relationship, we will now describe a general approach to the development and maintenance of the doctor-patient relationship that can best facilitate compliance as well as treatment in general.

First, the physician should be aware of factors related to compliance. The greater the number of factors present that can contribute to potential noncompliance, the greater the index of suspicion required on the part of the doctor. The doctor should communicate to the patient in a straightfoward noncritical manner his concern about compliance. He should convey the message that compliance with pharmacotherapy is not easy and that it is expected that difficulties will arise. He should share with the patient the expectation that the patient will discuss these difficulties with the doctor so that they can work together to achieve solutions to problems in carrying out the treatment regimen, either by altering the patients' attitudes and behavior or by changing the therapeutic regimen. Again, this should be done in a noncritical, accepting manner, or the patient may be discouraged from further disclosing information about compliance problems. The doctor should institute specific monitoring procedures for compliance and provide ongoing feedback to the patient about how the treatment is proceeding.

From the beginning of treatment, the doctor should establish an active collaboration with the patient, one which involves a reciprocity of roles. This may require significant adjustment on the part of the doctor and patient, as both may be accustomed to a more traditional relationship with less equality. The importance of such a relationship to the treatment should be presented to the patient, and open discussion should be oriented toward clarifying the expected roles and responsibilities involved in future work together. The patient should be allowed and encouraged to be as active in this process as is possible. This will facilitate his perception of control in the therapeutic interaction. The doctor should also let the patient know that his ideas, opinions and perspective are valued and are in fact crucial to the collaborative process. Patient dissatisfaction should be taken seriously and the etiology of it should be determined and addressed. Goals should be examined and compared, and where discrepancies exist, negotiation should take place. Every attempt should be made to tailor the therapeutic program to the patient's needs.

The doctor should actively inquire about the information the patient wishes or expects to receive in the therapeutic encounter and assess the patients' individual needs and abilities to comprehend the requested information. He should then determine the optimal type and amount of information to be presented and present this material in a clear, explicit and consistent fashion. The doctor should also keep in mind that general information about the illness may not be as relevant for the patient as specific information about the illness and the treatment that addresses the patient's needs and concerns. The doctor should remember that simply because material was communicated to the patient, it cannot be retained or assumed that the patient has assimilated this material. Conveyance of information should be followed by repeated inquiries to assess the patient's comprehension and by further explanation, clarification and discussion, if necessary.

The doctor should not remain aloof and distant under the guise of maintaining a "professional" relationship. He should convey, in a warm and friendly manner, a general attitude of concern, regard and support. This may not always be easy, as some patients may bring to the treatment situation anger and frustration about their illnesses, their need for treatment or their prior experiences with the mental health system. The physician should also communicate hopefulness to the patient through positive messages about the patient's prognosis, his belief in the efficacy of the treatment and his belief that the doctor-patient team can successfully work together to implement the treatment.

CLINICAL CASE DESCRIPTION

We will now present a clinical case to illustrate the principles we have outlined, and to demonstrate how these recommendations can be particularly useful with a "difficult" patient.

J.G. is a 30-year-old, white, single female professional who had been treated with weekly individual psychotherapy for approximately three years by a psychotherapist. She was referred for evaluation and potential drug treatment of her mood disorder. J.G. had been suffering from moderately severe and frequent mood swings for approximately five years. Although she had never been hospitalized, these depressive episodes had interfered with her work, interpersonal relationships and social functioning. Her therapist had strongly encouraged evaluation for medication on numerous occasions, but J.G. was adamantly opposed until the occurrence of the first clear episode of elevated mood, when she became alarmed and finally acquiesced.

From the outset it was clear that intense resistances were present. Upon contacting the psychiatrist to arrange an appointment, J.G. was overtly hostile and made clear her need for control. She stated that she did not really wish to take medication, expected no benefit from it and expected serious side effects as she invariably reacted poorly to even the most benign medications. In addition, it was difficult to find a mutually agreeable appointment time despite much flexibility on the part of the psychiatrist.

J.G. arrived 20 minutes late for the first session and was irritable and somewhat agitated. She began the session by railing about the medical profession and complaining about her fee, which she felt was exorbitant. The psychiatrist allowed her to vent her anger for a period of time and maintained an empathic attitude. He then proceeded with the history taking and clinical interview. As the interview proceeded, J.G. became less agitated and gradually began to reveal her anger about the unpredictability and lack of control over her mood swings, the way in which they disrupted her life and her resentment at needing treatment. The psychiatrist encouraged the expression of these feelings and acknowledged their legitimacy.

Toward the end of the interview the psychiatrist shared his impression about J.G.'s diagnosis (Bipolar illness, Type II) and his opinion that a trial of lithium therapy was warranted to see if clinical benefits might be achieved. A brief overview of affective disorders and their treatment was presented, with particular attention to the issue of drug treatment. Potential benefits, as well as dangers, such as side effects or complications, were discussed. At this point, J.G. stated that she was not yet ready to accept the idea of drug therapy and requested a list of "every research article ever written on lithium." Arrangements were made to provide her with several monographs and publications on affective disorder which are written for the lay public yet present relatively sophisticated information. It was mutually agreed that J.G. would read the written material and return for further discussion and questions. She was not willing to commit herself to another appointment, but did agree to arrange an appointment with her internist for the medical evaluation and laboratory studies necessary prior to lithium therapy. J.G.'s psychotherapist was informed about the issues and resistences that had arisen during the consultation and suggested that these would continue to be addressed in the psychotherapy.

Two weeks later J.G. called to make a second appointment. She had completed her medical evaluation and had read the material provided. She was less hostile and the session was spent productively discussing questions that had arisen since the last session, and addressing J.G.'s need for control and her fears of being out of control. At this time the psychiatrist gave a much more detailed explanation of the course of treatment, including dosages and dosage increases, blood level monitoring, side effects, and so forth. At several points, J.G. again became angry about certain of the potential side effects and about the necessary blood tests and her fear of needles. After further discussion and reassurance, she somewhat reluctantly stated that she would like to proceed with a trial of lithium therapy.

The psychiatrist advised J.G. that carrying out the trial would require a great deal of collaborative effort and that the patient would have important responsibilities. He also emphasized that close communication would be required, especially in the early phase of treatment. J.G. and the psychiatrist mutually agreed to begin the lithium at a low dosage and increase the dosage very slowly, allowing plenty of time for J.G. to accommodate. It was agreed that the dosage would not be increased until J.G. felt comfortable with an increase. In addition, it was made clear that if at any time she wished to discontinue the medication she should discuss this with the psychiatrist and they would stop the trial.

J.G. was instructed to monitor herself closely for the appearance of side effects, and it was agreed that she would phone the psychiatrist at the first sign of a problem. She was reassured that if problems arose they would be immediately attended to and appropriate interventions would be made. The psychiatrist arranged to call J.G. every other day for the first week to check on her condition. Since J.G. only felt comfortable having blood drawn at her internist's office, arrangements were made for the blood level to be drawn there instead of at a local laboratory. Her psychotherapist was notified of the planned course of treatment and J.G.'s concerns and resistances.

During the first week, J.G. noted the gradual onset of fatigue and decreased energy, which caused her to feel drowsy in the late afternoon and interfered with physical exertion. The psychiatrist inquired as to whether J.G. felt she could tolerate the effects for another week to see if their intensity might decrease, and J.G. agreed. After another week of treatment, the side effects decreased and she agreed to increase the medication to 600 mg per day. After several days on 600 mg of lithium, the fatigue returned and J.G. began complaining of memory problems and a feeling of motor incoordination. These symptoms did not lessen with time and during the second session a week later, J.G. was again angry and verbally abusive, expressing her frustration over the unpleasant symptoms she was experiencing. The psychiatrist encouraged J.G. to try a decreased dosage of 450 mg, suggesting that perhaps the increase was too rapid. However, over the next week, the symptoms persisted, and the dosage was further reduced. After several weeks on 300 mg of lithium, another unsuccessful attempt was made to increase the dosage. Since the lithium blood level on 300 mg was only .26 meg/l it was decided to terminate the drug trial. Again, there was close communication with J.G.'s psychotherapist about the course of treatment.

At the final session, both parties agreed that J.G. had made a sincere effort during the medication trial. J.G. expressed regret that she was unable to achieve a dosage level that would determine whether she could really benefit from the drug. The psychiatrist suggested that perhaps during the next depressive episode, an antidepressant might be tried and J.G. agreed. She thanked the psychiatrist and departed on congenial terms, stating that her attitudes about doctors and medication had changed for the better.

FUTURE WORK

Future work should focus on further describing and clarifying the nature of the therapeutic relationship in the context of psychopharmacologic treatment. Many unanswered questions exist regarding the ways in which the alliance in psychopharmacotherapy is similar to or different from the alliance that occurs in a medical pharmacotherapy situation, or in a psychotherapy situation where pharmacotherapy is not involved. Thus, the unique aspects of the "psychopharmacotherapeutic alliance" need further explication.

Recent methodological developments in the area of psychotherapy research may allow more sophisticated investigations to be carried out in this area. The Treatment of Depression Collaborative Research Project, NIMH, represents the first time a specified "clinical management" intervention has been developed for the pharmacotherapy condition. Various aspects of the pharmacotherapy intervention, including techniques specific to the condition of pill giving and receiving, as well as more general aspects of developing and maintaining a "pharmacotherapeutic alliance" (which would ideally promote optimal response to the active or pill-placebo) have been standardized and manualized. Having a standardized format for pharmacotherapy intervention represents a major step in facilitating future investigations of the nature of the therapeutic relationship in psychopharmacology, and should also facilitate the comparison of the therapeutic relationship in pharmacotherapy to that in other therapies.

REFERENCES

Asburn L: Patient compliance with medication regimens, in Biobehavioral Medicine. Edited by Sheppard J. Lidcombe, NSW, Cumberland College of Health Sciences, 1981

Auerbach A, Johnson M: Research on the therapist's level of experience, in Effective Psychotherapy. Edited by Gurman AS, Razin AM. New York, Pergamon Press, 1977

Baekeland F, Lundwall L: Dropping out of treatment: a critical review. Psychol Bull 82:738-783, 1975

Barrett-Lennard GT: Dimensions of therapist response as causal factors in therapeutic change. Psychological Monographs 76:43 (Whole No. 562), 1-36, 1962

Becker MH: The health belief model and personal health behavior. Health Education Monographs 2:324, 1974

Becker MH: Sociobehavioral determinants of compliance, in Compliance with Therapeutic Regimens. Edited by Sackett DL, Haynes RB. Baltimore MD, The Johns Hopkins University Press, 1976

Becker MH: Understanding patient compliance: the contributions of attitudes and other psychosocial factors, in New Directions in Patient Compliance. Edited by Cohen SJ. Lexington MA, Heath and Company, 1979

Becker MH, Maiman LA: Strategies for enhancing compliance. J Community Health 6:113-135, 1980

Becker MH, Maiman LA, Kirscht JP, et al: Patient perceptions and compliance: recent studies of the health belief model, in Compliance in Health Care. Edited by Haynes RB, Taylor DW, Sackett DL. Baltimore MD, The Johns Hopkins University Press, 1979

Beery J: Therapists' responses as a function of level of therapist experience and attitude of the patient. J Consult Clin Psychol 34:239-243, 1970

Berzins JI: Therapist-patient matching, in Effective Psychotherapy. Edited by Gurman AS, Razin AM. New York, Pergamon Press, 1977

Blackwell B: The drug defaulter. Clin Pharmacol Ther 13:841-848, 1972

Blackwell B: Drug therapy: patient compliance. N Engl J Med 289:249-252, 1973

Blackwell B: Treatment adherence. Br J Psychiatry 129:513-531, 1976

Blackwell B: The drug regimen and treatment compliance, in Compliance in Health Care. Edited by Haynes RB, Taylor DW, Sackett DL. Baltimore MD, The Johns Hopkins University Press, 1979

Bordin, E: Myths, realities and alternatives to clinical trials. Paper presented at International Conference on Psychotherapy, Bogota, Colombia, February 1983

Boyd JR, Covington TR, Stanaszek WF, et al: Drug defaulting: II. Analysis of noncompliance patterns. Am J Hosp Pharm 31:485-491, 1974

Caplan RD: Patient, provider and organization: hypothesized determinants of adherence, in New Directions in Patient Compliance. Edited by Cohen SJ. Lexington MA, Heath and Company

Cartwright R, Lerner B: Empathy, need to change and improvement with psychotherapy. Journal of Consulting Psychology 27:138-144, 1963

Charney E, Bynam R, Eldredge D, et al: How well do patients take oral penicillin? a collaborative study in private practice. Pediatrics 40:188-195, 1967

Christensen DB: Drug-taking compliance: a review and synthesis. Health Services Research 13:171-187, 1978

Davis MS: Variations in patients' compliance with doctors' advice: analysis of congruence between survey responses and results of empirical investigations. J Med Educ 41:1037-1048, 1966

Davis MS: Variations in patients' compliance with doctors' advice: an empirical analysis of patterns of communication. Am J Public Health 48:274-288, 1968

Davis MS: Variation in patients' compliance with doctors' orders: medical practice and doctor-patient interaction. Psychiatry in Medicine 2:31-54, 1971

Davis MS, Eichhorn R: Compliance with medical regimens: a panel study. Journal of Health and Human Behavior 4:240-249, 1963

Davis MS, VonderLippe RP: Discharge from hospital against medical advice: a study of reciprocity in the doctor-patient relationship. Soc Sci Med 1:336-344, 1968

DiNicolla DD, DiMatteo MR: Communication, interpersonal influence and resistance to medical treatment, in Basic Processes in Helping Relationships. Edited by Wills TA. New York, Academic Press, 1982

Downing RW, Rickels K, King L, et al: Factors influencing dosage deviation and attrition in placebo treated neurotic outpatients. J Psychiatr Res 12:239-256, 1975

Duehn WD, Proctor EK: Initial clinical interaction and premature discontinuance in treatment. Am J Orthopsychiatry 47:284-290, 1977

Eisenthal S, Emery R, Lazare A, et al: "Adherence" and the negotiated approach to patienthood. Arch Gen Psychiatry 36:393-398, 1979

Ettlinger PRA, Freedman GL: General practice compliance study: is it worth being a personal doctor? Br Med J 282:1192-1194, 1981

Evans L, Spelman M: The problem of noncompliance with drug therapy. Drugs 25:63-76, 1983

Fedder DO: Managing medication and compliance: physician-pharmacist-patient interactions. J American Geriatr Soc, 30(Suppl):S113-S117, 1982

Fiedler F: The concept of an ideal therapeutic relationship. Journal of Consulting Psychology 14:239-245, 1950a

Fiedler F: Factor analyses of psychoanalytic, nondirective and Adlerian therapy. Journal of Consulting Psychology 14:436-445, 1950b

Flesch R: A new readability yardstick. J Appl Psychol 32:221, 1948

Fox W: Self-administration of medications: a review of published work and study of problems. Bull Int Union Tuberc 32:307-331, 1962

Frank JD: Therapeutic factors in psychotherapy. Am J Psychother 25:350-361, 1971

Francis V, Korsch B, Morris M: Gaps in doctor-patient communication: patients' response to medical advice. N Engl J Med 280:535-540, 1969

Freedman N, Engelhardt DM, Hankoff LD, et al: Dropout from outpatient psychiatric treatment. Archives of Neurology and Psychiatry 80:657-666, 1958

Freemon B, Negrete VF, Davis M, et al: Gaps in doctor-patient communication: doctor-patient interaction analysis. Pediatr Res 5:298-311, 1971

Freud S: The technique of psychoanalysis, in Standard Edition of the Complete Works of Sigmund Freud, vol 23. Edited and translated by Strachey J. London, Hogarth, 1940, 1964

Garfield SL: Research on client variables in psychotherapy, in Handbook of Psychotherapy and Behavior Change: An Empirical Analysis. Second ed. Edited by Garfield SL, Bergin AE. New York, John Wiley & Sons, 1978

Garfield SL, Wolpin M: Expectations regarding psychotherapy. J Nerv Ment Dis 137:353-362, 1963

Garrity TF: Medical compliance and the doctor-patient relationship: a review. Soc Sci Med 15:215-222, 1981

Gillum RF, Barsky AJ: Diagnosis and management of patient noncompliance. JAMA 223:1563-1567, 1974

Glanz K: Dieticians' effectiveness and patient compliance with dietary regimens. J Am Diet Assoc 75:631-636, 1979

Gomes-Schwartz B: Effective ingredients in psychotherapy: prediction of outcome from process variables. J Consult Clin Psychol 46:1023-1035, 1978

Gordis L: Conceptual and methodological problems in measuring patient compliance, in Compliance in Health Care. Edited by Haynes RB, Taylor DW, Sackett DL. Baltimore MD, The Johns Hopkins University Press, 1979

Gottschalk LA, Mayerson P, Gottlieb AA: Prediction and evaluation of outcome in an emergency brief psychotherapy clinic. J Nerv Ment Dis 144:77-96, 1967

Gurman AS: The patients' perception of the therapeutic relationship, in Effective Psychotherapy. Edited by Gurman AS, Razin AR. New York, Pergamon Press, 1977

Haynes RB: A critical review of the determinants of patient compliance with therapeutic regimens, in Compliance with Therapeutic Regimens. Edited by Sackett DL, Haynes RB. Baltimore MD, The Johns Hopkins University Press, 1976

Haynes RB: Determinants of compliance: the disease and the mechanics of treatment, in Compliance in Health Care. Edited by Haynes RB, Taylor DW, Sackett DL. Baltimore MD, The Johns Hopkins University Press, 1979a

Haynes RB: Introduction, in Compliance in Health Care. Edited by Haynes RB, Taylor DW, Sackett DL. Baltimore MD, The Johns Hopkins University Press, 1979b

Heine RW, Trosman H: Initial expectations of the doctor-patient interaction as a factor in continuance in psychotherapy. Psychiatry 23:275-278, 1960

Howard KL, Orlinsky DE: Psychotherapeutic processes. Annu Rev of Psychol 23:615-668, 1972

Howard K, Rickels K, Mock JE, et al: Therapeutic style and attrition rate for psychiatric drug treatment. J Nerv Ment Dis 150:102-110, 1970

Hulka B: Patient-clinician interactions and compliance, in Compliance in Health Care.

Edited by Haynes RB, Taylor DW, Sackett DL. Baltimore MD, The Johns Hopkins University Press, 1979

Hulka B, Kupper L, Cassel J, et al: Doctor-patient communication and outcome among diabetic patients. J Community Health 1:15-27, 1975

Ivey A, Miller C, Gabbert K: Counselor assessment and client attitude: a systematic replication. Journal of Counseling Psychology 15:194-195, 1968

Jenkins, CB: An approach to the diagnosis and treatment of problems of health related behavior. Journal of Health Education 22 (Supplement):1, 1979

Kasl SV: Issues in patient adherence to health care regimens. Journal of Human Stress 1:5-17, 1975

Korsch B, Gozzi E, Francis V: Gaps in doctor-patient communication. I. Doctor-patient interaction and patient satisfaction. Pediatrics 42:855-871, 1968

Ley P: Primacy, rated importance and the recall of medical statements. J Health Soc Behav 13:311-317, 1972

Ley P: Memory for medical information. British Journal of Social and Clinical Psychology 18:245-254, 1979a

Ley P: The psychology of compliance, in Research in Psychology and Medicine, vol II. Edited by Osborne DJ, Gruneberg MM, Eiser JR. London, Academic Press, 1979b

Ley P: Satisfaction, compliance and communication. Br J Clin Psychol 21:241-254, 1982

Ley P, Jain V, Skilbeck C: A method for decreasing medication errors. Psychol Med 6:599-601 1976a

Ley P, Whitworth MA, Skilbeck CE, et al: Improving doctor-patient communication in general practice. Journal of the Royal College General Practitioners 26:720-724, 1976b

Levine DM, Green LW, Deeds SG, et al: Health education for hypertensive patients. JAMA 241:1700-1703, 1979

Lorr M: Client perceptions of therapists: a study of therapeutic relation. Journal of Consulting Psychology 29:146-149, 1965

Luborsky L, Chandler M, Auerbach AH, et al: Factors influencing the outcome of psychotherapy. Psychol Bull 75:145-185, 1971

Luborsky L, Crits-Christoph P, Alexander L, et al: Two helping alliance methods for predicting outcomes of psychotherapy: a counting signs vs. a global rating method. J Nerv Ment Disease 171:480-492, 1983

Malahy B: The effect of instruction and labeling on the number of medication errors made by patients at home. Am J Hosp Pharm 23:283-292, 1966

Marston M: Compliance with medical regimens: a review of the literature. Nursing Research 19:312-323, 1970

Marziali E, Marmar C, Krupnick J: Therapeutic alliance scales: development and relationship to psychotherapy outcome. Am J Psychiatry 138:361-364, 1981

Mazzullo JM, Lasagna LL: Take thou . . . but is your patient really taking what you prescribed? Drug Therapy 2:11-15, 1972

McKenney JM, Slining JM, Henderson HR, et al: The effect of clinical pharmacy service on patients with essential hypertension. Circulation 48:1104-1111, 1973

Mitchell JH: Compliance with medical regimens: an annotated bibliography. Health Education Monograph 2:75-87, 1974

Mitchell KM, Bozarth JD, Krauft CC: A reappraisal of the therapeutic effectiveness of accurate empathy, nonpossessive warmth and genuineness, in Effective Psychotherapy. Edited by Gurman AS, Razin AR. New York, Pergamon Press, 1977

Morgan R, Luborsky L, Crits-Christoph P, et al: Predicting the outcomes of psychotherapy by the Penn Helping Alliance Rating Method. Arch Gen Psychiatry 39:397-402, 1982

Muellen J, Abeles N: Relationship of liking, empathy and therapists' experience to outcome of psychotherapy. Journal of Counseling Psychology 18:39-43, 1971

Orlinsky DE, Howard KI: The therapist's experience of psychotherapy, in Effective Psychotherapy. Edited by Gurman AS, Razin AR. New York, Pergamon Press, 1977

Overall B, Aronson H: Expectations of psychotherapy in patients of lower socioeconomic class. Am J Orthopsychiatry 33:421-430, 1963

Parloff MB, Waskow IE, Wolfe BE: Research on therapist variables in relation to process and outcome, in Handbook of Psychotherapy and Behavior Change: An Empirical Analysis. Second ed. Edited by Garfield SL, Bergin AE. New York, John Wiley & Sons, 1978

Raskin A: A comparison of acceptors and resistors of drug treatment as an adjunct to psychotherapy. J Consult Clin Psychol 25:366, 1961

Reynolds E, Joyce CRB, Swift JL, et al: Psychological and clinical investigation of the treatment of anxious outpatient with three barbiturates and placebo. Br J Psychiatry 111:84-95, 1965

Richards AD: Attitude and drug acceptance. Br J Psychiatry 110:46-52, 1964

Rickels K, Cattell RB: Drug and placebo response as a function of doctor and patient type, in Psychotropic Drug Responses. Edited by May PRA, Wittenhorn JR. Springfield IL, Charles C Thomas, 1969

Rogers CR: The necessary and sufficient conditions of therapeutic personality change. Journal of Consulting Psychology 21:95-103, 1957

Roter D: Patient participation in the patient-provider interaction: the effects of patient question asking on the quality of interaction, satisfaction and compliance. Health Education Monograph 55:281, 1977

Sackett DL: The magnitude of compliance and noncompliance, in Compliance with Therapeutic Regimens. Edited by Sackett DL, Haynes RB. Baltimore MD, The Johns Hopkins University Press, 1976

Sackett DL, Snow JC: The magnitude of compliance and noncompliance, in Compliance in Health Care. Edited by Haynes RB, Taylor DW, Sackett DL. Baltimore MD, The Johns Hopkins University Press, 1979

Saltzman C, Luetgert M, Roth C, et al: Formation of a therapeutic relationship: experiences during the initial phase of psychotherapy as predictors of treatment duration and outcome. J Consult Clin Psychol 44:546-555, 1976

Schorr D, Rodin J: The role of perceived control in practitioner-patient relationships, in Basic Processes in Helping Relationships. Edited by Wills TA. New York, Academic Press, 1982

Schulman B: Active patient orientation and outcomes in hypertensive treatment. Medical Care 17:267-280, 1979

Shapiro RJ: Therapist attitudes and premature termination in family and individual therapy. J Nerv Ment Dis 159:101-107, 1974

Stimson GV: Obeying doctors' orders: a view from the other side. Soc Sci Med 8:97-104, 1974

Stoler N: Client likability: a variable in the study of psychotherapy. Journal of Consulting Psychology 27:175-178, 1963

Strupp HH, Wallach MS, Jenkins JW, et al: Psychotherapists' assessments of former patients. J Nerv Ment Dis 137:222-230, 1963

Svarstad B: The doctor-patient encounter: an observational study of communication and outcome. Doctoral dissertation, University of Wisconsin, 1974

Szasz T, Hollender MA: A contribution to the philosophy of medicine: the basic models of the doctor-patient relationships. Archives of Internal Medicine 97:585-592, 1956

Tagliacozzo DM, Ima K: Knowledge of illness as a predictor of patient behavior. J Chronic Dis 22:766-775, 1970

Tracy J: Impact of intake procedures upon client attrition in a community mental health center. J Consult Clin Psychol 45:192-195, 1977

VanPutten T: Drug refusal in schizophrenia: causes and prescribing units. Hosp Community Psychiatry 29:110-112, 1978

Wartman SA, Morlock LL, Malitz FE, et al: Patient understanding and satisfaction as predictors of compliance. Medical Care 21:886-891, 1983

Wilcox DRC, Gilan R, Hare EH: Do psychiatric outpatients take their drugs? Br Med J 2:790-792, 1965

Wilson JD, Enoch MD: Estimation of drug rejection in schizophrenic in-patients with analysis of clinical factors. Br J Psychiatry 113:209-211, 1967

Afterword

by John P. Docherty, M.D.

In Chapter 27, "Research on the Therapeutic Alliance in Psychotherapy," Dr. Dianna E. Hartley has provided an excellent review and overview of the conceptual development, the context and specific current research on the therapeutic alliance. Her review also raises several important questions for future research consideration. Dr. Hartley strongly implies that our current working definition of therapeutic alliance is still quite a simple one. It is clear that more conceptual and theoretical work must be undertaken to adequately articulate the complexities of the therapeutic relationship within the context of a conceptual structure. One example of such an articulation is the specification of other dimensions of the therapeutic relationship in addition to affiliation, such as dominance/submission, which should be included in an assessment of the therapeutic alliance. Even a simple elaboration such as this raises additional questions, such as, "What dimension of relatedness is most central to an effective therapeutic alliance?"

Dr. Hartley's chapter also makes us aware that we need clearer and more precise definitions of the specific therapist characteristics that enhance or impede the formation of the therapeutic alliance. The identification of such characteristics could significantly accelerate the effective training of psychotherapists. Her review further points out the necessity of delineating the mechanisms by which important therapist characteristics express themselves in the therapy, and the ways in which they enhance the formation and maintenance of the therapeutic alliance. "How do therapists who possess these characteristics behave in therapy? How are their differential helpful actions linked to their thoughts and feelings about the patient and about the transactions in question?"

This review also clearly provides a background for posing another important question: "What are the differential influences of patient diagnostic category and type of psychotherapy on the role and course of the therapeutic alliance in successful treatment?" Advances in the methodology of diagnosis and the assessment of the therapeutic alliance now make it possible to investigate such issues.

It is clear from Chapter 28 as well as from Chapter 29 that patient characteristics assume an especially important role in determining the success of short-term directive psychotherapy. The limited nature of the contact, as well as the specific task requirements of this form of psychotherapy, demand certain capabilities on the part of the patient. It is thus extremely important that empirical research be carried out to determine the precise description and differential predictive weight of patient characteristics for successful participation in this form of therapy.

This Afterword was written by Dr. Docherty in his private capacity. No official support or endorsement by NIMH is intended or should be inferred.

In Chapter 28, "The Therapeutic Relationship in Psychodynamic Psychotherapy: The Research Evidence and Its Meaning for Practice," Drs. Lester Luborsky and Arthur H. Auerbach briefly review and highlight some of the most clinically important findings in research on the therapeutic relationship. They point out that the concept of the therapeutic relationship is a broad one that encompasses the more restricted concept of the therapeutic alliance, which refers to a particular structure within the therapeutic relationship. Their review clearly indicates the reasons for the inherent interest and focus on the therapeutic alliance by noting that among the variables assessed in the relationship per se, the alliance variable seems at this point to be the most powerful predictor of outcome. The review raises several important points which should be specifically noted.

This chapter emphasizes the need for intensive investigation of patient "capacity for therapy" variables. Very few of these variables have been investigated, yet clinical experience suggests that there are certain affective, cognitive and personality characteristics in a patient that can severely limit his or her ability to engage in a useful therapy; this may be especially true for particular types of therapy. With regard to this issue, it is clear that future research will require studies of the complex linkage among patient or therapist variables, and the formation of the therapeutic alliance and outcome.

This chapter also highlights an important and still tentative finding in the field. It appears that the greater the degree to which a therapist adheres to a specific type of therapy in the conduct of a treatment, the better the outcome will be. This finding, while still under investigation, does raise other questions. For example, is this finding simply an artifact of patient difficulty (that is, the "more difficult" a patient is, the harder it is to maintain the integrity of the therapeutic approach), or is it an artifact of a more general therapist capability factor? Is the ability to control interventions with more focus and precision the salient variable that is simply reflected in an ability to maintain adherence to a particular set of prescribed therapeutic techniques?

Drs. Luborsky and Auerbach raise a question also raised in Chapter 27: namely, "Are different patient, therapist or relationship variables important in the conduct of different therapies?" The authors also note, as does Dr. Rush in Chapter 29, the differential findings with regard to the patient capacity for "experiencing" in client-centered versus primarily psychodynamic forms of psychotherapy.

This chapter raises an issue which may well be a critical one for the field in the next several years. This is the implication of the rapidly developing methodologies for the standardization of psychotherapy and the assessment of therapist competency for clinical training. These technologies, which stand in contrast to the inefficiency of much prior clinical training, have important and serious implications for the future design of educational programs.

In Chapter 29, "The Therapeutic Alliance in Short-Term Directive Therapies," Dr. A. John Rush reviews a number of important clinical issues that require attention in effecting a positive therapeutic alliance for the purpose of short-term directive psychotherapy.

Chapter 29 implicitly addresses a distinction between short-term and long-term psychotherapy. There are at least three issues involved in the differential construction of the therapeutic alliance in these two approaches to psychotherapy. First is the issue of sequencing: That is, what steps should be undertaken to develop a therapeutic alliance in these two forms of therapy, and what is the ordering of those steps? Second is the issue of differential goals: That is, to the extent that the goals of these two therapies differ, do they require different forms of therapeutic alliance? Dr. Bordin's (1983) conceptualization of the nature of the therapeutic alliance suggests that differential goals always require and give rise to different forms of therapeutic alliance. Third, does the therapeutic alliance for long-term psychotherapy need to be grounded in a different way than that for short-term psychotherapy? That is, must there be a more stable and permanent foundation laid for the therapeutic alliance in the context of a therapy that will last over a long period of time?

What is the proper role of emotional and evocative techniques for the facilitation of a short-term psychotherapy? Although we might not expect such techniques to have a profound impact for long-term therapy, might such techniques in the first encounter of patient and therapist facilitate a strengthened therapeutic alliance for short-term work?

Dr. Rush's clinical examples implicitly raise the question of the role of inpatient treatment in the preparation of patients for psychotherapy, particularly the effect of previous or intercurrent inpatient treatment on the therapeutic alliance. A research approach to this question probably best derives from placing it in the broader context of the role of the social and cultural influences on the development of a therapeutic alliance. To what extent is the therapeutic alliance hindered or facilitated by particular aspects of the patient's social resources and social network? What differential techniques for the facilitation of a therapeutic alliance will be required, depending upon the nature of the patient's social network and social resources? In the case of inpatient treatment, what variables in the inpatient setting can be called upon to strengthen the therapeutic alliance? These issues arise principally in the context of the discussion of short-term therapy, because underlying them is the question: "What other variables may be called upon to rapidly strengthen a therapeutic relationship and permit effective work to be carried out over a relatively short period of time?"

Chapter 30, "The Therapeutic Alliance With Difficult Patients," is a clinically rich and informative chapter, in which Drs. Mardi Horowitz and Charles Marmar vividly describe the problems encountered in the formation of a therapeutic alliance with "difficult" patients. Their work not only demonstrates a perceptive clinical appreciation of the central problem of treatment in such cases, but also reflects the considerable development of methods for quantifying and measuring the major components of this clinical problem. There are two other clinically relevant aspects of the problem of "difficult" patients which should be noted. The first of these is a consideration of the usefulness of borrowing techniques from other therapeutic approaches in order to resolve therapeutic "impasses." For example, with at least some of the dilemmas that are outlined in this chapter, the therapeutic situation might be resolvable through the use of a version of the gestalt "two chair" technique, in which the patient is asked to establish a dialogue with himself in which he articulates both sides of the dilemma. Yet other techniques might be particularly useful in dealing with such problems as they are experienced within a psychodynamic framework.

The second major issue, from a clinician's point of view, relates to the question, "When do you call a stop to the therapy?" This is a complex issue involving the recognition that the therapy has reached an impasse, at which point the likelihood of future therapeutic work is virtually nonexistent; and the clinical process through which such a determination may best be made and discussed with the patient. This is a central clinical issue, because it is at this point that the therapist must experience for himself or herself the patient's experience of the dilemma in the therapy. This is a central consideration also because it is not infrequent that a resolution is reached at this very point. Could it be that "beginning with the end" may be a useful strategy for approaching the problem of the "difficult" patient in psychodynamically oriented brief psychotherapy?

In Chapter 31, "The Influence of Gender and Race on the Therapeutic Alliance," Drs. Susan J. Blumenthal, Enrico E. Jones and Ms. Janice L. Krupnick demonstrate that there are many variables requiring further investigation in order to fully understand the structure and control of the therapeutic alliance. It is critical that we bear in mind that our knowledge of this important component of psychotherapy is still in its embryonic state. Gender and race variables, as well as other salient variables such as age, social class and occupational experience, affect the formation of the therapeutic alliance. If we consider only two of the tentative findings reported in this chapter, we can begin to see the potential for deepened understanding of the therapeutic process. For example, it appears that women may more readily establish more positive therapeutic alliances. If this is true, why is it true? Can we isolate salient differences in technique? Is it due to a gender effect on patient perception? Why is outcome not more discernibly affected? Second, a significant impact of the racial variable appears to be an impediment to establishing a lasting therapeutic contact. How is this effect exerted? What changes in technique could reverse this effect? This chapter illustrates the importance of developing a systematic understanding of those variables that both impede and facilitate the development of the therapeutic alliance.

In Chapter 32, "The Therapeutic Alliance and Compliance With Psychopharmacology," Drs. John P. Docherty and Susan J. Fiester have examined the influence of the psychosocial state on the conduct of psychopharmacology. However, it is important in considering the issue of therapeutic alliance to begin to consider the effect of drugs on psychosocial processes. David Janowsky, M.D., has termed this area of research "psychopharmacology of interpersonal processes." Current developments in the technology for assessing the therapeutic alliance now make clinical progress possible. It is now possible to ask such a critical clinical question as, "What is the effect of drug treatment on the development of a therapeutic alliance?" This is a simple, feasible study which (controlling for the drug and its administration, symptom severity, and diagnosis) can be practically and usefully carried out.

In addition, this chapter raises several other important questions for future research:

What is the nature of the relationship among the four major components of the clinician-patient relationship (role relationships, expectations, communication and effective time); for example, are there stages or phases in the development of the therapeutic relationship where particular components are most important? And how do individual doctor and patient factors interact with each other and with these other elements of the relationship?

The review notes that several factors, such as patient control, motivation and satisfaction may be involved as mediating factors between the basic elements of the relationships and compliance. Research is needed in order to further specify the processes and mechanisms by which these components have their effect on compliance.

Research is needed to further describe and understand the nature of the therapeutic alliance and compare it to the medical doctor-patient relationship, the psychotherapeutic doctor-patient relationship and the psychopharmacologic doctor-patient relationship. In particular, when psychotherapy and pharmacotherapy are carried out by the same clinician, is the type of alliance required for each type of treatment the same, different or complementary? Might they be at odds? Finally, does psychopharmacotherapy change the nature of the therapeutic relationship?

REFERENCES

Bordin E: Myths, realities and alternatives to clinical trials. Paper presented at International Conference on Psychotherapy, Bogota, Colombia, February 1983

Afterword

Afterword

by Robert E. Hales, M.D. and Allen J. Frances, M.D.

The faithful reader deserves our congratulations and gratitude. This is not a Volume that lends itself to digestion in big, easy bites. We hope that the time and concentration required has been sufficiently rewarded in expanded knowledge and in a shared sense of wonder at the rapid progress our field is enjoying.

Although Volume 4 has just been published, we have been at work on Volume 5 since the Fall of 1983. We wish to preview this Volume with you at this time.

The introduction will be written by Carol C. Nadelson, M.D., currently President-Elect of the American Psychiatric Association. We have expanded Volume 5 to include six sections. The first section, edited by Nancy C. Andreasen, M.D., Ph.D., will review recent developments in "Schizophrenia." Dr. Andreasen's section will discuss diagnosis and classification, cognitive aspects, neurobiology, genetics, psychosocial interventions and somatic therapy. Dr. Robert B. Millman will edit a section entitled, "Drug Abuse and Drug Dependence." This section will include five chapters concerning opiates, cocaine and amphetamines, depressants, marijuana and psychedelics. Each chapter will discuss the following topics: general description and origins, epidemiology, pharmacology and patterns of abuse, adverse effects and management. Next, Drs. Carolyn Robinowitz and Jeanne Spurlock will edit a section entitled, "Adolescent Psychiatry." This will include chapters on normality and development, legal issues, alcoholism and substance abuse, adolescence and illness, conduct disorders and adolescent depression.

Dr. Robert M. A. Hirschfeld's section will provide an overview of the recent developments in the diagnosis and treatment of personality disorders. Among the chapters will be discussions of the methods of classifying and treating personality disorders and the interaction between personality and Axis I symptomatic disorders. Drs. David Spiegel and W. Stewart Agras will edit a section entitled, "Psychotherapeutic Management of Medical Disorders." This section will include chapters in the following areas: a general discussion of behavioral modalities and theoretical considerations, inpatient care for combined medical and psychiatric disorders, gastrointestinal disorders, cardiovascular disease, habit disorders, and oncological and pain syndromes. Finally, Dr. Irvin D. Yalom will organize a section on "Group Psychotherapy" that includes discussions on therapeutic factors and interpersonal learning in therapy groups, and also chapters on homogeneous, inpatient and self-help groups.

We hope that this brief description of Volume 5 whets your appetite and we look forward to renewing our acquaintance with you next year, when we will present Volume 5 of *The American Psychiatric Association Annual Review*.

Index

Alcoholism:
    in parents of anorexics, 484–485
    and bulimia, 471, 497
Alexia, 123
Alexithymia, 371
Alienation, experiences of, 115, 131, 132
Alkalosis, from self-induced vomiting, 471
Alpha-adrenoreceptors, 40
Alpha methyldopa, 107
Aluminum toxicity, 222
Alzheimer's disease, see Dementia of the
    Alzheimer type
Alzheimer's Disease and Related Disorder
    Association (ADRDA), 221
Ambition, gender-linking, by therapist,
    589
Ambivalence, patient, 576
Amenorrhea, 446, 512
    in anorexia nervosa, 402, 439, 442–443,
        445, 453, 490, 517
    in normal-weight bulimia, 402
American Anorexia Nervosa Association
    (AANA), 520
American Cancer Society, 387
American Psychopathological Association,
    anxiety symposium, 356
Amino acids, neurotransmitter, 11, 13–14,
        39, 67–68
    defined, 83
    See also Neuropeptides
Amitriptyline, for bulimia, 476
Amnesia:
    in DAT, 215
    in temporal lobe patients, 193
Amphetamines:
    abuse of, 16, 17, 234
    for narcolepsy, 333
    schizophrenia-like psychosis induction,
        17–26
    stereotyped rat motor behavior and, 24
Amusia, 126
Amygdala, 163
ANAD, see National Association of
    Anorexia Nervosa and Associated
    Disorders
Anger:
    borderline personality, 357
    during interictal period, 193–194
Angiotensin, 11
Animal models, 37, 44
    of eating disorders, 517
    for obesity studies, 419, 424
    for sleep–wake cycle research, 277
    to test antipsychotic drugs, 17–21, 24
Anomia, 122
Anorexia nervosa, 438–456
    age of onset, 482
    amenorrhea, 402, 439, 445, 446, 452,
        490, 512, 517

atypical, 440
classic signs, 444-445
clinical characteristics, 441–446
confusion about needs in, 505–506
cultural predisposition, 448
in dancers and models, 448, 517
diagnosing, 438–440
effects of improvement, 453, 488–489,
    512–513
etiology, 503
expression of affect, 482, 489, 490, 493,
    495
family aspects, 448, 481–485, 488, 490,
    517
high negative expressed emotion and,
    491, 518
hospitalization, and afterwards, 449,
    453–454, 495, 519
incidence in first-degree relatives, 483
individual predispositions, 447
initial contact with therapist, 511
legal and ethical questions, 519
LH secretion patterns, 331
in males, 448–449
medical complications, 454–455
operant conditioning for, 450
parental personalities, 481–482, 485–486
personality characteristics, 509–510
pathogenesis, 481
pharmacotherapies for, 451–453
physical and lab abnormalities, 403
postmenopausal, 441
potassium depletion, 449, 454–455
psychotherapy strategies, 450–451, 510–
    513
restricting versus bulimic, 402, 440, 443–
    444, 452, 456, 464–465, 484, 490, 509
subtypes and typologies, 508–510, 516
symptoms, 441–443, 508–509
theories about, 447, 503, 505–507
therapist's countertransference, 519
in upper-class women, 420
Anorexia Nervosa and Related Eating
    Disorders, Inc. (ANRED), 520
Anorexoids, 482, 510
Anosognosia, 130–131
ANRED, see Anorexia Nervosa and
    Related Eating Disorders, Inc.
Antiarrhythmic drugs, organic mental
    disorders from, 229
Anticholinergics, 58–59
    toxicity, 107, 227
Anticonvulsants, 107
    for bulimia, 475
    for manic–depressive and affective
        disorders, 242
    side effects, 229–230
Antidepressants:
    for bulimia, 470, 475–476

for insomnia, 379, 380
Barrett–Lennard Relationship Inventory,
    536, 552
Basal forebrain cholinergic complex, 57–58
Basal ganglia:
    anatomy and physiology, 161, 163
    calcification of, 168
    disorders of, 58–60, 79, 105, 162, 217
    GABA concentrations, 70
    innervation to, 56
    motor symptoms and, 60
Basal metabolism, physical activity, and
    obesity, 425
Bayley Scales of Mental Development,
    and REM storms, 330
BBS, see Bombesin
Beck Depression Inventory, 569
Behavior therapy, 540, 563
    for anorexia nervosa, 504
    cognitive, 527
    emphasis on technique, 533
    for obesity, 428, 430, 431
Belladonna, 58, 227
Benzodiazepines:
    to control seizures, 78
    effect on GABA transmission, 70
    evidence of link between GABA and
        anxiety, 74
    for insomnia, 370, 380
    Librium, 76
    mechanism of action, 76
    and respiration, 387–388
    short-acting, 385, 388
    side effects, 384
    site, on $GABA_A$ receptors, 71
    and stimulants, 363
    Valium, 76
Benztropine, 107
Beta-adrenoceptors, 41
Beta-endorphin, 11, 85, 90–94, 408
Bicuculline, effect on GABA transmission,
    70
Binding, radioligand, 21–27
    nonspecific, 21–22
Binding sites:
    ^{3}H-spiroperidol, 22, 27, 32
    imipramine, 39
Binge-eating, 449, 464–465, 467
    antidepressants for, 475–477
    defining, 466
    in males, 466, 468
    and pimozide, 410
    after surgery, 427
Biofeedback, for insomnia, 365–366
Biogenic amines, 11, 13–14, 39
    uptake system, in depression, 39–40
Blood pressure:
    and cognitive impairment, 212
    during sleep, 272

and stroke, 152
Blood sugar, increases, effects on
    cognitive functioning, 212
Body image:
    in anorexia nervosa, 438, 439, 441, 447,
        505
    in bulimics, 470
    disparagement, 422–423, 427, 434
    in eating disorders, 508
    and psychosocial maturity, 505
    and self-esteem, 508
Bombesin (BBS), 11, 412, 413, 415
Bonding, between patient and therapist,
    534, 544
Borderline personality, 357–358, 506–507,
    565, 566, 574
    and bulimia, 509
    psychotherapeutic techniques for, 583
    sleep studies, 346
Bordin, E., 528–529
Boston Collaborative Drug Surveillance
    Study, 227, 382
Boundaries:
    family and individual, 488, 495
    open external, 496
    therapeutic, 535, 594
Bouton, neural, 9
Bradykinesia, 160
Bradykinin, 11
Brain:
    areas or regional systems, linked
        behaviors, 109–111, 115–117
    circulation, in sleep, 273–274
    cortical mapping, 116-117
    damage, in schizophrenia, 27
    disease, coarse, 114–115, 129, 133–135
    endocrinology, 107, 243–244
    imaging, 108, 110, 112, 134, 163, 217,
        241, 247–249
    injury to, 105, 142–155
    stroke-related damage, 146
    tumors, 148–149
Brain electrical area mapping (BEAM), 135
Brainstem, reticular core, 13
Breuer, J., 532
Broca, Paul, 255
Broca's area, 121, 122, 146
Bromocriptine, for anorexia, 452
Bruxism, sleep-related, 325
Buccolingual dyspraxia, 121, 128
Bulimarexia, 443, 465, 467, 469
Bulimia:
    addictive or impulsive behaviors, 509
    and anorexia nervosa, 402, 443–444,
        452, 456
    calories consumed, 468
    causes of, 505
    clinical characteristics, 468, 470–472
    cultural context, 473

discovery of, 6
Cholecystokinin (CCK), 11, 61, 412, 415
  increased doses, 413
  satiety action, 414
Choline, 49–50
Choline acetyltransferase, 49–50
  in basal forebrain cholinergic complex, 57–58
  in DAT, 222
Cholinergic compounds:
  dysphoriogenic effects, 349
  and sleep, in depression, 344, 348
Cholinergic REM Induction test, 353
Cholinergic systems, 49–65
Chorea, 160
Choreoathetosis, 160, 173
Chronobiology, 275, 371
  of depression, 349
Chronotherapy, 324, 372
Chubby Puffer syndrome, 333
Chunking, thought, for insomniacs, 367
Circadian rhythms, 275–276, 301–302, 308, 362
  in children, 329–331
  and depression, 349
  desynchronization, 373
  flattening, 353, 445, 446
  of LH production, 445
  unusual, 372
Circumplex concept, 540
Class, social:
  and anorexia nervosa, 441, 491
  issues, in therapy, 586, 597
  and obesity, 420
  and racial bias, 597
  similarities, between patient and therapist, 553, 554
Client-centered therapy, 536, 537, 540, 551, 552, 555, 556
Clinging:
  in anorexics, 506–507
  in temporal lobe patients, 195
Clomiphine, effect on LH, 445
Cloning, in RNA, 85, 87
Clozapine, 28–31
CNS, see Central nervous system
Coarse brain disease, 114–115, 129, 133–134
  EEG indications, 135
Cocaine:
  abuse, 234
  monoamine oxidase inhibitor side effects, 228
Cognition:
  impairment, in medical patients, 104
  techniques for testing, 115–117
  See also Thinking
Cognitive stages, and anorexia, 505–506
Cognitive therapy, 540, 563

cognitive restructuring, for eating disorders, 429, 475
  treatment package, 527
Collaboration, patient's, in work appropriate to therapy, 538
Co-localization, or cotransmitters, 14–15, 243–244
Coma:
  from brain tumor, 149
  psychosis on emerging from, 144
Command messages, from patient, 576–577
Communication:
  in families of anorexics, 482, 489, 490, 493, 495
  gender differences, 594
  and therapeutic alliance, 566
Competence, development of, in anorexics, 495
Competition, gender-linked, 588
Compliance:
  assessing, 607–609
  defined, 607–608
  determinants of, 609–612
  psychological factors, 610
Comprehension, auditory, 116, 122
Comprehensive Psychiatric Rating Scale, obsessional subscale, 352
Compulsion, defined, 160
Computerized axial tomography (CAT) scan, 108, 110, 112, 134, 163, 217, 241, 247
Computers, living-tissue interfacing, 249–250
Concentration, 137, 301, 567
  cortical mapping, 116–117
  effects of head injury, 143
Concussion, 134
Conditioning:
  operant, for anorexics, 450
  in sleep disorders, 302, 316–317
Confidentiality, therapeutic, 535
Configurational analysis, of impasses, 578–581
Conflict, family, in eating disorders, 488, 493, 495, 505
Consciousness, impaired level of, 148–149
Consensus Development Conference on Drugs and Insomnia (NIMH), 297, 388–389
Contact, unproductive, 576
Contract, therapeutic, 533
Control axis, in circumplex concept, 540
Controlled/controlling dilemma, 577
Conversion disorder, 176
  distinguishing from anorexia, 440
Convexity syndrome, 128
Cooperation, patient's, 537
Coping With Depression, 563

Dependency:
  in anorexics, 490, 493–494, 504, 506–507
  and pathogenic therapist, 535
  on therapist, 537, 576
Depressants, 75–76
Depression:
  ACTH levels, 93
  and aging, 349
  anergic, 341
  and anorexia, 442
  antihypertensive-induced, 107
  bipolar, 342, 345–346
  and borderline personality, 358
  and brain trauma, 144
  and bulimia, 470, 497
  and circadian time-keeping, 276
  cortisol secretion regulation in, 91, 445
  during dieting, 426
  differential diagnosis, 344–347
  endogenous, 38, 91–94, 344
  opiate-associated, 107
  pathophysiology of, 348–349
  prediction of treatment response, 347
  similarities with obsessive–compulsive
    disorder, 352
  and sleep, 341–350, 352
  somatic symptoms of, 317
  and somatostatin, 108, 244
  severe, and therapeutic alliance, 571
  stroke-associated, 105, 145–146
  subtypes, 345–347
Depth of Exploration Scale, 537
Depth/Value dimension, of session
  assessment, 539
Derogation, 562
  escalation of, 564
Detoxification, of patients with opiate
  addictions, 107
Development, gender-linked, 594–596
  See also Children
Dexamethasone suppression test (DST),
  83, 91–92, 146, 345
  for anorexics, 445
  on bulemics, 470
  obsessive–compulsive disorder study,
    353
Dextrals, 110
2-DG, see 2-Deoxy-D-glucose
Diabetes:
  and anorexia, 440
  and obesity, 421, 426
  in psychosomatic families, 488
Diagnosis, 180
  of anorexia nervosa, 438–440
  of black patients, 597
  of brain tumor, 148, 149
  of bulimia, 464–465
  clinical judgment in, 312
  of dementia syndrome, 219–220

with EEG sleep studies, 344
illegal drug use and, 233–236
of sleep disorders, 294–326
specific, 112
*Diagnostic and Statistical Manual of Mental
  Disorders, 3rd edition (DSM-III)*, 145,
  147, 164
  anorexia nervosa criteria, 439
  on bulimia, 464–465, 468
  classification of sleep disorders, 304
  on dementia, 212–213
Diagnostic Interview for Borderlines
  (DIB), 358
Diazepam:
  effects on normals, 385
  side effects, 384
Dichotomizations, 442, 504, 577
Dietary chaos syndrome, 443, 465
Dieting, 430–431
  and bulimia, 472
  complications of, 422, 426
  for moderate obesity, 428
  and physical activity, 425
Difficulty, in therapeutic alliance, 573–584
  psychotherapist's experience of, 573–574
Diffusion, blocking, 495
Digitalis toxicity, 229
Dilemmas, therapeutic:
  handling, 583–584
  impasses, 577–581
  sample, 580–581
  simple model of, 579
  zone of safety, between horns of, 579,
    580, 583
Disinhibition syndrome, *see* Organic
  aggressive syndrome
Disorders of excessive somnolence
  (DOES), 305–306, 308, 320–324
  long sleepers, 323
  percentage of patients with, 310
  psychophysiological, 320–321
Disorders of initiating and maintaining
  sleep (DIMS), 305, 307–308, 315–320,
  380
  associated with psychiatric disorders,
    317
  childhood-onset, 319
  differential diagnosis, 311, 314
  drug or alcohol abuse-related, 317–318
  persistent psychophysiological, 305,
    315–317
  short sleepers, 320
  short-term, 315
  situational, 305, 315
  transient, 315
  See also Insomnia
Disruptions, in therapeutic relationship,
  539
Dissociative states, interictal, 199–200

Distance/closeness dilemma, 577
Distrust, in anorexics, 439
DNA, *see* Deoxyribonucleic acid
DOES, *see* Disorders of excessive
    somnolence
Dominance, brain hemisphere, 110–111,
    116–117
    dysfunctions, and schizophrenic or
      affective disorders, 135
    and hypergraphia, 197
    language-related functions, 123
Domperidone, for anorexia, 455
Dopamine, 11, 15–16
    acetylcholine balance, and motor
      control, 29, 57
    and the antipsychotics, 17–33
    D-1 receptors, 24, 27
    D-2 receptors, 24–27, 32
    effects of antidepressants, 40–41
    food-reinforcing properties, 409–410
    and Huntington's, 163
    influence on sleep–wake cycle, 277, 281
    neuron depolarization block, 31
    radioligand studies, 21–27
    receptors, 22, 24–27, 32, 40–41
    supersensitivity, 24–26
Dopaminergic system, 166
    anatomy, 19–21
    and anorexia, 452
    hyperactivity in, 26, 452
Doppelganger phenomenon, 131
Double binds, between patient and
    therapist, 576–581
Down's syndrome:
    Alzheimer's-type pathology, 63
    cholinergic neurons in, 49
Doxepin, 568
Dream anxiety attacks, 325
Dreaming, ontogeny of, 329–331
Dressing praxis, 116, 120–121
Drivelling, 117
    in Wernicke's aphasia, 122
Drugs:
    accumulation, 386
    alcohol interactions, 77, 380
    antiarrhythmic, 107, 229
    anticholinergic, 29, 59, 107, 222, 227
    anticonvulsant, 107, 229–230, 242, 475
    antidepressant, 37–45, 64, 107, 172, 336,
      379, 384, 470, 475–476
    antiepileptic, 77–78, 452
    antihypertensive, 107, 228–229
    antipsychotic, 17–20, 23–24, 37, 107,
      227–228
    appetite suppressant, 429
    belladonna alkaloids, 107
    blood pressure effects, 151
    DIMS and, 317–318
    DOES associated with use of, 305, 321

dopaminergic-neurotransmission
    altering, 15
dosage, 7, 23, 31–32, 144, 220, 389
EEG sleep study monitoring, 347–348
effects of chronic treatment, 24–27, 38,
    41–44, 60, 75, 107
effects on GABAergic transmission, 70
for enuresis, 336, 347
experimental, 22
hypnotics, 380–390
illicit, 107
individual variation in effects of, 608
interactions with neurotransmitter
    receptors, 27–31
medication side effects, 227–231
overdose, 380
patient compliance, 607–626
poly abuse, 235–236
prescription, 107
psychotropic, 5–7, 15–16, 63–64, 107,
    227–228, 386
receptor theory, 18–19
See also Side effects
DST, *see* Dexamethasone suppression test
Dynorphin, 11, 85, 409
Dysgraphia, 123
Dyskinesias, 60, 160
    acute, 173
    spontaneous, 170
    tardive, 24–33, 60, 106, 170–172, 354
Dyslexia, 123, 132, 170
Dysmegalopsia, 115
Dysnomia, 122
Dysplasias, congenital, 199
Dyspraxias, 117, 120–122, 128, 132
Dysprosodia, 123–124
Dystonia, 160, 173
Dystonia musculorum deformans, 175
    anticholinergic drugs for, 60

Eating:
    deviant family patterns, 490
    habits, 427, 431
    rate of (binge), 428
Eating disorders, 401–521
    and affective disorders, 484
    age of onset, 456, 469
    assessment of, 403
    clinics and treatment units, 401
    common non-food or -weight issues,
      513
    dentition problems, 472
    diagnosis, 516–517
    dysfunctional weight-preoccupied
      families, 490
    in families of bulimics, 497
    names and addresses of national
      groups, 520
    parent–child interactions, 485–486

pathogenesis, 517–518
psychopathology, 518
social and cultural issues, 520
subgroups of patients, 508–510
transmission of, 483–484
treatment, 510–513, 518–520
Echopraxia, 117, 119
ECS, see Electroconvulsive seizures
Edema, peripheral, in anorexics, 444
EEG, see Electroencephalogram
EEG of Human Sleep: Clinical Applications,
  269
Ego:
  defects, in development of anorexics,
    447, 450
  functioning, and success of therapy, 532
Elderly:
  cholinergic function in, 64
  compliance, 609
  dementia in, 211–212
  flurazepam study, 382
  moderate wine use for, 387
  normal and abnormal sleep patterns,
    329, 349, 395
  use of hypnotics with, 386–387
Electrochemical communication, within
  nerve cells, 10
Electroconvulsive seizures (ECS), 242
Electroconvulsive therapy (ECT):
  anticonvulsant effects, 242
  antidepressant activity, 37
  blood pressure during, 152
  for depression, 107
  origins, 197, 241
  in the presence of brain tumor, 149
  serotonin-mediated behavior
    enhancement, 44
  time lag before therapeutic effect, 41, 42
Electroencephalograms (EEG), 110, 248
  abnormalities, in those with eating
    disorders, 472
  of anorexics, 452
  anxiety disorder studies, 356–357
  borderline personality studies, 357
  children's sleep patterns, 330
  in depression, 342–345
  development of, 267
  in hypnotics studies, 381–383
  in schizophrenics, 134–135
  sleep, 268–271
  in temporal lobe epilepsy, 106, 201
  in utero, 269
Electrolyte imbalance:
  in anorexics, 449, 454–455
  in bulimics, 471, 473
Electrosleep, 367
Emetics, ingestion by anorexics, 455
Emotion:
  high negative expressed, in families of

anorexics, 491, 518
  outward expression in insomniacs, 371
Emotional blunting, 124
  in schizophrenia, 114
Empathic holding treatment, 583
Empathy, therapist's, 551, 555, 556, 596
  defined, 595
  female therapists' capacity for, 595
  and racial differences, 600
Encephalitis, and organic aggressive
  syndrome, 147
Endocrinology:
  of anorexia nervosa, 445–446
  brain, 107–108, 243–244
  See also Hormones
Endorphins, 49
  levels, in anorexia nervosa, 446
Energy:
  balance, long-term, 406
  excess, in anorexics, 442
Enkephalins, 85
  and food intake, 409
Enmeshment, family:
  among anorexics, 487, 488, 493, 495
  in bulimics, 497
  in obese, 498
Enuresis:
  antidepressants for, 336, 347
  and sleep disorder, 335–336
Ependymomas, 148
Epilepsy, 107, 125
  anticonvulsant side effects, 229
  defense, in violent crime, 194
  and GABAergic function, 74–75,
    77–78
  grand mal, 205
  psychomotor, 113
  sleep-related, 314, 325, 373
  temporal lobe, 106, 125, 190–207
  See also Seizures
Epinephrine, 11
  adrenal-mediated, 407
Episodic dyscontrol syndrome, *see*
  Organic aggressive syndrome
Erections, sleep-induced, 268, 274–275,
  326
Ergots, dopaminergic, 32
Erotization, conflictual, 576
Escherichia coli, in mRNA cloning, 86–87
Estrogens, feedback systems, 445
Ethnocentricity, in therapist, 597–598
Euphoria, in MS, 178
Evaluation, neuropsychiatric, 104, 108–137
  alcohol use and driving patterns, 150
  eating disorders, 403
  goals, 109
  after medication washout period, 227
  neurologic history, 133–134, 143
  sleep disorders, 294–326, 369

inhibition, 78
Glycine, 11, 67
Goals:
  of psychotherapy research, 545
  of therapy, 533, 534
Golgi, phosphorylation in, 89
Gonadotropin:
  in anorexic males, 449
  levels, and amenorrhea, 445
Gonadotropin-releasing hormones, 517
Graphesthesias, 116, 129, 130
Grasp reflex, 133
Group therapy;
  for anorexia nervosa, 451
  for bulimia, 474–475, 497
  multiple-family, 494, 497
Growth hormone (GH):
  in anorexics, 445, 446
  circadian cycle, 276
  and hypopituitarism, 445
Guilt, in families of anorexics, 494

Habit spasms, 172
Hallervorden–Spatz disease, 162
Hallucinations, 114–115
  anticonvulsant-derived, 229
  auditory, 115, 125
  from flurazepam, 386
  from stroke, injury, or disease, 125
  after temporal region stroke, 146
  upon withdrawal from hypnotics, 388
Halstead–Reitan Battery, 136–137
Hamartomas, 201
  and temporal lobe epilepsy, 199
Hamilton Depression Rating Scale, 352,
  358, 569
Handedness, 110, 120
Head, injuries to, psychological
  manifestations, 125
  See also Brain
Headaches, 148
  cluster, 326
Health Belief Model, 610
Helping alliance:
  defined, 553
  types of, 554
Helping Alliance Questionnaire, 556
Hemichorea, 160
Hemispheres, brain, 110–111, 116–117
  connections between, 111, 130
  effect of stroke on, 146–147
  interhemispheric dysconnection, 120
  involved in language and memory
    disfunctions, 110, 121, 123, 135–126
  mental rotation and, 127–128
  nondominant brain disease, 114
  and speech, 123
  trauma to, 145
Hepatolenticular degeneration, 168

Heredity, see Genetic factors
Heroin, hypersomnia from, 321
Herpes, delusions, hallucinations, or
  mood disturbances of, 125
Hippocrates, 607
Histamine, 11
Histochemical techniques, to visualize
  acetylcholinesterase, 53
Homework, patient's, 566
Homocysteine, 11
Homosexuality, gender-matching
  therapist, 590
Honeymoon phenomena, in therapeutic
  alliance, 554
Hormones, 243–244
  changes, in anorexia nervosa, 445–446
  gastric satiety signal, 412
  interactions with antidepressants, 44
  peptides as, 84
  TRH and TSH, 11, 243, 445–446, 472
  See also Endocrinology
Hospitalization, as result of
  noncompliance, 607
Hostility:
  covert, patient, 610
  expression of, toward therapist, 538–539
HPA, see Hypothalamic–pituitary–adrenal
  axis
Hunger:
  awareness, in infant, 505–506
  center, in hypothalamus, 408
  gastric contractions, 406–407
  and human sham feeding, 412
  and insomnia, 362–363
  learned cues, 409
  physiology of, 406–416
  and pleasure, 409–410
  post-ingestive feedback, 409
Huntington's disease, 63, 105–106, 161–
  164
  chronic neuroleptics and D-2 increase,
    27
  and GABA, 73, 74
  genetic influence, 161, 163, 221
  motor symptoms, 60
  progressive dementia, 63
  psychiatric diagnosis, 106
  and somatostatin, 108, 244
  suicide concerns, 106
Hygiene, sleep, 301–302, 324, 333, 362–
  363, 389
Hyperactivity, 128
  anorexic, 442, 448, 450, 490, 517
  and sleep disorder, 334–335, 362, 363
Hyperglycemia, 407
Hypergraphia, 195–197
Hyperkinesia, 160
Hyperlipidemia, and obesity, 421, 426
Hyperphagia, evening, 422

and white noise, 362, 367
See also Disorders of initiating and
maintaining sleep
Institutionalization, sleep disturbances in
elderly and, 386
Insulin, for anorexics, 451
Integrative function, of mind, 578
Interactions, patient–therapist, in session,
539
Interests, similarity of, patient–therapist,
552–555
Interictal changes, in temporal lobe
epilepsy, 190–207
emotional and intellectual, 194–197
Intermittent explosive disorder, *see*
Organic aggressive syndrome
*International Classification of Diseases, 9th
Revision, Clinical Modifications (ICD-9-
CM)*, 307
International Journal of Eating Disorders,
401
Interpersonal behavior, patient's, 537, 539
Interpersonal Process Recall, 544
Interpersonal psychotherapy, 533, 563
treatment package, 527
Interpretation:
excessive, 583
significant, and transference changes,
544
Interruptions, during therapy,
minimizing, 535
Intestinal bypass surgery, 425–426
Intestine, satiety signals, 410–412
Intoxication, alcohol, 235
Intrusiveness, of parent, 574
Irritability:
as early manifestation of brain tumor,
149
postictal, 193
and right hemispheric lesions, 146–147
Ischemic score (IS), 215
Isolation, in families of anorexics, 489
Isonicotinic acid, effect on GABA
transmission, 70
Isonicotinic acid hydrazide (INH), GAD
and GABA-T inhibition, 69

Janowsky, David, 530
Jet lag, 372–373, 389
Jews, Ashkenazi, dystonia musculorum
deformans in, 175

Kernberg, Otto, 562
Kinesthetic dyspraxia, 132
Kinesthetic praxis, 116, 120
Klein, Donald, 527
Klein, Melanie, 562

L-aspartic acid, 67

L-glutamic acid, neurotransmitter activity,
67
Language:
clinical assessment, 114
cortical mapping, 116–117
disorders of, 125–126, 132
function, evaluating, 104, 121–125
hemispheric dominance for, 110, 121,
123
parietal lobe functions, 129
Lanugo, in anorexics, 444
Laxatives, for weight control, 402, 443,
449, 450, 452, 456, 464, 468, 471, 474,
511
Lay-led weight control groups, 430, 431
Left-handedness, 110
Leg-jerking, *see* Myoclonus
Lethargic syndrome, 267
Leucine-enkephalin, 11
Leukodystrophies, 178–179
Levodopa (L-dopa), 166
as dopamine precursor, 59
movement disorders induced by, 172
Parkinson's alleviation with, 25
side effects, 230
usefulness in dopamine receptor down-
regulation, 26
LH, *see* Luteinizing hormone
Librium, 76
Ligand-binding autoradiographic
techniques, muscarinic receptor
localization, 52
Likeability, patient's, 550–551, 555
Limbic system:
association cortex for, 126
epileptic discharge, 205
during temporal lobe epilepsy ictal
period, 190
Literal-mindedness, of anorexics, 506
Lithium:
for anorexia nervosa, 452–453
chronic administration, 75
discovery of, 6
mechanism of action, 45
movement disorders from, 172, 173
toxicity, 228, 452
treatment, concurrent with
neuroleptics, 26
Liver:
hepatic microsomal oxidizing systems,
380, 381
hepatic vagotomy, 415
Living systems theory, 491
Lobectomy, temporal, 204–205
Lobes, brain, 104
frontal, 109, 111, 113, 114, 116–119, 121–
123, 126–129, 132, 146, 149
occipital, 116–117, 132, 146, 149

parietal, 111, 113, 115–118, 120–122, 129–132, 149
temporal, 106, 116–117, 121–123, 125–126, 146, 149, 190–207, 248
Lock-and-key theory, of drug action, 18
Lock Wallace short marital adjustment test, 489
LSD, 234
Luria–Nebraska Battery, 135, 136
Luteinizing hormone (LH), 445
release during sleep, 331

Male world view, effects on therapy, 594
Mania, related to brain trauma, 144, 146
Mannerisms, 160
Manuals, psychotherapy, for training, 556–557
Mapping:
brain electrical area (BEAM), 135
cortical, 116–117
Marijuana, 233–234
Marriages, stable, chronic discord in, 488
Maturity:
development of, 489
physical, fears of anorexics, 506
psychosocial, fears of, 447, 505
of therapist, 535
Meal termination, physiology of, 410–414
Medial-orbital syndrome, 128–129
Medication, see Drugs
Medullablastoma, 148
Meige syndrome, 175
Melatonin, and circadian rhythms, 276
MEMA, see Middle ear muscle activity
Membrane, neuronal, 10, 49–52
barbiturate attachment, 76
ion permeability, 71, 72
Memory:
cortical mapping, 116–117
effects of starvation, 446
in the elderly, 211–212
function, evaluating, 104, 124
impairment, 567
long-term, 385
and REM sleep, 354
semantic, 384
short-term, 37
visual, 116, 125, 126
working, 57–58, 62
Memory-for-Designs test, 125
Men, see Gender
Meningiomas, 148
Menninger Foundation, 538
Therapeutic Alliance Scales, 543
Menopause, hormone changes of, and antidepressant efficacy, 44
Menstrual-associated syndrome, hypersomnia from, 323

Menstruation:
and eating disorders, 402, 442–443, 453
Mental illness:
organic, substance-induced, 107
racial differences in concept of, 599
Mental status:
examination, 104, 109–137
neuropsychiatric, 112–115
Mental Status Questionnaire, 219
Mesial temporal sclerosis, 201
Mesocortical system, dopamine pathway in, 20–21
Mesolimbic system, 29
dopamine pathways in, 20–21, 75
Metabolic emergency, 407
Metabolism, cellular, 407
Metachromatic leukodystrophy (MLD), 178–179
Metals, heavy, toxicity, 232–233
Methionine-enkephalin, 11
3-Methoxy, 4 hydroxy-phenylglycol (MHPG), 446
MID, See Multiple-infarct dementia
Middle ear muscle activity (MEMA), 355
Migraine, in mothers of anorexics, 485
Minerals, toxicity, 232
Mini-Mental State Examination, 112, 135, 219
Minnesota Multiphasic Personality Inventory (MMPI), 136, 167, 178
anorexia nervosa patients and their families, 489, 510
on bulimics and substance abusers, 471
insomniac profiles, 297, 356
Minorities:
psychotherapies for, 586, 596–601
training clinicians and researchers, 600
Mistrust, roots in early development, 574
Mitgehen, 119
Mitochondria:
in bouton, 9
phenothiazine effects, 7
Mixed messages, in families of anorexics, 495
See also Dilemmas
MMPI, see Minnesota Multiphasic Personality Inventory
Models, anorexia nervosa in, 448, 517
Monoamine oxidase inhibitors:
antidepressant effects, 38
behavioral side effects, 228
for bulimia, 477
development of, 6
time lag before therapeutic effect, 41
and tyramine foods, 151–152
Mood:
disturbances of, 148
poststroke disorders, 146
quality, intensity, appropriateness, 113

Office of Medical Applications of Research (OMAR), NIH, 262
Oligodendrogliomas, 148
Oligomenorrhea, and normal-weight bulimia, 402
OMS, see Dementia syndrome
Opiates, 231, 234
  antagonists, 409
  endogenous, 446
  similarity to GABA agonists, 78
Opioids, 83–95
Orality, 419
Orbitomedial syndrome, 128–129
Organic affective syndrome, 347
Organic aggressive syndrome/Intermittent explosive disorder/Episodic dyscontrol, 105, 144, 147–148
  treatment, 153–154
Organic hallucinosis, 145
Organic mental disorders, substance-induced, 227–236
Orientation, 137
  east–west, 131
  global, 116–117, 131
  to interpersonal relationships, patient–therapist, 553–555
  left–right, 129–131
  to time, place and person, 127–128
Outcome research, 528
Overblaming, self, in mothers of anorexics, 489
Overeating, 422
Overprotectiveness:
  and anorexia nervosa, 493
  in psychosomatic families, 488
Overstimulation, of child, 574
Ovulation, relation to critical body weight or fat, 443
  See also Amenorrhea

Pacemakers, circadian, 275–276
Paired Associate Learning Test, 112, 124
Palmar-mental reflex, 132–133
Pancreatic glucagon, 415
Panhypopituitarism, 440
Paradoxical prescription, 496
  for insomnia, 366, 369
Paragnosia, 131
Parallel processing, 578, 582
Paralysis, 160
Paramnesia, reduplicative, 131
Paranoia, in temporal lobe epilepsy, 106
Parasomnias, 306, 309, 325–326
Parasympathetic nervous system, acetylcholine neurotransmission, 54
Paraventricular nucleus, 408
Parentectomy, for anorexics, 492
Paresis, 160
Paresthesias, 133

Parietal lobes, see Lobes, brain
Parkinson's disease, 25, 58–59, 105, 128, 162, 164–166
  cholinergic neurons, 49
  dementia development, 63, 106
  depression in, 106
  dopamine loss, 20–21
  extrapyramidal GAD, 73
  GABA and, 73, 74
  psychiatric symptoms, 165–166
  and schizophrenia, 166
Pathogenicity, of therapist, 535
Patient:
  ability to imagine therapeutic alliance, 583
  adherence to agenda-setting, 565
  appropriate for gender-matching, 590
  cognitive set, 566
  compliance, 609–611
  defenses against trust, 562
  difficult, 573–584
  double binds in, 576–581
  factors contributing to therapeutic alliance, 536–539, 550
  fear of symptom exacerbation, 564
  female, 586–596
  medical or surgical, deliria in, 109
  noncompliers, 608
  perception of therapist, 535–536
  race of, 596–601
  role relationship models, 573–576
  selective response to same- or opposite-sex therapists, 595
  similarities with therapist, 552–555, 586
Patient involvement measure, 538, 539
PCP, see Phencyclidine
PDD, see Dementia, primary degenerative
Peers, patient's, as role-relationship models, 581
Penile tumescence, sleep-related, 268, 274–275, 326
Penn Helping Alliance Rating Method, 541, 542
Penn Psychotherapy Research Project, 537, 538, 555, 557
Pentobarbital, 380
Peptic ulcer, and anorexia, 440
Peptide bond, 83–84
  See also Neuropeptides
Perceptions:
  active, 127
  delusional, 115
  disturbances of, 114–115
  nondominant lobe coordination, 129
Perfectionism, in anorexics, 439, 447, 504, 508, 512
Perseveration:
  motor, 118
  number, 129

Psychotropics:
anticholinergic effects, 63–64
classes of, 6–7
half-life of, 386
lipophilic properties, 7
mechanism of action, 15–16
organic mental disorders from, 227–228
Pyramidal tract, 9, 111

Rabbit syndrome, 160
Race:
influence on therapeutic alliance, 586, 596–601
in mental status exam, 112
and therapeutic milieu, 598
training issues, 600–601
See also Socioeconomic status
Radioactive labeling, of neurotransmitters or drugs, 21–27
Radioligand binding technique, 33
Radioreceptor assay, of blood neuroleptic levels, 31–33
Rage, dyscontrol of, 147
See also Organic aggressive syndrome
Rapid eye movement (REM) sleep, 268, 284, 359
abnormal, 322, 333
and anxiety disorder, 356
cholinergic basis, 348–349
computer-assisted analysis, 346
in dementia, 354
in depression, 342–343
deprivation of, antidepressant effects, 42, 344
discovery of, 268
headaches, 326
latency, 174, 299, 342–344, 352, 355, 357–358
MEMA, 355
and NPR episodes, 274
in OCD patients, 174
REM storms, 330
repeated interruptions, 42, 319–320
in schizophrenics, 354–355
suppression, drug-induced, 347
Reading, 121
cortical mapping, 116
in mental status testing, 123
parietal lobe coordination, 129
See also Language
Real relationship, psychotherapeutic, 533, 575
Reality testing, impaired, 557, 567
Reasoning:
assessing, 126–127
dichotomous, or all-or-nothing, 442, 577
moral, gender-linked values, 594
See also Thinking

Receptor-binding/drug screening techniques, 21–22
Receptor theory, of drug action, 18–19
Receptors, neurotransmitter, 11–12, 18–19
acetylcholine, 51–53
alpha-adrenergic, 28–29, 408
beta-adrenergic and serotonergic, 41–44, 276
dopamine, 19–32, 40–41, 75
$GABA_A$, 71, 73, 75, 77
$GABA_B$, 71–73
interactions among, 27–31
muscarinic-cholinergic, 29–31
neuropeptide receptor proteins, 84
norepinephrine, 72
postsynaptic, disturbance of, 26–27
testing system, 6–7, 21–22, 24
Recognition, of the familiar, abnormalities in, 130–131
Recognition site, neurotransmitter-receptor, 11
Regional blood flow measures, 247–248
Regression:
allowing, 576
neural substrates, 246
and obesity, 434
and role-relationship models, 578
Rehabilitation:
after stroke, 146
Halstead–Reitan feedback for, 136
Reitan–Indiana Aphasia Screening Test, 135, 136
Relationship:
absence of supraordinate concept, 582
developing capacities for, 576
evaluating relatedness, 113–114
inner models of, in difficult patient, 574
intimate, equal, and therapeutic alliance, 581
psychotherapy training concerning relational bonds, 596
versus understanding, 557
See also Therapeutic alliance
Relaxation training, for insomnia, 365
Reliance, on hypnotics, 388
REM, *see* Rapid eye movement sleep
Repertory grid technique, 577
RER, *see* Rough endoplasmic reticulum
Research, psychotherapeutic, 527–529
into patient's behavior, 537
process studies, on gender, 589–590
on psychodynamic therapy, 550–553
Reserpine, 228
in animal models, 44
depression syndrome, 38, 107
Resistance, 532, 571
active, 538
in insomniacs, 370
social alliance as, 575

among bulimics, 443–444
Self-disclosure, by patient, 537
  effect of therapist's gender on, 589
Self-esteem:
  and anorexia nervosa, 438, 441–442,
    447, 450–451, 453, 493, 504, 505, 512
  and body image, in eating disorders,
    508
  female patient's, and female therapists,
    594
  impact of therapist's behavior on, 556
Self-fulfilling prophecy, 551
Self-monitoring, 537
  in behavioral treatment of obesity, 428
Self-organization, defect in, 507
Self psychology, application to anorexia,
  507
Sensitivity, of EEG sleep studies, 344
Sensory motor rhythm (SMR) training,
  365
Separation-individuation process, and
  anorexia, 506
Serotonin, 11, 61
  antidepressant effects on receptors, 40–
    41
  central function, drugs that increase, 43
  influence on sleep–wake cycle, 277–279
  and tryptophan, 446
  uptake inhibition, 38, 39
Sessions, therapy:
  good or bad, 539–541
  observer's viewpoint, 537, 539, 541
Set point:
  body temperature, 446
  body weight, 423, 427, 429, 447, 511,
    518
Sex-role bias, in psychotherapy, 586, 588–
  589
  research on, 591–592
  See also Gender
Sex-Role Stereotype Questionnaire, 588
Sexuality, during interictal period, 191–
  192
Sham feeding, 410
  CCK suppression, 413
  human, 412
Shell concept, of difficult patients, 573–
  574, 576
Shift work, and insomnia, 372–373
Side effects, 230–231, 608
  of antiarrhythmic drugs, 229
  of anticholinergics, 58–59, 63
  of anticonvulsants, 229-230
  of antidepressants, 37, 64
  of antihypertensive agents, 228–229
  of antipsychotics, 153–154
  in elderly patients, 354
  extrapyramidal, 63
  of GABAergic drugs, 71

of hypnotics, 384–387
from low drug dosages, 144
of neuroleptics, 20–21, 24–31, 59–60, 63
parkinsonian, 29, 58–59
of the phenothiazines, 18
psychosis, 106, 144
of psychotropics, 227–228
Similarities, between patient and
  therapist, 552–556, 586
  gender, 590
  racial, 596–601
Sinistrals, 110
Skin, changes in anorexia, 444
Sleep:
  in affective illness, 243
  alpha, 320
  conditioned associations to bed and
    bedroom, 302, 316–317, 368
  delta, 342, 355, 356
  and depression, 341–350
  and exercise, 362
  facilitation, versus induction, 277
  hygiene, 301–302, 324, 333, 362–363, 389
  and hyperactivity, 334–335
  monitoring, 299–300
  NREM (stages 1-4), 268–269, 283, 330,
    342, 353, 355, 364
  ontogeny of, 268–269, 329–331, 349–350
  physiology and neurochemistry of, 266–
    284
  and protein synthesis, 283
  regulation, two-process model, 349
  REM, see Rapid eye movement sleep
  requirements for, 300–301
  restriction, 367
  sleep evaluation laboratory, 263
  slow-wave (SWS), 269, 342, 343, 349
  stages, 267–269, 306, 309, 314, 342, 343,
    353–354
  terrors, 325, 332
  trying to, 316
  in utero, 269–270
Sleep disorders, 262–394
  ASDC nosology, 304–310
  centers, 298–299
  in children, 395
  of concern to psychiatrists, 309–310,
    313–326
  conditioned arousal, 302, 316–317, 368
  DIMS, see Disorders of initiating and
    maintaining sleep
  DOES, see Disorders of excessive
    somnolence
  in the elderly, 386–387
  evaluation and diagnosis, 294–326
  history, 303–304
  misprescription of hypnotics for, 386–
    387
  nonpharmacological treatment, 361–375

organic, 298–299
and starvation, 442
time spent in bed, 301–302
types of, 300–302, 307–309
Sleep-promoting substance (SPS), 283
Sleep–wake cycle, 275–276
  adolescent disturbances, 373
  Alzheimer's disruptions, 353, 359
  in borderline personality, 357
  in children, 329–331
  in depressives, 347, 349
  desynchronization, 372
  disorders of, 306, 308–310, 324–325,
    371–373
  neurotransmitter and peptide
    regulation, 276–284, 362
  setting, 301–302, 353, 362, 366
Sleeping pills, see Hypnotics
Slow-wave sleep, see Sleep, slow-wave
Smoothness/Ease dimension, in session
  assessment, 539
Snags, in psychotherapy, defined, 577
Snoring:
  in apneic patient, 318, 321
  in children, 334
Snout reflex, 133
Social alliance, 574–576, 578, 579
Social grace, loss of, 143
Social psychology, research on patient–
  therapist relations, 556
Society for Psychotherapy Research, 529
Socioeconomic status:
  in anorexia nervosa, 441, 491
  issues of, in therapy, 586, 597
  and obesity, 420
  similarities between patient and
    therapist, 553, 554
  See also Race
Sodium:
  GABA transport sites dependent on,
    68–69
  neuronal sodium/potassium balance, 10
Soft signs, neurologic, 112, 115, 119, 128,
  129, 132–134, 172
Soma, neural, 8
Somatization, of psychological distress,
  316, 361, 371, 571
  by anorexics, 448, 450
Somatostatin, 11, 61, 415
  and neuropsychiatric illness, 244
Somnambulism, 309
Spasticity, 160
Specificity:
  of EEG sleep studies, 344
  isomeric, 21–22
Speech:
  affective components, 116, 121, 137
  telegraphic, 121, 122
  See also Language

Sports, brain injuries from, 142, 144
  and risk taking, 151
Spouse, of obese person, 498–499
Standardization, of psychotherapeutic
  treatment, 527
Stanford–Binet, Verbal and Pictorial
  Absurdities, 112
Starvation:
  clinical characteristics, 441
  describing effects of, to anorexics, 511
  effects on thyroid gland, 445
  emotional disturbances of, 422, 440
  endogenous opiate production, 446
  hunger and satiety sensations, 442
  See also Anorexia nervosa
Stereognosis, 116, 130
Stereotyping, in psychotherapy, 586, 588–
  589
  research on, 591–592
Stereotypy, 160
Stimulants, abuse of, 16, 17
Stimulation, monotonous, for insomniacs,
  367
Stimulus-bound behavior, 117–119, 128
Stimulus control therapy, for insomnia,
  366
Stomach, satiety signals, 412
  See also Gastric...
Story Recall test, 124–125
Stress:
  and binge-eating, 470
  family response patterns, anorexics,
    486–487
  non-specific, 446
  and sleep disorders, 370
Striatonigral pathway, 20, 24–25, 30,
  56–57
  degeneration, 58, 59, 73–74, 162, 166
Striatum, 58
  dopaminergic denervation, 59
Stroke, 145–147, 151–152
  in and around Broca's area, 146
  delusions, hallucinations, or mood
    disturbances, 125
  emotional and cognitive changes, 145–
    146
  prevention, 151–152
  psychiatric aspects, 105
Structural Analysis of Social Behavior
  (SASB), 540
Subdiaphragmatic vagotomy, 415
Submissiveness, gender-linked, 588
Substance-P, 11
Substantia nigra, 163
  GABA receptors in, 73
Sudden Infant Death Syndrome, and
  sleep apnea, 334
Suicide, 151
  in bulimics, 443–444, 509